An Uncertain Safety

Thomas Wenzel · Boris Drožđek
Editors

An Uncertain Safety

Integrative Health Care for the 21st Century Refugees

Springer

Editors
Thomas Wenzel
World Psychiatric Association Scientific Section, Psychological Aspects of Persecution and Torture
Geneva
Switzerland

Boris Droždek
PsyQ/Parnassia Group
Rosmalen/Eindhoven
The Netherlands

ISBN 978-3-030-10286-9 ISBN 978-3-319-72914-5 (eBook)
https://doi.org/10.1007/978-3-319-72914-5

Printed on acid-free paper

This Springer imprint is published by the registered company Springer International Publishing AG part of Springer Nature.
The registered company address is: Gewerbestrasse 11, 6330 Cham, Switzerland

Foreword

Continuity and Shifts in Contemporary Refugee History

Human beings are and have always been both a territorial species, defending aggressively what they consider as their land, and a migratory species, exploring and investing new territories according to complexly entangled push and pull factors. Across millenaries and centuries, human groups have fled adverse environments: extreme climate, infertile lands, wars, and extermination by other human groups [1]. They have also always searched (like all other living beings) for better opportunities, in particular when local resources were not sufficient to meet the needs of a growing population.

Myths, tales, history, and fiction testify to the richness of migration trajectories and to the multiple obstacles associated with fleeing persecution or war. Mirroring both human generosity and our capacity for cruelty, all these narratives also reflect the multitude of discursive strategies that people in search of asylum have employed across ages [2, 3].

During the twentieth century the two worldwide conflicts have brought forward the contradictions between the emerging human right discourse and the appalling reality of asylum. The story of the St-Louis, this transatlantic ship carrying 800 Jews fleeing Nazi Germany, which was refused landing in Cuba, United States, and Canada before returning its passenger to their death in Europe, is exemplary.

The 1951 Geneva Convention was the first international agreement defining who is a refugee and outlining what is the basic protection which states should offer to the persons they welcome as refugees. This international convention stipulates that refugees who flee persecution because of political, ethnic, or religious reasons should not be expelled and returned to countries where their life and freedom would be threatened. According to the United Nations High Commissioner for Refugees (UNHCR), refugee protection includes access to fair asylum procedures and living conditions that allow refugees to live in dignity and safety. With time and social transformations in European and North American countries, gender and sexual orientations have progressively been recognized as legitimate reasons to be granted asylum.

One of the important, and ongoing, debates about asylum has been the tension between resettlement in the country of asylum and longer term solutions decided either by the states or by the refugees themselves. According to Chimni [4] the history of durable solutions to refugee movements after the Second World War can be divided into two distinct phases. From 1945 to 1985, resettlement in the country of asylum was promoted, although voluntary repatriation was considered as a better solution. In the second phase, repatriation became the overall objective. From 1985 to 1993, voluntary repatriation was advocated as the durable solution, while still insisting on the voluntary nature of the move. The notion of safe return, introduced in 1993, comforted the temporary protection regimes established in Western Europe. From then on, the doctrine of imposed return gradually gained credence, while the reality of involuntary repatriation grew.

Chimni [4] argues that involuntary repatriation is now the favored solution for the northern states because in the post-Cold War era there are no more geopolitical reasons to share the burden represented by the southern refugees, which require important resources. The relatively recent distinction between migrant and refugees is both interesting, because it helps to secure protection and limit abusess toward groups in very precarious situations, and problematic because the emphasis on vulnerability tends to minimize refugee resiliency and agency and it does not represent adequately the heterogeneity across migrant and refuge groups (UNHCR, 2016). Refugees are, by definition, individuals fleeing armed conflict or persecution, while migrants are often believed to migrate mainly to improve their lives through better job opportunities or education. Although this is partially true, the reality is much more complex and the two groups overlap widely: increasingly migrants change country because of political and social turmoil, and a significant number have experienced persecution or witnessed organized violence [5]. On the other hand, many refugees flee very adverse economic conditions, the absence of life perspectives, and (increasingly) climate change adversity associated with hunger and poverty.

From Being "At Risk" to Becoming "A Risk"

The contribution of growing migration waves with difficult socio-economic conditions in receiving countries has sharply shifted the perceptions about migrants and refugees. The representation of refugees as vulnerable because of their exposure to war trauma and their multiple experiences of losses and separation has been progressively replaced by representations of the potentially criminal refugee, perceived as abusing the benevolence from naïve host countries. This shift in discourses around refugees takes different forms. For example, it includes a transformation of representations of refugee children who become suspect of being disguised adults (with the battle around age determination) or of manipulating host country professional in benefit of their parents asylum claim in the case of the pervasive refusal syndrome [6]. Children and women are also frequently portrayed as victims of their own families, which are perceived as the barbaric other [7].

In this context the social rights associated with asylum have shrunk. Concepts of privilege and deservingness are progressively replacing the notion of rights in the field of education and of health care. In some countries access to services is limited or has been reduced directly through legislation [8]. But entitlement is not linearly associated with access to services. Numerous obstacles at the institutional and clinical levels, from lack of information to negative attitudes of health professionals toward refugees, can interfere with access [9, 10]. On the refugee side fear, lack of information, and past experiences of discrimination may also prevent them from accessing care [11].

A Public Health Challenge

The physical and mental health needs of refugees differ from those of host country residents. The prevalence of disease can differ because of higher exposure to infectious agents in unsafe environments or prolonged lack of access to health care [12]. Premigratory stress, complex and stressful migration trajectories, living conditions in host country, and genetic predispositions also play an important role. In addition, language and cultural differences, along with distrust toward institutions and discrimination experiences in the resettlement environment, have been repeatedly shown to interfere with appropriate access to health care services [12].

A review of the evidence on mental health care for refugees, asylum seekers, and irregular migrants [13] underlines that the increasing number of these vulnerable migrants is a challenge for mental health services in Europe. As was emphasized in prior reviews [14] refugee and asylum seekers have higher rates of stress-related disorders than the generals population. They may also have more depression than host country residents if they still live in poverty five years after resettlement [13]. They have no more other specific mental health disorders then the general population, although they may present clinically their distress in ways which are unfamiliar to host country professionals.

Most mental health problems in refugees can be addressed in primary care. Training of health professionals and availability of interpreters and cultural brokers are helpful to overcome linguistic and cultural differences and improve communication and mutual understanding [15]. The usefulness of a systematic screening for post-traumatic stress disorder (PTSD) in refugees is debatable. In Canada, the Canadian Medical Association has chosen to recommend against screening for PTSD in refugees because of the absence of proven benefits and of the possible harm associated with re-traumatization through screening procedures [16]. Assessment should however maintain a high index of suspicion about the possibility of trauma in refugees, particularly in presence of any behavioral and emotional symptoms and in case of unexplained medical symptoms. A comprehensive assessment includes considerations for premigration exposures, migration-related stresses, and uncertainties and resettlement experiences that may influence health outcomes [15].

In the present context of growing xenophobia and negative representations about refugees, the situation of refugees may sometimes best represented as an ongoing trauma rather than a post-trauma setting. This has be important implications in terms of intervention because promoting specialized trauma intervention, in particular trauma-focused approaches, without ensuring emotional safety, may be questionable. A phased approach, in line with UK National Institute for Clinical Excellence recommendations [17], may thus be, more than ever, a good way to address the present insecurity by emphasizing practical and social support and the establishment of a certain feeling of safety.

In this tense context, prevention must be intersectorial and include efforts to support refugees' social integration in their local environments through education, housing, and employment. It also entails advocating for migratory policy respectful of human rights (limiting detention among others) and non-segregatory resettlement policies.

As professionals working with refugees, history teaches us that we may need to prepare ourselves for a prolonged period of working against the current in a context of scarce resources and relatively negative public opinion. Although the results of this work may often be beyond our expectations and the refugee needs, this work is essential to promote an ethos of solidarity.

References

1. Bibeau. Généalogie de la violence. Le terrorisme: piège pour la pensée Montreal; 2015.
2. Fassin D. La Supplique - Stratégies rhétoriques et constructions identitaires dans les demandes d'aide d'urgence. Annales HHS. 2000;Septembre-octobre(5):953–81.
3. Barsky RF. Arguing and justifying: assessing the Convention Refugee's choice of movement, motive and host country. New York: Ashgate; 2001.
4. Chimni BS. From resettlement to involuntary repatriation: towards a critical history of durable solutions to refugee problems. Refug. Surv. Q. 2004;23(3):55–73.
5. Rousseau C. Le jeu des différences. In: Colin C, editor. Une juste place pour tous les enfants: Plaidoyer pour l'action. Montréal: Éditions de l'Hôpital Sainte-Justine - Centre hospitalier universitaire mère-enfant; 2004. p. 119–31.
6. Bodegård G. Life-threatening loss of function in refugee children: another expression of pervasive refusal syndrome? Clin Child Psychol Psychiatry. 2005;10(3):337–50.
7. Kronick R, Rousseau C. Rights, compassion and invisible children: a critical discourse analysis of the parliamentary debates on the mandatory detention of migrant children in Canada. J Refug Stud. 2015;28(4):544–69.
8. Ruiz-Casares M, Rousseau C, Currie JL, Heymann J. "I hold on to my teddy bear really tight": results from a child online survey on being home alone. Am J Orthopsychiatry. 2012;82(1):97–103.
9. Ruiz-Casares M, Cleveland J, Oulhote Y, Dunkley-Hickin C, Rousseau C. Knowledge of healthcare coverage for refugee claimants: results from a survey of health service providers in Montreal. PLoS One. 2016;11(1):e0146798.
10. Rousseau C, Oulhote Y, Ruiz-Casares M, Cleveland J, Greenaway C. Encouraging understanding or increasing prejudices: a cross-sectional survey of institutional influence on health personnel attitudes about refugee claimant' access to health care. PLoS One. 2017;12(2):e01709.
11. Chase LE, Cleveland J, Beatson J, Rousseau C. The gap between entitlement and access to healthcare: an analysis of "candidacy" in the help-seeking trajectories of asylum seekers in Montreal. Soc Sci Med. 2017;182:52–9.
12. Pottie K, Greenaway C, Feightner J, Welch V, Swinkels H, Rashid M, Rousseau C, Tugwell P; coauthors of the Canadian Collaboration for Immigrant and Refugee Health. Evidence-based clinical guidelines for immigrants and refugees. CMAJ. 2011;183(12):E824–925.
13. Priebe S, Giacco D, El-Nagib R. Public health aspects of mental health among migrants and refugees: a review of the evidence on mental health care for refugees, asylum seekers and

irregular migrants in the WHO European region. Copenhagen: WHO Regional Office for Europe; 2016.
14. Fazel M, Reed RV, Panter-Brick C, Stein A. Mental health of displaced and refugee children resettled in high-income countries: risk and protective factors. The Lancet. 2012;379(9812):266–82.
15. Kirmayer LJ, Narasiah L, Munoz M, Rashid M, Ryder AG, Guzder J, et al. Common mental health problems in immigrants and refugees: general approach in primary care. Can Med Assoc J. 2011;183(12):E959–67.
16. Rousseau C, Pottie K, Thombs B, Munoz M, Jurcki T. Post traumatic stress disorder: evidence review for newly arriving immigrants and refugees. Can Med Assoc J. 2011. www.cmaj.ca/lookup/suppl/doi:10.1503/cmaj.090313/-/DC1.
17. National Collaborating Centre for Mental Health, Royal College of Psychiatrists' Research Unit. Post-traumatic stress disorder. The management of PTSD in adults and children in primary and secondary care. In: Excellence NIfC, editor. London: Gaskell and the British Psychological Society; 2005.

Cécile Rousseau
Professor, Division of Social and Cultural Psychiatry
McGill University, Montreal, Canada

Preface

From a Certain Unsafety to an Uncertain Safety: An Overview of the Book

Migratory processes have always been an integral part of human history. In the twenty-first century we are, yet again, facing large movements of people due to armed conflicts, economic and ecological challenges, in particular in the Middle East and Africa. We are witnessing endless cohorts of refugees moving through Europe from its Mediterranean shores to the north and rubber boats full with refugees capsizing in front of the Italian and Greek coasts on a daily basis, causing deaths of thousands. Hundreds of thousands of refugees are now populating camps in the south of Turkey, Syrians seeking refuge in Lebanon form by now one fourth of that Middle Eastern country's population, and many of these camps are becoming long-term or permanent accommodations due to the ongoing conflicts in countries of origin. At the same time, citizens in the EU countries receiving refugees are polarized, with the ones welcoming them with respect and genuine interest for their existential needs and uncertainties on the one side, and those fearing cultural and political destabilization in Europe and therefore rejecting refugees on the other. They are reported to fear terrorist attacks and loss of economic privileges, although there are economists arguing that the influx of refugees may contribute to economic growth of the host countries in the western world in a positive way, and most terrorist attacks are not committed by asylum seekers and refugees. Consequently, we witness building of walls, like in Calais, France, and fences, like in Hungary, in an attempt of the nations to "protect" themselves from the arrival of "the others." We also witness practices of detention of refugees on remote islands like on Nauru and Manus (Australia), where "the others" seeking refuge because of human rights violations in their home countries get confronted with similar violations inflicted by the "host" society. In our globalized world, the omnipresent media suggest that we are facing a "refugee crisis," uncomparable to the earlier ones in the history of humankind. Yet, we may ask ourselves: is this a crisis caused by large numbers of refugees alone or also, or even mainly, by a crisis of solidarity, coordination, and respect for humanitarian ethics in the "host" societies?

Earlier experiences with a large influx of refugees, as for example the one during the war in former Yugoslavia, have demonstrated that high numbers of refugees in a context of a major humanitarian crisis can be well handled by host societies, if there is political willingness, coordination, and an adequate and integrative interdisciplinary response is applied. Experiences accumulated in the past decades with a number of humanitarian disasters that have caused substantial local, regional, and international displacement have led to a better understanding of severe psychological and social impacts of displacement, and to creation of effective support models and general standards by international organizations. These can be, nowadays, seen as the best practice guidelines, which integrate different social, legal, medical, and psychological needs of refugee populations. The complexity of an adequate response by medical, mental health, and other leading professionals should follow an overall plan reflecting collaboration of all involved agencies and stakeholders, as proposed, for example, in the Interagency Standing Committee (IASC) models. However, since the "refugee experience" is of utmost complexity, one should be aware that the strategies applied in assisting these populations should not unduly medicalize socio-political problems or psychologize human rights violations, and that they must be "person-centered" in their final, practical implementation. Refugees may not only suffer from general and/or mental health problems, but they very often face accumulated losses in all areas of their existence impacting family relationships, and their social, economic, and spiritual well-being.

Health professionals throughout the world, active in conflict, post-conflict, or host country settings, are trying to assist refugees to the best of their abilities. This book is written for them and by them.

It aims at collecting and presenting the state-of-the-art knowledge on the support for refugees facing general health, psychological, and mental health challenges, and at revealing innovative portals of entry toward understanding of the complexity surrounding refugeehood and forced migration in the twenty-first century.

Therefore, all contributions in this volume follow an interdisciplinary and context-sensitive approach to the health of refugees.

The largest part of this book concentrates on general approaches to assisting refugees in the host countries of the industrialized western world. Why did we decide on this main focus? It is well known that the largest part of the globally displaced population is surviving as internally or regionally "displaced persons" in temporary reception camps, like for example in the Middle East. Otherwise, they survive on the streets, or by grace and humanity of individual hosts. However, responses in developing countries require a different set of resources and special approaches to long-term planning. Also, these approaches may vary according to substantial regional differences and are, therefore, not covered in more detail in this volume. Another topic, which is covered only partially, is the one regarding conditions for a return of refugees to their respective home countries and their reintegration, as these processes require various, context-dependent, long-term, and complex social, political, and economic measures, as well. These areas will be addressed in a follow-up volume to this book.

Chapter by Chapter: Why Read This Book?

The first part of this book covers general background topics depicting social, psychological, and legal aspects of the "refugee experience," and some universal issues regarding assessment and assistance to refugees with their general health and mental health problems. Also, interventions in emergency settings and in conflict regions, presenting both the common approach to designing large-scale, health-based humanitarian interventions and a critical analysis, are presented.

In the second part of the book, chapters discuss assistance to refugees in the context of industrialized, western host countries. They will elaborate on a range of topics: from contextual determinants and moderators of the refugees' mental health to specific considerations regarding refugee children and adolescents and both verbal and experiential interventions in the mental health domain. Last but not least, protection of refugees in places of detention, the use of interpreters in assisting refugees, and the "care-for-caregivers"—the important issue of protection of helpers—are covered, as well.

The third part of the book focusses on physical health of refugees in different settings. Both medical care for refugees in refugee camps and integration of refugee care in public health systems of the host countries are discussed.

In the foreword to this volume, *Cécile Rousseau* discusses refugeehood from a historical perspective and sketches the shift in perception of refugees by the host environments throughout time.

Brandon Hamber focuses on the impact of social violence on refugees and presents it as a central factor forcing most refugees to leave their homes and social networks and seek an insecure new future in other countries. He also stresses the importance of a contextual perspective, necessary for understanding of how refugees are being exposed to violence, and of the promotion of social change as a way to deal with a violent past.

Vamik Volkan uses a psychoanalytic approach to understand the key aspects of challenges faced by refugees and elaborates on the large-group identity processes, both in the refugee and in the host communities. He explores bereavement, loss, and mourning as the key determinants of the "refugee experience".

Adel-Naim Reyhani introduces the legal framework of international protection mechanisms and the status of refugees summarizing the development of asylum and refugee law throughout time. The author further presents the current international legal and humanitarian framework and addresses challenges in accessing the right to asylum and refugee protection.

Thomas Wenzel, Sabine Völkl-Kernstock, Tatiana Urdaneta Wittek, and David Baron discuss different aspects of recognizing, understanding, and assessing problems in refugees and how to address them within a multidisciplinary interventions framework. They present the sets of tools developed by international networks and organizations, which help planning of interventions and include continuous monitoring. Mental health assessment, the identification of vulnerable groups, and the use of medical forensic expertise to support protection of refugees are covered, too.

Hanna Kienzler, Cameron Spence, and Thomas Wenzel present strategies developed in order to recognize, conceptualize, and integrate cultural background in assessment and treatment of refugees.

Inka Weissbecker, Fahmy Hanna, Mohamed El Shazly, James Gao, and Peter Ventevogel elaborate on complex challenges in addressing mental health and psychosocial support needs of refugees. They present the key global guidelines in the sector and a variety of mental health intervention modalities applicable in large-scale humanitarian crises.

Nimisha Patel provides an introduction to the international framework of agencies, politics, and ethical challenges forming the background of the global humanitarian response in support of refugees. Moreover, she presents a critique of current approaches from the perspective of power differences and elaborates upon alternative ways to improve assistance to refugees rooted in the ethics of international intervention strategies in humanitarian disasters.

Branka Agic, Lisa Andermann, Kwame McKenzie, and Andrew Tuck describe the "seven D's" model, which provides a good overview and guidance regarding the main psychosocial stresses negatively impacting mental health of refugees. These stresses should be recognized and addressed adequately by the health care networks.

Ilse Derluyn, Elisa van Ee, and Sofie Vindevogel introduce the topic of resilience in refugee health, a topic that has become a major focus in the international discourse. Further, they discuss special considerations regarding vulnerable groups of refugees, like child soldiers, children born out of rape, unaccompanied minors and elderly. They present the pitfalls regarding labeling of certain refugee groups as vulnerable and its consequences for allocation of resources.

Trudy Mooren, Julia Bala, and Marieke Sleijpen build further on the subject of the importance of resilience factors in assisting unaccompanied refugee minors and present at large the specific characteristics of refugee adolescents from developmental, culture-sensitive, and contextual perspectives.

Boris Droždek and Derrick Silove elaborate further on complexity of the "refugee experience," introduce different models and frameworks for understanding of the impact of contextual variables on refugees' mental health, and provide an overview of the present state-of-the-art approaches in psychotherapy with refugees.

Joost Jan den Otter, Thomas Wenzel, Bernadette McGrath, Andres Leal Osorio, and Boris Droždek discuss the issue of detention of refugees in the industrialized, western host countries. Detention is used by governments with the aim to assert control over the influx of refugees, but at the same time it seriously violates basic human rights and has severe negative short- and long-term impacts on refugees' health. This discussion is illustrated with examples from Australia and the EU.

Clemens Ley and María Rato Barrio present a resource-oriented, trauma-sensitive approach to sport and physical activity, aiming at promoting health and psychosocial support among refugees. They also discuss implementation of this approach both in refugee camps in post-conflict zones and in the context of host countries in the western industrialized world.

Maria Kletečka-Pulker, Sabine Parrag, Boris Droždek, and Thomas Wenzel focus on another major aspect of the daily work with refugees, that of working together with interpreters. The use of trained interpreters and awareness of special challenges, like the issue of confidentiality, need to be integrated in different areas of the refugee care in order to enable efficient communication. The authors present case examples for practical solutions, including video translation and the UNHCR training model.

Rosa Izquierdo, Nino Makhashvili, Boris Droždek, and Thomas Wenzel address the important topic of protecting helpers from psychological impacts of the work with refugees. The helpers, whether volunteers or professionals, can be confronted both with refugees' disclosures of the traumatic past and with insecure, difficult, and sometimes even dangerous life circumstances. This may take a heavy toll on them and can affect their mental health well-being and functioning in the professional and private domains.

In the part of the book dealing with physical health of refugees, *Michael Kühnel, Boris Droždek, and Thomas Wenzel* cover the most common general health issues and outline the principles of medical care and public health, like those provided by the International Red Cross services, in the setting of refugee camps.

Last but not least, *Maria van den Muijsenbergh* discusses general health issues and intervention models aiming at integrating refugee care in public health systems of the host countries.

In conclusion, we live in times when those seeking refuge in the industrialized, western world are forced to substitute their fears for annihilation with uncertainty and not with the much needed protection and safety. In the present public discourse refugees shift from being a population "at risk" to becoming "a risk" for the host societies. These processes aggravate the "refugee experience" and may negatively impact the health of refugees. Therefore, all chapters in this book form a strong plea for a broad interdisciplinary and context-sensitive rehabilitation framework, the one being multidimensional instead of reductionist, culture-sensitive instead of culture-blind, the one being socio-politically engaged and firmly rooted in the human rights perspective to assisting those in need.

Rosmalen/Eindhoven, The Netherlands — Boris Droždek
Geneva, Switzerland — Thomas Wenzel

Endorsements

"An uncertain safety"–is an apt title that captures the challenges that refugees continue to face once they reach safety. The publication is both informative and instructive–setting out existing practices in psychosocial and mental health programmes for refugees, while pointing very frankly at the gaps. The authors do not claim to have solutions to all of these, but offer constructive ideas on how to address them, and identify clear priorities for further research. Finally, and most importantly, the contributions are grounded in extensive professional experience and research, but are infused with a strong sense of compassion and humanity, conveying that refugees are fellow human beings, and not just statistics. I hope that many mental health professionals, organisations, donors and partners will take advantage of this publication and respond to its call for engagement in ensuring that mental health of refugees is given the importance it deserves."

Filippo Grandi
United Nations High Commissioner for Refugees

"This book describes the needs and rights of traumatized refugees to safety, physical and mental rehabilitation as well as the many challenges faced by health care providers in host countries. Written by medical, psychological, and other experts, based on a broad range of experience with refugees, the authors make an important contribution toward better understanding and assisting the twenty-first century refugees."

Manfred Nowak
Professor for International Human Rights at the University of Vienna and former UN Special Rapporteur on Torture

"An uncertain safety" is both a timely exploration of the paradoxes and contradictions that characterize the so-called refugee crisis of the twenty-first century, and a guide to much of what is new and innovative in the field of looking after the health, mental health, and psychosocial needs of refugees. With chapters written by active practitioners in the fields of medicine, law, and mental health of refugees, this book is ripe with the freshness and legitimacy that only actual lived experience at the forefront of refugee care can confer. This volume is a recommended reading for experienced practitioners, those venturing into this most demanding and rewarding field, and of course, anyone interested in developing a better understanding of refugee issues and refugee recovery.

Jorge Aroche
Clinical Psychologist, CEO STARTTS, Sydney, Australia President of the International Rehabilitation Council for Torture Victims (IRCT)

Acknowledgments

We want to extend our gratitude to Springer and especially to Sylvana Freyberg for their patient and kind support during the course of putting this book together, to all contributors for their thoughtful insights in the course of the process, and last but not least, to our families and friends for support, inspiration, and understanding. Further, we want to gratefully acknowledge the advice and support of our friends at UNHCR, and UNICEF, especially Annika Bergunde, Johannes Wedenig, and Beate Dastel.

Finally, we dedicate this book to the memory of Bent Soerensen, who has recently passed away and was a friend and inspiration for many members of the global community working on human rights, torture, and the protection of refugees, and to a late friend, a long-term collaborator in earlier publications, and one of the pioneers in the world of psychotraumatology Professor John P. Wilson.

Contents

About the Editors

Thomas Wenzel, MD is a psychiatrist and psychotherapist, and professor of psychiatry at the Medical University of Vienna, Austria, working with refugees and victims of torture and other violent crimes since 1986. He is co-founder of the Hemayat and Wellcome treatment centers for torture survivors in Vienna, of the transcultural outpatient department at his University. Moreover, he is co-founder and past chair of the World Psychiatric Association scientific section on Psychological Aspects of Persecution and Torture, past medical director of the IRCT (International Rehabilitation Council for Torture Victims). He served as Secretary General of the International Academy of Law and Mental Health, and is presently chair of the working groups on refugees and pluricultural therapies of the European Association for Psychotherapy and the World Council for Psychotherapy. He is involved in international research, publications and teaching, especially on the UN Istanbul-protocol and transcultural medicine, and is a scientific coordinator of several EU projects related to stress, trauma, and resilience.

Boris Drožđek, MD, PhD is a psychiatrist and psychotherapist with over 25 years of experience in treating victims of war and political violence. He is currently associated with PsyQ/Parnassia group, Netherlands. In addition, he works in his private practice De Hemisfeer and is the international director of the Summer School of Psychotrauma in Dubrovnik, Croatia. Dr. Drožđek publishes in the fields of psychotraumatology and transcultural psychiatry, and teaches and gives training and workshops on a regular basis worldwide. Together with John P. Wilson he has edited the books *Broken Spirits: The Treatment of Traumatized Asylum Seekers and Refugees, War and Torture Victims* (Brunner-Routledge, New York, 2004) and *Voices of Trauma: Treating Survivors across Cultures* (Springer, New York, 2007). He is the former board member of NtVP (The Dutch Psychotrauma Society), IRCT (International Rehabilitation Council for Torture Victims) Executive Committee member, and currently a board member of the ISHHR (International Society for Health and Human Rights).

About the Contributors

Branka Agic, MD, PhD is the Manager of Health Equity at the Centre for Addiction and Mental Health (CAMH). She is an assistant professor in the Department of Clinical Public Health and Associate Field Director of the Master of Science in Community Health (MScCH) in Addictions and Mental Health at the University of Toronto, Canada.

Lisa Andermann, MPhil, MD, CM, FRCPC is an assistant professor in the Department of Psychiatry, University of Toronto, Canada, and psychiatrist at Mount Sinai Hospital, where she works in the Psychological Trauma Clinic and the Ethnocultural Assertive Community Treatment Team. She is also a consultant psychiatrist and Health Committee member at the Canadian Centre for Victims of Torture and a former Board Member. Her main areas of interest in research and teaching focus on cultural psychiatry.

Julia Bala, PhD is a licensed clinical psychologist and psychotherapist working for Foundation Centrum '45/Arq Psychotrauma Expert Group in the Netherlands. Specialized in the diagnosis and therapy of traumatized refugee children and families, she has been involved in the development of treatment methodologies, preventive programs, research, and transfer of expertise. Her main fields of interest are the family consequences of traumatic experiences, strengthening resilience, and the preventive potentials of multifamily therapy.

David Baron is a professor and chief of psychiatry at the Keck Hospital of the University of Southern California (USC), Los Angeles, USA. Further, he is Director of the Global Center for Exercise, Psychiatry and Sport at USC, Keck School of Medicine at USC, a Co-Chair of the World Psychiatric Association Scientific Section on Sport and Exercise Psychiatry, and a Chair of the World Psychiatric Association Scientific Section on Psychiatry, Medicine & Primary Care.

María Rato Barrio, PhD is affiliated with the Asociación para la cooperación, la convivencia y la investigación (ACCI), Madrid, Spain. She lectures, researches, and publishes mainly in the fields of the so-called sport for development and peace, intercultural living together, and research methods. She is involved in different research and social projects in a range of countries throughout Africa and Latin America, and recently worked as a postdoctoral fellow in South Africa conducting an ethnographic study on violence, otherness, and urban spaces.

Ilse Derluyn, PhD is affiliated as lecturer to the Department of Social Work and Social Pedagogy of Ghent University, Belgium, where she teaches courses in migration and refugee studies. Her main research topics concern psychosocial well-being of unaccompanied refugee minors, migrant and refugee children, war-affected children, victims of trafficking, and child soldiers. She is also heading the Centre for the

Social Study of Migration and Refugees (CESSMIR) and is co-director of the Centre for Children in Vulnerable Situations (CCVS).

Elisa van Ee, PhD, LLM is affiliated as clinical psychologist and researcher with the Psychotraumacentrum Zuid-Nederland and with the Radboud University Nijmegen, the Netherlands, as director of the Psychotherapy Residency of the Radboud Center of Social Sciences. Her main interest is psychodiagnostics and treatment of the complex consequences of trauma on families, in particular refugee families, veteran families, and children born of sexual violence.

Mohamed Elshazly, MD, MSc, ABPsych is a consultant psychiatrist with more than a decade of experience in clinical mental health services, capacity building, and mental health and psychosocial support programs in Middle East emergencies. He is working now as a Mental Health and Psychosocial Support officer for United Nations High Commissioner for Refugees in Iraq.

James Gao is a postgraduate medical student on the MSc Global Mental Health course taught by the Centre for Global Mental Health, London. He has previously interned for the WHO and International Medical Corps. He has collaborated on a number of projects for MSF UK and has conducted research on specialized psychiatric care in the West Bank.

Brandon Hamber professor, is the John Hume and Thomas P. O'Neill Chair in Peace based at the, International Conflict Research Institute (INCORE) at Ulster University, Belfast, Northern Ireland. He is also a member of the Transitional Justice Institute at the university and is an honorary professor of the African Centre for Migration and Society at the University of the Witwatersrand in South Africa.

Fahmy Hanna, MD psychiatrist, is a technical officer in the WHO Department of Mental Health and Substance Abuse in Geneva. He has more than a decade of experience in mental health service development in low and middle income settings and has previously served at the WHO offices in Syria and Libya. He contributed to supporting WHO mental health in emergency operations during Ebola and Zika viruses outbreak responses. In addition to his work in emergencies, he supports WHO work in the areas of monitoring mental health global indicators and mhGAP implementation.

Rosa Izquierdo psychologist, is an expert in migrations, human rights, and human resources/staff support. She has dedicated her career to the United Nations at headquarters, regional offices, and field locations, both in contexts where emergencies and displacement occur or and providing guidance to decision-making bodies. Currently, she serves as an independent external expert to international organizations, like the European Commission, and to national governments on crisis, security, protection, and mental health. She is also the founder and CEO of GLOCARIS-GLOCAl Minds Rosa Izquierdo.

Hanna Kienzler, PhD is a senior lecturer (assistant professor) in the Department of Global Health & Social Medicine at King's College London, UK. She has a longstanding academic interest in the field of global health, in connection with organized violence, ethnic conflict, and complex emergencies, and their health and mental health outcomes. She conducts ethnographic research on the impact of war and trauma on women in Kosovo, on new mental health treatment options for torture survivors in Nepal, and on humanitarian and mental health interventions in the occupied Palestinian territory and Kosovo.

Maria Kletečka-Pulker, PhD is a Doctor of Juridical Science and a research associate at the Medical University of Vienna, Austria. Besides, she is managing director and deputy head of the Institute for Ethics and Law in Medicine (University of Vienna), and a member of the Bioethics Committee of the Federal Chancellery of the Republic of Austria.

Michael Kuehnel, MD is a general practitioner and a specialist in Water, Sanitation and Hygiene (WASH), Public Health and Tropical Medicine. He has been involved in a number of disaster response missions for the Red Cross. During the refugee crisis in 2015/2016 he worked in refugee camps and rescue missions in Austria, Greece, and on the Mediterranean Sea.

Clemens Ley, PhD is affiliated with the Institute of Sport Science, University of Vienna, Austria. He conducted postdoc research in South Africa in the field of community sport, exercise, and HIV and undertook fieldwork in various post-conflict contexts, e.g., in Guatemala with women and children suffering from violence; in African countries, including the Kakuma Refugee Camp; and in Austria with war and torture survivors.

Nino Makhashvili is associate professor and head of the Mental Health Resource Center at the Ilia State University, Tbilisi, Georgia. Also, as a Director of the foundation Global Initiative on Psychiatry-Tbilisi (GIP-T), she works on structural changes of the mental health field in countries of the Caucasus region, in Central Asia, and in Ukraine. Since the mid-1990s she has been involved in the fields of social psychiatry and psycho-trauma with refugees and IDPs, prisoners, victims of interpersonal violence, and torture survivors.

Bernadette McGrath has almost 20 years of experience in leading and managing non-profit community-based organizations in Australia. She was the Director of STTARS, the South Australian torture and trauma service, for 12 years and is currently CEO of the Australian based Overseas Services to Survivors of Torture and Trauma.

Kwame McKenzie, MD, MRCPsych is CEO of the Wellesley Institute. He is an international expert on the social causes of illness, suicide, and the development of effective, equitable health systems. In addition, he is the Director of Clinical Health

Equity at CAMH, and a full Professor and the Co-Director of the Division of Equity Gender and Population in the Department of Psychiatry, University of Toronto, Canada.

Trudy Mooren, PhD works as a clinical psychologist at Foundation Centrum'45, part of Arq Psychotrauma Expert Group in the Netherlands. She is an associate professor affiliated with the Department of Clinical Psychology of Utrecht University. She is a licensed therapist in cognitive behavioral therapy, EMDR, and family therapy, gives trainings, and supervises trainees. In her research she focuses on consequences of violence and migration for children, adolescents, and families. She studies the sequelae of traumatic events on subsequent lifetime development.

Maria van den Muijsenbergh, MD, PhD is a general practitioner and senior researcher at Pharos, Centre of Expertise on Health Disparities, Utrecht, the Netherlands, and at the Radboud University Medical Centre, Department of Primary and Community Care, Nijmegen, the Netherlands.

Andres Leal Osorio received his master's degree in social work in 2011 and since then has been working closely with refugees and asylum seekers and specifically, survivors of torture and trauma. He has worked within a number of different immigration detention facilities in Australia and is a member of the Harvard Program in Refugee Trauma.

Joost Jan den Otter is a public health specialist who has been working in the field of health and human rights for several decades. Currently, he is detention doctor at the International Committee of the Red Cross (ICRC) and is secretary of the World Psychiatric Associations' Scientific Section for Psychological Consequences of Torture and Persecution. The views in his chapter reflect the authors' opinion and not necessarily those of the ICRC.

Sabine Parrag is university assistant at the Institute for Ethics and Law in Medicine at the University of Vienna, Austria, and a PhD student in social sciences.

Nimisha Patel is a consultant clinical psychologist in the UK. She is the Executive Director of the International Centre for Health and Human Rights, a UK-based NGO, and Professor of Clinical Psychology on the Professional Doctorate in Clinical Psychology at the University of East London. She has worked in human rights NGOs, the British national health service, and in many countries as a consultant for a range of international organizations, including United Nations agencies.

Adel-Naim Reyhani is a lawyer and a researcher affiliated with the Ludwig Boltzmann Institute of Human Rights in Vienna, Austria. Previously, he has been a legal adviser at the Diakonie Refugee Service, lawyer at the Austrian Asylum Court, and has participated in different studies and reports on asylum and migration for the European Migration Network (International Organization for Migration).

Cécile Rousseau, MD is professor of psychiatry at McGill University and scientific Director of the Research Institute on health and cultural diversity SHERPA. She has worked extensively with immigrant and refugee communities, developing specific school-based interventions and leading policy-oriented research. Presently her research focuses on the evaluation of collaborative mental health care models for youth in multiethnic neighborhoods and on intervention and prevention programs to address youth radicalization.

Derrick Silove is a scientia professor of psychiatry at the University of New South Wales, Sydney, Australia. He has a long history extending over 30 years working in training, service development, and research with refugees and societies affected by mass conflict and persecution. He has focused specifically on work in his geographical region, particularly in Timor-Leste, Vietnam, Bougainville, and among West Papuan refugees in Papua New Guinea.

Marieke Sleijpen, PhD is a psychologist and researcher at Foundation Centrum '45, partner in Arq Psychotrauma Expert Group, and a lecturer at the Department of Clinical Psychology, Utrecht University, the Netherlands. Her main research interest is related to resilience in adolescent refugees and asylum seekers. Currently she is the project leader of a study on resilience in unaccompanied adolescents from Eritrea in the Netherlands, a collaboration with NIDOS Foundation.

Cameron Spence is a Canadian PhD candidate at the Department of Global Health & Social Medicine, King's College London. He is a medical anthropologist currently working on "an ethnography of home treatment in psychiatry." His work investigates the intersection between the practice and experience of community mental health in local economies and landscapes of care.

Andrew Tuck, MA is a research coordinator in the Health Equity Department at the Centre for Addiction and Mental Health (CAMH), Toronto, Canada. He was a member on two Mental Health Commission of Canada project teams that conducted research, hosted pan-Canadian consultations, and authored reports for bettering the mental health of immigrants, refugees, and ethno-cultural and racialized populations in Canada.

Pieter Ventevogel, MD, PhD is a psychiatrist and medical anthropologist with more than 15 years of work experience in humanitarian settings. Since 2013, he is the Senior Mental Health Officer with UNHCR, the Refugee Agency of the United Nations.

Tatiana Urdaneta Wittek is a lawyer, specialized in Human and Victims Rights. She is collaborating with the Boltzmann Institute for Human Rights, Vienna, Austria, and with Professor Manfred Nowak (former UN Special Rapporteur on Torture).

Sofie Vindevogel is a lecturer in the Department of Orthopedagogy and researcher at the Expertise Centre on Quality of Life (E-QUAL) at University College Ghent in Belgium. Her current research explores the ways children, youth, families, and communities in (post-)conflict situations deal with adversity and which resources contribute to their resilience.

Vamik Volkan is professor emeritus of psychiatry at the University of Virginia, Charlottesville, VA, USA. Also, he is President Emeritus of the International Dialogue Initiative and Past President of the Virginia Psychoanalytic Society, Turkish-American Neuropsychiatric Society, International Society of Political Psychology, and American College of Psychoanalysts.

Sabine Völkl-Kernstock is Head of the Outpatient Unit for Trauma Assessment and Child Protection Unit at the Medical University of Vienna/Department of Child and Youth Psychiatry, Austria. She is a licensed clinical and health psychologist and psychotherapist with a long-standing experience in the work with traumatized children with different ethnic backgrounds.

Inka Weissbecker, PhD, MPH is the Senior Global Mental Health and Psychosocial Advisor for the International Medical Corps and has provided remote and on-site technical oversight and support in the areas of assessment, program design, project implementation, and evaluation of mental health and psychosocial programs to over 15 conflict and crisis affected countries.

Part I

General Aspects and the Interdisciplinary Mental Health Care Emergency Response

1 Changing Context and Changing Lenses: A Contextual Approach to Understanding the Impact of Violence on Refugees

Brandon Hamber

Abstract

Refugees can face a range of social, political, cultural, existential and spiritual challenges that extend beyond the impact of discrete events or direct psychological and physical harms. Such suffering can only be understood relative to and dependent upon the context in which it is experienced. Context is a major, not a tangential, component of conceptualising assistance to refugees. Hans Keilson's approach of sequential traumatisation shows that interventions to assist refugees need to extend to understanding the role of the context over time and that past experiences are always reinterpreted through the prism of the present. Different community and individual processes (such as testimony and social activism) can create new contextual meaning for refugees. Changing the context is a psychological intervention. There is a responsibility on mental health workers and practitioners to find ways to change and influence the socio-political context.

1.1 Introduction

> As soon as this bruised population makes its appearance, fear, compassion and blame jostle together with their cargo of blinding stereotypes: a world of victims, dirty like the wars that have produced it, a violent and unjust world in which people kill each other for no reason in some far-off place. ([1], p. 1)

B. Hamber
John Hume and Thomas P. O'Neill Chair, International Conflict Research Institute (INCORE), Ulster University, Belfast, Northern Ireland

African Centre for Migration and Society, University of the Witwatersrand, Johannesburg, South Africa
e-mail: b.hamber@ulster.ac.uk

T. Wenzel, B. Droždek (eds.), *An Uncertain Safety*,
https://doi.org/10.1007/978-3-319-72914-5_1

This chapter focuses on how dealing with the legacy of violent pasts can impact upon refugees.[1] Drawing on my previous work with victims of political violence more broadly,[2] I outline a generic framework for understanding the impact of political violence on refugees. I first explain how the impact of large-scale political violence can be understood and the needs this creates for victims of political violence and refugees in particular. I then discuss a theoretical model that can be used to understand the impact of political violence and apply it to the context of refugees. Thereafter I address, at a macro level, what this model practically means for the nature of the interventions that can be considered appropriate for addressing the psychological, social and political needs of refugees. I conclude with some reflections on the role of psychologists and mental health workers in addressing such needs.

1.2 The Impact of Mass Violence

The assumption behind this chapter is that we are talking about a certain type of context. While all contexts differ, this chapter reflects on cases in which large-scale armed conflict has taken place or is taking place. Such conflict results in the loss of life and a range of other human rights violations (e.g. torture), but also the destruction of infrastructure and livelihoods. A further result can be the internal displacement of peoples and refugees fleeing across borders and/or individuals being forced into transitory camps as the conflict unfolds and finally ends. Typically these conflicts result in the breakdown of intercommunity relationships and social connections on top of other destructive impacts. The initial context of destruction, and the migration process with its many facets, can be dominated by a feeling, and of course a reality, that nowhere is safe and where the line between death and extreme suffering on the one hand and ordinary living on the other is obliterated. Individual victims can become estranged from their families, communities and wider society. This undermines their sense of belonging to society [3, 5, 6], and the estrangement is often exacerbated by social conditions such as poverty, racism, gender discrimination, exclusion and physically moving away from one's perceived community or home. Extreme political violence therefore tell victims something about their place in society, but it can also dehumanises them through words (e.g. through the labelling of Tutsis as "cockroaches" during the Rwandan genocide or as calling refugees "makwerekwere",[3] derogatory slang for foreigners in South Africa). In the UK, the

[1] The definition of refugee is a complex issue. This is discussed elsewhere in this book. Broadly I would adopt a definition of the term as described by AOAV, i.e. refugee is best used as a term by those who self-describe as refugees which may include "those who are still seeking asylum. However, where it is referred to in the context of laws and policy, the term identifies those who have been granted asylum" ([2], p. 2).

[2] This chapter draws on two works [3, 4]. Parts of the text have been extracted from these works and in terms of [4] reproduced with permission of the Berghof Institute.

[3] The term is allegedly onomatopoeic, South Africans claim to hear "kwere, kwere" when immigrants open their mouths. The term is derogatory.

columnist in The Sun, Katie Hopkins, described refugees as a "feral humans", "spreading like the norovirus" and "cockroaches", among other slurs [2]. Such stereotyping has been found across Europe in the press and in political statements and often conflates refugees and economic migrants [2].

Agier reminds us that terms such as displaced and refugee say little about the essential facts behind the labels, that is:

> These people escaped a massacre, fled from direct threats to their lives, surviving by chance the bombardment of their village, the machine-gunning of their building, or the destruction of their town. ([1], p. 14)

Reflecting on refugees in recent camps in Greece, Morgan notes:

> This is a population who have lived through years of violent conflict, been forced to flee, and are now living in cramped, overcrowded, and unhygienic conditions and facing an uncertain future. ([7], p. 896)

Even when considering physical injuries these have social and community ramifications that move beyond the physical. A recent Action on Armed Violence (AOAV) report notes:

> Refugees may also face additional stresses as a result of physical injuries obtained from explosive weapons, with many facing a range of temporary or permanent impairments. Some have undergone dramatic changes in appearance or experienced the traumatic amputation of a limb, whilst many others have life-changing injuries such as loss of hearing or sight. As a result, affected persons may feel that their independence has been taken away, and that they no longer could play a useful part in family or community life, leading to feelings of detachment, withdrawal and hopelessness. ([2], p. 6)

In other words, political violence experienced by many refugees is not only about harm to the body as the social fabric, structures and institutions are damaged [8, 9]. The extreme nature of the violence alters the normative order, as well as individual and social meaning systems, social relations and ways of life [10, 11]. As with political violence more generally, at a social level, trust and a sense of connection between groups, normally a key part of well-being, are destroyed, and the concept of the negative "other" often emerges or hardens [12–14]. All these processes can place during a conflict that leads to flight and within transitory spaces and new host countries.

Although not developed to look at refugees in the particular but rather authoritarian state violence, the notion of extreme traumatisation nonetheless captures the type of contexts I have outlined above [15–17]. Elsewhere I have argued [3] that what one could call "extreme political traumatisation" is made up of four elements:

1. Structural violence cut through by race, ethnicity, gender, age and class
2. Direct violence inflicted through physical harm that is laden with social meaning; psychological destruction and alteration of individual and community meaning systems through extreme violence and through dislocating ("uncanny") acts such as targeting civilians, torture, killings or disappearance and displacement, among other things

3. Discursive distortion marked by a rhetoric of dehumanisation, deceptive public discourse and lies; exclusionary language aimed at creating a lack of social belonging and in some cases inflaming direct violence
4. Destruction of social ties and relationships, not only between victims and their place in society (their country or citizenship) and also physical dislocation but also between individuals, groups and communities in that society

The context of extreme traumatisation therefore conveys an environment where thinking about trauma as a series of individual events, with a beginning, middle and end, is inadequate. The traumatic experience is substantially more totalising. Put another way, for refugees the fissures are human, material and environmental ([1], p. 8), and needs are multidimensional having medical, psychological, social, political, cultural and legal dimensions [18]. Therefore, the models we use to understand the impact of such processes, and the interventions that follow, need to be more robust than seeing refugees as survivors of discrete acts of political violence.

1.3 Linking Context and Traumatic Processes

The theory of Hans Keilson can be useful in thinking about how best to understand the type of traumatic processes for survivors of political conflict or refugee communities fleeing political persecution [19].[4] Keilson sought, by focusing on Jewish World War II orphans in the Netherlands in a longitudinal study over 25 years, to understand the impact on the orphans of the experience in full and over time. Keilson, in his study, identified three sequences that had an impact of the children's present and future well-being: the occupation of the Netherlands by the Nazis and the direct threats to family and community integrity, direct persecution resulting in experiences of hiding and/or concentration camps and other experiences and, finally, the post-war period of remaining in foster families or returning home and related events [19].

Recently, Michel Agier used a similar mapping process to outline three (slightly different) sequences experienced for contemporary refugees:

> First of all, the stage of destruction—land, house and towns ravaged by war, as well as broken trajectories of lives and the irreducible mark of physical and moral wounds. Then that of confinement—months of waiting, years or whole life-cycles spent in transit on the fringes of cities or in camps that seem trying to become towns without ever managing to do so. Finally, the moment of action, still uncertain and hesitant: the search for a right to life and speech which, in the disturbed context of war and exodus, often emerges in a context of illegality may eventually give birth to new form of political commitment. ([1], p. 4)

[4] I would like to thank Dr. David Becker for introducing me to the work of Keilson and explaining its significance. What I present here is built on his initial insights, and I am deeply grateful.

Others too have noted that the migration trajectory can be divided into three components: premigration, migration and postmigration resettlement. Each phase is associated with specific risks and exposures ([20], p. 961).

Traumatisation of the children, according to Keilson, differed relative to the different traumatic sequences to which they were exposed. This meant that some orphans who objectively may have had a terrible experience in the war, but a fairly satisfactory post-war situation such as being adopted by a caring family, might have in the long run psychologically been better off than those who had a relatively "better" experience during the war but a worse post-war experience. The trauma was not static but depended on different experiences over a period time as well as sequences of experience. What Keilson's study, therefore, shows us—albeit obvious on some levels—is that different sequences, or contexts and situations, can impact on the development of trauma in different ways. In other words, it is not only the physical or psychological stress which victims or survivors endured that is important (say in Keilson's sequence one and two) but also how this was mediated contextually at different points over time. Simply put, Keilson's theory suggests that being part of an objectively terrible traumatic incident is not the simple or linear predictor of a trauma reaction. Someone could suffer immeasurably, but be well supported emotionally and by their community, resulting in them coping better and emerging in a relatively healthy psychologically state. Another individual could cope fairly well after the incident and have objectively, and relatively speaking, a less traumatic history, but live in a hostile impoverished environment with no support. This can result in them suffering more developmentally and psychologically speaking than the person who experienced a greater direct traumatic or persecutory incident.

If we apply Keilson's theory to say Vietnam veterans, we would have to ask what was the mediating variable in their current psychological state: the experiences of the war or the experiences of coming home to a hostile society? Obviously both but mainstream traumatic stress models often excessively focus on the experiences of the war rather than other social and political sequences such as coming home. In a similar way, if one thinks of refugees, it can be their experiences in a country in to which they move or settle that determines how their different prior experiences are interpreted and understood, not simply what happened in causing them to flee. Suffering therefore does not end when moving to a new country or away from direct persecution—the original experiences are reinterpreted through the prism of the new sequence.

Keilson argues that the description of the changing traumatic situation should be the framework within which we understand any trauma and is the best predictor of whether mental health problems will indeed develop. Thinking of trauma in relation to the context, and sequentially across time as Keilson proposes, implies that there is no "post" in thinking about trauma [5], there is no universal response to a traumatic situation and there is no logical presumption that everyone in a traumatic situation will experience trauma. Trauma can only be understood relative to and dependent upon the context in which it is experienced. If the theory of sequential traumatisation is right, we can expect people to experience different mental health impacts at different moments in time.

From another angle, there is a debate within the psychological literature concerning the concept of trauma and its relationship to time and sequence. Allan Young points out that making a diagnosis of PTSD "presumes that time moves from the etiological event to the post-traumatic symptoms" ([21], p. 135). He argues that all that is visible in the present is the individual's psychological state, and time is assumed to run backwards to the so-called traumatic incident, even though this may not be the case. Yet diagnosticians use a range of technologies (such as diagnosis using criteria) to try to get traumatic time to run from the assumed etiological event to the so-called post-traumatic symptom; to this end a diagnosis such as post-traumatic stress disorder is essentially "invented" [21].

My core argument here is that medicalised and essentially linear understandings of trauma overemphasise the role played by the traumatic incident in the individual's current psychological state, rather than trying to understand the context and subjective meaning of that psychological state relative to what has happened and the current context [3]. As Drožđek has written "Perceiving the 'individual survivor as a patient,' one individualizes and medicalizes social destruction and collective suffering" ([22], p. 9). This is of profound importance: in short political violence is a social phenomenon, and to expect to deal with its consequences outside of the social context is to misread its impact.

What is the significance of this? Primarily, it has implications for how and where we target interventions aimed at dealing with trauma experienced by refugees, and this, in turn, is important for how we conceptualise the role of mental health workers, as well as politicians and anyone who can shape the social context. What it means directly for those forced from their homes or resettling in a new society following political violence is that the context in which they find themselves is integrally linked to whether a traumatic reaction is likely.

Refugees, Keilson tells us, will across their lifespans continually interpret past experiences of violence or suffering (say in the country from which they fled) through the lens of the current context. Ongoing socio-economic marginalisation in new country, or experiences of racial abuse or xenophobia, does not have static or discrete consequences but will affect how refugees ascribe meaning to their original and hence ongoing suffering. Sequential traumatisation or, more to the point, an ongoing harmful social context (even if a new country and less directly harmful than say direct experiences of war from which refugees fled) accounts for a continual re-evaluating of original traumas and alters the meaning given to it. This is not the same as the idea that repressed traumas can resurface after an event at a later time, but, rather, building on Keilson's theory, we need to understand trauma as intertwined with the particular context of the present and not only about experiences of the past.

The new sequence (say resettlement) might offer physical safety from political violence. A so-called successful flight from "an environment of insecurity, exposure to violence, and destroyed homes" ([23], p. 903) can have positive mental health effects or limit the potential for harm. But equally resettlement, even if considered "successful", can, for example, result in other conflicts of loyalty or guilt to those left behind, not to mention wider existential issues, cultural and language problems hampering belonging and/or questions about the long-term future for self, family or friends. An individual who objectively experienced less direct persecution prior to fleeing but on arrives in a new country experiences xenophobia or racism could have a worse long-term prognosis, than someone who experienced more direct violence in the country from which they fled but has a more positive post-persecution experience. Suffering is therefore linked with the "polarised debate and inflammatory political posturing" ([2], p. 18) that often surrounds issues of migration in the contemporary world. Equally, being in a refugee camp can create a psychological sense of liminality and indefinite life separated from context [1] exacerbating previous experiences and merging in a traumatic process that is not made up of isolated events.

Ongoing social issues after resettlement often account for why initial mental health indicators after resettlement tend to decline over time. As has been noted:

> Once future status is decided, resettlement usually brings hope and optimism, which can have an initially positive effect on well-being. Disillusionment, demoralization and depression can occur early as a result of migration-associated losses, or later, when initial hopes and expectations are not realized and when immigrants and their families face enduring obstacles to advancement in their new home because of structural barriers and inequalities aggravated by exclusionary policies, racism and discrimination. ([20], p. 961)

As AOAV notes after studying recent refugees in the UK, Germany and Greece:

> …despite the trauma many refugees had already faced, they were forced to endure further stress when they reached Europe. Many refugees are forced to live in poor condition and face the frustration of waiting for their responses for years that, after having witnessed the effects of brutal violence and war, exacerbates mental conditions. Refugees from Syria, Iraq and Afghanistan already suffer from collective, trans-generational trauma and are in dire need of support. ([2], p. 36)

Patterns of dehumanisation and a lack of empathy for refugees [2], as well the often difficult legal and social environment in which they find themselves, can compound psychosocial challenges. Reflecting on refugees experiences in the UK, it has been noted:

> Not only was the law itself confused but the asylum process itself was reported to be traumatic—a place where empathy was rarely shown and where those trying to navigate the process felt dehumanised. Many of the respondents spoke English fairly well and were not otherwise vulnerable, but they expressed particular concern for others that were vulnerable who would have to navigate the same process. ([2], p. 30)

The nature of support in an environment of supposed security can therefore assist or aggravate mental health issues. For example, admission of families with children on flight into so-called safe countries can be an effective way to reduce negative mental health symptoms [23].

Therefore attempting to categorise the impact of violence as a set of standard psychological responses is theoretically inadequate and misses that trauma is essentially a contextual process. The concept of post-traumatic stress disorder (PTSD) and the word "trauma" itself have become a shorthand that tells us little about the context of violence, its cultural specificities and how dealing with violence is linked with the socio-economic, political and cultural context ([24], for a wider discussion for further limits of the concept of PTSD). The concept pathologises a social phenomenon (political violence or being forced from your home), and "trauma" has begun to change the language of suffering. Victims end up expressing themselves in medical language ("I am suffering from PTSD", "I am traumatised"), masking the detail of the full nature of interlocking suffering where direct harm from violence that takes place in different sequences intersects with class (generally poverty and inequality) and other forms of social exclusion that are interconnected with gender, age or race, among other factors [3].

As a concept, trauma, and PTSD specifically, drives thinking towards homogeneity, as if all experiences of violence have the same outcome or need the same treatment, whether caused by domestic violence, political acts or natural disasters. This strips away the meaning individuals attach to violence in different contexts and the impact of temporal realities. To an advocate of PTSD a nightmare is a symptom, but for one individual a nightmare might be immaterial, to another it might be a reason to seek medical help and to yet another it might be the ancestors passing on a message or sign of spiritual discord [8, 25, 26]. Much distress among communities of migrants and refugees in South Africa, for example, has been found to emanate from their material existence with its poverty, joblessness, experiences of social dislocation in their newly settled country, ongoing forms of violence embedded in the community and home, as well as the way this existence is interpreted through the metaphysical realm (e.g. as the result of ancestors, community disruption or the consequences of sin) [25].

Extreme levels of political violence, therefore, disrupt meaning systems, ways of life and everyday existence. Different violent and political incidents have distinctive political, social and cultural meanings over time and, thus, specific impacts. Understanding the different sequences of experiences, as well as the attributed meanings, is integral to recovery and adjustment in a new setting after displacement. We should therefore not forget that how we define and conceptualise suffering can impact on well-being [27]. As Bittenbinder notes, if refugees (seeking help) are:

> …simply defined as "disturbed" or "ill" it can aggravate their situation. If their suffering is only seen as social or political, it ignores their real problems on the individual mental and psychical health level. Thus the definitions that are used to describe problems of refugees themselves can influence their mental health. ([27], p. 33)

1.4 Macro Models of Intervention

Drawing from the model outlined above, we can conclude that the nature of all experiences over time are therefore critical to how the original suffering is understood. It also means greater attention needs to be paid to understanding and describing different social contexts. The specific question it raises is what does this mean for the types of interventions that might be used. Different authors (as is evident throughout this book), as well as agencies, have proposed different ways of thinking about interventions in such complicated contexts. One of the most well-known of these is the Inter-Agency Standing Committee (IASC) Guidelines on Mental Health and Psychosocial Support in Emergency Settings [28]. This model, although it has its limits (discussed later) and is not directly aimed at dealing with refugee issues, is helpful in its ability to acknowledge the needs the wider context creates beyond individual psychological need with humanitarian emergencies creating a wide range of problems experienced at the individual, family, community and societal levels [28] (see also the chapter by Wenzel et al. in this book).

At a practical level, the IASC guidelines identify four broad categories or types of interventions that could improve the psychosocial well-being of those in the midst of humanitarian and political emergencies. These can be thought of as a pyramid (see Fig. 1.1).

Needs listed at the bottom of the pyramid require the most intervention (from external agencies generally speaking), and those identified thereafter need progressively less, although all layers are important and require implementation concurrently [28]. The most extensive task, according to the IASC guidelines, is to (re) establish security, adequate governance and services that address basic physical needs (food, water, basic health care, control of communicable diseases, etc.). Secondly, help needs to be offered in accessing key community and family support (family tracing and reunification, assisted mourning and communal healing ceremonies, etc.). Thirdly, nonspecialised supports (these can include emotional and livelihood support) for the still smaller number of people who additionally require more focused individual, family or group interventions by trained and supervised workers should be ensured. Finally, the specialised services of psychologists, psychiatrists or other trained individuals should be offered to people with severe mental disorders whenever their needs exceed the capacities of existing primary/general health services [28].

There are many different types of intervention implicit in the four levels outlined above. Less clinical and community-driven approaches (at the community and family level, as well as nonspecialised support) could include activities such as group sharing of problems, community dialogue, traditional healing rituals, art

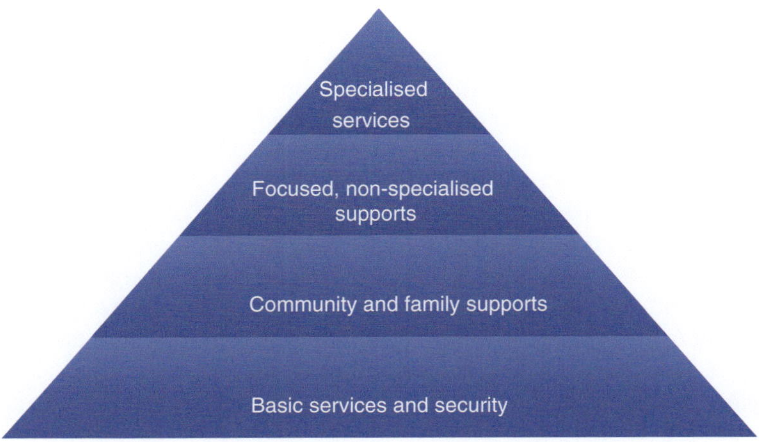

Fig. 1.1 Intervention pyramid for mental health and psychosocial support in emergencies ([28], p. 12)

projects, theatre initiatives, interpersonal skills development, training on issues such as human rights and mediation and engagement in livelihood projects. The umbrella category of psychosocial interventions is often used to describe such approaches, although what specifically constitutes a psychosocial project is not always clear [29].

Some of the key questions concern how the levels relate to each other. For example, are individual interventions such as counselling effective in a context where structural injustice remains, or can group interventions that may be judged valuable by individuals (such as a drama programme with victims of violence) have a scalable impact on wider society? There are also difficulties concerning who drives such programmes, for example, "outsiders", local NGOs and/or global NGOs, as well as how one captures processes (e.g. community rituals) outside of the formal intervention level (meaning NGO or state programmes). More recently the term "psychosocial practices" has been used to capture strategies driven locally and within society that contribute to well-being, such as the use of rituals, religious ceremonies, mourning practices, processes that mix trauma language with different approaches (as in some religious counselling), familial support and the support of friends and peer networks, among many other methods [30]. These are, in fact, the main ways individuals seek support, survive and deal with complex issues with a sense of agency and resilience, yet they receive little focus in the psychosocial fields [30, 31].

The psychosocial method also approaches well-being largely from the perspective of the individual and only minimally considers the impact of psychosocial approaches on peacebuilding and social change more broadly [30]. A further challenge of this approach is that the psychological and social dimensions of well-being are not separate categories of experience. The individual (psycho) and collective (social) dimensions of well-being are clearly seen as interrelated and experienced holistically. In other words, a key relationship exists between individual healing processes and collective strategies including interventions at the social level and the context more widely. The IASC pyramid does not in itself show sufficient interrelationship between different needs and levels. It states this is important, however, and those who use the model in interventions are also clear that goal of intervention should be to restore human, social and cultural capital in the first instance, that is, a process of "transformation, involving new relationships between the capacities, linkages, values and resources of that community" ([32], p. 163). It is also not another form of Maslow's Hierarchy of Needs [33–35] (and I believe they do not mean it in that way either), although it is easy to see how it can be read as such.

In my more recent work, however, I and others have criticised the notion of psychosocial as it still largely implies a mechanistic interaction between the "psycho" and the "social", and the IASC pyramid does the same to some degree [36]. I concur with Becker that the binary between social and psychological is essentially an "illusion" [37]. One cannot compartmentalise mental and emotional issues as distinct from physical and material issues; they are not only interrelated but also indistinguishable [14]. Michel Agier makes a similar point about the refugee experience, that is, any sequential way of understanding the refugee experience can only be illustrative as sequences are "so interwoven that to ignore one of them means losing a sense of the whole" ([1], p. 4).

Therefore, although the concept of psychosocial is helpful and extends the boundaries of theory and practice beyond the individual, it misses key dimensions of human experience [36], as does any mechanistic model that tries to fully described the refugee experience or the ever changing social context. The emotional and psychological, and the material and social, cannot be separated out, and interventions that focus on one side of the "psycho" or "social" equation or the other (although useful at times for individuals), or models that imply the "psycho" or "social" affects the other in a linear or even dynamic way, do not conceptually grasp how people live their lives and how their sense of well-being is constructed [36].

That said, to find the words to capture this composite reality is not easy. For many organisations offering support to refugees, even though they might have a wider contextual analysis of the problems faced by refugees, their approach still seems to be dominated by psychological and medical service models due to limited resources and the political challenges of approaching refugee issues more widely [18]. Much work remains to fully understand how psychosocial interventions integrate, interact or are linked to the social context and to potentially transformative changes for both individuals and societies. In my and others' recent work, we have started to consider this difficult question and develop more integrated contextual approaches and frameworks [18, 30, 38]. Such frameworks are difficult to implement as they also need to take account of dynamic life-long contexts and processes. Extreme political violence, as argued earlier, is not just about moments of the exceptionality (meaning human rights violations such as murder, torture and disappearance) but ongoing long-term processes and interrelated sequences.

This is not to say that direct human rights violations are not devastating, but in most cases violence is not a once off or isolated event, but equally social problems are not merely variables affecting mental health that come and go with governments or when individuals cross borders. Many refugees (as well as those that support them) face an "intercultural experience" every day having to react to different and varied cultures, as well as variety of political and ethical realities that change constantly [27]. Whatever the context, life is a series of daily stressors of different kinds and magnitudes that cannot be disentangled easily or experienced in some sort of isolated way; they also generally persist long into the future [25]. Such experiences cannot be captured by or fully represented by a series of projects or programmes, or one or even multidimensional models, as coming to terms with the past and human rights violations is essentially a personal life-long project that will require different approaches and social practices at different moments that will shift and change with time and location. To fully capture this process, I quote from a recent work [25]:

> Clearly, a holistic approach would be best, but what this means in the complex world… is almost impossible to define—but what we now know…is that the everyday experience of life, psychological wellbeing, spiritual enrichment, and material existence are interconnected, interlinked and often indistinguishable. No healing approach…fully capture(s) this. In the final instance however what seems to be at the core of the distress which is used as the driving force to seek out healing of some sort, is a desire to make

> sense of what is happening in the precarious world…To this end…it all shows the importance of meaning making within the healing process no matter how it is finally addressed. (p. 178)

Melanie Klein notes harm inflicted can never be completely "made good" [39]. We need to accept that we cannot repair the irreparable (bring back those who were killed or reconstruct the sense of home destroyed by conflict and following displacement) and that the future is always going to be an ambiguous place haunted by the ghosts of the past while we try to move forward [3]. Coming to terms with the past, especially with relation to mass atrocity and displacement, is a dynamic lifelong process that is context dependent. In addition, those affected by violence are also active agents in such processes. As Horst notes, refugees are:

> Often depicted as vulnerable victims or cunning crooks. These images do no justice to the multifaceted and fluid humanness that characterise individual refugees, or to the agency…agency involves power: the power of doing things or leaving them, thus making a difference…agency of actors is both enabled through and constrained by the structural properties of social systems, while simultaneously leading to their reproduction. ([40], p. 11–12)

What Hans Keilson's teaches us is that the context continues to be part of this process and this raises important questions for the issue of refugees at different stages including the impact of the liminal spaces they end up in or the society in which they may find themselves, even if these are considered safer than the place they left. Built on the experience of numerous centres across Europe working with refugees, it has been concluded that any treatment strategy will only be effective if the rights of clients attending such centres lead to self-determination and empowerment and if approaches also facilitate cultural diversity and affiliations between refugees themselves and with the host community [18]. Put another way, attempts at rehabilitation of refugees need to pay attention to past sequences but also coping in exile in the transcultural context in which individuals might find themselves [27].

1.5 Changing Context and Changing Lenses

In line with the approach taken above, therefore coming to terms with a legacy of violence and displacement is both an individual and a social task and deeply contextual. Issues of context—social, political and cultural—are primary, not secondary, factors in the psychological process of a victim's response to violence suffered [41]. Context is a major, not a tangential, component of conceptualising assistance to victims of extreme political traumatisation whether refugees or as general survivors of political violence. The importance of context and the approach outlined in this chapter is (at least) twofold, that is, the ability of the context to create meaning through different community and individual processes and how social change can promote psychological resolution and the role of mental health workers in this.

1.5.1 Meaning Making

It is often the meaning of political violence within a social and political context that is paramount to survivors. The dominant approach to dealing with political trauma is a cognitive one [42], along with others methods (Drožđek and Silove is this volume). Although some approaches are more contextually and narrative oriented [38, 43], most are preoccupied with the individual in the therapy room and narrow psychopathological approaches.

However, in line with the broader notion of harms outlined in this chapter, the bigger question is how meaning systems are altered by extreme contexts, and what the relationship is between intrapsychic processes and social change at different points in time. This is profoundly significant for refugee communities who often find themselves, and their plight, at the centre of public discussion—generally from a negative perspective in political and popular discourse. This is not to say that various approaches do not consider the social meaning of events [44, 45], but the question is what type of processes can be used to recreate meaning for refugees.

Testimony, as one method, in the clinical setting has been found to be of benefit to refugees and alleviate suffering as it changes the meanings people attach to political violence [46]. Testimony, often shared in public or through projects that capture experiences, can help to reconstitute individuals and create an existential community based shared experience [1]. Furthermore, testimony can also be critical to deliver rights, titles and documents to refugees that can be essential to survival [1].

Ndlovu in her research focuses on Zimbabwean migrants (some of the members are refugees, some are economic migrants) in South Africa who share their experiences of the Gukurahundi[5] through a group called the Zimbabwe Action Movement (ZAM) [48]. ZAM uses the public process of composing and performing songs, poetry and drama and speaking about their experiences to challenge dominant narratives [48]. The public testimony of these Zimbabweans serves two functions, that is, to:

> Navigate their lives in Johannesburg and negotiate between the nostalgia and the complex histories of “home”. By engaging in activities to correct the past, the migrants use the migrant space to engage in work that imagines a better “home”...and serves...a dual purpose, raising awareness amongst South Africans of their plight while at the same time working towards a different future in Zimbabwe. They address the past as well as present ills in their lives. ([48], p. 75)

A similar initiative is the suitcase project, which involves decorating old suitcases as a vehicle for storytelling in a deliberate and attentive way, that was developed with unaccompanied child refugees settling in South Africa [49, 50]. Interestingly, one of the challenges with the project is that in the beginning many of the young people feel compelled to “perform” a certain type of vulnerability

---

[5] A period of political violence, orchestrated by Mugabe’s army against political opponents, between 1982 and 1987 that is still silenced in contemporary Zimbabwe [47].

associated with a global discourse on the plight of refugees [49]. It is only with time that they shed the desire to perform certain vulnerabilities. In this particular project, it culminated in the group of young people developing into a formal group and displaying their decorated suitcases in a public art process and in so doing gained back agency over their refugee experiences ([49], p. 17). They saw displaying of their art as a way of countering the everyday xenophobia "so people can see we didn't choose to come here" ([49], p. 17).

That said, public testimony can also be associated with other political rather than individual agendas [3]. This, for example, can be the case in macro political processes such as truth commissions, which might have a reconciliatory agenda whereas some survivors might strive of retributive justice [51]. Stevan Weine also notes that there are risks with regard to testimonies becoming "depersonalized, decontextualized, objectified and reduced" losing their meaning and importance to the individual and wider society (46, p. xiii). Speaking out can also be associated, particularly for those in a challenging position and feeling they are reliant on others as refugees, with pressure to tell stories and please others perceived in more powerful positions [49]. Clacherty [49] quotes from child refugees experiences of therapy:

> When we told them (the counsellors) something, they forced their way to ask about things we didn't want to say. [15]

> This one time I felt sad, and this woman was pressurising me to talk, talk, talk, and I felt pressurised. [14]

> She the psychologist just wanted me to cry about it. I got bored so I did, and then she the psychologist felt better. [16]

These quotes, despite showing incredible empathy and resilience from the young people, speak to the often acontextual desire of certain therapies (and testimony projects) to simplistically assume speaking out is helpful in some linear way. For those in transitionary spaces (say refugee camps), all this becomes even more challenging. For the Zimbabwean ZAM group mentioned above, it has been a challenging process as they are still seeking apology and reparations from the Zimbabwean government who does not acknowledge their suffering [48]. They also live in an environment in South Africa where there is hostility to Zimbabwean refugees and migrants, and in some cases violent xenophobia, from the local population. Although they see their efforts to publicise their plight as extremely beneficial, every day is also a struggle economically and socially. Nonetheless, using the South African truth and reconciliation process to confer legitimacy on the value of speaking out, the members of the group feel it is central to coping with the after effects of the massacres decades later, particularly the value of connecting with others with similar experiences and the solidarity that flows from working together on creative processes [48]. Connecting refugees to community groups and structures has been identified by others too as critical to the mental health of refugees:

> The presence of welcoming links within ethnic communities or religious congregations can buffer the effects of migration losses, isolation and discrimination. Migrant youth living in communities with a high proportion of immigrants from the same background are better adjusted, partly because they have positive role models, a stronger sense of ethnic pride and social support, which can help them deal with the stressors of poverty, discrimination and racism. Becoming familiar with existing community and religious organizations can help practitioners identify and mobilize psychosocial support and other resources when needed. ([20], p. 964)

Supporting victims of political violence (in this case refugees being hosted in a new country), to be active agents within their environment, is therefore critically important. In so doing, individuals can be empowered to change the contexts in which they live, at least to a degree, and feel some reconnection socially—the very process extreme trauma undermines. The meaning of extreme political traumatisation cannot be reworked and integrated psychologically in isolation of connection with others, society and community because extreme political traumatisation involves destroying meaning and relationship to community life, as was noted earlier. Connecting with others in society, and those in a similar position, can align inner reality with what is happening externally. Profound loss is not only about dislocation or mislocation within the individual psyche but is also about the disconnection between inner and social reality [52]. Dialogue with different groups and new social interactions are often necessary to create a wider context of understanding. It is though such activity that the development of new narratives, as well as the creation a meaning structure of what has taken place for the refugee, can take place.

It is for this reason that individual interventions (such as therapy) should, at the very least, be complemented by other culturally appropriate individual, social and group support strategies. Mental health professionals still however tend to overemphasise the need for therapy and the importance of overt symptoms when dealing with refugees who are victims of political violence. Medicalised models give limited scope for including a focus on meaning and context [53]. This focus can also further limit professionals' own horizons in terms of what support work they themselves feel they can engage in, such as supporting the development of support groups or campaigning activity, or actively linking the survivor with different types of support and activities including those in civil society; for example, legal advice, education programmes, community storytelling and community development projects. Other interventions are also needed including structures for mentoring, voluntary work to support integration as well as interventions in political decision-making processes by those working with refugees [27].

That said, for many refugees (say hosted in a new country) the types of approaches outlined above may be necessary but are also in themselves often not sufficient. Negative social stereotyping often drives refugees back into their own communities, and their legal status can often prevent them from speaking out or drawing attention to themselves. There is clearly a need to target, in a culturally appropriate way, the personal needs of a survivor, but we also need to pay attention to the collective and societal level [22]. Local meanings of distress and healing from non-Western populations that have experience political violence need to be part of how we think about any context and structure interventions [24]. The wider context needs to be addressed beyond what organised and active survivors can do themselves.

1.5.2 Promoting Social Change

Keilson's sequential traumatisation or contextual model, as has been shown, implies that social context, or what he would call traumatic sequences over different time periods, shapes the traumatic outcome often more profoundly than the original violation. The corollary of this, stated plainly, is presumably that changing the social context influences the traumatic outcome. If this is correct then it intimates a responsibility. If we are concerned with the well-being of survivors and families of refugees who have suffered political violence, we need to consider changes in the context as a psychological intervention, not merely a social or political concern. This implies ongoing responsibilities for those with a duty to care for individuals over the long term, but also all those who can change the context, such as politicians and practitioners.

This is not a completely new finding because others too, most notably Ignacio Martín-Baró and others [54], have argued that human beings can be transformed by changing their reality [55]. This not only means changing physical and social structures but also involves changing mental structures through an active process of dialogue and "conscientisation" to decode the world and grasp the mechanisms of oppression and dehumanisation [54, 55]. Community development, building on existing resilience and creating social capital are key to these processes [32]. This itself can lead to empowerment and active involvement in social processes.

Thus, a responsibility exists for mental health workers, and arguably practitioners and those with the power to change social structures, to change the context in the present—this could include sharing accurate information about refugees to challenge social stereotyping, challenging unfair legal practices or deportations, advocating for human rights-driven approaches to refugees and education about issues at various levels. We all need to find the courage to speak the truth about the societies in which they live and the way they, through structure, discourse and praxis, perpetuate or create social conditions that prevent psychological recovery for refugees. This is of course easier said than done given the highly political nature of refugee issues in many countries. In addition, many of those organisations are offering support to refugees facing their own sustainability problems, funding shortages and high level of organisational and political stress due to the work they undertake [27].

Of course, psychologists and mental health workers cannot solve all the social and political problems facing refugees, but we can ask "whether psychological knowledge will be placed in the service of constructing a new society" ([56], p. 46). We could start by challenging ourselves as top-down therapeutic experts. We should ask how can our knowledge be used to accompany others and support social change. This needs to be done with an acute awareness of bolstering community support structures already in place and natural support systems rather than seeking to control or displace them [57]. In other words, one needs to walk alongside survivors and with them, assisting with the skills one has. Maritza Montero has spoken about this as working "along with the people, facilitating discussions, providing information, helping people to develop aspects concerning their self-esteem, their prejudices, and their stereotypes, and fostering democratic dialoguing, so multiple voices are heard" and in so doing "rescuing their potential and resources for transformation" ([58], p. 525). Accompaniment can include engaging with survivors in social processes and programmes, dialogue, reconnection with others and processes of change from speaking out or public testimony to using one's privileged position to impart information and knowledge that can be used and appropriated to assist survivors to better advocate for social change. As Suarez notes "a key task for the future is to connect the trauma paradigm with larger global structures, processes, and movements of social transformation" ([24], p. 150).

Conclusions

There is no medical solution to political trauma. The concerns refugees facing cannot be counselled away. We may be able to treat its effects therapeutically in some cases, but political trauma is always caused by, and finally addressed, in relation to a political and social context. If we want less trauma in the world, we need to not only assist those suffering but also prevent suffering in the first place and to the best of our abilities understand and transform the environments in which some are attempting to recover. The socio-political context, in this regard, is the prism through which all support should flow. As Jonny Steinberg, writing about Asad Abdullahi, a Somali migrant, who travelled to South Africa via Kenya and Ethiopia reminds us:

> Something momentous can happen to a person we barely know, yet we will understand intuitively what he is going through simply because we, too, are human. But there are moments in a person's life one will never understand if one does not know something about his world. ([59], p. 13)

References

1. Agier M. On the margins of the world: the refugee experience today. Cambridge: Polity Press; 2008.
2. Dathan J, Waszkewitz H, Hart M. The refugee explosion: how Europe treats refugees fleeing explosive violence. London: Action on Armed Violence; 2017.
3. Hamber B. Transforming societies after political violence: truth, reconciliation and mental health, Peace psychology book series. New York: Springer; 2009.
4. Hamber B. Dealing with painful memories and violent pasts: towards a framework for contextual understanding. In: Austin B, Fischer M, editors. Berghof dialogue series 11. Berlin: Berghof Centre; 2015.
5. Becker D. Dealing with the consequences of organized violence. In: Berghof handbook for conflict transformation. Berlin: Berghof Research Center for Constructive Conflict Management; 2001.
6. Becker D. Confronting the truth of the erinyes: the illusion of harmony in the healing of trauma. In: Borer TA, editor. Telling the truths: truth telling and peace building in post-conflict societies. Indiana: Notre Dame Press; 2006. p. 231–58.

7. Morgan J. Disability—a neglected issue in Greece's refugee camps. Lancet. 2017; 389(10072):896.
8. Summerfield D. The Impact of war and atrocity on civilian populations. In: Black D, Harris HG, et al., editors. Psychological trauma: a developmental approach. London: Royal College of Psychiatry, Gaskell; 1996. p. 148–55.
9. Lykes MB, Mersky M. Reparations and mental health: psychosocial interventions towards healing, human agency, and rethreading social realities. In: De Greiff P, editor. The handbook of reparations. Oxford: Oxford University Press; 2006. p. 589–622.
10. Humphrey M. The politics of atrocity and reconciliation: from terror to trauma. Routledge studies in social and political thought. London: Routledge; 2002.
11. Martín-Baró I. War and mental health. In: Writings for a liberation psychology. Dallas: Harvard University Press; 1996. p. 108–21.
12. Beneduce R, Jourdan L, Raeymaekers T, Vlassenroot K. Violence with a purpose: exploring the functions and meaning of violence in the Democratic Republic of Congo. Intervention. 2006;4(1):32–46.
13. Staub E. Reconciliation after genocide, mass killing, or intractable conflict: understanding the roots of violence, psychological recovery, and steps toward a general theory. Polit Psychol. 2006;27(6):867–94.
14. Williamson J, Robinson M. Psychosocial interventions, or integrated programming for well-being? Intervention. 2006;4(1):4–25.
15. Becker D. The deficiency of the concept of post-traumatic stress disorder when dealing with victims of human rights violations. In: Kelber RJ, Figley CR, Gersons BPR, editors. Beyond trauma: cultural and societal dynamics. New York: Plenum Press; 1995. p. 99–114.
16. Becker D, Castillo MI, Gomez E, Kovalskys J, Lira E. Subjectivity and politics - the psychotherapy of extreme traumatization in Chile. Int J Ment Heal Syst. 1989;18(2):80–97.
17. Kornfeld LE. The development of treatment approaches for victims of human rights violations. In: Kelber RJ, Figley CR, Gersons BPR, editors. Beyond trauma: cultural and societal dynamics. New York: Plenum Press; 1995. p. 115–31.
18. Bittenbinder E, editor. Beyond statistics: sharing, learning and developing good practice in the care of victims of torture. Berlin: von Loeper Literaturverlag; 2012.
19. Keilson H. Sequential Traumatization in Children: a clinical and statistical follow-up study on the fate of the Jewish war orphans in the Netherlands. English edn. Jerusalem: The Magnes Press; 1992.
20. Kirmayer LJ, Narasiah L, Munoz M, Rashid M, Ryder AG, Guzder J, et al. Common mental health problems in immigrants and refugees: general approach in primary care. Can Med Assoc J. 2011;183(12):E959–E67. https://doi.org/10.1503/cmaj.090292.
21. Young A. The Harmony of illusions: inventing post-traumatic stress disorder. Princeton: Princeton University Press; 1995. p. 327.
22. Drožđek B. How do we salve our wounds? Intercultural perspectives on individual and collective strategies of making peace with own past. Traumatology. 2010;16(4):5–16. https://doi.org/10.1177/1534765610362800.
23. Soykoek S, Mall V, Nehring I, Henningsen P, Aberl S. Post-traumatic stress disorder in Syrian children of a German refugee camp. Lancet. 2017;389(10072):903–4. https://doi.org/10.1016/S0140-6736(17)30595-0.
24. Suarez EB. Trauma in global contexts: integrating local practices and socio-cultural meanings into new explanatory frameworks of trauma. Int Soc Work. 2016;59(1):141–53. https://doi.org/10.1177/0020872813503859.
25. Palmary I, Hamber B, Nunez L, editors. Healing and change in the city of gold: case studies of coping and support in Johannesburg. New York: Springer; 2014.
26. Wessells M, Monterio C. Healing wounds of war in Angola. In: Donald D, Dawes A, Louw J, editors. Addressing childhood adversity. Cape Town: David Philip; 2000. p. 176–201.
27. Bittenbinder E, editor. Good practice in the care of victims of torture. Berlin: von Loeper Literaturverlag; 2010.
28. Inter-Agency Standing Committee (IASC). IASC guidelines on mental health and psychosocial support in emergency settings. Geneva: Inter-Agency Standing Committee; 2007.

29. Galappatti A. What is a psychosocial intervention? Mapping the field in Sri Lanka. Int J Ment Health, Psychosoc Work Counselling Areas Armed Conflict. 2003;1(2):3–17.
30. Hamber B, Gallagher E, editors. Psychosocial perspectives on peacebuilding. New York: Springer; 2015.
31. Hamber B, Palmary I, Nunez L. Healing and deliverance in the city of gold. In: Palmary I, Hamber B, Nunez L, editors. Healing and change in the city of gold: case studies of coping and support in Johannesburg. New York: Springer; 2015. p. 169–80.
32. Ager A, Strang A, Abebe B. Conceptualizing community development in war-affected populations: illustrations from Tigray. Commun Dev J. 2005;40(2):158–68. https://doi.org/10.1093/cdj/bsi024.
33. Maslow AH. A theory of human motivation. Psychol Rev. 1943;50(4):370–96.
34. Maslow AH. Motivation and personality. New York: Harper and Row; 1954.
35. Maslow AH. Toward a psychology of being. New York: D. Van Nostrand; 1968.
36. Hamber B, Gallagher E, Weine S, Agger I, Bava S, Gaborit M, et al. Exploring how context matters in addressing the impact of armed conflict. In: Hamber B, Gallagher E, editors. Psychosocial perspectives on peacebuilding. New York: Springer; 2015. p. 1–32.
37. Becker D. Working on the psychosocial gap: challenges, hopes, perspectives. In: Austin B, Fischer M, editors. Bergh of handbook dialogue series no. 11. Berlin: Bergh of Foundation; 2015.
38. Drožđek B. Challenges in treatment of posttraumatic stress disorder in refugees: towards integration of evidence-based treatments with contextual and culture-sensitive perspectives. Eur J Psychotraumatol. 2015;6(1):24750. https://doi.org/10.3402/ejpt.v6.24750.
39. Klein M, Riviere J. Love, hate, and reparation. The Norton library. New York: Norton; 1964.
40. Horst C. Transnational nomads: how Somalis Cope with refugees life in the daab camps of Kenya. New York: Berghahn Books; 2006.
41. Bracken PJ, Petty C. Rethinking the trauma of war. London: Free Association Books; 1998.
42. National Collaborating Centre for Mental Health. Post-traumatic stress disorder: the management of PTSD in adults and children in primary and secondary care. National Clinical Practice Guideline Number 26. London: British Psychological Society & Gaskell; 2005.
43. Miller KE, Kulkarni M, Kushner H. Beyond trauma-focused psychiatric epidemiology: bridging research and practice with war-affected populations. Am J Orthopsychiatry. 2006;76(4):409–22. https://doi.org/10.1037/0002-9432.76.4.409.
44. Eagle GT. An integrative model for brief term intervention in the treatment of psychological trauma. Int J Psychother. 1998;3(2):135–46.
45. Silove D. The ADAPT model. Intervention. 2013;11(3):237–48.
46. Weine S. Testimony after catastophe: narrating the traumas of political violence. Evanston: Northwestern University Press; 2006.
47. CCJP LRF. Gukurahundi in Zimbabwe: a report into the disturbances in Matabeleland and the Midlands 1980 - 1988. Johannesburg: Jacana; 2006.
48. Ndlovu DS. Violence and memory in breaking the silence of Gukurahundi: a case study of the ZAM in Johannesburg, South Africa. In: Palmary I, Hamber B, Nunez L, editors. Healing and change in the city of gold: case studies of coping and support in Johannesburg. New York: Springer; 2014. p. 59–77.
49. Clacherty G. The suitcase project: working with unaccompanied child refugees in new ways. In: Palmary I, Hamber B, Nunez L, editors. Healing and change in the city of gold: case studies of coping and support in Johannesburg. New York: Springer; 2014. p. 13–31.
50. Clacherty G, Welvering WTSSAD. The suitcase stories: refugee children reclaim their identities. Cape Town: Double Storey; 2006.
51. Hamber B, Wilson R, editors. Symbolic closure through memory, reparation and revenge in post-conflict societies. In: Traumatic Stress in South Africa Conference; 1999, 27–29 January; Parktonian Hotel, Johannesburg, South Africa.
52. Klass D. Continuing conversation about continuing bonds. Death Stud. 2006;30(9):843–59.
53. de Vries MW. Cultural aspects in traumatic stress. In: van der Kolk BA, McFarlane A, Weisaeth L, editors. Traumatic stress. The effects of overwhelming experience on mind, body, and society. New York: Guilford; 1996. p. 398–413.
54. Martín-Baró I. Writings for a liberation psychology. Dallas: Harvard University Press; 1996.

55. Burton M, Kagan C. Liberation social psychology: learning from Latin America. J Community Appl Soc Psychol. 2005;15(1):63–78.
56. Martín-Baró I. The role of the psychologist. Writings for a liberation psychology. Dallas: Harvard University Press; 1996. p. 33–46.
57. Landau J, Saul J. Facilitating family and community resilience in response to major disaster. In: Walsh F, McGoldrick M, editors. Living beyond loss: death in the family. New York: Norton; 2004. p. 285–309.
58. Montero M. The political psychology of liberation: from politics to ethics and back. Polit Psychol. 2007;28(5):517–33.
59. Steinberg J. A man of good hope: one man's extraordinary journey from Mogadishu to Tin Can Town. London: Vintage; 2015.

Mourning, Large-Group Identity, and the Refugee Experience

2

Vamık D. Volkan

Abstract

The refugee experience varies tremendously. I have interviewed some who barely escaped to safety by literally running over dead bodies. In October 2016, the Associated Press stated that at least 3800 refugees had died in the Mediterranean Sea so far that year in an attempt to reach Europe. We can easily imagine the "survival guilt" experienced by their relatives or friends who did not lose their lives. I also have interviewed children who were babies when they were saved and taken to a foreign place, and as they grew up they had no recollection of their parents who had been killed. Other refugees face less traumatic but still impactful conditions.

The initial care of the newcomers also varies from one host area to another. Some are kept behind barbed wires while others receive sophisticated and humane care. In this chapter I will not focus on initial care, but rather on two psychological phenomena all refugees share after their dislocations: an obligatory mourning process due to loss and its complications and a struggle with national, ethnic, religious, and other large-group identity issues. The very act of settling in a new place where natives have different shared sentiments and speak a different language inflames the newcomers' large-group identity issues. Meanwhile, a huge number of individuals in host countries perceive the mass of refugees as "the Other" and develop hostile prejudice against them. This chapter also examines refugees as the Other.

V. D. Volkan
University of Virginia, Charlottesville, VA, USA
e-mail: omervamik@aol.com

T. Wenzel, B. Drožđek (eds.), *An Uncertain Safety*,
https://doi.org/10.1007/978-3-319-72914-5_2

2.1 Psychoanalytic Observations

Psychoanalysts have presented observations and theories concerning voluntary or forced newcomers to another country, and descriptions of their experiences range from newcomers facing "culture shock" [1, 2], to developing guilt for surviving while others did not [3], to becoming "bicultural persons" without conflict [4, 5]. Other psychoanalysts who had escaped from the Holocaust wrote their memoirs (e.g., see: [6–10]). I reviewed psychoanalytic observations of what newcomers face in host countries and theories related to them in my book on immigrants and refugees [11]. Sometimes people are dislocated within the same country and are settled in a new place where the natives also belong to their ethnic group and speak the same language. For example, after the collapse of the Soviet Union, ethnic conflicts erupted in the Republic of Georgia. Georgians living in the Abkhazia section of the country were forced to flee elsewhere in the country. Under such situations the newcomers' and hosts' adjustments, in general, follow similar processes to those of newcomers who settle in a location where natives have different language, religion, and other cultural amplifiers. For example, when I was working with Georgians who had escaped from Abkhazia in 1993, I noticed the newcomers' hesitation to mix with the local people, and on many occasions I noted "Refugee Go Home" signs in the streets of Tbilisi [11].

2.2 Refugees' Mourning

There is one obligatory, common element that refugees initially share, to one degree or the other, for the rest of their lives. Since moving from one location to a foreign location involves losses—loss of family members and friends; loss of ancestors' burial grounds; loss of familiar language, songs, smells, and food; loss of previous support systems—all dislocation experiences can be examined in terms of the refugees', and even voluntary immigrants', ability to mourn and/or resistance against the mourning process.

Adult-type responses to meaningful losses can be divided into two phases: (1) the grief reaction and (2) the work of mourning. The grief reaction includes responses such as shock, denial and bargaining to reverse the outcome, pain, and anger, all of which, especially anger, eventually lead to the beginning of an emotional "knowledge" that the lost object is indeed gone. Before grief is completed, the work of mourning, as Sigmund Freud [12] described, begins. Mourning refers to a long-time process that involves revisiting, reviewing, and transforming the mourner's emotional investment in the images of the lost object. It comes to a practical end when such preoccupations, with associated affects, lose their intensity. Mental health workers who are assigned to care for refugees at the time of their dislocations usually observe the newcomers' grief reactions. In this chapter my focus is the mourning processes. However, I have observed individuals who are stuck in repeating their grief reactions, even many years after experiencing their significant loss [13].

The mourning process results in the mourner's identification with images of such lost persons or things and their realistic and/or fantasized psychological functions [12]. There can be enriching identifications: The indolent son of a lawyer has an urge to enroll in law school after his father's death. A refugee some years after settling in a new country may become a novelist telling stories of her grandfather or other persons or things lost during forced dislocation, thereby earning money and fame. Disruptive identifications that are invested with deep ambivalence cause "melancholia" [12]. Some refugees who continue to have contradictory perceptions and affects about the place and people they left behind and about conditions in the new location experience depressive affects for a long time.

For all practical purposes, the mourning process comes to an end when the images of lost items in the mourner's mind become "futureless" [14]. In other words, the mourner's internal relationship with such images no longer preoccupies the mourner's mind. Since individuals retain images of lost persons or things in their minds during their lifetimes, theoretically speaking we can say that the mourning process never ends until the mourner dies [13]. In examining refugees' adjustments, we need to access their ability to make the images of what was lost "futureless."

Many refugees become "perennial mourners" [11, 15] to one degree or another depending on their personality organization, severity of traumas associated with their dislocation, the degree of support system and acceptance in the host country, and the availability and the nature of connection with persons and things at the location left behind. Perennial mourners experience their mourning without bringing it to a practical conclusion or developing melancholia.

2.3 Linking Objects and Linking Phenomena

Perennial mourners create linking objects or linking phenomena. A linking object is an item such as a coin or photograph from the old country that the perennial mourner makes *magical.* This linking object unconsciously connects the lost persons' or things' mental representations with the mourner's corresponding self-representation *out there.* It becomes a psychological meeting ground for both. The linking object in the external world contains the tension between ambivalence and anger pertaining to the narcissistic hurt inflicted on the refugee by his losses.

By *controlling* the linking object, the refugee controls his confusing affects pertaining to a wish to recapture some elements left behind and affects related to this wish and other affects related to his other wish to completely say goodbye to his losses. Thus the refugee avoids the psychological consequences if any of these two wishes are gratified. When a refugee "locks up" in a drawer a coin that has become a linking object, he also "hides" his complicated mourning process in the same drawer. All such a person needs is to know where the coin is and how it is safely tucked away. Such a refugee may unlock the drawer during an anniversary of the dislocation and look at the coin or touch it. But as soon as he feels anxious, the coin is locked up again. Since the linking object or phenomenon is "out there," the mourner's mourning process too is *externalized.* This way the refugee finds a way of escaping from feeling the painful struggle within himself. Through the creation of a linking object or phenomenon, the refugee makes an "adjustment" to the complication within the mourning process; the refugee makes the mourning process "unending" so as not to face the conflict pertaining to the relationship with the images of what was left behind and new images he is facing in the new location.

Sometimes a linking object is a living being. A Georgian refugee family left their beloved pet dog behind when they fled from Abkhazia and settled at an internally displaced persons' location near Tbilisi. At their new location they saw a black dog roaming this refugee camp, took the new dog into their crowded room, and adopted him. The animal evolved as their living linking object; it became "magical." It represented their wish to go back to Abkhazia and their wish to accept their loss "out there." Since the dog was psychologically so important, the family became preoccupied with caring for and protecting this animal in an exaggerated fashion in their miserable refugee camp [11].

A linking phenomenon refers to a song, a smell, a gesture, an action, or an affect that functions as a linking object. For example, whenever a refugee feels internal pressure to complete her mourning, a song from the old country comes to her mind, and she utilizes this song as a linking phenomenon. An affect, especially nostalgia [16], can also function as a linking object.

Linking objects and phenomena should not be confused with childhood transitional objects and phenomena that are reactivated in adulthood. A transitional object represents the first not-me, but it is never totally not-me. It links not-me with mother-me, and it is a temporary construction toward a sense of reality and security [17, 18]. Linking objects and phenomena must be thought of as tightly packed symbols whose significance is bound up in the conscious and unconscious nuances of the internal relationship that preceded a significant loss such as a forced dislocation. Linking objects and linking phenomena also should not be confused with keepsakes. A keepsake does not function as a repository where a complicated mourning process is externalized. A typical keepsake provides continuity between the time before the loss and the time after the loss or generational continuity if the lost person or item belonged to a previous generation.

Some refugees become pathologically preoccupied with their linking object or phenomenon to the degree that they do not have much energy left to spend on finding new ways of living. I noted in more than a few cases how a psychological struggle over losing and wishing to refind what was left behind was generalized. For example, they would talk about a persistent habit of losing keys for their apartment or car, when such luxury was available to them, and then finding the lost items in unexpected places. On the other hand, other refugees with perennial mourning gain useful time through their utilization of linking objects and phenomena. Keeping a sense of belonging to the past as well as a foot in the future (where the images of lost things, relatives, and friends will be futureless) can provide a helpful gradual transition for these individuals over a period of years. Then these refugees begin to function as healthy mourners as their linking objects and linking phenomena stop being magical. They become able to recognize both the distinction and the continuity between the past, present, and future and develop healthy biculturalism.

On many occasions refugees, without being fully aware of it, may develop their linking objects and linking phenomena as they are escaping from a dangerous place and coming to a safe location. Mental health workers assigned to look after the refugees at the time of their dislocations should have knowledge about linking objects and phenomena [13, 15] and their meanings for the newcomers.

2.4 Age Factor

Some of the refuges are babies or young children who cannot mourn like adults, but later their parents and other psychologically important persons in their environment pass their complicated issues to the youngsters. Becoming a refugee during adolescence incurs extra problems [5, 11]. During the adolescent passage, youngsters loosen their attachments to and internal relationships with their childhood object images, modify them, replace them, or even give them up [19]. As stated by Martha Wolfenstein [20], the adolescent passage is the crucial process that separates one's ability or inability to genuinely mourn in an adult fashion. Dislocation from a familiar place to a foreign one leads to youngsters' combining their internal and external turmoil; they face what Amsterdam psychoanalyst Jelly van Essen called, "double mourning" [21].

2.5 Large-Group Identity

During the adolescence passage youngsters' large-group identity also becomes crystallized [22]. By the term "large group," I refer to hundreds of thousands or millions of individuals who share the same tribal, ethnic, religious, national, historical, and ideological sentiments, even though they will not meet each other in their lifetimes. Large-group identities are the end-result of myths and realities of common beginnings, historical continuities, geographical realities, and other shared linguistic, societal, religious, cultural, and ideological factors. In common language large-group identities are expressed by saying "I am Basque," "I am Lithuanian Jew," "I am Syrian," "I am German," or "I am Catholic."

Being a refugee during adolescence passage often brings the young displaced person's large-group identity problems to the surface. German psychoanalyst Annette Streeck-Fischer's [23] presentation of the stories of three adolescents who were rather recent comers to Germany illustrates these youngsters' large-group identity issues. The first patient was the 15-year-old son of a Polish-German mother and a Turkish father, both of whom came to Germany as adolescents. The teenager's maladjustment to being a newcomer included his glorification of militant ideologies of his father's native country. The second patient was 1 year older than the first one; she had lived in Moscow with her parents until she was 11 years old, where she experienced increasing anti-Semitism. Through her symptoms and actions in a hospital setting, she managed to make her caretakers feel as if they were Nazi torturers or concentration camp guards. The third patient was 15 and a half, the daughter of a

German mother and a black African father. In her case, boundaries between the mother's and the father's large-group identities were blurred, creating severe confusion and difficulty with reality testing.

Not only youngsters going through adolescent passage or completing it but all refugees—except very small children who are still unaware that they belong to a specific large group—face large-group identity problems following their dislocations. Let me now very briefly look at what is personal identity and how shared large-group identity develops. The concept of personal "identity" is defined as, "a persistent sameness within oneself... [and] a persistent sharing of some kind of essential character with others" [24]. There is a consensus that an individual's "identity" refers to a *subjective experience*. It is differentiated from related concepts such as an individual's "character" and "personality," which are usually used interchangeably. The latter terms describe others' impressions of the individual's emotional expressions, modes of speech, typical actions, and habitual ways of thinking and behaving. If we observe someone to be habitually clean, orderly, or greedy, or if he uses excessive intellectualization and shows excessive ambivalence and controlled emotional expressions, we say that this person has an obsessional character. If we observe someone who is overtly suspicious and cautious, and whose physical demeanor suggests that she is constantly scanning the environment for possible danger, we say that this person has a paranoid personality. Unlike the terms "character" and "personality," "identity" refers to an individual's inner working model—he or she, not an outsider, senses and experiences it.

Scientific observations of infants in recent decades have taught us that an infant's mind is more active than we originally thought [25–27]. We now know that there is a psychobiological potential for we-ness and bias toward our own kind. However, because the environment of an infant and very small child is restricted to family and other caregivers, the extent of "we-ness" does not include a distinct intellectual and emotional dimension of large-group identity. Infants and very small children are *generalists* [24] as far as tribal affiliation, nationality, ethnicity, and religion are concerned; the subjective experience and deep intellectual knowledge of belonging to a large-group identity develops later in childhood. Such sharing of sentiments applies as well to those who are members of a politically ideological group to whose ideology their parents and the important people in their childhood environment subscribed.

There is a well-known term in psychoanalysis known as *stranger anxiety* [28]: infants' recognition that not all the faces around them belong to their caregivers. At 8 months of life, the baby fears the stranger/Other who, in reality, has done nothing harmful to the baby. A normal phenomenon in human development, stranger anxiety is a response to the stranger/Other in the infant's mind and becomes the foundation for the evolution of future "normal" prejudice. We realize that the infant starts differentiating between stranger/Other and familiar/Other. However, an 8-month-old baby has no idea of large-group identity; she is a "generalist."

Freud [29] held that parents are the representatives of society to their child.

Individuation and identification processes slowly force children to give up being "generalists." After psychologically separating themselves from the mother and mothering caregivers [30], children identify with realistic, fantasized, wished-for, or scary aspects of important individuals in their environment and their psychological functions, including these individuals' investments in cultural amplifiers and other large-group investments such as historical images. Sometimes adults "teach" children in indirect ways what large-group identity is. In Cyprus, Greeks and Turks lived side by side before the two communities were divided physically starting in early 1963 and de facto in 1974. As pork is part of the Greek diet, Greek farmers often raise pigs. Although all children are drawn to farm animals, a Turkish child would be discouraged from touching a piglet, as it would be perceived as "dirty" since Muslim Turks do not eat pork. Pigs do not belong in the Turks' large group, and for the Turkish child the pig will be regarded as a cultural amplifier for the Greeks. Children also identify with parents' and other important persons' prejudicial attitudes.

Now let me focus on another concept I call "depositing" [31–34]. In identification, the child is the primary active partner in taking in and assimilating an adult's mental images and owning this person's ego and superego functions. In depositing, the adult person more actively pushes his or her specific images into the developing self-representation of the child and transfers psychological tasks. In other words, the adult person uses the child (mostly unconsciously) as a permanent reservoir for certain self- and other images and psychological tasks belonging to that adult. In addition to children's identifications with adults around them, such adults' depositing images such as historical images with which the child never had an experiential connection, the child starts owning his or her large-group identity.

When refugees find themselves in a location where people have a different large-group identity and start a new life, their large-group identity issues appear, like those observed in Annette Streeck-Fischer's three teenage patients. Many circumstances influence how refugees will handle these large-group identity issues. If their original language evolves as their linking phenomenon, they will have a hard time learning a new language and their adaptation will be very difficult.

2.6 Border Psychology

When there is a surge of refugees, a host country's large-group identity and other large-group concerns also become visible, and huge numbers of individuals may perceive the refugees as the Other. The concept of "the Other" is at least as old as the Biblical confrontation between the Israelites coming out of Egypt and entering what would become the Holy Land where they encountered the Canaanites, the prototypical Others. We do not know what the Canaanites at first blush thought of these intruders into their space, which immediately illuminates one of the problems with the concept of the Other—we usually only see it from one side—side A considers side B as the Other, without our knowing what B thought of A. There is also the problem of the demonization of the Other, as I will illustrate.

We can imagine the unprecedented surge of refugees flooding into Europe and other locations as representing the Other who are threatening the stability of "host" countries' psychological borders. In order to examine this threat, think in terms of how individuals learn to wear two main layers, like fabric, from the time they are children.

The first layer, the individual layer, fits each of them snugly, like clothing. It is one's core personal identity that provides an inner sense of persistent sameness for the individual. The second layer is like the canvas of a big tent, which is loose fitting, but allows a huge number of individuals to share a sense of sameness with others under the same large-group tent. We can visualize large-group identity markers, such as shared images of ancestors' historical events, which I named "chosen traumas" or "chosen glories" [35, 36], as different colorful designs stitched on the canvas of each large group's metaphorical tent. Chosen glories are shared mental images of pride- and pleasure-evoking past events and heroes that are recollected ritualistically. Chosen traumas are the shared mental images of an event in a large group's history in which the group suffered a catastrophic loss, humiliation, and helplessness at the hands of enemies, plus an inability to mourn. Often chosen traumas and chosen glories appear as intertwined. Utilizing chosen traumas and chosen glories for increasing large-group narcissism and conservatism is not dangerous by itself. But its exaggeration and contamination with malignant prejudice against the Other or racism certainly creates severe problems.

Under a huge large-group tent, there are subgroups and subgroup identities, such as professional and political identities. While it is the tent pole—the political leader and the governing body—that holds the tent erect, the tent's canvas psychologically protects the leader, other persons with authority, and all members of the large group. From the view of individual psychology, a person may perceive the pole as a father figure and the canvas as a nurturing mother. From a large-group psychology point of view, the canvas represents the *psychological border* of large-group identity that is shared by tens, hundreds of thousands, or millions of people.

Many individuals in the host countries where mass refugee issues are present or expected are concerned and even terrified that their country's social customs and economies will be damaged and that they will not be able to support the massive influx of the newcomers. But, psychologically speaking, the main fear is the contamination of their large-group identity by the identity of the Other.

Those who are able to keep their individual identities separate from the impact of large-group sentiments become willing to open the tent's gate and accept the huge number of newcomers. Those who perceive the newcomers as tearing holes in, thus damaging, the metaphorical large-group tent's canvas—the border of large-group identity—become anxious and defensively perceive the huge immigrant population as a threat. Earlier I mentioned that our having "normal" prejudicial feelings starts in childhood. Now many persons in the host country may develop hostile, even malignant, shared prejudice. The polarization in the "host" country leads to new political and social concerns and complications. Refugee problems are closely connected with present-day world affairs.

2.7 A Look at Today's World

Globalization and incredible developments in communication and travel, alongside their positive aspects, have brought confrontations and conflicts among populations with different cultural, religious, historical, and geographical investments. The existence of vast numbers of refugees in many locations of the world has added to and complicated such confrontations and conflicts. Kenya has been known as the home of the largest refugee camp in the world on the Kenya-Somalia border. Most refugees there come from Somalia, which has been torn by civil war. Cambodia is filled with refugees from the Khmer Rouge; in fact the whole country is a refugee from the years of slaughter. Over two and a half million persons in Turkey who escaped from Syria have created huge practical, as well as political and cultural, problems for that country. News about Europe's present refugee crisis and its link to terrorism since the 13 November 2015 terrorist attacks in Paris is broadcasted daily. After the Paris attacks, some people in France put graffiti on the walls of mosques or "dirtied" them with pork blood, and there were random attacks in the streets on people who looked "Arab." Terrorism has become connected with newcomers and in turn with refugees.

Let me return to my tent metaphor. I already mentioned subgroups under such a tent. Being a leader or employee of a big business, for example, makes such persons invest intensely in the identity of their business subgroup. However, such business leaders or employees do not lose their first type of large-group identity that was established in childhood. Terrorist organizations, such as Al-Qaeda and ISIS, however, truly illustrate the formation of a large group and large-group identity *in adulthood* [37]. Members of such organizations or lone wolves connected to them function under the dominant impact of this second-type large-group identity. They lose the influence the large-group identity they developed in their childhood—such as their personal moral attitudes—had on their behavior patterns. Terrorists or suicide bombers perform their inhumane acts not simply because of problems their individual identities started to develop in childhood, but primarily because psychologically, they totally become representatives of their adulthood's large groups, and they perceive their horrible acts as a duty to protect or bring attention to their second-type large-group identity.

We have entered 2017 by further linking terrorism with newcomers and, by generalizing it, with refugees. A newcomer murdered people in a well-known nightclub in Istanbul a couple of hours into the year 2017. It is expected that more newcomers, as lone wolves or members of terrorist organizations such as ISIS and Al-Qaeda, will carry out inhumane activities. Shared perceptions of refugees, in general, will continue to frighten large numbers of people in host countries where such shared fear has already led to societal divisions.

I had a chance to examine the beginning of such a division in Finland in late 2016. My knowledge about the situation in Finland comes from my interviews with Finnish colleagues in the mental health field and some academicians in other fields. In the 1970s some refugees from Chile and Vietnam came to Finland. These refugees easily adapted to the Finnish society and their numbers were relatively low. In the 1980s there were not many refugees in Finland, and there was not much interest among Finnish mental health workers about the psychology of refugees and the local population's perception of them. Beginning in the early 1990s however, Finland began receiving more and more refugees from Somalia, the Balkan countries, Afghanistan, the Middle East, and other places. Somalis had more difficulty adapting to their new location. There are about 11,000 Somalis in Finland, and only around 15% of them are employed. Somalis have darker skin color, are Muslims, and many still wear traditional garments. A center for torture victims was established in Helsinki, and many mental health workers did a good job helping these people. Nevertheless Finland's acceptance of Somali refugees' as newcomers has been complicated.

Over the last few years, thousands of new refugees, mostly from Syria, Iraq, and Afghanistan, have arrived in Finland, creating unexpected emotional chaos. Refugees from the Middle East were also Muslims and most of them were men. Some Finns perceived them as "deserters" and developed stereotypical prejudicial perceptions of them. In late September 2016, Finnish officials published a plan to create a special center for those refugees who are considered security threats in order to keep them under control. At that time it was not clear if this plan would be accepted. Some individuals whom I interviewed seemed shocked and embarrassed upon hearing news about the Finnish authorities' intent to use a small island that belonged to Finland to locate newcomers who were perceived as dangerous, even though there was uncertainty about whether or not these perceptions were true. These interviewees thought of themselves, and other Finns who thought like them, as separate from those who had hostile prejudice against the refugees.

Many counties are busy with political, social, economic, legal, cultural, religious, and medical aspects of present-day refugee issues and with finding solutions to border crossing problems, settlement programs, and security matters. Large numbers of people in these locations wish to respond to troubled people from other countries in humane and practical ways. At the same time, another large group of natives are experiencing realistic and fantasized fear of refugees and hostile prejudice against them and are trying to keep their large-group identities from contamination by the Other's large-group identity. Such sentiments become exaggerated by political manipulations and political propaganda.

Brexit, a political movement, is closely related to large-group identity issues. The idea of having an ethnically pure national identity or being a "synthetic nation" [38] composed of only *selected* people from *selected* locations is an illusion in our present-day world. But by supporting Brexit, in a sense, a huge number of persons in England have declared the following: "We can choose newcomers to our country. We can accept people from Canada, for example, but the unwanted Others from unwanted locations cannot disturb our glorious large-group identity." We also know that several political parties in different countries in Europe have become influential not only by supporting conservatism and nationalism but also by exhibiting xenophobia. During the last presidential election campaign in the United States, the now president of the United States Donald Trump even called himself "Mr. Brexit." Trumps' "wall," accompanied by his remarks to keep Muslims out of the country, became a symbol of a protective border of the American large-group identity for a substantial number of persons in the United States.

2.8 Last Comments

In this chapter I focused on refugees' mourning over their losses and the inflammation of large-group identity issues among both refugees and people in host countries. Such psychological information may open doors for dialogue between mental health workers and those authorities in charge of refugee issues and perhaps even with some politicians who may have their own thoughts about dealing with refugee problems. Without making a list here, I wish to express my appreciation for the increasing number of efforts in recent decades by psychotherapists, psychoanalysts, social workers, and other mental health professionals to understand and deal with these issues in communities worldwide.

For some time I have been urging more education about large-group psychology in its own right. Considering large-group psychology in its own right means making formulations as to a large groups' conscious and unconscious shared psychological experiences and motivations that initiate specific social, cultural, political, or ideological processes [32, 33]. Present-day massive refugee problems, and the realistic as well as fantasized ways they are being linked to terrorism and religion, require applications of large-group psychology concepts if we are to understand inflammations of large-group identity issues, various types of border psychology, and the leader-followers interactions associated with them. Meanwhile, I should state that it is beyond my expertise to examine the real, practical aspects of having huge numbers of "outsiders" settling in "host" countries in so many locations in the world. Obviously, credible, realistic, and practical issues and security concerns need to be addressed in the best way possible by authorities assigned to handle them.

Refugees' challenges are not all the same. They arrive from a variety of locations with different availability of funds and other practical matters that must be dealt with. The best and most practical interventions and the nature of difficulties encountered can evolve with circumstances, and interventions would be best considered according to the existing realities of each location. At the present time, I am familiar with the psychologically informed intervention strategy sponsored by the International Psychoanalytic University in Berlin. I met with eight bright and dedicated students in their mid-twenties who have been working in Berlin with refugees from northern Africa, Syria, Iran, and elsewhere for some time. These students are educated about mourning and large-group identity issues, and their work is supervised by two well-known German psychoanalysts. They regularly meet with certain refugees and help them with their language problems, learning German, finding jobs, and adjusting to their new environments. At the same time they try to inform the authorities dealing with these refugees about the newcomers' psychology. What they have been doing is impressive. After some hours with them, I noted that intense transference manifestations of refugees with whom they have been working were directed to the students. For example, a student was regularly meeting with a couple from North Africa. When the wife realized that the student knew French, she began speaking to her in French, a language that her husband did not understand. She told the student how her husband was abusing her physically, and she wanted the student to do something about this situation. The student did not have the necessary education and experience to be a therapist and was burdened with this situation that was above and beyond her assigned task to help newcomers adjust to their new country. Another student was the daughter of Iranian parents who had settled in Germany before she was born. She knew the Iranian language and had an emotional connection with her parents' original country. The Iranian newcomers "selected" this student as their savior, and, in turn, she developed a burdensome countertransference expectation of herself as a "savior." Fortunately, the German psychoanalyst supervisors were aware of the situation and helped her.

The more I learned about the newcomers in Berlin who were involved in this project, I was reminded of my work in South Ossetia in the early 1990s with youngsters who had escaped from war zones in the Republic of Georgia and become internally displaced youth in Tskhinvali, the capital of South Ossetia. At that time there was not a single person trained as a psychologist in South Ossetia, but intervention with the psychological problems of these children and youngsters was being recommended by outsider psychologists, visitors in Tskhinvali, with only sporadic financial help from Europe.

It is clear that we cannot devise a universal intervention recipe to deal with refugees. For host countries intervention focus should be on developing strategies to lower anxiety within the native population and to find ways to avoid malignant rituals against the newcomers. In efforts to deal with polarization in a host country, focus should not be on "normal" shared prejudices; it should be on preventing political/societal/historical factors that inflame large-group identity sentiments, so that such prejudices do not take hostile or malignant forms.

References

1. Ticho G. Cultural aspects of transference and countertransference. Bull Menn Clin. 1971;35:313–34.
2. Garza-Guerrero AC. Culture shock: its mourning and vicissitudes of identity. J Am Psychoanal Assoc. 1974;22:400–29.
3. Grinberg L, Grinberg R. Psychoanalytic perspectives on migration and exile. N. Festinger, Trans. New Haven: Yale University Press; 1989.
4. Julius DA. Biculturalism and international interdependence. Mind Hum Interact. 1992;3:53–6.
5. Akhtar S. Immigration and identity: turmoil, treatment and transformation. Northvale: Jason Aronson; 1999.
6. Parens H. Renewal of life: healing from the Holocaust. Schreiber: Rockville, MD; 2004.
7. Ornstein A, Goldman S. My mother's eyes: Holocaust memories of a young girl. Covington: Clerisy Press; 2004.
8. Muller-Paisner V. Broken chain: Catholics uncover the Holocaust's hidden legacy and discover their Jewish roots. Charlottesville: Pitchstone; 2005.
9. Kahn C. Undeterred, I made it in America. Bloomington: Author House; 2008.
10. Ornstein P, Epstein H. Looking back: memoirs of a psychoanalyst. Lexington: Plunkett Lake Press; 2015.
11. Volkan VD. Immigrants and refugees: trauma, perennial mourning, prejudice, and border psychology. London: Karnac; 2017.
12. Freud S. Mourning and melancholia. Standard ed. London: Hogarth Press, 1957. vol. 14, pp. 237–58.

13. Volkan VD, Zintl E. Life after loss: lessons of grief. New York: Charles Scribner's Sons; 1993.
14. Tähkä V. Dealing with object loss. Scand Psychoanal Rev. 1984;7:13–33.
15. Volkan VD. Linking objects and linking phenomena: a study of the forms, symptoms, metapsychology, and therapy of complicated mourning. New York: International Universities Press; 1981.
16. Volkan VD. Nostalgia as a linking phenomenon. J Appl Psychoanal Stud. 1999;1:169–79.
17. Winnicott DW. Transitional objects and transitional phenomena: a study of the first not-me possession. Int J Psychoanal. 1953;34:89–97.
18. Greenacre P. The transitional object and the fetish: with special reference to the role of illusion. Int J Psychoanal. 1970;51:447–56.
19. Blos P. The adolescent passage: developmental issues. New York: International Universities Press; 1979.
20. Wolfenstein M. How mourning is possible. Psychoanal Study Child. 1966;21:93–123.
21. Van Essen J. The capacity to live alone: unaccompanied refugee minors in the Netherlands. Mind Hum Interact. 1999;10:26–34.
22. Volkan VD. The need to have enemies and allies: from clinical practice to international relationships. Northvale: Jason Aronson; 1988.
23. Streeck-Fischer A. Identity formation difficulties in immigrant adolescents: three cases from Germany. Am J Psychoanal. 2015;75:438–53.
24. Erikson EH. The problem of ego identity. J Am Psychoanal Assoc. 1956;4:56–121.
25. Stern DN. The interpersonal world of the infant: a view from psychoanalysis and developmental psychology. New York: Basic Books; 1985.
26. Bloom P. How pleasure works: the new science of why we like what we like. New York: W. W. Norton; 2010.
27. Lehtonen J. The matrix of mind: the networks of the brain, and the principle of transformation in art therapy for psychosis. In: Killick K, editor. Art therapy for psychosis. London: Routledge; 2016.
28. Spitz R. The first year of life. New York: International Universities Press; 1965.
29. Freud S. An outline of psycho-analysis. Standard ed. London: Hogarth Press. vol. 23, pp. 211–53; 1957; 1939 [1940].
30. Mahler MS. On human symbiosis and the vicissitudes of individuation. New York: International Universities Press; 1968.
31. Volkan VD. Psychoanalytic technique expanded: a textbook of psychoanalytic treatment. Istanbul: OA Press; 2010.
32. Volkan VD. Enemies on the couch: a psychopolitical journey through war and peace. Pitchstone: Durham; 2013.
33. Volkan VD. Psychoanalysis, international relations, and diplomacy: a sourcebook on large-group psychology. London: Karnac; 2014.
34. Volkan VD. A Nazi Legacy: a study of depositing, transgenerational transmission, dissociation and remembering through action. London: Karnac; 2015.
35. Volkan VD. On chosen trauma. Mind Hum Interact. 1991;4:3–19.
36. Volkan VD. Bloodlines: from ethnic pride to ethnic terrorism. New York: Farrar, Straus and Giroux; 1997.
37. Suistola J, Volkan VD. Religious Knives: historical and psychological dimensions of international terrorism. Durham: Pitchstone; 2017.
38. Loewenberg P. Fantasy and reality in history. London: Oxford University Press; 1995.

Asylum and Refugee Law: Ancient Roots and Modern Challenges

3

Adel-Naim Reyhani

Abstract

Today, terms like 'asylum', 'asylum seeker', 'refugee', 'refugee protection', or 'Refugee Convention' are increasingly used in different spaces of public discourse, while often the precise substance of the concepts underlying these terms is not addressed and remains rather vague or even inaccurate. To contribute to a clearer understanding of the foundations of asylum and refugee law, this text provides introductory remarks from a historical and conceptual perspective.

As a first step, the text briefly sketches out the historic development of asylum, from the early sources in religious texts and legal practice, to the emergence of the 1951 Refugee Convention and its 1967 Protocol, and the regional developments that followed. On this basis, it discusses the notion of a right to asylum and underlying thoughts in political theory, as well as the definition of 'refugee' and the rights of refugees. Finally, the text will refer to current challenges in accessing the right to asylum and refugee protection in the European context.

3.1 Introduction: The Development of Asylum and Refugee Law

Humanity has a long history of asylum. References to protection provided to individuals by sovereigns or higher powers are found in the oldest religious scriptures as well as in the (legal) practices of our most ancient civilizations.

An early Jewish conception of asylum can be found in passages such as Exodus 21:13 and Book of Kings 1:50–53 or 2:28–34, where asylum was granted to the

A.-N. Reyhani
Ludwig Boltzmann Institute of Human Rights, Vienna, Austria
e-mail: adel-naim.reyhani@univie.ac.at

T. Wenzel, B. Drožđek (eds.), *An Uncertain Safety*,
https://doi.org/10.1007/978-3-319-72914-5_3

innocent who took refuge at the altar. In the following, cities were established by law as places for refuge [1]. These references can be understood as the first roots of the normative nature of asylum as we know it today [1]. The religious tradition of asylum later found its continuation in the New Testament,[1] the Quran,[2] and more recently in the scriptures of the Bahá'í Faith.[3]

In legal practice, asylum has considerable parallel tradition. The oldest international agreement for which content is documented, the Egyptian-Hittite peace treaty ('Kadesh Treaty'), already contained clauses addressing the protection of individuals [1]. The text was ratified (1258 BC) and held that populations should be exchanged between the two powers under the condition of amnesty [2]. In ancient Greece, asylum was an expression of divine power, where human justice led to unsatisfactory situations and the temples served as refuge. In Rome, the temple provided protection to those outside the pale of law [1, 3].

These instances of protection constitute the early sources of our modern conception of asylum. During the Age of Enlightenment, a significant shift occurred towards the notion of asylum as an institution for the protection of the politically persecuted [1]. For the longest time, asylum was mostly understood as an expression of sovereignty by a state or state-like entity and a respected exception to the principle of a state's sovereignty over its own nationals [1, 4]. Although still contested, a notable development in establishing the notion of a right of individuals to asylum has been accomplished in the end of the last century.[4]

Our understanding of asylum has additionally largely been shaped by political developments in the first half of the twentieth century and the plight of refugees and exiles experienced during and between the World Wars. This period brought a formulation of a right to seek and enjoy asylum in the 1948 Universal Declaration of Human Rights (UDHR).[5] More importantly, the processes since the early 1920s culminated in legally binding international agreements on the 1951 Refugee Convention[6] and later its 1967 Protocol.[7]

These developments have had such encompassing consequences for the use of the term asylum that, although historically and conceptually inaccurate, the category of a refugee, as defined in the Convention, is today equated with asylum status, e.g. in the legislation of many European states [5]. Viewed aright, while asylum should be more broadly understood as the protection a state grants to a non-citizen,

---

[1] Matthew 1, 13–15; 25, 35.

[2] Quran 8, 74; 9, 6.

[3] Bahá'u'lláh, The Summons of the Lord of Hosts.

[4] It is worth noting, however, that already early scholars of international law, such as Hugo Grotius, mentioned a right to asylum in the first half of the seventeenth century [24].

[5] The drafting process on Article 14 [1] of the UDHR reveals that there was a tension between states that regarded asylum as their sovereign right and those which saw it as a duty [4].

[6] Convention Relating to the Status of Refugees, further referred to as the 1951 Convention

[7] Protocol relating to the Status of Refugees, further referred to as the 1967 Protocol.

the 'refugee', as legally defined by the Convention, is a category of individuals that should receive such protection.[8]

The immediate developments leading to the 1951 Convention (now ratified by 145 states) can be traced back to the 1920s, after Western countries started imposing restrictions on immigration during and after World War I [6].[9] Over one million Russians and Greeks and hundreds of thousands of Magyars and in the 1930s half a million fleeing Nazi Germany and hundreds of thousands of Spanish Republicans were forced to move elsewhere to seek protection [6]. The development of modern refugee law can be understood as a response to these instances of injustice and suffering.

The first legal developments in the process leading to an international treaty governing the relationship between states and refugees took place with the appointment of Fridtjof Nansen as High Commissioner for Russian Refugees in 1921 and the introduction of the Nansen Passport System, providing Russian refugees an identity certificate under the so-called 1922 Arrangement[10] and thus facilitating the access to residence rights [6]. The interwar period further saw an extension of the Passport System to other refugees, the first definitions of the term 'refugee', the milestone of the 1933 Refugee Convention[11] as the first binding multilateral instrument to provide legal protection to refugees and the 1938 Convention[12] addressing the situation of German refugees [6].

This legal framework—particularly the 1933 Convention—created in the interwar period for the protection of refugees, albeit still rudimentary and later impaired by the war, served as a basis for the formulation of the 1951 Convention [6]. From a juridical perspective, this framework and particularly the conception of the refugee it entailed was designed as a response to the breakdown in the international order and the phenomenon that individuals did not longer enjoy the protection of any state. The process of drafting the Convention started with a United Nations General Assembly resolution in February 1946 and was concluded through the adoption of the Convention at the UN Conference of Plenipotentiaries in July 1951 [7].[13]

The centrepiece of the 1951 Convention is certainly the definition of the term 'refugee' in Article 1 A. It serves as a key to the scope of rights and duties formulated in the Convention. And already in the drafting process, this Article received most attention [7]. Its interpretation is since the object of a dynamic debate on various levels and will also be discussed later in this contribution.

Almost two centuries later, the scope of the Convention was extended through the adoption of a successive treaty, the 1967 Protocol. The purpose of the Protocol

---

[8] The term 'refugee', beyond its legal definition in international law, has its etymological roots in the word 'refuge' in Old French, meaning 'hiding place'.

[9] Up to the early twentieth century, displaced or persecuted individuals and groups in Europe were able to move quite freely to other places and regions.

[10] Arrangement with Respect to the Issue of Certificates of Identity to Russian Refugees.

[11] Convention relating to the International Status of Refugees, further referred to as the 1933 Convention.

[12] Convention concerning the Status of Refugees Coming from Germany.

[13] See also GA Resolution 8 (I) of 12 February 1946.

was to remove the effects of the limitations of the Convention in its temporal and geographical scope to events occurring in Europe before 1 January 1951, as provided by Article 1 B of the Convention.

The 1951 Convention with its definition of the 'refugee' does not essentially contribute to a different conception of the notion of asylum, as it only establishes a category of individuals to which asylum or protection shall be granted. Despite this, the Convention is the strongest international legal document that contains rights related to the notion of asylum.

Parallel to the establishment of the Convention, the broader concept of asylum itself (referring to the protection a state grants to a non-citizen) was the subject of developments in relation to the 1967 United Nations Declaration on Territorial Asylum. This declaration was a result of the lack of an agreement among governments to include a 'right to asylum' in the International Covenant on Civil and Political Rights (ICCPR) [4, 8]. Until today, international law lacks a clear definition of the term asylum [4].[14]

3.2 Regional Contexts

Against the backdrop of the overall history of the notion of asylum and the development of modern refugee law as described above, asylum and refugee law took distinct but interrelated developments in different places.

3.2.1 Europe

In Europe, where the 1951 Convention and its 1967 Protocol apply throughout the region, the Council of Europe (CoE) and the European Union (EU) have both shaped the reality of asylum, creating a sophisticated legal framework that addresses the protection of refugees. Notwithstanding this worldwide unique system, national asylum systems remain in need of harmonization and reform, and the goal of a well-functioning common system is currently not within immediate reach.

The overall situation in Europe is characterized by its complexity and the overlap of different legal systems. Already in the 1960s, different bodies within the CoE started to address refugee protection [9]. Since then, the CoE has influenced European

[14] It has been even argued that the meaning of the word 'asylum' tends to be assumed by those who use it. According to UNHCR, the 'institution of asylum is not however limited only to the prohibition on refoulement. It includes, inter alia, (1) access of asylum-seekers to fair and effective processes for determining status and protection needs, consistent with the 1951 Convention and its 1967 Protocol; (2) the need to admit refugees to the territories of States; (3) the need for rapid, unimpeded and safe UNHCR access to persons of concern; (4) the need to apply scrupulously the exclusion clauses stipulated in Article 1F of the 1951 Convention; (5) the obligation to treat asylum-seekers and refugees in accordance with applicable human rights and refugee law standards; (6) the responsibility of host States to safeguard the civilian and peaceful nature of asylum; and (7) the duty of refugees and asylum-seekers to respect and abide by the laws of host States' [15].

asylum law on different levels, most notably through the jurisprudence of the European Court of Human Rights (ECtHR) on the European Convention on Human Rights (ECHR) [9]. The ECHR and its supplementary protocols do not include a right to asylum or provisions on the protection of refugees. However, the ECtHR established that asylum seekers and refugees fall under the scope of the ECHR [9]. Moving beyond this initial recognition, its case law on the principle of *non-refoulement* under Article 3 ECHR as well as the development of standards in procedures and treatments, provided by Articles 5 (liberty and security), 8 (private and family life), and 13 (effective remedy), have significantly influenced the reality of asylum in Europe today [9].

Unlike the CoE that had human rights as a core element of their foundation, the EU's approach was initially primarily guided by economic motives and the goal of creating a common market, which placed a focus on immigration control concerns [9]. A shift on the way to a 'Common European Asylum System' came through the 1999 Tampere Conclusions, emphasizing the respect for the right to asylum and the 1951 Convention. The direct link to questions of border control was however never lost [9]. The EU's legal framework, including primary and secondary law as well as the interpretation through the Court of Justice of the European Union (CJEU), today addresses in detail all aspects of the state's relationship with asylum seekers and refugees, including sanctions for carriers, border control mechanisms, a system to determine the responsible Member State, reception conditions, the asylum procedure itself, as well as the question of who qualifies for international protection, a term used to include both refugee and subsidiary protection (based on Article 3 ECHR) status [9]. On the human rights level, the inclusion of a 'right to asylum' in Article 18 of the EU's Fundamental Rights Charter marked an important milestone for the development of the concept of asylum. The exact range and scope of this right, however, remains still undetermined [1].

3.2.2 Asia

Asia is, besides Africa, the region with the largest scale of refugee movements worldwide, with a vast and complex geographic area. It is also the region with the least number of states that accept the 1951 Convention [10]. Persistent conflicts in many countries, including Afghanistan, Pakistan, Iraq, Syria, Yemen, as well as Bangladesh, Sri Lanka, Myanmar, Vietnam, Cambodia, and Laos, continuously generate more forced migration [10]. Despite a lack in the ratification and implementation of the 1951 Convention in the region, most states are parties to central human rights documents that impose significant obligations on states in their relationship with refugees.[15] Moreover, within national legislation, many states that are not parties to the 1951 Convention provide temporary refuge for asylum seekers under different frameworks [10].

[15] Such as the International Covenant on Civil and Political Rights, the International Covenant on Economic, Social and Cultural Rights, the International Convention on the Elimination of all Forms of Racial Discrimination, the Convention Against Torture and Cruel, Inhuman or Degrading Treatment or Punishment, as well as the Convention for the Elimination of all Forms of Discrimination Against Women.

3.2.3 Africa

In 1969 the Organisation of African Unity (OAU) adopted its own Refugee Convention, the OAU Convention Governing the Specific Aspects of Refugee Problems in Africa. Despite the lofty ideals expressed in this treaty, invoking a spirit of solidarity and international cooperation and enhancing the scope of the 1951 Convention, the reality of asylum in Africa remains a considerable challenge. Forced migration, produced by the still high number of lasting conflicts, is a major concern for the region [11].

3.2.4 The Americas

In the Americas, already in 1954, the Caracas Convention on Territorial Asylum affirmed the principle of asylum within Latin America. In the early 1980s, the Cartagena Declaration on Refugees was adopted by 10 countries and later integrated into several Latin American states' legislation [12]. In 2004, the Mexico Plan of Action to Strengthen International Protection of Refugees in America emerged. Meanwhile and notwithstanding political developments, the United States of America and Canada remain of central importance for the reception of refugees in the region [12].

3.3 The 1951 Refugee Convention and Its 1967 Protocol

The 1951 Convention and its 1967 Protocol are rightfully considered the centrepiece of international refugee law. First and foremost, they contain a binding definition of the category 'refugee' as well as related rights of individuals and obligations of 148 states that are currently party to one of the two instruments.

3.3.1 The Definition of 'Refugee'

Pursuant to Article 1 A [2] of the Convention, a person to whom the following criteria apply is to be considered a refugee[16]:

- Is outside his or her country of nationality or habitual residence
- Has a well-founded fear of being persecuted because of his or her race, religion, nationality, membership of a particular social group, or political opinion
- And is unable or unwilling to avail him- or herself of the protection of that country, or to return there, for fear of persecution

[16] Article 1 A [1] deals with 'Statutory Refugees', i.e. persons considered to be refugees under the provisions of international instruments preceding the Convention.

3.3.1.1 Well-Founded Fear of Persecution

According to the Office of the United Nations High Commissioner for Refugees (UNHCR), whose interpretation is most important to the understanding of the Convention, the phrase ‘well-founded fear of being persecuted’ is key to the understanding of the definition. It contains both a subjective and an objective element. On the one hand, it refers to the person applying for protection and his or her subjective perspective. On the other hand, the frame of mind of the individual must be supported by an objective situation [13].[17]

The term ‘persecution’ is not further defined by the Convention itself. In a nutshell, it can be understood as a severe human rights violation, combined with the failure of a state to protect the individual concerned [13]. In principle, either the state itself (or persons/entities acting on behalf of a state) or private actors can be the agents of persecution. In cases where the agent of persecution cannot be attributed to the state, the question arises whether the act can constitute persecution in the meaning of the Convention. In general, it can be said that the persecution originating from private actors qualifies as persecution under the Convention if one of the following scenarios apply: the state is unwilling, or the state is unable to protect against non-state actors, or government authority has fallen apart and one can speak of a ‘failed state’ [13].

3.3.1.2 Persecution Grounds

The Convention requires that the persecution has a nexus to one or more of the five enumerated grounds mentioned therein, namely, race, religion, nationality, membership of a particular social group, or political opinion.

The term *race* is considered problematic, as it runs counter to the principle of the unity of the human race [13]. Despite this fundamental criticism, the term can be understood as covering groups that can be divided according to differences concerning certain physiological parameters or groups sharing the same culture, language, history, or similar identities [13, 14].

The notion of *religion* is closely tied to the right to freedom of religion and belief as protected by, inter alia, Article 9 ECHR or Article 18 ICCPR. According to the UNHCR, the term can include religion as belief (forum internum), religion as identity, and religion as a way of life (forum externum) [13, 14].

The term *nationality* also constitutes a legal term, as compared to the other Convention grounds. It refers to a legal tie between an individual and a state, by which the individual is subject to the jurisdiction of that state. However, it can also be used to encompass groups with the same language, culture, and history who form part of a political union, thus overlapping with the notion of race [13, 14].

The category *membership of a particular social group* has the least clarity as regards its exact scope and meaning. It has, however, significant practical importance in individual asylum cases. One of the most comprehensive descriptions is provided by the Qualification Directive of the EU (2011/95/EU), stating in Article 10 that ‘a group shall be considered to form a particular social group where in particular: members of that group share an innate characteristic, or a common

[17] Some scholars argue, however, that the definition only requires an objective element [13].

background that cannot be changed, or share a characteristic or belief that is so fundamental to identity or conscience that a person should not be forced to renounce it, *and* that group has a distinct identity in the relevant country, because it is perceived as being different by the surrounding society'. In other legal frameworks, by UNHCR, and parts of academia, however, only one of these two elements, namely, the protected characteristics or the social perception, are being required [13–15].

The term 'political opinion' can be understood as covering 'any opinion on any matter in which the machinery of State, government, and policy may be engaged' [13]. According to UNHCR, also cases where a political opinion is (only) attributed by the agent of persecution to the applicant can fall under this ground [14].

3.3.1.3 Further Conditions

In addition to the requirement of well-founded fear of being persecuted for the reasons mentioned above, the Convention asks for further conditions to come within the scope of the protection provided. The person must be outside the country of his or her nationality (or former habitual residence in case of stateless persons) and either unable or unwilling to avail him- or herself of the protection of that country. In the latter context, although not explicitly mentioned in the Convention, the concept of 'internal flight alternative' has been developed. According to this principle, individuals can only qualify as refugees under the Convention, if they cannot reasonably find safe alternatives[18] within their own home country [13].

3.3.1.4 Determining Refugee Status

The consequences that derive from the definition of refugee status are, in practice, regularly predicated upon determination by an authority that the individual or group concerned fulfils the criteria of Article 1 A of the Convention. A person becomes a refugee, however, not through determination, but the moment he or she falls under the definition of a refugee. Thus, the determination of refugee status by an authority has a declaratory character [4]. Given the definition of the Convention, determining refugee status involves subjective and objective factors and the concern for the individual situation of the person concerned as well as within the country of origin [4]. In principle, a decision always requires a case-by-case attempt to prophesy what would happen in case the individual is sent back to his or her home country. Against this backdrop, the question of standard of proof gains importance. It can be said that the onus of establishing well-founded fear of persecution is on the applicant and that objective evidence is called for. However, given the fact that documentary corroboration is often unavailable, the applicant is essentially asked to demonstrate the likelihood of persecution [4], and the 'duty to ascertain and evaluate all the relevant facts is shared between the applicant and the examiner', as UNHCR [14] notes.

[18] According to UNHCR, the internal flight alternative can only be applied if the area of relocation is practically, safely, and legally accessible to the individual, if the agent of persecution is not the state itself, if a non-state agent cannot persecute the claimant in that area, if there is no risk of being persecuted or being subject to other serious harm upon relocation, and the claimant can lead a relatively normal life without facing undue hardship in the proposed area [14].

3.3.2 The Rights of Refugees

Connected to the definition of a refugee and the determination of refugee status by a competent authority, the Convention provides a series of rights to those who qualify as refugees and stipulates obligations of states receiving refugees. Traditionally, the duty of *non-refoulement*, as stipulated in Article 33 of the Convention, has received most attention and has been understood as the core right or duty that the Convention establishes [15]. However, the Convention itself entails further essential rights and obligations. And, these rights are complemented by regional and international human rights instruments, such as the ECHR.

The rights stipulated in the Convention can be categorized, according to the specific group they address and the level of attachment to the asylum state, as rights of refugees physically present, lawfully present, and lawfully staying [16].[19] Among the rights enjoyed by those individuals who qualify as refugees, even though this has not yet been recognized by the state in which they are physically present, are the right to enter and remain in the asylum state (*non-refoulement*); freedom from arbitrary detention and penalization for illegal entry; physical security (right to life); the necessities of life, property, family unity, freedom of thought, conscience, and religion; education; documentation of identity and status; as well as judicial and administrative assistance. The rights of those refugees who are lawfully present in the country of asylum, e.g. asylum seekers, increase by the right to protection against expulsion, freedom of internal movement, and self-employment. If refugees are lawfully staying in a country, for example, when they have been granted asylum status, the right to work, freedom of association, access to housing and welfare, labour and social security rights, intellectual property rights, and the entitlement to receive travel documentation are added. Furthermore, the so-called rights to a durable solution have been attached to the refugee status, including repatriation and voluntary return/reestablishment, local integration (citizenship), and resettlement [16].

3.4 A Right to Asylum

While the questions of who qualifies as a refugee and what rights are connected to refugee states have a relatively solid legal foundation, the status of international asylum law as such, as it goes beyond the protection provided to refugees by the Convention, remains unclear. At the international level, there indeed exists no legal text of universal scope that explicitly deals with a right to asylum, and the UDHR, in Art 14, merely recognizes a right to seek and enjoy asylum, but not a right to be granted asylum. However, particularly through the impact of the 1951 Convention and its 1967 Protocol as well as international human rights norms, such as the International Covenant on Civil and Political Rights (ICCPR) and the ECHR, the assumption that asylum is an exclusive right of states has been challenged. Moreover,

[19] In some cases, where the refugee will be under the control and authority of a state party, specific rights can already inhere even though he or she is not even present in the territory of that state [16].

the principle of asylum is reflected in many constitutions around the world [1].[20] This may even suggest that asylum can be understood as a general principle of international law [1].

As mentioned, asylum was for the longest time viewed as a right of states rather than then a right of individuals. This latter notion has only recently gained momentum in legal literature. The legal nature of asylum as a right of individuals is a controversial issue among scholars in refugee law.

At a time, when the consensus was that individuals were not to be considered legal personas in international law, Grahl-Madsen concluded that 'the idea that States might agree on a binding convention guaranteeing the individual a right to be granted asylum is not entirely utopian' [17]. He further stated that 'our generation has witnessed an impressive development towards an internationally guaranteed right for the individual to be granted asylum' [18] and that the principle of *non-refoulement* in the Refugee Convention[21] imposed an obligation on states to grant asylum if no other country was ready to receive them after a reasonable time [18]. However, following the failure of the 1977 Conference on Territorial Asylum, the focus of the debate was put on the content of the 1951 Convention rather than the status and nature of asylum [1].

The basic ambiguity with respect to 'asylum' is particularly obvious in respect of the debate on Article 18 of the Charter of Fundamental Rights of the European Union which stipulates a right to asylum. With respect to the 'vagueness of the institution' [4], Article 18 has been described as 'linguistically vague' [19]. Some scholars hold that Article 18 does only refer to the procedural right to seek asylum. Others, including UNHCR,[22] have convincingly argued for a broader understanding of this provision [4, 20].

Connected to these legal developments and status of a right to asylum is the crucial question of the foundation of the concept of asylum in philosophy and political theory. Against the backdrop of the current organizational and structural arrangement

[20] According to Gil-Bazo, the constitutions of Angola, Benin, Bolivia, Bulgaria, Burundi, Brazil, Cape Verde, Chad, China, Colombia, Costa Rica, Cuba, Democratic Republic of Congo, the Dominican Republic, Ecuador, Egypt, El Salvador, France, Germany, Guatemala, Guinea-Conakry, Honduras, Hungary, Italy, Ivory Coast, Mali, Mozambique, Nicaragua, Paraguay, Peru, Portugal, Spain, and Venezuela all include a notion of asylum. Their definitions of asylum vary, however, as does their understanding of who qualifies for the protection of asylum [1].

[21] As UNHCR has stated 'The principle of non-refoulement applies to any conduct resulting in the removal, expulsion, deportation, return, extradition, rejection at the frontier or non-admission, etc. that would place a refugee at risk' [14].

[22] UNHCR has noted 'that the right to asylum in Article 18 of the EU Charter contains the following elements: (1) protection from refoulement, including non-rejection at the frontier; (2) access to territories for the purpose of admission to fair and effective processes for determining status and international protection needs; (3) assessment of an asylum claim in fair and efficient asylum processes (with qualified interpreters and trained responsible authorities and access to legal representation and other organizations providing information and support)) and an effective remedy (with appropriate legal aid) in the receiving state; (4) access to UNHCR (or its partner organizations); and (5) treatment in accordance with adequate reception conditions; (6) the grant of refugee or subsidiary protection status when the criteria are met; (7) ensuring refugees and asylum-seekers the exercise of fundamental rights and freedoms; and (8) the attainment of a secure status' [15].

of the worldwide human society in sovereign nation states, the perspective based on Hannah Arendt's analysis of the plight of refugees and the stateless has gained continuous attention. For Arendt, the crisis in the protection of the rights of refugees is grounded in the observation that the idealistic notion of human rights is not more than an empty shell, if the individuals concerned are not embedded in a political community in which their actions and opinions become meaningful. The principal dilemma facing refugees in their (asymmetrical) relationship towards states, then, is the lack of a 'place of their own', where they are regarded as equals. They are, in a legal sense, 'nowhere in this world' [21], which has led Arendt to postulate 'the right to have rights' as the only human right [22]. Bearing in mind the deplorable results that the modern order with its insistence on national sovereignty in an increasingly interdependent world [23] has brought for refugees, it thus becomes a most urgent concern to strengthen the right to asylum and to accelerate processes that can overcome the nation state-centric perspectives on refugee protection.

3.5 Accessing Asylum

Today, despite the encompassing legal developments in human rights, asylum, and refugee law, one of the major challenges facing the international community as well as regional political organizations and nation states in their relationship with those who lose their effective link to their home countries relates to the access to asylum.[23] These developments are particularly striking when it comes to liberal democracies that are theoretically based on a commitment towards the protection of human rights.

For instance, in Europe[24]—the cradle of modern refugee protection—the debate on the so-called refugee crisis ties into the legal and political developments aimed at further restricting the access of refugees to the territory of EU Member States and to proper asylum procedures. [25]

Amongst these, the externalization of migration control – the attempt to prevent migrants, including asylum-seekers, from entering the legal jurisdiction or territory of the EU – is most critical, as it strives to fully eschew the responsibility to guarantee the right to asylum. The EU's efforts to relocate its own borders to third countries through specific extraterritorial measures of pre-border control comply with an underlying logic of fighting illegal immigration and securing borders, emphasizing constant surveillance and insinuating that migrants intend to circumvent border checks. Thus, if they apply to migrants and asylum-seekers alike, the right to asylum is severely damaged. For example, the attempt of raising the policing capacities

[23] In this context, inter alia, questions of extraterritoriality or the legal encounter of a state with an individual asylum seeker attempts to extend migration control well beyond the borders of the state, as well as the involvement of private actors plays crucial roles [25].

[24] Obstacles to accessing asylum are not only a European phenomenon but a considerable international challenge; see, e.g. the OHCHR's criticism of Australia's refugee policy, http://www.ohchr.org/en/NewsEvents/Pages/DisplayNews.aspx?NewsID=20889&LangID=E.

[25] The current rapid and alarming developments in policies and political discourse as regards the EU's cooperation with Libya cannot be adequately addressed here.

of authorities in third countries to prevent asylum-seekers from departing towards the EU – while the same authorities are unable to protect the most fundamental human rights and freedoms of migrants – has perpetuated an intolerable situation of gross human rights violations in the direct neighbourhood of the EU.

Despite this, calls for legal pathways to access asylum in Europe have remained unanswered, also by the CJEU. In its Judgment C-638/16 PPU X and X of 7 March 2017, the Court determined there is no obligation of Member States to grant humanitarian visas, even if refusing a visa would result in inhuman and degrading treatment of the applicant. Deviating from the Advocate General's opinion, the Court ruled that such applications do not fall within the scope of the Visa Code.

Conclusions

The ancient roots of asylum in legal practice and religious scriptures as well as the development of the principle of asylum in the history of mankind serve as a reminder of its normative nature. The legal framework in place and most notably the 1951 Convention and its 1967 Protocol have answered to the protection needs of millions of asylum seekers. However, the modern context and the current structural arrangement of our global society, with its insistence in upholding the principle of national sovereignty and belonging despite increasing global interdependencies, still bear unresolved challenges for this field of law. It is striking how the right to access asylum is under severe pressure in the cradle of modern refugee law. Keeping in mind the traditional character of asylum as an instrument to compensate for situations of perceived injustice and severe human rights violations, the importance of significant progress in a practical and informed discourse on the concept of asylum must be recognized.

References

1. Gil-Bazo M. Asylum as a general principle of international law. International Journal of Refugee Law. 2015;27:3–28.
2. Hull E, Plaut W. Asylum: a moral dilemma. International Migration Review. 1996;30:1096.
3. Bau I. This ground is holy. 1st ed. New York: Paulist Press; 1985.
4. Goodwin-Gill G, McAdam J. The refugee in international law. 1st ed. New York: Oxford University Press; 2011.
5. Gil-Bazo M. Refugee status and subsidiary protection under EC law: the qualification directive and the right to be granted asylum. In: Whose freedom, security and justice? EU immigration and asylum law and policy. Oxford: Hart Publishing; 2007.
6. Skran C. Historical development of international refugee law. The 1951 convention relating to the status of refugees and its 1967 protocol. New York: Oxford University Press; 2011.
7. Einarsen T. Drafting history of the convention/New York protocol. The 1951 convention relating to the status of refugees and its 1967 protocol. New York: Oxford University Press; 2011.
8. Edwards A. Human rights, refugees, and the right 'to enjoy' asylum. International Journal of Refugee Law. 2005;17:293–330.

9. Klug A. Regional developments: Europe. The 1951 convention relating to the status of refugees and its 1967 protocol. New York: Oxford University Press; 2011.
10. Blay S. Regional developments: Asia. The 1951 convention relating to the status of Refugees and its 1967 protocol. New York: Oxford University Press; 2011.
11. Van Garderen J, Ebenstein J. Regional developments: Africa. The 1951 convention relating to the status of refugees and its 1967 protocol. New York: Oxford University Press; 2011.
12. Piovesan F, Jubilut L. Regional developments: Americas. The 1951 convention relating to the status of refugees and its 1967 protocol. New York: Oxford University Press; 2011.
13. Zimmermann A, Mahler C. Article 1A. The 1951 convention relating to the status of refugees and its 1967 protocol. New York: Oxford University Press; 2011.
14. UNHCR, editor. Handbook and guidelines on procedures and criteria for determining refugee status. 1st ed. Geneva: UNHCR; 2011.
15. UNHCR (2012) Public statement in relation to Zuheyr Freyeh Halaf v. the Bulgarian State Agency for Refugees pending before the Court of Justice of the European Union. http://www.refworld.org/docid/5017fc202.html. Accessed 21 Apr 2017.
16. Hathaway J. The rights of refugees under international law. 1st ed. Cambridge: Cambridge University Press; 2005.
17. Grahl-Madsen A. The status of refugees in international law. 1st ed. Leiden: Sijthoff; 1972.
18. Grahl-Madsen A. Territorial asylum. 1st ed. Stockholm: Almqvist & Wiksell International; 1980.
19. Noll G. Seeking asylum at embassies: a right to entry under international law? International Journal of Refugee Law. 2005;17:542–73.
20. Gil-Bazo M. The charter of fundamental rights of the European Union and the right to be granted asylum in the union's law. Refugee Survey Quarterly. 2008;27:33–52.
21. Oudejans N. The right to have rights as the right to asylum. Netherlands Journal of Legal Philosophy. 2014;43:7–26.
22. Arendt H. Es gibt nur ein einziges Menschenrecht. Die Wandlung. 1949;4:754–70.
23. Karlberg M. Beyond the culture of contest. 1st ed. Oxford: George Ronald; 2004.
24. Weis P. The development of refugee law: transnational legal problems of refugees. 1st ed. New York: C. Boardman Co.; 1982.
25. Gammeltoft-Hansen T. Access to asylum. 1st ed. New York: Cambridge University Press; 2013.
26. European Union Agency for Fundamental Rights. FRA Opinion on fundamental rights in the 'hotspots' set up in Greece and Italy. 2016. http://fra.europa.eu/sites/default/files/fra_uploads/fra-opinion-5-2016-hotspots_en.pdf. Accessed 21 Apr 2017.
27. Boltzmann Institute of Human Rights. Stellungnahme zur Verordnung der Bundesregierung zur Feststellung der Gefährdung der Aufrechterhaltung der öffentlichen Ordnung und des Schutzes der inneren Sicherheit. 2016. http://bim.lbg.ac.at/sites/files/bim/attachments/stellungnahme_verordnung_ludwig_boltzmann_institut_fuer_menschenrechte_2016-10_corr.pdf. Accessed 21 Apr 2017.
28. Frühwirth R. Die Sonderbestimmungen zum sogenannten "Notverordnungsrecht". Asyl- und Fremdenrecht, WEKA, Wien; 2016.

Identifying Needs, Vulnerabilities and Resources in Refugee Persons and Groups

4

Thomas Wenzel, Sabine Völkl-Kernstock, Tatiana Urdaneta Wittek, and David Baron

Abstract

The global increase in refugees has led to a number of critical challenges, which should be addressed by an interdisciplinary approach to permit identification and understanding of the complex needs and vulnerabilities of the diverse refugee groups, and guide both emergency aid and long-term planning.

The approach chosen would be guided by the priorities in a specific situation, and the professional background of the helper. In an emergency setting a comprehensive assessment of mental health might for example not be possible or even necessary. Therefore, we recommend the reader selects the sections of the following chapter that are most relevant to his or her work.

Part I of the chapter will introduce the subject with a short overview of general assessment models and tools, developed by UN organisations and international NGOs that should be considered in any humanitarian disaster and displacement of large population groups. The authors also address specifics that are frequently neglected, including considerations of ethics and data protection in shared data.

T. Wenzel (✉)
World Psychiatric Association Scientific Section,
Psychological Aspects of Persecution and Torture, Geneva, Switzerland
e-mail: drthomaswenzel@web.de

S. Völkl-Kernstock
Trauma Assessment and Child Protection Unit, Medical University of Vienna, Vienna, Austria

Department of Child- and Youth Psychiatry, Medical University of Vienna, Vienna, Austria
e-mail: sabine.voelkl-kernstock@meduniwien.ac.at

T. U. Wittek
Ludwig Boltzmann Institute of Human Rights, Vienna, Austria
e-mail: Tatiana.Wittek@lansky.at

D. Baron
Psychiatry, Keck Hospital of USC, Keck School of Medicine at USC, Los Angeles, CA, USA
e-mail: Dave.Baron@med.usc.edu

T. Wenzel, B. Drožđek (eds.), *An Uncertain Safety*,
https://doi.org/10.1007/978-3-319-72914-5_4

Part II of the chapter explores the identification and primary protection of vulnerable groups. As an example of the complex interdisciplinary situation encountered in highly vulnerable groups, this chapter also elaborates on the specific steps relevant to the support and protection of survivors of torture. These include legal, medical, social and psychological aspects, and can be linked to developing strategies like universal jurisdiction contributing to long-term justice and the recovery of a civil society.

Identification of resources and resilience factors is also important to counter the risk of a too narrow focus on vulnerabilities in the assessment of refugee groups and will be covered in this part of the chapter.

Parts III and IV of this chapter focus on the specific aspect of mental health assessment in adults and children including specific toolboxes and instruments that can be used for the evaluation of mental health-related factors in communities, groups and individuals.

4.1 Part I: General Considerations: Assessment as a Continuous Process

In a major humanitarian disaster, such as a war with large numbers of displaced persons, existing "universal" intervention strategies and pre-prepared emergency plans or checklists [1] can only serve as general guidelines, because situational and culturally specific factors for every incident and group need to be recognised and addressed in any intervention plan. A first step towards early intervention and long-term planning is the recognition of actual needs and vulnerabilities of a displaced or asylum-seeking population.

Within such complex situations, needs in different groups of refugees have to be viewed as dynamic due to frequent and often dramatic changes in the population composition, interaction with the environment, new life events, health risks and/or political developments affecting the individuals, their family members or the group as a whole [2]. Additional changes are brought about by the longitudinal processes of social adaptation to refugee camp situations or host countries and their respective sociocultural organisations. This requires a continuous monitoring and assessment process to avoid missing critical developments and changes. For example, during the war in Syria, an adaptation of screening and vaccination efforts was necessary because of the transition from a pre-war well-vaccinated population to a growing number of younger refugees who had not benefitted from a vaccination programme [3, 4]. Priorities while in transit and shortly after arrival in host countries were primarily basic protection, housing, food and contact with family members, but these changed over time to become long-term rehabilitation needs, development of a new life plan, eventual return after improvement of the situation in their country of origin or integration into host societies as time progresses. Finally, it is necessary to monitor outcomes of earlier interventions. Short feedback loops to guide modification of interventions can play an important role, especially during large-scale emergency responses.

Strategic planning of assessment and crisis responses is a task that requires interdisciplinary collaboration and an effective coordination between different stakeholders. Since a crisis response most often includes the work of many organisations and agencies, responsibility for efficient use of resources and adequacy of care offered requires a joint approach to the situation, a shared understanding of intervention models and priorities and sharing of information as proposed by the Inter-Agency Standing Committee (IASC) (see also Weissbecker et al. and Patel et al. in this book).

Assessment strategies must fit the characteristics of the target groups and their cultural and social backgrounds, as well as the aforementioned integrative strategic concepts and standards required by the respective organisations and governmental agencies involved. These include not only the collection of data on individuals and groups, but also the analysis of existing research in order to determine the quality of existing intervention models and emergency plans. Therefore, humanitarian and UN organisations frequently provide assessment tools embedded in their field manuals, which are designed for use with groups or individuals to identify their vulnerabilities and needs and to guide planning and intervention activities. In the long-term, all results should feed into a "lessons-learned" model to contribute to evidence-based conclusions that can be used in similar situations and in long-term strategic planning in the global network of humanitarian organisations.

4.1.1 WHO, UNHCR and UNICEF Models for General Assessment and Monitoring in Larger Groups

In the following part of the chapter, we give a short overview and examples of common models and instruments that can guide assessment and a comprehensive understanding of any particular situation. These tools support the steps to be taken, from a very general first response framework to more specific components of assessment and monitoring models, and have been developed by international organisations and UN agencies as part of a continuous process. They should be considered in any humanitarian disaster that leads to displacement of large population groups, and usually share common characteristics such as the increasing usage of a participatory approach that includes members of the refugee population.

The *World Health Organisation*, in collaboration with UNHCR and the International Organisation for Migration (IOM), has developed a special tool for situational assessment: the "Toolkit for assessing health system capacity to manage large influxes of refugees, asylum-seekers and migrants".[1] It is designed to help health authorities and their partners, particularly in Europe, to "identify gaps, build on existing capacities and develop informed health interventions for arrivals of large groups of migrants". It also offers support for intersectoral "coordination and collaboration in the development and implementation of the health sector response".

[1] Toolkit for assessing health system capacity to manage large influxes of refugees, asylum-seekers and migrants, World Health Organization 2016, online at www.who.org.

The toolkit consists of three parts: Part I offers a broad background on health and refugee movements towards and within Europe, Part II is a guide for assessors, and Part III contains specific interview guidelines for semi-structured interviews with various stakeholders. The toolkit also provides practical information about how to deal with the general health needs (as outlined also by Kühnel et al. and van den Muijsenbergh et al. in this book) and can be used for identification of the areas that should be included in a comprehensive assessment of overall needs.

UNHCR provides another comprehensive set of tools for assessment of different aspects of the work with refugee populations. The UNHCR "Tool for Participatory Assessment in Operations"[2] is also based on a participatory approach, which is defined in this case as "a process of building partnerships with refugee women and men of all ages and backgrounds by promoting meaningful participation through structured dialogue" in order to "gather accurate information on the specific protection risks they face and the underlying causes, to understand their capacities, and to hear their proposed solutions". This strategy is expected to mobilize communities to "take collective action to enhance their own protection and [it also] forms the basis for the implementation of a rights and community-based approach" [3]. Participatory strategies are not only part of the assessment, but can also be seen as an intervention influencing the basic situation encountered and activating community members, thereby confirming the well-known notion that any observation changes that which it observes (Fig. 4.1).

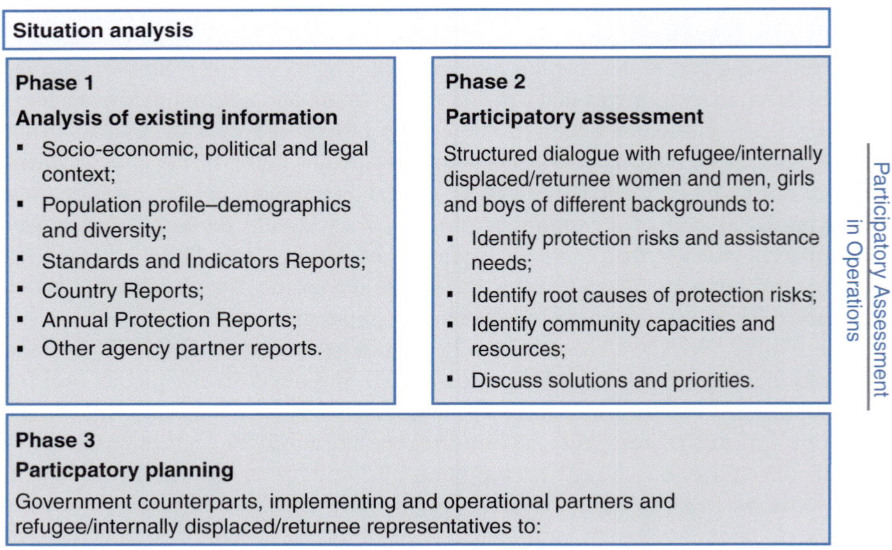

Fig. 4.1 UNHCR situation analysis and participatory assessment model

[2] http://www.unhcr.org/publications/legal/450e963f2/unhcr-tool-participatory-assessment-operations.html.

A version to guide the work with children is also available by UNHCR (see later in this chapter).

UNICEF proposes a strategy addressing the needs of children that should be considered by all organisations. This approach is called "Core Commitments for Children (CCCs) in Humanitarian Action". It was reviewed several times and is considered to be a "global framework" for humanitarian action directed at children.[3] The handbook includes an integrated assessment model and several monitoring strategies that integrate a risk management strategy and (see Sect. 4.1.16 of the manual) and outcome monitoring. It is a good example of the integration of the necessary assessment steps in an overall intervention plan and the institutional guiding principles. The well-designed action steps are based on an interdisciplinary approach encompassing legal, social, health and general safety factors.

The *IASC guidelines*[4] (see also Chap. 6 in this book) on mental health and psychosocial issues further differentiate between an emergency response, a minimum response and a comprehensive response. The guidelines provide recommendations using action sheets. Action Sheet 2.2 deals with assessment and further underlines the need of a comprehensive situational analysis and information to be gathered in an integrated approach, including all "relevant demographic and contextual information, people's experiences of the emergency, mental health and psychosocial problems, existing sources of psychosocial well-being and mental health, organisational capacities and activities, programming needs and opportunities". Participatory systems should be used and involve groups of beneficiaries in an inclusive and culturally sensitive manner. Specific outcome indicators must be defined to help monitor the set of interventions applied. They should follow the "SMART" (specific, measurable, achievable, relevant and time-bound) model. Further models to explore mental health needs will be discussed later in this chapter.

4.1.2 Ethical and Legal Aspects in Collecting and Sharing Information on Refugee People

Establishing trust between the different actors involved, as well as between helpers and refugee people, is necessary for an efficient collaboration. A strategy to exchange information must, as noted before, be implemented between organisations, and confidentiality must be addressed throughout the process of data gathering, storing and sharing. Safeguards need to be put in place to protect sensitive social and health data against abuse and use for other gains than those agreed on, including political ones (see also ([5]), p. 29).

[3] https://www.unicef.org/publications/files/CCC_042010.pdf. Accessed 1 Apr 2017.

[4] Inter-Agency Standing Committee (IASC) (2007). IASC Guidelines on Mental Health and Psychosocial Support in Emergency Settings. Geneva: IASC. Available from http://www.humanitarianinfo.org/iasc/content/products.

[5] WHO/UNHCR: assessing mental health and psychosocial needs and resources: toolkit for humanitarian settings, 2012. Available www.apps.who.int/iris/bitstream/10665/.../9789241548533_eng.pdf. Accessed 1 Jun 2017.

Privacy, in general, should be protected according to the United Nations Universal Declaration of Human Rights 1948. Article 12 confirms that “No one shall be subjected to arbitrary interference with his privacy, family, home or correspondence, nor to attacks upon his honour and reputation. Everyone has the right to the protection of the law against such interference or attacks”.

Article 8 of the EU Charter of Fundamental Rights further states that “1. Everyone has the right to the protection of personal data concerning him or her. 2. Such data must be processed fairly for specified purposes and based on the consent of the person concerned or some other legitimate basis laid down by law. Everyone has the right of access to data, which have been collected concerning him or her, and the right to have it rectified. 3. Compliance with these rules shall be subject to control by an independent authority”. The above-mentioned standards must also be respected in refugee persons.

ISO standards that can be used to guide specific steps in protection and serve as points of reference include ISO/IEC 27001:2013, ISO/IEC 27005 and ISO 29100. The new EU General Data Protection Regulation (GDPR) (EU) 2016/679 should also be considered in this context.

UNHCR has taken special efforts in this area and published comprehensive guidelines for data protection in 2015,[6] as well as detailed analyses of their application in complex situations like cash-based interventions.[7] Sensitive data in refugee care include but are not limited to information about healthcare, housing, leisure time, social and legal aid, legal questions and personal information pertaining to items such as asylum procedures and the monitoring of human rights abuses. Leaking of this information to a country of origin or political groups might endanger the refugee person, his/her family members and possibly entire communities.

Data protection policies need to include legal, technical and organisational safeguards; organisations have to be aware of new strategies that might violate the above-mentioned rights, for example, by profiling or by accessing data carriers including printers and cloud systems. Confidentiality in medical settings and treatment must be respected and protected and should include an agreement to data collection and further use of data. Collection of data for healthcare research must comply with international standards, especially with the World Medical Association Declaration of Helsinki (as last revised 19 October 2013) and related documents [5]. This is of special importance in vulnerable groups like refugees [6] and requires careful consideration and respect for culture specific factors, especially when sensitive areas are addressed [7]. Ownership of research data is another important aspect which has been discussed in fields like cultural anthropology. It should be given more attention in the future, especially in research on refugees [8].

On the other hand, dissemination of non-sensitive information, anonymous data and data obtained with informed consent should not be restricted by interagency

[6] UN High Commissioner for Refugees (UNHCR), Policy on the Protection of Personal Data of Persons of Concern to UNHCR, Geneva, May 2015. www.refworld.org/docid/55643c1d4.html. Accessed 1 Jun 2017.

[7] Privacy impact assessment of UNHCR cash-based interventions, UNHCR, December 2015, online at www.globalprotectioncluster.org/…f-unhcr-cbi_en.pdf. Accessed 1 Jun 2017.

competition or considerations like that of later academic publication. Instead, its use ought to be dictated by its relevance for monitoring, identification of crucial factors and comprehensive planning of the to-be-executed actions [9].

All stakeholders involved should be made aware of these issues, including interpreters that play an important role in most settings. Ethical standards must be respected and should guide all levels of interventions as binding frameworks (see also Patel et al. in this book) and must be included in training of all involved groups.[8]

4.2 Part II: Identification and Basic Protection of Vulnerable Groups and Identification of Individual and Group Resources: Integrating Medical and Legal Aspects

4.2.1 Identification of Vulnerable Groups

Refugee people can be seen as a potentially vulnerable group in general, at risk for both health-related problems and for severe human rights violations, including trafficking, sexual abuse [10–12] or even specific dangers such as organ trading [13–15]. Subgroups with especially high vulnerability due to exposure to those risks and other factors such as prior persecution, age or gender need to be identified and should receive special support and protection, especially when large numbers of refugee people require attention or the number of those receiving asylum or other forms of protection is limited (see also Chaps. 9 and 10 in this book).

4.2.1.1 The UNHCR Vulnerability Screening Tool

UNHCR has recently developed a rather comprehensive screening tool, entitled "Identifying and addressing vulnerability: a tool for asylum and migration system",[9] and developed in collaboration with the International Detention Coalition (IDC) as part of the Vulnerability Assessment Framework.[10] It is well-constructed and provides guidelines for concrete help in different steps of the reception and asylum system. It follows accepted international standards and is based on extensive experience and field-testing. UNHCR follows a definition of vulnerabilities that is not limited to medical aspects, but is based on an interdisciplinary approach and a screening system with a broader focus. It gives orientation by providing main categories, using the concept of "domains" (Table 4.1).

Further, the manual underlines the importance of alternative placements of vulnerable individuals, for example, avoiding detention (p. 9; see also Chap. 12 in this book). In addition to this, it stresses that the adequate training and capacity building of staff and helpers cannot be replaced by the use of screening instruments. The

[8] See http://www.ohchr.org/english/law/index.htm for an overview.

[9] The tool is available, for example, from www.refworld.org/pdfid/57f21f6b4.pdf. Accessed 1 Jun 2017.

[10] http://www.unhcr.org/innovation/labs_post/vulnerability-assessment-framework/. Accessed 1 Jun 2017.

Table 4.1 UNHCR vulnerability domains

Child	• Unaccompanied or separated child • Child accompanied by parent(s), other family members or guardians
Sex, gender, gender identity, sexual orientation	• Pregnant woman or girl or nursing mother • Sole or primary carer(s) (of dependent child, elderly person or person with a disability) • Woman at risk of sexual or gender-based violence or adult or child experiencing family violence, exploitation or abuse • Person at risk of violence due to their sexual orientation and/or gender identity, LGBTI (lesbian, gay, bisexual, transgender or intersex persons)
Health and welfare concerns	• Physical and mental health • Risk of suicide • Disability • Elderly person • Substance addiction • Destitution
Protection needs	• Refugee and asylum seeker • Survivor of torture and trauma • Survivor of sexual or gender-based violence or other violent crimes • Victim of trafficking in persons • Stateless person
Other	• The interviewer has an opportunity to identify vulnerability factors not captured by the previous domains

impact of the "human factor" on the quality of outcomes is addressed in the definition of a number of values and attitudes, foundational knowledge and skills presented in the manual. For specific target groups, such as victims of domestic violence, more detailed instruments can be applied. The "Heightened Risk Identification Tool", also published by UNHCR, at present in version 2,[11] is intended for priority assessment in critical situations. This instrument, together with the user guide, offers a risk assessment yielding an estimate for a "high", "medium" or "low" risk with follow-up time windows and identification of priority risks.

Early recognition of torture survivors, as an especially vulnerable group, will be covered later on in this chapter.

4.2.2 Vulnerability in the EU Framework Reception Directive and in Asylum Interviews

In host countries like the EU, the USA or Australia, special systems, including asylum procedures, are designed and put in place to regulate migration and guide reception of asylum seekers. These are implemented with a substantial administrative effort. In the EU, the recast Reception Conditions Directive (2013/33EU),[12] that

[11] www.refworld.org/pdfid/4c46c6860.pdf.

[12] http://eur-lex.europa.eu/legal-content/EN/TXT/?uri=CELEX:32013L0033.

in turn also defines vulnerable groups, has been developed as an important framework to guide the reception of asylum seekers.

4.2.2.1 Asylum Interviews and Vulnerable Groups

Granting or denying asylum or other forms of residence providing a person with a transient or permanent protection (as outlined in more detail in Chap. 3 in this book) requires a highly demanding evaluation process and special training not limited to knowledge of legal and humanitarian standards. This is particularly the case where decisions can directly impact safety or even the life of persons escaping persecution and their dependents. Besides country information (provided, e.g. by the freely accessible online ECOI Database (European Country of Origin Information Network)),[13] documents and legal research, medical and psychological evaluation can be of major importance in the course of asylum interviews and in the identification of vulnerable groups as they can confirm factors related to persecution and torture or other indicators of vulnerability relevant to the asylum process and protection. They might also be necessary as psychological and mental health problems in refugees can interfere with their memory functions or with disclosure of the personal history and consequently hinder the full and consistent reporting required during the legal evaluation of the case. This issue will be explored in detail later in this chapter. Obviously, care must be taken to choose only objective, reliable and recent sources and to validate conclusions wherever possible.

Training of officials involved in the asylum process, provided in many countries in collaboration with the UNHCR, needs to create awareness of the steps necessary to cope with these challenges and acquire the comprehensive set of skills needed. This should include teaching of special interview skills to recognise and deal with traumatised or otherwise vulnerable clients and prevent re-traumatisation in those groups, train intercultural awareness and skills but also help to implement strategies to prevent bias and burnout in those conducting interviews. Participants should further understand the need to involve independent and qualified experts for medical, psychological, cultural or legal expertise where necessary. Interpreters must also receive special training (see Chap. 14 in this book and the special training programme developed by UNHCR[14]).

4.2.2.2 The "EASO Quality Tool on Identification of Persons with Special Needs"

A complex online tool was developed by the European Asylum Support Office (EASO)[15] to provide information for protection and identification of persons with special needs (IPSN).[16] It is presented as a "support tool for officials involved in the asylum procedure and reception" and assumes no specific medical or psychological

[13] https://www.ecoi.net/.

[14] Project QUADA, at present available in Austria, international version of the handbook in preparation, www.bfa.gv.at/files/broschueren/Trainingsprogramm_WEB_15032016.pdf. Accessed 20 Jun 2017.

[15] https://www.easo.europa.eu/. Accessed 20 Jun 2017.

[16] https://ipsn.easo.europa.eu/. Accessed 20 Jun 2017.

Table 4.2 IPSN EASO tool for identification of persons with special needs: main groups identified

• Accompanied minors
• Unaccompanied minors
• Disabled people
• Elderly people
• Pregnant women
• Single parents with minor children
• Victims of human trafficking
• Persons with serious illnesses
• Persons with mental disorders
• Persons who have been subjected to torture
• Persons who have been subjected to rape
• Persons who have been subjected to other serious forms of psychological, physical or sexual violence
• LGBTI (lesbian, gay, bisexual, transgender or intersex persons)
• People with gender-related special needs

background qualification in those who apply it. It distinguishes 14 selected categories of applicants with special needs that are seen as a "non-exhaustive" listing and should not replace individual assessment. It is similar to but not identical to the already mentioned UNHCR model (Table 4.2).

The authors describe the specific steps in the procedure covered by the tool: "first contact - making an application; lodging the application; personal interview; end of the first-instance asylum procedure; and reception support". They underline the importance of embedding the instrument in the existing EASO training standards and point out a number of important ethical considerations including the need for confidentiality and the use of detention only as a last resort ("ultima ratio"). The at-present obvious disregard for the cautions against detention at least in the EU and Australia is discussed in a separate chapter of this book (Chap. 12).

As mentioned earlier, a continuous process of reassessment is necessary because needs might only arise or be identified at later stages; for example, new stressors or risk factors such as news received concerning the death of family members due to war or persecution, or additional relevant information might be brought up with delay because of trauma-related shame or posttraumatic stress disorder (PTSD).

The instrument leans heavily on the use of the internet, gives little detailed guidance, such as questions that could be used, and must be considered with caution. In addition, many of the items included, such as the taking of a nearly complete psychopathological status including affect and thought processes, would require the experience of a well-trained mental health professional. However, this expertise is commonly not integrated in the refugee reception screening or asylum procedures. Therefore, quality of training in the use of this instrument and additional expertise involved in the course of an assessment are important, as the instrument is often used by officials who lack sufficient training. To our knowledge, no scientific evaluation of the sensitivity of this instrument has been published so far.

4.2.2.3 The EU Dublin III System and Vulnerable Groups

The highly controversial European "Dublin III" system (see EU directive Nr. 604/2013) provides for the first step in the decision-making process and determines whether an asylum seeker should be returned to a country where she/he first entered the EU (the "Schengen" system) to conduct the evaluation of the asylum application. This may contain a major risk, particularly for vulnerable groups, as the quality of protection and measures related to the asylum process differs substantially between the EU countries. The UNHCR and other organisations have observed a rising number of violations of basic standards with the use of this system.[17] Continuous monitoring, especially by the UNHCR and NGOs, has confirmed that return to some EU countries leads to a loss of basic provisions due to inadequate asylum procedures[18] and an increased risk of other human rights violations in asylum applicants. While safeguards should, in general, never be put at risk, vulnerable groups always need special protection also against the potentially adverse impact of the Dublin III-based measures. These might separate family members from each other leading to the loss of the respective support given to sick or otherwise vulnerable family members, might interrupt or endanger ongoing necessary medical and psychological treatments and lead to additional suffering and secondary victimisation.

4.2.3 Torture Survivors as a Highly Vulnerable Group

Legal and humanitarian standards as well as medical and psychological aspects must be considered to provide for identification and the specific support needs of each vulnerable group. The challenge of the protection and needs of torture survivors can be seen as a good example for the complex interdisciplinary aspects to be included in the identification and first-line support and protection not only of this but also of similarly highly vulnerable and usually distressed groups.

Refugees who have been exposed to severe persecution and torture should receive special protection and support based on the above-mentioned EU directive

[17] UN High Commissioner for Refugees (UNHCR), *Hungary as a country of asylum. Observations on restrictive legal measures and subsequent practice implemented between July 2015 and March 2016*, May 2016. Available at: http://www.refworld.org/docid/57319d514.html. Accessed 6 July 2017.

[18] See for example Amnesty International, report 06.07.2015 "Europe's Borderlands: Violations against refugees and migrants in Macedonia, Serbia and Hungary" at https://www.amnesty.org/en/documents/eur70/1579/2015/en/. Accessed 6 July 2017.

but also on the UN Convention against Torture (CAT[19]). The universal prohibition against torture and similar acts of violence (see, e.g. Article 3 European Convention on Human Rights, Article 16 CAT: "Other Cruel, Inhuman or Degrading Treatment or Punishment" (IDT) [16] as a preventive tool) is a key human rights standard and "non-derogable", i.e. it cannot be suspended under any circumstances, including so-called national emergencies.[20] Despite these legal provisions, torture and IDT remain prevalent with high exposure risks in many countries where refugees originate from [17] and also in transit countries [38]. Torture is frequently not recognised as part of the personal background in refugees and migrants [24, 25] and must receive more attention.

Torture can be limited to psychological torture in cases when perpetrators try to avoid evidence of torture from physical injuries. Physical and psychological torture both incur a risk for development of psychological symptoms [38]. A considerable number of studies with different groups of survivors have documented the severity of the impact of torture [18–21] that can even, in many cases, be treatment resistant, like in the case of chronic pain [22]. A risk for indirect trauma in family members or even transgenerational transmission of trauma in refugee families, as documented also in the second- and the third-generation family members of Holocaust survivors, should be considered as well [23, 24]. The UN CAT therefore also underlines the right to complete medical, psychological and social rehabilitation upon torture [42]. This right is not limited to the country where a survivor originates from.

In addition, safety and protection against renewed torture exposure by forced return is a key issue. The principle of non-refoulement is laid out inter alia by the UN Convention relating to the Status of Refugees 1951, which, in Article 33(1), provides that: "No Contracting State shall expel or return a refugee in any manner whatsoever to the frontiers of territories where his life or freedom would be threatened on account of his race, religion, nationality, membership of a particular social group or political opinion". Further, Article 3 of the UN CAT states that "No State Party shall expel, return or extradite a person to another State where there are substantial grounds for believing that he would be in danger of being subjected to torture". This non-refoulement principle of the UN CAT and of other international treaties complements the prohibition in absolute terms of torture or inhuman or degrading treatment or punishment expressed in Article 3 of the UN CAT. From this international legal obligation follows the duty of states to secure torture or IDT victims from renewed torture or IDT as a consequence of the repatriation.

[19] http://www.ohchr.org/EN/ProfessionalInterest/Pages/CAT.aspx. Accessed 25 Dec 2016.

[20] Convention against Torture and Other Cruel, Inhuman or Degrading Treatment or Punishment, entry into force 26 June 1987. http://www.ohchr.org/EN/ProfessionalInterest/Pages/CAT.aspx. Accessed 25 Dec 2016.

4.2.4 Forensic Assessment of Sequels to Torture and Violence and the "Istanbul Protocol" as an Interdisciplinary Standard

Medical proof of earlier torture is usually seen as sufficient evidence to confirm a risk of renewed torture or IDT. Forensic medical and psychological examination in asylum and humanitarian cases [53–56] is, as noted before, especially important when physical or psychological illness might impair the interview process or if they can serve as evidence for persecution or other factors relevant to protection needs, moreso if torture is alleged or suspected. General knowledge about the situation in a country of origin [52] and about the history of a specific person might provide sufficient ground to provide asylum or subsidiary protection without such medical proof. Neglect of proper investigative tools including the use of independent medical and psychological expertise can on the other hand not only lead to a flawed or invalid process, but also to a violation of the above protective principles, torture or death if an allegation of torture or IDT is not believed, and consequently protection would not be given. Providing such expertise is an obligation of governments and not of the applicant. This can also be linked to the obligation of initiating an investigation by the Istanbul Protocol standard[21] as outlined below. In addition, further important reasons to conduct a full medical and psychological evaluation and documentation as illustrated in Fig. 4.2 later in this chapter should be kept in mind.

The "Istanbul Protocol" (Manual on the Effective Investigation and Documentation of Torture and Other Cruel, Inhuman or Degrading Treatment or Punishment (IDT)) (IP, [25, 26]) is the relevant standard that must be used in medical and psychological assessment of alleged torture and in the later legal investigation, even if this last step is not usually taken up as part of the asylum process. It is supported by the UN bodies and medical and health-care umbrella organisations like the World Medical Association, the World Council for Psychotherapy and the World Psychiatric Association [27]. Adequate forensic documentation and reporting of findings that can be used in an independent investigation, court proceedings and asylum hearings are usually not included in medical or psychological education curricula. The IP should, therefore, become part of professional training including lifelong learning models in the legal and health-care professions.[22] It is not primarily intended for, but can also give helpful information in the assessment of, sequels of other forms of violence or persecution that do not fulfill the strict CAT definition of torture or IDT.

Timely, even if only basic, documentation of sequels to torture as a first step does not only provide guidance for treatment needs but also protects evidence before traces of torture vanish, especially when torture exposure has been recent. It can be performed by basic health-care services following general IP guidelines together with the identification of a person as a possible survivor. This helps in the later

[21] www.ohchr.org/Documents/Publications/training8Rev1en.pdf.

[22] Training models are provided, for example, in the EU-based ARTIP/ATIP approach (www.istanbulprotocol.info/) and by Physicians for Human Rights (http://physiciansforhumanrights.org/issues/torture/international-torture/istanbul-protocol-model-medical-curriculum.html).

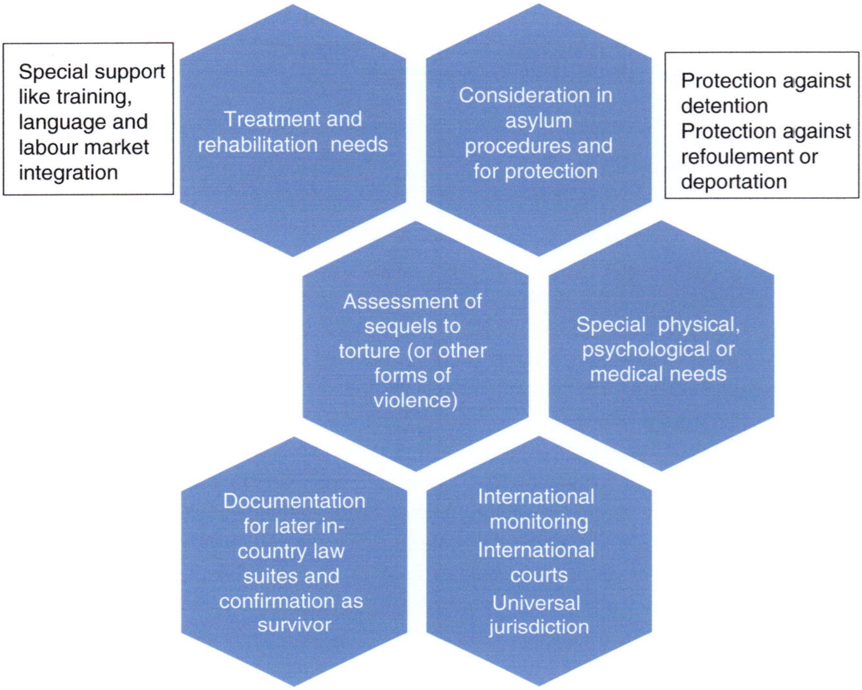

Fig. 4.2 Use of the results of the medical examination in cases of suspected violence, torture or Inhuman or degrading treatment (IDT)

preparation of a comprehensive IP report that will be provided by a forensically trained expert who is not always easily accessible. The IP draws attention to the fact that a negative finding must not contradict reports on torture by the survivor. Factors including but not limited to healing, a lack of sensitivity of diagnostic tools or impairment of memory or memory recall must be considered in this case (see also Table 4.3).

Besides providing evidence, the examination can also be used to support further aims such as prosecution of perpetrators and universal jurisdiction that will be covered in more detail later in this chapter.

The IP also provides strategies for protection against secondary victimisation or "re-traumatisation" of victims by inadequate procedures, such as forced memory recall, which can increase distress and lead to substantial suffering and a substantial increase in affective and anxiety symptoms. This must be considered not only by health professionals but also by lawyers and officials involved in asylum procedures and is in turn an important aspect in general guidelines for support of victims of crime, such as the EU directive.[23]

[23] Directive 2012/29/EU establishing minimum standards on the rights, support and protection of victims of crime was adopted on 25 October 2012 and entered into force on 15 November 2012. Accessed 20 Aug 2017.

It can further be argued that the substantial number of refugees that are victims of crimes, either in their homelands or in transit, or of trafficking, should receive the same quality and guarantees of support and protection as other victims that are outlined in this directive, be it criminal or asylum proceedings, action related to universal jurisdiction or in other situations. The recent (2012) revision includes a number of additional important rights of victims and obligations of member states and strengthens earlier rights that are at present only granted if a criminal case is handled by EU courts. They include, for example, the rights to accessible and understandable information, victim support or specialist support services. The framework also underlines the special care to be taken in identification and support of vulnerable groups:

"Individual assessment to identify vulnerability and special protection measures. All victims will be individually assessed to determine whether they are vulnerable to secondary or repeat victimisation or intimidation during criminal proceedings. If they have specific needs, a whole range of special measures will be put in place to protect them. Children are always presumed vulnerable and particular attention will be paid to some categories of victims such as victims of terrorism, organised crime, human trafficking, gender-based violence, violence in close-relationships, sexual violence or exploitation, hate crime and victims with disabilities".[24]

As already discussed, psychological symptoms or disorders and physical disorders with psychological impact resulting from torture or IDT as well as from other injuries or illness are of major relevance in the asylum interview. They are sometimes not only the most persistent evidence of persecution, violence or torture, but they can, and frequently do, interact with the legal process of seeking asylum. These symptoms and disorders may interfere with memory "storage" during torture, other traumatic events or in the aftermath, and if present during the interview, they may interfere with interaction, memory recall and reporting of events. In all such cases, this can result in incomplete, inadequate or self-contradictory answers and narratives that are frequently misunderstood as a sign of low credibility by legal professionals (Table 4.3).

A heightened sense of responsibility and a solid professional expertise are required to assess survivors of torture. This includes not only a substantial knowledge of transcultural medicine and psychiatry, trauma and forms of torture but also a training in the IP (e.g. in specialised centres of the International Rehabilitation Council for Torture Survivors (IRCT),[25] in curricula like the university-based EU ARTIP/ATIP[26] or in the German SBPM Standards) [28].

[24] http://ec.europa.eu/justice/criminal/victims/rights/index_en.htm. Accessed 15 July 3027.

[25] www.irct.org.

[26] www.istanbulprotocol.info.

Table 4.3 Factors interacting with concentration, disclosure, coherent reporting and memory recall in torture survivors, but also other refugee groups

Factor	Examples
Psychological symptoms related to (post)traumatic stress	Dissociation, shame, distrust, survivor guilt or shame feelings, psychogenic amnesia, concentration difficulties, intrusive memories (flashbacks)
Psychological symptoms as part of other mental health disorders	Psychosis, severe depression, dementia
Psychological symptoms related to physical factors	Diabetes, brain trauma, hunger strike, dehydration, use of medication or substances interfering with concentration or memory
Specific aspects of torture	Disorientation or disinformation used as a tool in psychological torture
Cultural factors	Shame related to sexual torture, fear of disclosure in the community or in front of an interpreter, differences in the understanding of legal or medical concepts and terms, gender related issues

4.2.5 The Next Immediate Steps: Necessary Actions to Protect and Support Vulnerable Groups

Upon identification of a vulnerable group or person, during the asylum-related interviews or other steps such as during a first medical examination, adequate actions should be taken in order to provide medical and psychological support and treatment, as well as practical, social and legal steps for protection.

An example are *gender* issues that must be taken seriously and should follow recommended standards as outlined in the IASC Gender Handbook in Humanitarian Action.[27] Close attention to these issues will, for example, help prevent putting single women or transgender persons at risk for discrimination or harassment in an inadequately guarded and insecure refugee camp area (see also Chaps. 9 and 16 in this book).

Although exposure to severely stressful life events is sometimes claimed to lead to increased hardiness or resilience in survivors of different forms of persecution and violence, existing data indicate that in most cases the opposite is true [29–32] and that both physical and psychological health of such individuals become affected [33], leading to a large subgroup of refugee persons that are vulnerable because they are distressed, traumatised or otherwise sensitive individuals (see also Chap. 11 in this book). A stable, protective environment, sufficient access to reliable information, avoidance of factors that would trigger earlier traumatic experiences and support given in social networking to reduce anxiety about the fate of dislocated family members can be seen as important aspects of a supportive environment for this group. Special programmes (see Chap. 13 in this book) and culture-sensitive psychotherapy can help to cope with impacts of both present and earlier stress. Support such as psychological help or treatment might also be needed during the asylum

[27] http://www.unhcr.org/protection/women/50f91c999/iasc-gender-handbook-humanitarian-action.html.

procedures, which should be conducted in a timely manner and within a framework of respectful interaction [34, 35].

Other *medical or mental health conditions* may also increase vulnerability. A person suffering from chronic psychosis, especially schizophrenia, will be more vulnerable to many stress factors, even when he or she is not at present suffering from an acute psychotic episode. A setting that avoids too much stress and provides a balance between avoiding information overload on one side (such as a crowded tent) and a lack of structure in daily activities and/or isolation on the other, consequently offering an adequate "stimulus window", can be an important tool to address this specific vulnerability [36]. The same obviously holds true for physical medical disorders that might be accompanied by other specific forms of psychological vulnerability and support needs, such as epilepsy. Disorders that are more prevalent in some migrant or refugee groups, like sickle cell disease [37] or pain that might be caused by familial Mediterranean fever [38], may require special support and protection in coordination with other family members as primary caregivers. Psychological impairment by a severe mental health problem or handicap might further require support by a legal representative, such as a guardian who needs to be appointed for legal procedures and the asylum process. Human rights standards relevant for groups with special needs should be respected in addition to the general safeguards for refugees.

4.2.5.1 Further Legal Steps After Identification of Victims of Human Rights Violations and the Question of Universal Jurisdiction: Challenging, Neglected, but Necessary

We want to reiterate the issues that survivors of torture and similar survivors of massive human rights violations face, to illustrate that in some vulnerable groups further legal steps should be taken besides providing protection and immediate social, medical and psychological support. These could serve for the prevention of further persecution, prevent impunity of perpetrators and might be a prerequisite for a return in a country of origin and contribute to the development of a civil society and rule of law. So far, this is rarely considered as a priority as compared to more immediate needs including protection, but can be seen as an important challenge in the next decades. The process of collecting important information evidencing ongoing human rights violations that would otherwise be difficult to obtain on-site in countries with repressive regimes or an ongoing war could be crucial in some situations. IP-based assessment can and should help to collect such evidence and support the monitoring activities of international EU and UN bodies, like the Committees against Torture or the International Criminal Courts.

Similar considerations apply, obviously, also for other victims of human rights violations such as trafficking or gender-based persecution.

4.2.6 Universal Jurisdiction: A Standard for the Future?

In national legislations, special steps such as a report to the public prosecutor are frequently required from the physician in cases of injuries caused by a third party, a step that is rarely taken in refugee cases if a crime such as torture was allegedly committed in a country of origin or countries in transit. This runs contrary to the duty of the forum state to investigate, for example, allegations of torture and inhuman or degrading treatment or punishment committed abroad. According to the respective national implementation of the UN CAT, prosecution may be subject to the presence of the alleged torturer on the territory. But according to Article 12 UN CAT, preliminary proceedings shall be initiated even without the presence of the perpetrator in the forum state.

However, effective mechanisms for international collection and reporting have yet to be established in many areas. One potential option may be the instigation of an international investigation in a host country, such as the collective case of Syrian survivors brought to court in Germany [39]. The complaints and investigations in host countries of the victims are grounded in the principle of universal jurisdiction [40]. This principle is "based on the notion that certain crimes are so harmful to international interests that states are obliged to bring proceedings against the perpetrator, regardless of the location of the crime and the nationality of the perpetrator or the victim" [41]. The principle of universal jurisdiction, therefore, does not require a territorial or personal link with the crime, the perpetrator or the victim. Universal jurisdiction allows for trial of international crimes committed by anybody, anywhere in the world, and it is justified by two main ideas: first, that the crimes to which it applies are so grave that they harm the entire international community and, second, that no safe haven should be available for those who committed them [42]. According to international convention, universal jurisdiction applies, inter alia, to genocide, crimes against humanity, extrajudicial executions, war crimes, torture and forced disappearances. In this context, it is worth highlighting the UN CAT specifying in its Article 5 that each state shall "take such measures as may be necessary to establish its jurisdiction over such offences in cases where the alleged offender is present in any territory under its jurisdiction and it does not extradite him". With this, Article 5 places an obligation on state parties to establish their jurisdiction over the crime of torture in a comprehensive manner in order to avoid providing safe havens for perpetrators of torture [43].

Universal jurisdiction is of crucial importance as it is a recognition that the crimes to which it applies are international crimes. International crimes are so egregious that they offend the sensibilities of the whole world, and therefore the international community has an interest in seeing that justice is done.[28] Today a huge number of domestic legislations provide for universal jurisdiction and empower national courts to investigate and prosecute persons suspected of international crimes. However, many of these definitions do not completely align with the strictest requirements of international law providing for universal jurisdiction. Therefore, the new complaints which have been brought for Syrian victims in different national states such as Spain, Sweden and Germany may contribute to filling the gap of impunity, which either exists due to a lack of implementation of the principle of universal jurisdiction into domestic legislations or due to unwillingness of domestic authorities to act. The existing instruments based on universal jurisdiction should be taken up by host countries, specifically as this would contribute to addressing factors that lead refugees to leave their homelands.

[28] http://www.redress.org/country-work/no-safe-havens-for-torturers-the-application-of-universal-jurisdiction.

4.2.6.1 Repatriation, Forced Return to Transit Countries and Vulnerable Groups

The influx of refugees in the European Union and Australia has led to dubious practices such as large-scale detention in general (see earlier in this chapter and Chap. 12 in this book) and to vigorous efforts of the governments to return or shift asylum seekers to third countries, frequently against their will and increasingly under violation of international human rights standards.[29] These countries might be transit countries, for example, those in the EU Dublin III system described before or countries of origin which are willing to accept a person back. Further, these efforts can also be accompanied by incentives for successful repatriation.

4.2.6.2 Legal Aspects

In this context, it has to be noted that the obligation of the refuge state or the asylum seeker's state of temporary stay extends a duty in respect to everyone within their jurisdiction not to expose them to an irremediable situation of objective danger even outside their jurisdiction. This obligation of the states arises from different international treaties, among others by the UN Convention relating to the Status of Refugees 1951, the ECHR and the UN CAT.

Forced repatriation, deportation, refoulement and even voluntary return can lead to substantial legal, health and social problems for the persons involved, even after immediate hostilities in war areas have ceased [44] not only in the case of torture survivors. The principle of non-refoulement is laid out by the UN Convention relating to the Status of Refugees 1951 (see also Chap. 3 in this book), which, in Article 33(1), provides that: "No Contracting State shall expel or return a refugee in any manner whatsoever to the frontiers of territories where his life or freedom would be threatened on account of his race, religion, nationality, membership of a particular social group or political opinion".

Interruption of ongoing treatment in survivors of torture or IDT, but also the return to a situation where either stress aggravates torture-related trauma or no sufficient effective rehabilitation is accessible, could be seen as a violation of the right to rehabilitation as outlined in the UN CAT: Article 14(1) UN CAT encompasses the right of a victim of an act of torture to obtain redress and an enforceable right to a fair and adequate compensation, including the means for as full a rehabilitation as possible.

In cases of persecution or torture-related trauma, treatment in a country of origin, even if available, should not be expected to generate adequate results, because of a permanent threat of further violence, trigger signals reactivating anxiety and flashbacks as well as re-exposure to impunity and persistence of perpetrators in positions of power. Even if treatment is available, a return against the will of the person would therefore not be justified.

In most transit countries but also countries of origin, access to medical treatment in general and to trauma-specific treatment in particular is highly limited or might not even be available at all because of financial, geographical or safety concerns and/or a lack of trained experts [45]. This is of relevance not only for torture survivors but for any vulnerable group in urgent need of treatment.

[29] https://www.unicef.org/.../SILENT_HARM_Eng_Web.pdf.

4.2.6.3 Medical and Psychological Aspects

The persistent threat of being returned, in combination with the often unclear length of a waiting time for execution of refoulement, is emotionally challenging for all refugees but particularly for vulnerable groups like those suffering from severe psychological trauma (see also again Chaps. 11 and 12 in this book). Moreover, refugee families that are an important protective factor may be torn apart by forced repatriation or refoulement.

In a study conducted for UNICEF on families returned to Kosovo from Germany and Austria upon a longer stay in the host countries, both the circumstances of forced return and social environment encountered in the country of origin were experienced as extremely stressful or even traumatic. Children reported that the "old home country" was foreign to them and that they became socially isolated upon return.[30] The experience of a procedure of forced return, involving police forces with dogs, taking place often at night, was described as their "worst experience in life" by many of the children. Further, substantial and specific trauma-related mental health needs were identified, in particular untreated PTSD in parents. These needs could not be met by the resources in Kosovo and must be expected to further reduce positive resources in the later development of the children or contribute to a transgenerational transmission of trauma.

Due to complexity of the challenges mentioned, each individual case should be carefully evaluated prior to the forced return. Even in cases where no stable legal and psychosocial situation in a host country can be expected, and no danger is attached to returning, voluntary return should be properly prepared and supported. The Dutch Pharos centre has published a helpful booklet for preparation of return to countries of origin.[31]

Those who cannot be returned or those who return but receive no official status in a home country become a stranded group without legal status and access to healthcare, work or social services [46], turning into a highly vulnerable and often desperate group. Because of this lack of a legal status, they will often not be identified in general surveys. Special models would have to be developed to address social and health risks and possible interventions in this group, and this will be a distinct challenge in future planning of refugee care.

4.2.7 Not Only Vulnerable: Identifying Resources

4.2.7.1 Individual Coping and Resources

Collecting information on available resources can be as important as the identification of problems, vulnerability or needs. Individual resources, positive coping skills [47] and other aspects of resilience are usually not covered in healthcare instruments. More work is required to develop instruments to identify these resources and salutogenic interventions that can re-enforce self-respect and confidence of an

[30] https://www.unicef.org/.../SILENT_HARM_Eng_Web.pdf.

[31] http://www.pharos.nl/nl/kenniscentrum/algemeen/webshop/product/34/facing-return. Accessed 2 May 2017.

individual or a group. A complex interaction of present social factors, culture, mental health and lifetime experiences should be considered in this context (see also Chaps. 10 and 13 in this book and in the UNHCR framework discussed later in this chapter), as simple models cannot cover all the factors involved, and both quantitative and qualitative research is necessary to develop a deeper understanding of the issue.

Panter-Brick et al., for example, used an Arabic version of the Child and Youth Resilience Measure (CYRM) in Jordan [27]. In a sample of Syrian refugees living in this country, the authors found no correlation of a person's earlier history, in this case lifetime trauma exposure, to individual resilience scores, but found them inversely associated with severity of mental health symptoms. Somasundaram conducted a comprehensive assessment of stressors and present protective factors in a major civil war zone in Sri Lanka using a qualitative approach and identified "families, female leadership and engagement, cultural and traditional beliefs, practices and rituals" to be protective in post-conflict recovery [48].

Positive coping skills and resilience can in turn be taught to refugees and helpers, as demonstrated by Chemali et al. with fieldworkers in a refugee programme [49]. These concepts are also used by the International Federation of Red Cross and Red Crescent Societies in their book on "Life Skills—Skills for Life" that provides special chapters—i.e. "Life skills needs assessments" and "Monitoring and evaluating life skills programmes"[32]—to help identify needs, resources and outcomes. Handbooks geared towards resilience teaching skills have been published by most organisations, including UNICEF[33] and WHO[34] (see also online resources like the "Resilience" resource database[35]). Religion and other meaning-giving frameworks, rituals and established social networks are an example of potential culture- and community-based resources [50–53] that can be extended or reconstructed to build individual or group resilience [48, 54].

4.2.8 Identification of Human Resources in Refugee Health Care

It could also be helpful to identify persons in a refugee community with basic nursing and other health care skills who could assist other group members with injuries, impairments and disabilities; identifying trusted persons in the community may also be important as they can help spreading critical information in the community. Trained health-care professionals among refugees, such as medical doctors or psychologists, can be another important resource [55, 56] to be identified. Legal and professional frameworks, bias or guidelines might limit the scope of work for such

[32] http://pscentre.org/resources/life-skills-skills-for-life-a-handbook/. Accessed 30 May 2017.

[33] http://unicef.org%2Feapro%2FLife_Skills__A_facilitator_guide_for_teenagers.pdf&usg=AFQjCNHbf6mxvdnuLiTacDy4PoL57Nkp5g&sig2=ECx3HL0ZOaih67czYsb7ow&cad=rja. Accessed 30 May.2017.

[34] www.who.int/school_youth_health/.../sch_skills4health_03.pdf. Accessed 3 Jun 2017.

[35] www.resilience-project.eu.

expert groups in a host country, and their involvement might require careful negotiation to provide an adequate definition of tasks and responsibilities [57–64]. Where feasible, changes in legislation and rules of the host country might be considered and offer possible solutions for solving of this problem. If a full integration of health professionals into medical services of the host country is not possible, their valuable experience with language and culture can still support and guide planning and programmes or can be taken up by participation, for example, in research activities. A focused training programme might be required to prepare them for their activities in the new legal and cultural environment [65–67], similar to the training programmes developed for interpreters in health care or in legal work (see Chap. 14 in this book).

While these refugees can be perceived as ideal participants in humanitarian work, it is crucial to be aware of their own vulnerabilities, including trauma, suffering and exhaustion, which require safeguards to be in place to protect them from developing burnout or forms of vicarious trauma (see also Chap. 15 in this book). These risks should be balanced with potential positive outcomes, like recovery of self-esteem, use of displacement time for learning, continued medical education (CME), capacity building, a positive influence on group dynamics in the refugee community and better cultural adaptation and acceptance of local services. In the long-term resettlement of healthcare experts in host countries, although advantageous for the local health care system, may cause "brain drain" of professionals from the country of origin and should be considered as a long-term risk [68].

4.3 Part III: General Assessment of Mental Health and Psychosocial Needs

4.3.1 Assessment in the WHO "Mental Health and Psychosocial Needs and Resources in Major Humanitarian Crises" Guidelines

The WHO promotes the "Mental Health and Psychosocial Support" (MHPSS) model which is based on the awareness of presence of different layers of psychosocial needs as defined in the broadest possible sense (see again Chaps. 6 and 7 in this book for an in-depth presentation of the concept). It contains a comprehensive set of recommendations and specific tools. These are developed for different tasks and cover areas from general coordination and advocacy to health care system and community-based factors.[36] The need of a continuous, repetitious and flexible assessment of the approach is also stressed, and a process outline is presented (Fig. 4.3):

This model underlines the importance of prevention and psychosocial support measures to address emergencies with the well-coordinated inclusion and training of helpers. Data on stress-related disorders confirm the assumption that adequate

[36] www.who.int/mental_health/emergencies/9781424334445/en. Accessed 20 May 2017.

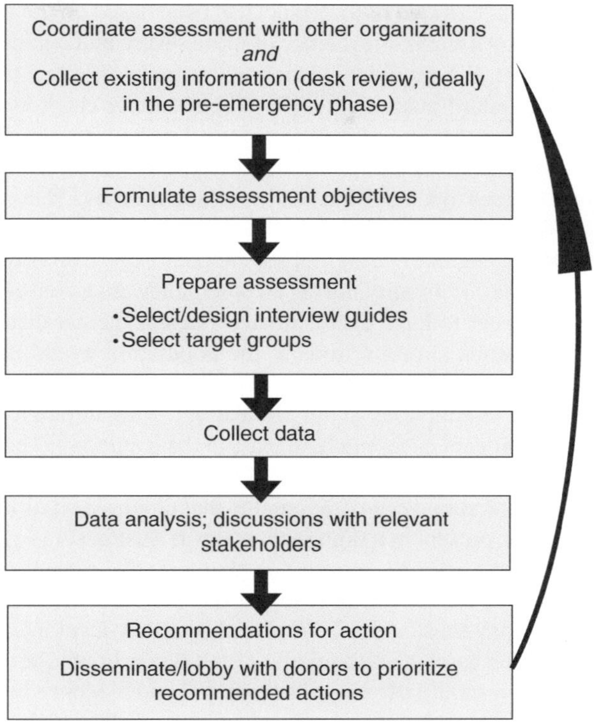

Fig. 4.3 Assessment, collection and use of data in the WHO MHPSS handbook

Table 4.4 Mental health and psychosocial needs and resources in major humanitarian crises layers

Layer I	Social considerations in basic services and security
Layer II	Strengthening community and family supports
Layer III	Focused psychosocial supports
Layer IV	Clinical services

social support is a major factor, for example, in prevention and longitudinal course of posttraumatic stress disorder (PTSD) [69, 70] (Table 4.4).

The model is justified also in light of the frequent lack of local professionals, the added resources necessary to offer trained interpreters, but also of the stigma attached to mental health problems in many cultures [45]. It has been promoted in a number of recent publications in the medical literature [71, 72], is firmly supported by umbrella organisations and can be seen as an important counter-model to overly clinical or biological approaches.

The authors of this chapter share this understanding, but also want to take up the recent discussion on some aspects of a potentially uncritical use of the MHPSS model that can serve to guide a continuous process of improvement of the complex approach. Critique of the model has been based on the fact that earlier research data have shown a high prevalence of more severe and clinical level disorders and related problems, like suicidal ideation and suicide, in many refugee populations assessed with standard instruments ([73–79] and other chapters in this book). Therefore, at least some groups of refugees may be expected to require more attention from trained mental health professionals. The WHO/IASC handbook on the MHPSS, in turn, argues that instruments used in such surveys "have usually been validated only outside emergency situations in help-seeking, clinical populations, for whom distress is more likely a sign of psychopathology than it would be for the average person in the community during an emergency. As a consequence, many surveys of this type appear to have overestimated rates of mental disorder, suggesting incorrectly that substantial proportions of the population would benefit from clinical psychological or psychiatric care" (p. 29). This argument contains a bias and a number of implicit assumptions about clinical and epidemiological studies not backed up by sufficient data or research, at least in the handbook. Though many instruments have indeed been developed with clinical populations, this is by no means true for all, and a substantial body of data remains that confirms significant mental health problems might be present in a high percentage at least in some groups (see also Chaps. 8 and 11 in this book and later in this chapter). The argument that in principle only very small numbers of refugees might require professional mental health interventions, which may mostly else be replaced by lower-level interventions, therefore requires further research and should be tested again in any new refugee group in question. Research should be well-differentiated and evidence based.

Tot et al. have recently conducted a major exploratory project to guide further research based on the MHPSS model [80]. The authors conducted semi-structured focus group discussions in three countries (Peru, Uganda and Nepal), including policymakers, academic researchers, humanitarian aid workers, governmental and UN agencies and non-governmental organisations to identify and comment on priority questions for MHPSS research. Results demonstrated differences in understanding of the research process but identified similar priority areas to be addressed as: (1) the prevalence and burden of mental health and psychosocial difficulties in humanitarian settings, (2) how MHPSS implementation can be improved, (3) evaluation of specific MHPSS interventions, (4) the determinants of mental health and psychological distress and (5) improved research methods and processes.

Updated resources including meetings can be found on the network sites of the MHPSS.[37]

Early identification of general needs and the needs of those most distressed or at risk is obviously a key challenge. Reliable screening instruments (see Sect. 4.3 of this chapter), adequate training of helpers and the use of effective and culture-sensitive instruments to recognise and refer those in need of expert interventions to the scarce highly trained professionals are of special importance (Table 4.5).

---

[37] See https://mhpss.net. It should be considered that the website is not an official WHO but supported by US AID.

Table 4.5 UNHCR/WHO assessment toolkit

Tool #	Title	Method	Why use this tool
		For coordination and advocacy	
1	Who is where, when, doing what (4Ws) in mental health and psychosocial support summary of manual with activity codes	Interviews with agency programme managers	For coordination, though mapping what mental health and psychosocial supports are available
2	WHO assessment schedule of serious symptoms in humanitarian settings (WASSS)	(Component of) Community household survey (representative sample)	For advocacy, by showing the prevalence of mental health problems in the community
		For MHPSS through health services	
3	Checklist for site visits at institutions in humanitarian settings	Site visit, interviews with staff and patients	For protection and care for people with mental or neurological disabilities in institutions
4	Checklist for integrating mental health in primary health care (PHC) in humanitarian	Site visit, interviews with PHC programme managers	For planning a mental health response in PHC
5	Neuropsychiatric component of the health information system (HIS)	Clinical epidemiology using health information system	For advocacy and for planning and monitoring a mental health response in PHC
6	Mental health system formal resources in humanitarian settings	Review of documents, interviews with managers of services	For planning (early) recovery/(re-)construction, through knowledge on formal resources in the regional/ national mental health system
		For MHPSS through diverse sectors, including through community support	
7	Checklist on obtaining general (non-MHPSS specific) information from sector leads	Review of documents by sector lead	For summarising general (non-MHPSS specific) information already known about the current humanitarian emergency (to avoid collecting new data on what is already known)
8	Template (or desk review of pre-existing information relevant to mental hearth and psychosocial support in the region/country)	Literature review	For summarising MHPSS information about this region/country—already known before the current humanitarian emergency (to avoid collecting new data on what is already known)

(continued)

Table 4.5 (continued)

Tool #	Title	Method	Why use this tool
9	Participatory assessment I: perceptions by general community members	Interviews with general community members (free listing with further questions)	For learning about local perspectives on problems and coping in a participatory manner to inform MHPSS response
10	Participatory assessment II: perceptions by community members with in-depth knowledge of the community	(Individual or group) Key informant interviews	
11	Participatory assessment III: perceptions by severely affected persons themselves	Interviews with severely affected persons (free listing with further questions)	
12	Humanitarian Emergency Settings Perceived Needs Scale (HESPER)	Community household survey (representative sample) (early in emergencies this method may also be adapted in convenience samples of key informants)	For informing response, through collecting data on the frequency in the community of physical, social and psychological *perceived* needs

The handbook summarising this model also includes specific mental health assessment and needs assessment tools, which are designed in such a way that they inform intervention planning in an integrated way, particularly in resource-scarce environments.[38]

The model follows the practice common in mixed method and qualitative scientific research. First, available data are collected in a desktop review, enabling preparation of further steps [81] that are to be implemented with participatory assessment that includes (at least) three groups: the general community members, experienced community members with special knowledge and those who are experiencing a problem. Finally, a household survey based on the Humanitarian Emergency Settings Perceived Needs Scale[39] can be performed that was also used successfully in a recent study by Jordans et al. [82]. A manual is again available to guide all steps of the process, from training of interviewers, through implementation of a survey, to analysis and reporting of results. UNHCR has published an evaluation of this approach in 2012 which included 42 countries and has identified health care concerns as the most frequently raised issue.[40]

---

[38] http://www.who.int/mental_health/en/.

[39] www.whqlibdoc.who.int/publications/2011/9789241548236_eng.pdf. Accessed 2 May 2017.

[40] www.alnap.org/pool/.../unhcr-participatory-assessments-2014.pdf.

4.4 Part IV: Mental Health Assessment in Refugee Populations

4.4.1 Medical Classification Systems and the DSM-5 as a Framework For Mental Health

4.4.1.1 The Diagnostic and Statistical Manual (DSM) and the WHO International Classification of Diseases (ICD)

It should again be emphasised that, in accordance with the WHO/UNHCR MHPSS models mentioned, many groups of refugee persons will only suffer from transient psychological reactions that are mainly a reflection of ongoing insecurity, stressors or mourning after bereavement. A psychiatric diagnosis might not have to be established and an intervention by an expert might therefore not be required, with the exception of minor interventions such as short-term medication in combination with non-pharmacological measures for problems like insomnia. Identifying factors leading to stress reactions can be more important than establishing a medical diagnosis. Improving the living conditions to avoid overcrowding and noise during the night or access to contact with family members in the home country might, for example, be more efficient than medical treatment, especially in long-term interventions.

Despite these general considerations, if problems develop or reach a particular level, further support or treatment might be required. Developing problems like suicidal ideation might be common in refugee populations as signs of general distress [79] and need early recognition as they might later be followed by increased rates of completed suicide, especially in the case of additional risk factors [83–85]. Hermans, for example, followed 2291 refugees for a total of 289 person years (py) in a long-stay camp in Greece. Besides upper respiratory tract infections (treatment rates (TR) 89.6/100py) and dental problems, the rates of suicide attempts (TR 1.4/100py) and psychological problems were high (TR 19.4/100py). Early recognition of trends and vulnerable groups can therefore be important, even if a problem has not yet reached the level requiring an expert intervention in the MHPSS model.

In humanitarian settings, it is important for health professionals and non-medical aid providers to also have a firm knowledge of the pitfalls in the use of standardised medical classification systems in order to avoid misunderstandings in the interpretation of quantitative data for clinical and research use, but also in long-term planning.

In general, the classification system provided by the World Health Organisation, i.e. the International Classification of Diseases (ICD),[41] has been accepted as the common standard, but alternative standards are used in specific areas, like mental health research or forensic assessment. In these areas the American Psychiatric Associations Diagnostic and Statistical Manual, at present in its fifth revision (DSM-5),[42] is frequently used and might in some countries be used even as the standard reference. However, this system is limited to mental health problems and is not always easy to integrate with the ICD-based approach. Efforts are taken to develop diagnostic com-

[41] www.who.int/whosis/icd10.

[42] www.dsm5.org/.

parison tables, though criteria and diseases to be recognised and coded can differ substantially at times. This is also the case with posttraumatic stress [86–92] discussed later on. Another challenge is the non-frequent, but usually substantial, general changes in the ICD system. The current 10th ICD version is globally used in health monitoring and planning, but the new 11th version has been already announced. It is expected that the new version will bring considerable changes in categories and definitions of disorders, which might also increase the divergence between ICD and DSM, at least in some areas [92].

Further, in some countries, specific or older versions, such as the ICD-10 CM (Clinical Modification) or the earlier CCD (Chinese Classification of Disease) [93], have been or are still being used due to factors such as a pre-existing local system of health care recompensation. Therefore, it should be considered that results from earlier research might not be comparable with new data based on recent modifications and that standard instruments need to be retranslated and revalidated (a process which is already well underway for the DSM-5).

Category-based systems such as the DSM have been criticised, especially in the context of war and trauma, as being culturally biased, providing "artificial" and insufficiently research-based categories and creating a dichotomous separation between the "normal" and "pathological" [94]. "Dimensional" models and new research models including the recent Research Domain Criteria [95–98] have been proposed. They underline a continuum between normal reaction and a "disorder" and should lead to a new reference framework for mental health care. DSM-5 has in this context been named a "book of woes" as it allows, for example, "grief" to be defined as a bereavement "disorder" which at least potentially might in practice carry the risk of distorting and pathologising a normal, culturally specific reaction to death [99]. Still, it now includes an advanced model of understanding cultural factors, which will be discussed separately in this book (see Chap. 5).

4.4.2 The Mental Health Gap Action Programme (mhGAP) and Comprehensive Diagnostic Assessment in Refugee Groups

Mental health is often considered to be one of the key areas in health care requiring improvement particularly, but not only, in developing countries. The "Mental Health Gap Action Programme" (mhGAP) addresses this issue specifically (see also Chap. 6 in this book). The WHO provides a recently updated general handbook titled "Guideline for Mental, Neurological and Substance Use Disorders"[43] to provide guidance in addressing different challenges that are given priority in this model. The book provides guidelines and flow charts for all steps, from general interaction and basic assessment to general evidence-based treatment in regard to common mental health problems. The assessment of quality of evidence is based on the "PICO" (population/intervention/comparison/outcome) model which helps avoiding inadequate generalisations and permits comparisons. Both medical treatment

[43] www.who.int, mhGAP intervention guide—version 2.0.

and psychosocial concepts are covered, and important resource-oriented and salutogenic-focused chapters, like recovery-oriented psychosocial strategies enhancing independent living and social skills, are included. Due to the focus and methodology used, the evidence base for respective interventions is evaluated much more strictly than in many other guidelines and meta-analytic review articles in the field. Specific trauma-related disorders common in refugee populations are not covered in detail, and the approach does not leave space for transcultural considerations or for interaction between general conditions and development of symptoms.

In the following discussion of specific assessment instruments, we will pay attention to both unspecific mental health problems, including those outlined in the mhGAP, and to specific mental health problems common in refugee groups.

Table 4.6 illustrates the importance of choosing the right tool to avoid an overly narrow focus that might neglect important signals, needs or vulnerabilities, like

Table 4.6 Potential mental health problems in refugee populations—an overview

Type	Example	Comment, key interventions
First episode of (chronic) disorder/vulnerability	Schizophrenia—acute episode	Requires thorough diagnostic steps and major treatment and rehabilitation efforts
Worsening or new episode of pre-existing (chronic) disorder	Episode of bipolar disorder	Might be triggered by stress or by break in medication schedule
Culture-specific reaction to stress (cultural (local) idioms of distress (IoD); see again Chap. 5 in this book)	Fainting spells, specific idioms of distress	Culture-sensitive psychosocial interventions
Specific stress-related disorders	Posttraumatic stress disorder	Might require support and potentially treatment (protection, psychosocial intervention, basic medication over a limited time, in some cases psychotherapy)
Symptoms or disorders as unspecific reaction to trauma or distress (unspecific as they also might be caused by other factors)	Depression, eating disorders, suicidal ideation, self-injurious behaviour	Might also require support and treatment, as above
Reactions to stress without pathological connotation	Mild non-clinical behaviour or reactions such as anxiety, hunger strike	Address stress factors, medical intervention rarely required (for hunger strike, see Chap. 12 in this book)
Secondary complications	Secondary alcohol/ substance abuse (e.g. in the self-"treatment" of PTSD-related sleep disorder)	Might require specific treatment, rehabilitation and also intervention for primary disorder
Physical disorders presenting with psychological symptoms	Thyroid disorders, diabetes, brain trauma, side effects of medication	Address physical problem, short-term symptom-oriented psychiatric treatment might be required

screening for posttraumatic stress disorder (PTSD) only. Mental health problems in refugees or displaced populations are by no means monodimensional, as they include a wide range of problems or disorders reflecting stress, but also pre-existing illness, transcultural factors, symptoms related to the impact of physical injuries after accidents, war, torture or physical disorders presenting with mental health symptoms. The last group includes disorders, such as diabetes or high blood pressure, which have a tendency to first manifest or worsen during a refugee experience, and more specific regional disorders like pain and musculoskeletal complaints (MSCs) in familial Mediterranean fever (MTF) [100]. Another specific factor is the use of traditional herbal medicines or other traditional medicine-based health models that might interact with treatment or lead to specific side effects ([101], see also Chap. 16 in this book).

Symptoms of blunt brain trauma and other forms of traumatic brain injury (TBI) can also be taken as an example as they may be frequent but are often not recognised in survivors of torture [102–104] or in those exposed to blasts and similar war-related events [105–110] or other acts of violence. They can be similar to or co-morbid with PTSD causing their misidentification in refugee people with PTSD [111]. “Shared” symptoms include concentration and memory problems, irritability, decreased stress tolerance and insomnia. However, a diagnosis of TBI or post-concussional symptoms [112] might be based on clinical symptoms alone if radiological examinations are inconclusive or unavailable. A different treatment approach [113] and special support is needed in cases of the presence of both disorders especially as this heightens the risk of suicide [114–116] and other adverse outcomes. The Harvard Trauma Questionnaire consequently explores possible brain trauma [117], but few studies in torture survivors so far also avoid this trap by specifically assessing for TBI or the presence of both PTSD and TBI [103, 118].

These examples underline the importance of particular knowledge and skills that physicians working with refugees who have been exposed to torture or war should have. However, this knowledge is not a part of common medical education curricula, as discussed in the context of the Istanbul Protocol and other chapters of this book.

4.5 Part V: Tools for *Individual- and Person-Centred* Mental Health Assessment and Research: A Short Primer

Standardised tools can be used in assessment of mental health problems in individuals and groups. They can be applied in addition to or instead of a clinical interview with a psychiatrist or a clinical psychologist. In the latter case, the assessment process should be supervised and results evaluated by such experts. However, understanding complex and specific cultural or individual needs of the person should, as noted, not be based on the results of such tools only, but the tools can help identifying major psychological problems or clinical symptoms. Culture-sensitive assessment in turn has been demonstrated to be a complex issue and will be addressed in a special chapter of this book (see Chap. 5).

4.5.1 General Mental Health Screening Instruments

Short screening instruments can detect a certain level of distress, but are usually insufficient for establishing of a DSM or ICD diagnosis, as the outcomes should be interpreted with care. A high level of anxiety identified by such a tool can suggest the presence of different mental health problems, such as general anxiety disorder, a psychotic disorder or a posttraumatic stress disorder, but this could also be caused by general distress due to difficult life circumstances in the absence of a clinical disorder.

4.5.1.1 The General Health Questionnaire (GHQ)

The General Health Questionnaire (GHQ) is probably the most frequently used and also the best validated general screening questionnaire used to identify persons that might require mental health interventions. It is available in a large number of languages and conveniently ranges from very short (GHQ 12) to much longer, more comprehensive versions. One such version is the GHQ 28, which has been successfully used in studies with refugees, like the one by de Jong in Rwandan and Burundese refugee camps [119]. This study carefully evaluated possible cut-off scores in the study sample and identified, in most cases, relatively high rates of subjects scoring beyond the cut-off scores for clinical "caseness", i.e. potentially in need of treatment. High rates of persons in potential need of treatment as identified by the instrument are found in a number of further studies [79, 82, 119–133] with different refugee populations, suggesting that different cut-off scores may be required in highly distressed but not clinically sick populations that might not require medical or psychological treatment, as mentioned in the earlier discussion of the MHPSS model. This finding is similar to those in the study by Kalafi with Afghan refugees in Iran (34.5%) [124] and by the study which authors of this chapter executed in Kosovo (41.7% for moderate to severe depression (see above)), while Getanda et al. found caseness at threshold level at 100% in 100 internally displaced persons in Kenya [132]. Subscales of the GHQ have been defined that give more specific information on problems like suicidal ideation [79, 132].

4.5.1.2 The Hopkins Symptom Checklist (HSCL)

The HSCL 25 [134] is another instrument frequently used in refugee populations. It has been translated into numerous languages, and recent studies have explored its adaptations for different cultures and settings in the HSCL 25 and HSCL 37 versions [135–139]. The HSCL measures symptoms of anxiety and depression, the total score is based on an average of 25 items and a depression score is based on the average of the 15 depression items. The depression score corresponds with the diagnosis of a depressive episode, while the general score corresponds to general distress.[44]

[44] http://hprt-cambridge.org/screening/hopkins-symptom-checklist/.

4.5.2 Non-verbal Screening

As non-verbal behaviour in human interactions can communicate important information, the capacity to decode it should be learned by the helpers during their training. However, specific assessment tools do not exist or are in a research and development phase and usually cannot be applied in a clinical setting.

4.5.2.1 (Semi-)Structured Interview Schedules to Identify DSM and ICD Disorders

Clinical interviews by a trained psychiatrist or clinical psychologist and (semi-) structured interview schedules are usually perceived as reference standards in psychiatric practice and research. For working with refugees, training must also include specific knowledge on culture and other factors relevant in a specific group. Semi-structured interview schedules usually consist of open questions providing room for individual differences in describing personal experiences of symptoms correlating to the standard diagnostic criteria defined by DSM or ICD classifications. These interviews often require more time, training and/or a higher level of expertise in the interviewer, but they provide the most reliable results if validated in a specific language and population. Adaptations of these instruments can be made in order to fit a specific culture and setting more adequately. For example, Brink et al. have used components of the SCID (see below) to develop and validate a questionnaire to assess Karen refugees from Burma, presently displaced in larger numbers to the USA [140].

4.5.2.2 WHO CIDI and World Mental Health Composite International Diagnostic Interview (WHO WMH-CIDI)

The WHO WMH-CIDI[45] [141, 142] has been developed based on the original World Health Organization's Composite International Diagnostic Interview (WHO CIDI [143]).

It is a fully structured interview that again requires prior training, but in contrast to the SCID (see below), it does not require to be applied by experts such as psychiatrists. The authors stress that it can be used both for epidemiological and cross-cultural studies and for clinical purposes. In addition to the diagnostic part included in the original CIDI, it can elicit important information relevant for public health and the assessment of service indicators and determine "the burden of these disorders, assess service use, the use of medications in treating these disorders, and who is treated, who remains untreated, and what are the barriers to treatment". This list of additional tools and modules indicate a strong focus on practical relevance and makes this instrument a much better fit for a comprehensive mental health assessment than the original CIDI. Within these additional tools and modules, the authors included an improved screening section, sections on distress and impairment, clinical severity, questions about a lifetime course and about 12-month persistence, on subthreshold diagnoses, the Sheehan Disability Scales, the WHO Disability

[45] https://www.hcp.med.harvard.edu/wmhcidi.

Schedule (DAS) and an extended section on "noncore" conditions. The last section contains an extended and improved PTSD section which is particularly relevant for refugee groups. In order to balance a comprehensive approach with an efficient use of tighter resources, this instrument is based on a modular approach that provides different versions and pathways to be selected depending on the setting and client characteristics. This CIDI version is perhaps the most comprehensive mental health assessment tool that can also be used in larger refugee populations. However, its use might be limited because of the effort and resources required to translate, obtain permission and train staff in the use of this instrument in an emergency setting. It also does not include a comprehensive culture-specific section, such as the DSM-5 Cultural Formulation Interview (CFI), that may be added in transcultural and migrant research. The most recent version (3.1 in 2017) presented online at the time when this chapter was written had not yet been updated for DSM-5 or ICD-11.

4.5.2.3 Structured Clinical Interview for DSM (SCID)

The structured clinical interview for DSM (SCID) [144] is often perceived as the reference standard in research, but it has also been used in clinical practice and in forensic evaluation, primarily in the USA. It covers all major (DSM) clinical disorders, but requires prior training by experts. It is a complex instrument and should be applied by a trained mental health expert. Despite these challenges, a number of studies using the SCID or parts of it in refugee populations have been published [145–149], or the SCID was used to support development of culture-specific instruments [140].

4.5.3 Screening for Trauma-Related Issues

Screening for trauma-related issues and in particular PTSD is one of the most common assessments performed in refugee populations. As discussed before, posttraumatic stress or even severe stress reactions in general are by no means limited to PTSD, but may include depression, other unspecific but relevant disorders and culture-based problems [150], and the PTSD diagnostic category has been criticised by many researchers in the field of cultural anthropology and transcultural psychiatry as a too limited concept (see Chap. 5 in this book on this subject and the concept of "cultural idioms of distress").

PTSD symptoms can best be understood in a model based on evolutionary psychology that explains PTSD as an adaptive and normal response to threat, developing into a clinical problem under adverse conditions [151–153]. They can and frequently lead to severe complications such as substance abuse, depression, suicidal behaviour and problems in everyday life, occupation and the family system [154–159] and should therefore be taken serious (see also Chap. 11 in this book) in spite of the care necessary in avoiding an overemphasis that would distract from other important problems and cultural background.

Recent and substantial changes in the DSM-5 such as the integration of "complex" symptoms and also in the upcoming ICD-11 PTSD criteria that apparently will include a new separate diagnosis of "complex" PTSD [160] should be considered when using an instrument in forensic evaluation [27] or when comparing already published research data. In a study using a US national community sample and two US Department of Veterans Affairs clinical samples [92], Wisco, for example, demonstrated prevalence of PTSD using ICD-11 draft criteria to be 10–30% lower than in DSM-5 and 25 and 50% lower than in ICD-10. This can be expected to lead also to problems in specific areas like forensic evaluation, for example, in the use of the Istanbul Protocol in refugee survivors of torture.

4.5.3.1 Clinician-Administered PTSD Scale (CAPS)

The Clinician-Administered PTSD Scale (CAPS) is frequently seen as the "gold" standard in PTSD research and also in forensic assessment of controversial cases [161]. This semi-structured interview schedule should be used by experts, preferably with prior training. A full evaluation can, in our experience, take up to 60–90 min. The CAPS includes "complex" PTSD symptoms, has been updated for DSM-5 [162], provides a severity index and permits—in contrast to questionnaires or cross-sectional interviews—assessment of the longitudinal development of symptoms over time at least in a retrospective way and of further important aspects. It has also been adapted for and tested in different cultures and in refugee groups (see, e.g. Malekzai et al. [163], Charney et al. [164]). Hinton et al. have used the CAPS as part of a well-designed combined strategy to explore trauma, PTSD symptoms and cultural idioms of distress in studies with Cambodian refugees [165–168]. Recent studies also used the CAPS as an outcome measure in treatment of PTSD in refugees. Halvorsen et al. have used the instrument to assess change in PTSD symptoms during narrative exposure therapy [169], Ter Heide used the HTQ (see below) and CAPS to evaluate eye movement desensitisation and reprocessing (EMDR) treatment outcomes [170] and Hensel-Dittmann et al. to compare stress inoculation training (SIT) with narrative exposure therapy (NET) [171].

4.5.4 Harvard Trauma Questionnaire (HTQ)

The Harvard Trauma Questionnaire (HTQ) is one of the most frequently used instruments for the evaluation of PTSD symptoms. The Medline standard database alone lists 81 publications either using or referring to the HTQ (as reviewed in 2017). This instrument was pioneering culture-based (re)validation [117, 172] of trauma-related symptoms. It includes a (slightly controversial) list of events that must be adapted to fit the respective target populations and questions inquiring into suspected brain trauma, and it already included symptoms of "complex" PTSD that have only now been integrated in the extended PTSD definition in DSM-5. Recent reanalysis of larger datasets indicated that the cut-off scores still might differ between ethnic groups [173]. The core items (without the events list) take in our experience about 6–10 min to answer, while the full tool takes about 20 min either as interview or as a pen-and-paper tool. Users should keep in mind that the original cut-off scores consist of a score for the core symptoms (DSM-III-R/DSM-IV) and an additional score for integrating the complex symptoms. A new version reflecting the changes to the PTSD diagnosis in DSM-5 has been developed and is already in use [91, 174]. The differences in subscales used and different versions circulating around should again be taken into consideration when comparing data from different researches.

4.5.4.1 Specific Topics

Common problems in distressed populations also can include more specific aspects, not limited to anxiety or depressed mood. Recommended instruments, for example, for the assessment of dissociation include the Peritraumatic Distress Inventory (PDI) [175, 176] and the Peritraumatic Dissociative Experiences Questionnaire (PDEQ) [177].

Suicidal ideation and suicide risk may be assessed with items or subscales from standard instruments, such as the Watson subscale in the GHQ [79, 132]. However, these scales cannot always reliably predict suicide risk, and a careful consideration of the cultural background needs to guide early recognition and interventions especially in these more specific areas.

4.5.5 Specific Instruments for Screening of Refugee Populations

4.5.5.1 The PROTECT Instrument

The PROTECT instrument was developed as part of an EU-funded project (Process of Recognition and Orientation of Torture Victims in European Countries to Facilitate Care and Treatment Questionnaire (PQ)). The multilingual ten-item PQ should identify subgroups being at a low, medium and high risk for trauma-related mental health disorders. The latter two subgroups should be seen by a healthcare professional.[46] Part of the questionnaire is rather general and not "trauma" specific, as it might yield positive responses also in clients with general physical or psychological problems. However, several items may help identifying common cultural idioms of distress. To our knowledge, only face-value validity was obtained for this instrument, and future research should be performed to assess sensitivity and specificity of the instrument in comparison to other tools.

4.5.5.2 The Refugee Health Screener (RHS-15)

The Refugee Health Screener (RHS-15) [178–182] is a well-documented instrument that has been translated into a number of different languages. It has been developed through participatory research with refugee people and has been argued to be particularly sensitive to culture and the refugee experience. In addition to screening for selected anxiety, depression and PTSD symptoms, it also includes questions on personal history and on coping strategies. The original questionnaire was evaluated in a new study which has indicated that the case sensitivity and specificity to DPs were acceptable ($\geq$0.87/0.77). Also, the study proposed that an even shorter, 13-item scale, might be "more efficient and as efficacious for case

[46] http://www.pharos.nl/information-in-english/protect-recognition-and-orientation-of-torture-victims.

identification" [180]. It is certainly one of the most promising refugee specific instruments. Polcher used the RHS with 178 adult refugees identifying 51 (28.6%) that were positive for a risk of emotional distress, with the highest rates in refugees from Iraq [181]. Johnson-Agbakwu used the RHS in 112 women from different countries seeking gynaecological help, with 26 (23.2%) scoring positive, again, mainly those coming from Iraq [179].

Other tools available may be highly culture specific, like the Afghan Symptom Checklist (AFCL), developed and used in several studies [120, 121], and a specific five-item screening instrument for Karen refugees [140].

4.5.6 Assessment of Psychological Problems in Children

Assessing the impact of distress or trauma on children or even of psychological health on a specific cultural background is a complex task, as it depends also on age and developmental stage of the child. Recent publications claim that children as young as 9 months old can suffer, for example, from posttraumatic stress reactions [10–17]. The DSM-5 has already extended the description of trauma-related disorders in children [183–185]. This will again, as in the case of adult PTSD, require updating and revalidation of the existing instruments. However, the complexity of impacts of stressful and traumatic events on children is still insufficiently defined in the DSM-5 model. Groups with special backgrounds, like those suffering from transgenerational trauma or former child soldiers, can also present with complex multilevel impacts of trauma on development, social skills, coping and behaviour. These groups require special models to understand their needs and design possible rehabilitation strategies [186, 187].

4.5.6.1 Participatory Assessment

UNHCR has developed a special handbook for *Participatory Assessment with Children and Adolescents* ("Listen and Learn")[47] as part of the development of a UNHCR Global Protection Agenda for Children. The material has been field-tested in India, Jordan, Kenya and Nepal. The model is based on workshops (similar to focus groups) and supported by a number of tools included in the manual. They include specific exercises to be used in workshops, guidelines on how to address children in distress, games like picture bingo cards, child-friendly feedback sheets and a manual on how to work with puppets. The handbook is user-friendly and easy to read and comprehensive in its approach and can be a key tool in understanding and addressing the specific perception and needs of children as important partners in a community or group coping process. The models proposed can be also considered as a first intervention. Further handbooks are the *Child Protection Rapid Assessment* handbook and toolkit by the Global Protection Cluster, Child Protection

[47] http://www.unhcr.org/protection/children/50f6d1259/listen-learn-participatory-assessment-children-adolescents.html. Accessed 10 Jun 17.

Working Group, published last December 2012,[48] and the comprehensive handbook on Children and Evaluation by "Save the Children".[49]

4.5.6.2 Creative and Visual Media

Depending on age, creative media [48, 188] can be the best tools in understanding experiences and needs of children as they trigger emotional processes more than questionnaires or other verbal instruments [189]. They can even be used in the documentation of human rights violations for courts. Members of the NGO "Waging Peace" were, for example, travelling through eastern Chad to collect facts about the humanitarian and human rights situation as well as information on security concerns in the region by conducting interviews with displaced persons and refugees. While a team member was interviewing adults, she decided to give paper and pencils to children living in the camp and ask them to illustrate their dreams and strongest memories. The resulting paintings gave a different version of the events than those given by the Sudanese government in Khartoum, who had always denied supporting Janjaweed paramilitary groups. In November 2007, the paintings were accepted as contextual evidence for the crimes committed in Darfur by the International Criminal Court in The Hague.[50]

Recently, a Danish group has published the cartoon-based "Darryl" instrument, built on the CAPS, that can be used as an example of how to create a bridge between visual media and questionnaire-based approaches in trauma assessment of children. However, further research will be required to evaluate its application in different cultures [190].

4.5.6.3 Standardised Diagnostic Tools

In the next section, some standardised diagnostic tools for children will be reviewed. Their use depends on age and literacy, besides the previously mentioned factors like culture. The tools presented in the following subchapter also are not limited to evaluation of formal diagnostic ICD or DSM categories such as PTSD, as other types of information including the presence of internalising or externalising reactions are also considered as relevant in children. Application might include questions that are posed to parents, which again would limit the use of an instrument, in groups like unaccompanied minors. Special care and a sensitive approach are required when interacting with traumatised children [191], and special training might be required even for experienced healthcare professionals.

The Mini-International Neuropsychiatric Interview for children and adolescents (M.I.N.I. Kid) [192] is a relatively short, structured diagnostic interview which assesses the current prevalence of child and adolescent psychiatric diagnoses for DSM-IV and ICD-10. The assessment includes evaluation of a lifetime (earlier) diagnosis of psychiatric disorders. When dealing with a culturally diverse group of

---

[48] http://cpwg.net/. Accessed 10 Jun 17.

[49] www.savethechildren.org.uk/.../children_and_partipation_1.pdf. Accessed 10 Jun 17.

[50] http://www.wagingpeace.info/index.php/the-drawings. Accessed 10 Mar 16.

individuals facing extreme stress, relative brevity of this assessment method makes it suitable for establishing a general overview of the individual's wellbeing.

4.5.6.4 The Youth Self-Report (YSR)

This prominent and well-established 112-item self-reporting, screening questionnaire assesses the individual's emotional and behavioural problems and has been used in migrant and refugee populations [193, 194]. Although it is designed for youth aged 11 to 18, evidence has demonstrated that younger children are also able to provide reliable reports within the Internalizing and Externalizing scales [195].

4.5.6.5 The UCLA PTSD Reaction Index for DSM-IV Revision I

This brief self-reported screening tool is used to assess trauma exposure and post-traumatic stress symptoms for all DSM-IV PTSD symptoms in school-age children and adolescents who report traumatic experiences. The 20-question item sheet indices are linked to the DSM-IV criteria and can provide preliminary PTSD diagnostic information, as well as a cut-off value reflecting the diagnostic criteria, as described in DSM-IV [196–198]. The tool was recently adapted for the DSM-5 classification [199]. It is important to note that the UCLA PTSD Reaction Index R is not intended to be used in place of a structured clinical interview. Instead, it functions as a quick and efficient screening tool providing information regarding the frequency of symptoms.

4.5.6.6 Children's Revised Impact of Event Scale (CRIES-8/CRIES-13)

The scales, designed for children aged 8+ (CRIES-8) or 13+ (CRIES-13), work efficiently in classifying children with and without PTSD. CRIES-8 lacks arousal items, while CRIES-13 includes them [200]. Available in a number of different languages, these scales consist of four items measuring intrusion and four items measuring avoidance. They are designed for the use with children who are able to read independently, but at least the CRIES-8 also has been used with reading support in refugee children, for example, by Salari, who found 76% of unaccompanied refugee children mainly from Afghanistan to be over the cut-off score for PTSD [201] in a study making use of this approach.

4.5.6.7 Child Posttraumatic Cognitions Inventory (CPTCI)

The CPTCI was adapted by Meiser-Stedman, Smith, et al. from the earlier adult version, and it consists of 25 age-appropriate items that make up two subscales [202]. As a well-validated and effective measure that is not specific to the type of trauma exposure, the questions cover the "permanent and disturbing change" subscale (CPTCI-PC) and the "fragile person in a scary world" subscale (CPTCI-SW). The CPTCI-PC focuses on the negative effects the frightening event may have had on the child and his/her perception of the future in the light of the frightening event. In contrast, the CPTCI-SW looks at the child's perception of the world, including those around him/her who are perceived as threatening and confirming their own sense of weakness.

4.5.6.8 The Child Behaviour Checklist (CBCL)

This parent/teacher report questionnaire is one of the most widely used measures in child and adolescent psychology. It analyses the individuals' various maladaptive behavioural and emotional problems and has been frequently used in refugee populations [194, 203, 204]. Although this standardised assessment tool gives a thorough overview of a child's internalising and externalising problems, it would only be applicable after the individual has become slightly more settled and has developed a relationship with a teacher or guardian who could reliably answer questions in case of unaccompanied refugee minors.

4.5.6.9 Hopkins Symptom Checklist-37 for Adolescents (HSCL-37A) [137]

The HSCL-37A is a 37-item self-report measure designed for unaccompanied asylum-seeking adolescents aged 12+ and has been used in a number of recent studies [138, 204, 205]. The 37-item question sheet measures symptoms of traumatic stress broken down into 10 anxiety items (e.g. feeling tense), 15 items measuring depression (e.g. crying easily) and 12 externalising items (e.g. arguing often). The answers are marked on a four-point subscale (1, never, to 4, always). Furthermore, Bean [137] has modified this checklist by adding increasing sizes of coloured circles to the terms of the Likert scale to make it more understandable and more accessible to culturally diverse groups. The instrument is flexible, and Mels et al. have consequently used the HSCL-37A to demonstrate a strategy for rapid adaptation of instruments in an emergency setting [139].

4.5.6.10 Strengths and Difficulties Questionnaire (SDQ12-15) [206]

Finally, Goodman's (1997) SDQ is a brief behavioural screening questionnaire for adolescents aged 11–17 years. Twenty-five attributes are divided into five subscales: emotional symptoms, conduct problems, inattention-hyperactivity, peer problems and prosocial behaviour. This screening questionnaire is probably one of the most widely used assessment tools for assessing childhood mental health disorders and is as such highly reliable [207]. It can also be used in exploring complex research questions in refugee groups, as demonstrated by Dalgaard in his study on trauma transmission [23].

Conclusions

The identification and comprehensive understanding of the needs and vulnerability of individuals, groups and communities in refugee populations is a complex challenge. Attention to this can be expected to contribute to better results in support and protection in general but also in targeted allocation and efficient use of resources. The models and tools available for general and community-based assessments as a central element in comprehensive multi-actor strategies provided by the IASC, WHO, UNHCR, UNICEF and the new model to be published by Medicines Sans Frontiers can be expected to be excellent guiding frameworks. They offer well-tested general tools, reflect decades of experience in numerous settings and should in our opinion be used whenever possible.

Special tools and strategies are available for the assessment of mental health on both the individual and on the community level.

Identification of vulnerable groups, including survivors of persecution and torture, is of special importance given the present politically motivated strategies denying refugees support and protection in host countries (as also described in Chap. 2). Basic human rights of all refugee groups and the special needs of vulnerable groups must be recognised and should receive adequate attention as requested by local legal and international humanitarian and human rights standards.

A well-planned and well-managed intervention programme, supported by international collaboration between governments, NGOs and the UN agencies, that is based on reliable data, and identification of needs and vulnerable groups, as outlined in this chapter, can be seen as a good alternative to measures reflecting political manipulation of group anxieties that have become increasingly popular as proposed by Volkan in this book.

References

1. Aladhrai SA, Djalali A, Della Corte F, Alsabri M, El-Bakri NK, Ingrassia PL. Impact of the 2011 revolution on hospital disaster preparedness in Yemen. Disaster Med Public Health Prep. 2015;9(4):396–402.
2. Bloch-Infanger C, Battig V, Kremo J, Widmer AF, Egli A, Bingisser R, et al. Increasing prevalence of infectious diseases in asylum seekers at a tertiary care hospital in Switzerland. PLoS One. 2017;12(6):e0179537.
3. Ismail SA, Abbara A, Collin SM, Orcutt M, Coutts AP, Maziak W, et al. Communicable disease surveillance and control in the context of conflict and mass displacement in Syria. Int J Infect Dis. 2016;47:15–22.
4. Ozaras R, Leblebicioglu H, Sunbul M, Tabak F, Balkan II, Yemisen M, et al. The Syrian conflict and infectious diseases. Expert Rev Anti-Infect Ther. 2016;14(6):547–55.
5. Rits IA. Declaration of Helsinki. Recommendations guidings doctors in clinical research. World Med J. 1964;11:281.
6. Tangwa GB. Research with vulnerable human beings. Acta Trop. 2009;112(Suppl 1):S16–20.
7. Culhane-Pera KA, Moua M, Vue P, Xiaaj K, Lo MX, Straka RJ. Leaves imitate trees: Minnesota Hmong concepts of heredity and applications to genomics research. J Community Genet. 2017;8(1):23–34.
8. Jaffe AE, Steel AL, DiLillo D, Hoffman L, Gratz KL, Messman-Moore TL. Victim alcohol intoxication during a sexual assault: relations with subsequent ptsd symptoms. Violence Vict. 2017;32(4):642–57.
9. Haskew C, Spiegel P, Tomczyk B, Cornier N, Hering H. A standardized health information system for refugee settings: rationale, challenges and the way forward. Bull World Health Organ. 2010;88(10):792–4.
10. Lay M, Papadopoulos I. Sexual maltreatment of unaccompanied asylum-seeking minors from the Horn of Africa: a mixed method study focusing on vulnerability and prevention. Child Abuse Negl. 2009;33(10):728–38.
11. Office of Refugee Resettlement (ORR), Administration for Children and Families (ACF), Department of Health and Human Services (HHS). Standards to prevent, detect, and respond to sexual abuse and sexual harassment involving unaccompanied children. Interim final rule (IFR). Fed Regist. 2014;79(247):77767–800.

12. Sipsma HL, Falb KL, Willie T, Bradley EH, Bienkowski L, Meerdink N, et al. Violence against Congolese refugee women in Rwanda and mental health: a cross-sectional study using latent class analysis. BMJ Open. 2015;5(4):e006299.
13. International Summit on Transplant Tourism and Organ Trafficking. The declaration of Istanbul on organ trafficking and transplant tourism. Clin J Am Soc Nephrol. 2008;3(5):1227–31.
14. Moszynski P. Organ traffickers are targeting refugees in Egypt, warns charity. BMJ. 2011;343:d8254.
15. Najafizadeh K, Ghorbani F, Rostami A, Ghobadi O, Barbati E, Rad SS, et al. Seeking consent in the country of origin for transplantation from a brain-dead refugee in the host country. Saudi J Kidney Dis Transpl. 2010;21(2):345–7.
16. Mautino KS. The convention against torture and other forms of cruel, inhuman and degrading treatment or punishment. J Immigr Health. 2000;2(4):179–81.
17. The Lancet. Torture and ill treatment in Syria's prisons. Lancet. 2016;388(10047):842.
18. Song SJ, Subica A, Kaplan C, Tol W, de Jong J. Predicting the mental health and functioning of torture survivors. J Nerv Ment Dis. 2017;206(1):33–9.
19. Wenzel T, Griengl H, Stompe T, Mirzaei S, Kieffer W. Psychological disorders in survivors of torture: exhaustion, impairment and depression. Psychopathology. 2000;33(6):292–6.
20. Wenzel T. Torture. Curr Opin Psychiatry. 2007;20(5):491–6.
21. Ghaddar A, Elsouri G, Abboud Z. Torture and long-term health effects among lebanese female political prisoners. J Interpers Violence. 2016;31(3):500–14.
22. Defrin R, Ginzburg K, Mikulincer M, Solomon Z. The long-term impact of tissue injury on pain processing and modulation: a study on ex-prisoners of war who underwent torture. Eur J Pain. 2014;18(4):548–58.
23. Dalgaard NT, Todd BK, Daniel SI, Montgomery E. The transmission of trauma in refugee families: associations between intra-family trauma communication style, children's attachment security and psychosocial adjustment. Attach Hum Dev. 2016;18(1):69–89.
24. Dalgaard NT, Montgomery E. Disclosure and silencing: a systematic review of the literature on patterns of trauma communication in refugee families. Transcult Psychiatry. 2015;52(5):579–93.
25. Iacopino V, Ozkalipci O, Schlar C. The Istanbul Protocol: international standards for the effective investigation and documentation of torture and ill treatment. Lancet. 1999;354(9184):1117.
26. Ucpinar H, Baykal T. An important step for prevention of torture. The Istanbul protocol and challenges. Torture. 2006;16(3):252–67.
27. Wenzel T, Frewer A, Mirzaei S. The DSM 5 and the Istanbul Protocol: diagnosis of psychological sequels of torture. Torture. 2015;25(1):51–61.
28. Hofmann M, Hagemeier I, Altenhain K, Kruse J. Evaluation of medical and psychological expert opinions in asylum and residence legislation. Psychother Psychosom Med Psychol. 2014;64(1):12–9.
29. Hauff NJ, Fry-McComish J, Chiodo LM. Cumulative trauma and partner conflict predict post-traumatic stress disorder in postpartum African-American women. J Clin Nurs. 2016;26(15-16):2372–83.
30. Levy-Gigi E, Richter-Levin G, Okon-Singer H, Keri S, Bonanno GA. The hidden price and possible benefit of repeated traumatic exposure. Stress. 2016;19(1):1–7.
31. Ponnamperuma T, Nicolson NA. Negative trauma appraisals and PTSD symptoms in Sri Lankan adolescents. J Abnorm Child Psychol. 2016;44(2):245–55.
32. Bottche M, Heeke C, Knaevelsrud C. Sequential traumatization, trauma-related disorders and psychotherapeutic approaches in war-traumatized adult refugees and asylum seekers in Germany. Bundesgesundheitsblatt Gesundheitsforschung Gesundheitsschutz. 2016;59(5):621–6.
33. Atwoli L, Stein DJ, King A, Petukhova M, Aguilar-Gaxiola S, Alonso J, et al. Posttraumatic stress disorder associated with unexpected death of a loved one: cross-national findings from the world mental health surveys. Depress Anxiety. 2017;34(4):315–26.
34. Schock K, Rosner R, Knaevelsrud C. Impact of asylum interviews on the mental health of traumatized asylum seekers. Eur J Psychotraumatol. 2015;6:26286.

35. Hainmueller J, Hangartner D, Lawrence D. When lives are put on hold: lengthy asylum processes decrease employment among refugees. Sci Adv. 2016;2(8):e1600432.
36. Takahashi H, Rissling AJ, Pascual-Marqui R, Kirihara K, Pela M, Sprock J, et al. Neural substrates of normal and impaired preattentive sensory discrimination in large cohorts of nonpsychiatric subjects and schizophrenia patients as indexed by MMN and P3a change detection responses. NeuroImage. 2013;66:594–603.
37. McMahon C, Callaghan CO, O'Brien D, Smith OP. The increasing prevalence of childhood sickle-cell disease in Ireland. Ir J Med Sci. 2001;170(3):183–5.
38. Backman O. Abdominal pain in a refugee. Duodecim. 2003;119(18):1779–81.
39. Brosch P. Here's how German courts are planning to prosecute Syrian war crimes. The Washington Post; 2017.
40. Levy D, Sznaider N. Sovereignty transformed: a sociology of human rights. Br J Sociol. 2006;57(4):657–76.
41. Robinson M. The Principles of universal jurisdiction. Princeton: Princeton University Press; 2001.
42. Philippe X. The principles of universal jurisdiction and complementarity: how do the two principles intermesh? Int Rev Red Cross. 2006;88(862):23.
43. Nowak M. Torture and enforced disappearance. In: CSM K, editor. International protection of human rights: a textbook. Turku: Institute for Human Rights, Åbo Akademi University; 2012. p. 153–87.
44. Calam R. Public health implications and risks for children and families resettled after exposure to armed conflict and displacement. Scand J Public Health. 2017;45(3):209–11.
45. Wenzel T, Kienzler H, Wollmann A. Facing violence - a global challenge. Psychiatr Clin North Am. 2015;38(3):529–42.
46. Mylius M, Bornschlegl W, Frewer A. Medizin für "Menschen ohne Papiere": Menschenrechte und Ethik in der Praxis des Gesundheitssystems. Göttingen: V&R Unipress; 2011. 276p.
47. Seguin M, Roberts B. Coping strategies among conflict-affected adults in low- and middle-income countries: a systematic literature review. Glob Public Health. 2017;12(7):811–29.
48. Somasundaram D, Sivayokan S. Rebuilding community resilience in a post-war context: developing insight and recommendations - a qualitative study in Northern Sri Lanka. Int J Ment Heal Syst. 2013;7(1):3.
49. Chemali Z, Borba CPC, Johnson K, Hock RS, Parnarouskis L, Henderson DC, et al. Humanitarian space and well-being: effectiveness of training on a psychosocial intervention for host community-refugee interaction. Med Confl Surviv. 2017;33(2):141–61.
50. Kristiansen M, Younis T, Hassani A, Sheikh A. Experiencing loss: a muslim widow's bereavement narrative. J Relig Health. 2016;55(1):226–40.
51. Hasanovic M, Pajevic I. Religious moral beliefs inversely related to trauma experiences severity and presented posttraumatic stress disorder among Bosnia and Herzegovina war Veterans. J Relig Health. 2015;54(4):1403–15.
52. Bryant-Davis T, Ullman S, Tsong Y, Anderson G, Counts P, Tillman S, et al. Healing pathways: longitudinal effects of religious coping and social support on PTSD symptoms in African American sexual assault survivors. J Trauma Dissociation. 2015;16(1):114–28.
53. Simmelink J, Lightfoot E, Dube A, Blevins J, Lum T. Understanding the health beliefs and practices of East African refugees. Am J Health Behav. 2013;37(2):155–61.
54. Bongartz D, Kraft S. Promoting resilience with rituals. Kinderkrankenschwester. 2013;32(3):97–9.
55. Lehmann V. Physicians who come to Norway as refugees. Tidsskr Nor Laegeforen. 1993;113(25):3165.
56. Wenzel T. Refugee doctors can do valuable work in European host countries. BMJ. 1999;318(7177):196.
57. Rumani G. Refugee doctors find it hard to get back into practice. BMJ. 2001;322(7290):862.
58. Cheeroth S, Ambrose L. A training programme for refugee doctors. Hosp Med. 2002;63(10):582–3.
59. Stewart E, Nicholas S. Refugee doctors in the United Kingdom. BMJ. 2002;325(7373):S166.

60. Leaver L. Overseas-trained refugee doctors. Med Educ. 2003;37(1):77.
61. Al-Dhahir L. Re-training refugee and other overseas doctors. Clin Med. 2006;6(2):217.
62. Hilton C. Refugee doctors and the development of psychiatry. Br J Psychiatry. 2006;189:383–4.
63. Arie S. Syrian doctors risk arrest and deportation for treating fellow refugees in Lebanon and Jordan. BMJ. 2015;350:h1699.
64. Abbara A, Orcutt M, Gabbar O. Syria's lost generation of doctors. BMJ. 2015;350:h3479.
65. Ong YL, Trafford P, Paice E, Jackson N. Investing in learning and training refugee doctors. Clin Teach. 2010;7(2):131–5.
66. Ong YL, Paice E. A successful initiative for getting refugee doctors back into medical employment: the PRIME project. Br J Hosp Med. 2006;67(5):264–6.
67. Ong YL, Gayen A. Helping refugee doctors get their first jobs: the pan-London clinical attachment scheme. Hosp Med. 2003;64(8):488–90.
68. Ferracioli L, De Lora P. Primum nocere: medical brain drain and the duty to stay. J Med Philos. 2015;40(5):601–19.
69. Zhou X, Wu X, Zhen R. Understanding the relationship between social support and post-traumatic stress disorder/posttraumatic growth among adolescents after Ya'an earthquake: the role of emotion regulation. Psychol Trauma. 2017;9(2):214–21.
70. Reavell J, Fazil Q. The epidemiology of PTSD and depression in refugee minors who have resettled in developed countries. J Ment Health. 2017;26(1):74–83.
71. de Jong JT, Berckmoes LH, Kohrt BA, Song SJ, Tol WA, Reis RA. public health approach to address the mental health burden of youth in situations of political violence and humanitarian emergencies. Curr Psychiatry Rep. 2015;17(7):60.
72. Tol WA, Purgato M, Bass JK, Galappatti A, Eaton W. Mental health and psychosocial support in humanitarian settings: a public mental health perspective. Epidemiol Psychiatr Sci. 2015;24(6):484–94.
73. Ao T, Shetty S, Sivilli T, Blanton C, Ellis H, Geltman PL, et al. Suicidal ideation and mental health of Bhutanese refugees in the United States. J Immigr Minor Health. 2016;18(4):828–35.
74. Centers for Disease Control and Prevention. Suicide and suicidal ideation among Bhutanese refugees--United States, 2009-2012. MMWR Morb Mortal Wkly Rep. 2013;62(26):533–6.
75. Falb KL, McCormick MC, Hemenway D, Anfinson K, Silverman JG. Suicide ideation and victimization among refugee women along the Thai-Burma border. J Trauma Stress. 2013;26(5):631–5.
76. Lerner E, Bonanno GA, Keatley E, Joscelyne A, Keller AS. Predictors of suicidal ideation in treatment-seeking survivors of torture. Psychol Trauma. 2016;8(1):17–24.
77. Reko A, Bech P, Wohlert C, Noerregaard C, Csillag C. Usage of psychiatric emergency services by asylum seekers: clinical implications based on a descriptive study in Denmark. Nord J Psychiatry. 2015;69(8):587–93.
78. Sundvall M, Tidemalm DH, Titelman DE, Runeson B, Baarnhielm S. Assessment and treatment of asylum seekers after a suicide attempt: a comparative study of people registered at mental health services in a Swedish location. BMC Psychiatry. 2015;15:235.
79. Wenzel T, Rushiti F, Aghani F, Diaconu G, Maxhuni B, Zitterl W. Suicidal ideation, post-traumatic stress and suicide statistics in Kosovo. An analysis five years after the war. Suicidal ideation in Kosovo. Torture. 2009;19(3):238–47.
80. Tol WA, Patel V, Tomlinson M, Baingana F, Galappatti A, Silove D, et al. Relevance or excellence? Setting research priorities for mental health and psychosocial support in humanitarian settings. Harv Rev Psychiatry. 2012;20(1):25–36.
81. Troya MI, Greene MC, Santos CG, Shultz JM. Conducting a desk review to inform the mental health and psychosocial support response to the 2016 Ecuador earthquake. Disaster Health. 2016;3(4):90–101.
82. Jordans MJ, Semrau M, Thornicroft G, van Ommeren M. Role of current perceived needs in explaining the association between past trauma exposure and distress in humanitarian settings in Jordan and Nepal. Br J Psychiatry. 2012;201(4):276–81.
83. Fellmeth G, Paw MK, Wiladphaingern J, Charunwatthana P, Nosten FH, McGready R. Maternal suicide risk among refugees and migrants. Int J Gynaecol Obstet. 2016;134(2):223–4.

84. Vijayakumar L. Suicide among refugees--a mockery of humanity. Crisis. 2016;37(1):1–4.
85. Colucci E, Too LS, Minas H. A suicide research agenda for people from immigrant and refugee backgrounds. Death Stud. 2017;41(8):502–11.
86. Cyniak-Cieciura M, Staniaszek K, Popiel A, Praglowska E, Zawadzki B. The structure of PTSD symptoms according to DSM-5 and IDC-11 proposal: a multi-sample analysis. Eur Psychiatry. 2017;44:179–86.
87. Danzi BA, La Greca AM. DSM-IV, DSM-5, and ICD-11: identifying children with posttraumatic stress disorder after disasters. J Child Psychol Psychiatry. 2016;57(12):1444–52.
88. Hansen M, Hyland P, Armour C, Shevlin M, Elklit A. Less is more? Assessing the validity of the ICD-11 model of PTSD across multiple trauma samples. Eur J Psychotraumatol. 2015;6:28766.
89. Haravuori H, Kiviruusu O, Suomalainen L, Marttunen M. An evaluation of ICD-11 posttraumatic stress disorder criteria in two samples of adolescents and young adults exposed to mass shootings: factor analysis and comparisons to ICD-10 and DSM-IV. BMC Psychiatry. 2016;16:140.
90. Sachser C, Goldbeck L. Consequences of the diagnostic criteria proposed for the ICD-11 on the prevalence of PTSD in children and adolescents. J Trauma Stress. 2016;29(2):120–3.
91. Tay AK, Mohsin M, Rees S, Steel Z, Tam N, Soares Z, et al. The factor structures and correlates of PTSD in post-conflict Timor-Leste: an analysis of the Harvard Trauma Questionnaire. BMC Psychiatry. 2017;17(1):191.
92. Wisco BE, Miller MW, Wolf EJ, Kilpatrick D, Resnick HS, Badour CL, et al. The impact of proposed changes to ICD-11 on estimates of PTSD prevalence and comorbidity. Psychiatry Res. 2016;240:226–33.
93. Chen YF. Chinese classification of mental disorders (CCMD-3): towards integration in international classification. Psychopathology. 2002;35(2-3):171–5.
94. Bracken PJ, Giller JE, Summerfield D. Psychological responses to war and atrocity: the limitations of current concepts. Soc Sci Med. 1995;40(8):1073–82.
95. Zambrano-Vazquez L, Levy HC, Belleau EL, Dworkin ER, Howard Sharp KM, Pittenger SL, et al. Using the research domain criteria framework to track domains of change in comorbid PTSD and SUD. Psychol Trauma. 2017;9(6):679–87.
96. McTeague LM. Reconciling RDoC and DSM approaches in clinical psychophysiology and neuroscience. Psychophysiology. 2016;53(3):323–7.
97. Krueger RF, Hopwood CJ, Wright AG, Markon KE. Challenges and strategies in helping the DSM become more dimensional and empirically based. Curr Psychiatry Rep. 2014;16(12):515.
98. Franklin JC, Jamieson JP, Glenn CR, Nock MK. How developmental psychopathology theory and research can inform the research domain criteria (RDoC) project. J Clin Child Adolesc Psychol. 2015;44(2):280–90.
99. Tay AK, Rees S, Chen J, Kareth M, Silove D. Factorial structure of complicated grief: associations with loss-related traumatic events and psychosocial impacts of mass conflict amongst West Papuan refugees. Soc Psychiatry Psychiatr Epidemiol. 2016;51(3):395–406.
100. Cavkaytar O, Duzova A, Teksam O, Karabulut E, Derman O, Kale G, et al. Final diagnosis of children and adolescents with musculoskeletal complaints. Minerva Pediatr. 2017;69(1):50–8.
101. Lin SY, Hou SJ, WH W, Chen SM, Young TK. Effect of traditional Chinese herbal medicines on the pharmacokinetics of western drugs in SD rats of different ages. I. Aminophylline-Tin chuan Tang and aminophylline-Hsiao Ching Long Tang. J Pharmacobiodyn. 1991;14(4):201–6.
102. Keatley E, d'Alfonso A, Abeare C, Keller A, Bertelsen NS. Health outcomes of traumatic brain injury among refugee survivors of torture. J Head Trauma Rehabil. 2015;30(6):E1–8.
103. Mollica RF, Chernoff MC, Megan Berthold S, Lavelle J, Lyoo IK, Renshaw P. The mental health sequelae of traumatic head injury in South Vietnamese ex-political detainees who survived torture. Compr Psychiatry. 2014;55(7):1626–38.
104. Keatley E, Ashman T, Im B, Rasmussen A. Self-reported head injury among refugee survivors of torture. J Head Trauma Rehabil. 2013;28(6):E8–E13.

105. Junaid M, Mamoon-ur R, Afsheen A, Tahir A, Bukhari SS, Kalsoom A. Changing spectrum of traumatic head injuries: demographics and outcome analysis in a tertiary care referral center. J Pak Med Assoc. 2016;66(7):864–8.
106. Stemper BD, Pintar FA. Biomechanics of concussion. Prog Neurol Surg. 2014;28:14–27.
107. Fares Y, Fares J, Gebeily S. Head and facial injuries due to cluster munitions. Neurol Sci. 2014;35(6):905–10.
108. Xie K, Kuang H, Tsien JZ. Mild blast events alter anxiety, memory, and neural activity patterns in the anterior cingulate cortex. PLoS One. 2013;8(5):e64907.
109. Rosenfeld JV, McFarlane AC, Bragge P, Armonda RA, Grimes JB, Ling GS. Blast-related traumatic brain injury. Lancet Neurol. 2013;12(9):882–93.
110. Rosenfeld JV, Ford NL. Bomb blast, mild traumatic brain injury and psychiatric morbidity: a review. Injury. 2010;41(5):437–43.
111. Doherty SM, Craig R, Gardani M, McMillan TM. Head injury in asylum seekers and refugees referred with psychological trauma. Glob Ment Health. 2016;3:e28.
112. Radhakrishnan R, Garakani A, Gross LS, Goin MK, Pine J, Slaby AE, et al. Neuropsychiatric aspects of concussion. Lancet Psychiatry. 2016;3(12):1166–75.
113. Stein DM, Feather CB, Napolitano LM. Traumatic brain injury advances. Crit Care Clin. 2017;33(1):1–13.
114. Brenner LA, Betthauser LM, Homaifar BY, Villarreal E, Harwood JE, Staves PJ, et al. Posttraumatic stress disorder, traumatic brain injury, and suicide attempt history among veterans receiving mental health services. Suicide Life Threat Behav. 2011;41(4):416–23.
115. Bryan CJ, Clemans TA. Repetitive traumatic brain injury, psychological symptoms, and suicide risk in a clinical sample of deployed military personnel. JAMA Psychiat. 2013;70(7):686–91.
116. Finley EP, Bollinger M, Noel PH, Amuan ME, Copeland LA, Pugh JA, et al. A national cohort study of the association between the polytrauma clinical triad and suicide-related behavior among US Veterans who served in Iraq and Afghanistan. Am J Public Health. 2015;105(2):380–7.
117. Mollica RF, Caspi-Yavin Y, Bollini P, Truong T, Tor S, Lavelle J. The Harvard Trauma Questionnaire. Validating a cross-cultural instrument for measuring torture, trauma, and posttraumatic stress disorder in Indochinese refugees. J Nerv Ment Dis. 1992;180(2):111–6.
118. Nickerson A, Garber B, Ahmed O, Asnaani A, Cheung J, Hofmann SG, et al. Emotional suppression in torture survivors: relationship to posttraumatic stress symptoms and trauma-related negative affect. Psychiatry Res. 2016;242:233–9.
119. de Jong JP, Scholte WF, Koeter MW, Hart AA. The prevalence of mental health problems in Rwandan and Burundese refugee camps. Acta Psychiatr Scand. 2000;102(3):171–7.
120. Cheung P. Posttraumatic stress disorder among Cambodian refugees in New Zealand. Int J Soc Psychiatry. 1994;40(1):17–26.
121. Cheung P, Spears G. Psychiatric morbidity among New Zealand Cambodians: the role of psychosocial factors. Soc Psychiatry Psychiatr Epidemiol. 1995;30(2):92–7.
122. Khavarpour F, Rissel C. Mental health status of Iranian migrants in Sydney. Aust N Z J Psychiatry. 1997;31(6):828–34.
123. Thabet AA, Abed Y, Vostanis P. Effect of trauma on the mental health of Palestinian children and mothers in the Gaza Strip. East Mediterr Health J. 2001;7(3):413–21.
124. Kalafi Y, Hagh-Shenas H, Ostovar A. Mental health among Afghan refugees settled in Shiraz, Iran. Psychol Rep. 2002;90(1):262–6.
125. Chou KL. Psychological distress in migrants in Australia over 50 years old: a longitudinal investigation. J Affect Disord. 2007;98(1-2):99–108.
126. Pernice R, Trlin A, Henderson A, North N, Skinner M. Employment status, duration of residence and mental health among skilled migrants to New Zealand: results of a longitudinal study. Int J Soc Psychiatry. 2009;55(3):272–87.
127. Tremblay J, Pedersen D, Errazuriz C. Assessing mental health outcomes of political violence and civil unrest in Peru. Int J Soc Psychiatry. 2009;55(5):449–63.

128. Hamid AA, Musa SA. Mental health problems among internally displaced persons in Darfur. Int J Psychol. 2010;45(4):278–85.
129. Idemudia ES, William JK, Boehnke K, Wyatt G. Gender differences in trauma and post-traumatic stress symptoms among displaced Zimbabweans in South Africa. J Trauma Stress Disord Treat. 2013;2(3):1340.
130. Idemudia ES, Williams JK, Madu SN, Wyatt GE. Trauma exposures and posttraumatic stress among Zimbabwean refugees in South Africa. Life Sci J. 2013;10(3):349.
131. Dick M, Fennig S, Lurie I. Identification of emotional distress among asylum seekers and migrant workers by primary care physicians: a brief report. Isr J Psychiatry Relat Sci. 2015;52(3):14–8.
132. Getanda EM, Papadopoulos C, Evans H. The mental health, quality of life and life satisfaction of internally displaced persons living in Nakuru County, Kenya. BMC Public Health. 2015;15:755.
133. Idemudia ES. Trauma and PTSS of Zimbabwean refugees in South Africa: a summary of published studies. Psychol Trauma. 2017;9(3):252–7.
134. Derogatis LR, Lipman RS, Rickels K, Uhlenhuth EH, Covi L. The Hopkins Symptom Checklist (HSCL): a self-report symptom inventory. Behav Sci. 1974;19(1):1–15.
135. Hinton WL, Du N, Chen YC, Tran CG, Newman TB, Lu FG. Screening for major depression in Vietnamese refugees: a validation and comparison of two instruments in a health screening population. J Gen Intern Med. 1994;9(4):202–6.
136. Kleijn WC, Hovens JE, Rodenburg JJ. Posttraumatic stress symptoms in refugees: assessments with the Harvard Trauma Questionnaire and the Hopkins symptom Checklist-25 in different languages. Psychol Rep. 2001;88(2):527–32.
137. Bean T, Derluyn I, Eurelings-Bontekoe E, Broekaert E, Spinhoven P. Validation of the multiple language versions of the Hopkins Symptom Checklist-37 for refugee adolescents. Adolescence. 2007;42(165):51–71.
138. Mels C, Derluyn I, Broekaert E, Rosseel Y. The psychological impact of forced displacement and related risk factors on Eastern Congolese adolescents affected by war. J Child Psychol Psychiatry. 2010;51(10):1096–104.
139. Mels C, Derluyn I, Broekaert E, Rosseel Y. Community-based cross-cultural adaptation of mental health measures in emergency settings: validating the IES-R and HSCL-37A in Eastern Democratic Republic of Congo. Soc Psychiatry Psychiatr Epidemiol. 2010;45(9):899–910.
140. Brink DR, Shannon PJ, Vinson GA. Validation of a brief mental health screener for Karen refugees in primary care. Fam Pract. 2016;33(1):107–11.
141. Alonso J, Angermeyer MC, Bernert S, Bruffaerts R, Brugha TS, Bryson H, et al. Sampling and methods of the European Study of the Epidemiology of Mental Disorders (ESEMeD) project. Acta Psychiatr Scand Suppl. 2004;420:8–20.
142. Kessler RC, Ustun TB. The World Mental Health (WMH) survey initiative version of the World Health Organization (WHO) composite international diagnostic interview (CIDI). Int J Methods Psychiatr Res. 2004;13(2):93–121.
143. Janca A, Ustun TB, Sartorius N. New versions of World Health Organization instruments for the assessment of mental disorders. Acta Psychiatr Scand. 1994;90(2):73–83.
144. Kosten TR, Bryant K, Rounsaville BJ. The SCID: a clinical instrument for assessing psychiatric disorders. NIDA Res Monogr. 1990;105:213–9.
145. Silove DM, Steel Z, Susljik J, Frommer N, Lonergan C, Chey T, et al. The impact of the refugee decision on the trajectory of PTSD, anxiety, and depressive symptoms among asylum seekers: a longitudinal study. Am J Disaster Med. 2007;2(6):321.
146. Roth G, Ekblad S, Prochazka H. A study of aggression among mass-evacuated Kosovo Albanians. Torture. 2009;19(3):227–37.
147. Teodorescu DS, Heir T, Hauff E, Wentzel-Larsen T, Lien L. Mental health problems and post-migration stress among multi-traumatized refugees attending outpatient clinics upon resettlement to Norway. Scand J Psychol. 2012;53(4):316–32.
148. Elhabiby MM, Radwan DN, Okasha TA, El-Desouky ED. Psychiatric disorders among a sample of internally displaced persons in South Darfur. Int J Soc Psychiatry. 2015;61(4):358–62.

149. Teodorescu DS, Heir T, Siqveland J, Hauff E, Wentzel-Larsen T, Lien L. Chronic pain in multi-traumatized outpatients with a refugee background resettled in Norway: a cross-sectional study. BMC Psychol. 2015;3(1):7.
150. Kaiser BN, Haroz EE, Kohrt BA, Bolton PA, Bass JK, Hinton DE. "Thinking too much": a systematic review of a common idiom of distress. Soc Sci Med. 2015;147:170–83.
151. Diamond DM, Zoladz PR. Dysfunctional or hyperfunctional? The amygdala in posttraumatic stress disorder is the bull in the evolutionary China shop. J Neurosci Res. 2016;94(6):437–44.
152. Sipahi L, Uddin M, Hou ZC, Aiello AE, Koenen KC, Galea S, et al. Ancient evolutionary origins of epigenetic regulation associated with posttraumatic stress disorder. Front Hum Neurosci. 2014;8:284.
153. Silove D. Is posttraumatic stress disorder an overlearned survival response? An evolutionary-learning hypothesis. Psychiatry. 1998;61(2):181–90.
154. Haagen JF, Ter Heide FJ, Mooren TM, Knipscheer JW, Kleber RJ. Predicting post-traumatic stress disorder treatment response in refugees: multilevel analysis. Br J Clin Psychol. 2017;56(1):69–83.
155. Sullivan TP, Weiss NH, Flanagan JC, Willie TC, Armeli S, Tennen H. PTSD and daily co-occurrence of drug and alcohol use among women experiencing intimate partner violence. J Dual Diagn. 2016;12(1):36–42.
156. Yehuda R, Lehrner A, Rosenbaum TY. PTSD and sexual dysfunction in men and women. J Sex Med. 2015;12(5):1107–19.
157. Weiss NH, Tull MT, Sullivan TP, Dixon-Gordon KL, Gratz KL. Posttraumatic stress disorder symptoms and risky behaviors among trauma-exposed inpatients with substance dependence: the influence of negative and positive urgency. Drug Alcohol Depend. 2015;155:147–53.
158. Wahlstrom LC, Scott JP, Tuliao AP, DiLillo D, McChargue DE. Posttraumatic stress disorder symptoms, emotion dysregulation, and aggressive behavior among incarcerated methamphetamine users. J Dual Diagn. 2015;11(2):118–27.
159. Ramsawh HJ, Fullerton CS, Mash HB, Ng TH, Kessler RC, Stein MB, et al. Risk for suicidal behaviors associated with PTSD, depression, and their comorbidity in the U.S. Army. J Affect Disord. 2014;161:116–22.
160. Shevlin M, Hyland P, Karatzias T, Fyvie C, Roberts N, Bisson JI, et al. Alternative models of disorders of traumatic stress based on the new ICD-11 proposals. Acta Psychiatr Scand. 2017;135(5):419–28.
161. Young GPTSD, in Court III. Malingering, assessment, and the law. Int J Law Psychiatry. 2017;52:81–102.
162. Weathers FW, Bovin MJ, Lee DJ, Sloan DM, Schnurr PP, Kaloupek DG, et al. The clinician-administered PTSD scale for DSM-5 (CAPS-5): development and initial psychometric evaluation in military Veterans. Psychol Assess. 2017. https://doi.org/10.1037/pas0000486.
163. Malekzai AS, Niazi JM, Paige SR, Hendricks SE, Fitzpatrick D, Leuschen MP, et al. Modification of CAPS-1 for diagnosis of PTSD in Afghan refugees. J Trauma Stress. 1996;9(4):891–8.
164. Charney ME, Keane TM. Psychometric analyses of the Clinician-Administered PTSD Scale (CAPS)--Bosnian translation. Cultur Divers Ethnic Minor Psychol. 2007;13(2):161–8.
165. Hinton DE, Chhean D, Fama JM, Pollack MH, McNally RJ. Gastrointestinal-focused panic attacks among Cambodian refugees: associated psychopathology, flashbacks, and catastrophic cognitions. J Anxiety Disord. 2007;21(1):42–58.
166. Hinton DE, Chhean D, Pich V, Um K, Fama JM, Pollack MH. Neck-focused panic attacks among Cambodian refugees; a logistic and linear regression analysis. J Anxiety Disord. 2006;20(2):119–38.
167. Hinton DE, Chhean D, Pich V, Pollack MH, Orr SP, Pitman RK. Assessment of posttraumatic stress disorder in Cambodian refugees using the clinician-administered PTSD scale: psychometric properties and symptom severity. J Trauma Stress. 2006;19(3):405–9.
168. Hinton DE, Chhean D, Pich V, Hofmann SG, Barlow DH. Tinnitus among Cambodian refugees: relationship to PTSD severity. J Trauma Stress. 2006;19(4):541–6.

169. Halvorsen JO, Stenmark H. Narrative exposure therapy for posttraumatic stress disorder in tortured refugees: a preliminary uncontrolled trial. Scand J Psychol. 2010;51(6):495–502.
170. Ter Heide FJ, Mooren TM, van de Schoot R, de Jongh A, Kleber RJ. Eye movement desensitisation and reprocessing therapy v. stabilisation as usual for refugees: randomised controlled trial. Br J Psychiatry. 2016;209(4):311–8.
171. Hensel-Dittmann D, Schauer M, Ruf M, Catani C, Odenwald M, Elbert T, et al. Treatment of traumatized victims of war and torture: a randomized controlled comparison of narrative exposure therapy and stress inoculation training. Psychother Psychosom. 2011;80(6):345–52.
172. Halepota AA, Wasif SA. Harvard Trauma Questionnaire Urdu translation: the only cross-culturally validated screening instrument for the assessment of trauma and torture and their sequelae. J Pak Med Assoc. 2001;51(8):285–90.
173. Rasmussen A, Verkuilen J, Ho E, Fan Y. Posttraumatic stress disorder among refugees: measurement invariance of Harvard Trauma Questionnaire scores across global regions and response patterns. Psychol Assess. 2015;27(4):1160–70.
174. Tay AK, Jayasuriya R, Jayasuriya D, Silove D. Assessing the factorial structure and measurement invariance of PTSD by gender and ethnic groups in Sri Lanka: an analysis of the modified Harvard Trauma Questionnaire (HTQ). J Anxiety Disord. 2017;47:45–53.
175. Brunet A, Weiss DS, Metzler TJ, Best SR, Neylan TC, Rogers C, et al. The peritraumatic distress inventory: a proposed measure of PTSD criterion A2. Am J Psychiatry. 2001;158(9):1480–5.
176. Thomas E, Saumier D, Brunet A. Peritraumatic distress and the course of posttraumatic stress disorder symptoms: a meta-analysis. Can J Psychiatr. 2012;57(2):122–9.
177. Blanc J, Rahill GJ, Laconi S, Mouchenik Y. Religious beliefs, PTSD, depression and resilience in survivors of the 2010 Haiti earthquake. J Affect Disord. 2016;190:697–703.
178. Hollifield M, Verbillis-Kolp S, Farmer B, Toolson EC, Woldehaimanot T, Yamazaki J, et al. The Refugee Health Screener-15 (RHS-15): development and validation of an instrument for anxiety, depression, and PTSD in refugees. Gen Hosp Psychiatry. 2013;35(2):202–9.
179. Johnson-Agbakwu CE, Allen J, Nizigiyimana JF, Ramirez G, Hollifield M. Mental health screening among newly arrived refugees seeking routine obstetric and gynecologic care. Psychol Serv. 2014;11(4):470–6.
180. Hollifield M, Toolson EC, Verbillis-Kolp S, Farmer B, Yamazaki J, Woldehaimanot T, et al. Effective screening for emotional distress in refugees: the refugee health screener. J Nerv Ment Dis. 2016;204(4):247–53.
181. Polcher K, Calloway S. Addressing the need for mental health screening of newly resettled refugees: a pilot project. J Prim Care Community Health. 2016;7(3):199–203.
182. Salt RJ, Costantino ME, Dotson EL, Paper BM. "You are not alone" strategies for addressing mental health and health promotion with a refugee women's sewing group. Issues Ment Health Nurs. 2017;38(4):337–43.
183. Tedeschi FK, Billick SB. Pediatric PTSD in the DSM-5 and the forensic interview of traumatized youth. J Am Acad Psychiatry Law. 2017;45(2):175–83.
184. Tedeschi FK, Billick SB, Pediatric PTSD. Clinical, forensic, and diagnostic understanding. J Am Acad Psychiatry Law. 2017;45(2):161–9.
185. La Greca AM, Danzi BA, Chan SF. DSM-5 and ICD-11 as competing models of PTSD in preadolescent children exposed to a natural disaster: assessing validity and co-occurring symptomatology. Eur J Psychotraumatol. 2017;8(1):1310591.
186. Winkler N, Ruf-Leuschner M, Ertl V, Pfeiffer A, Schalinski I, Ovuga E, et al. From war to classroom: PTSD and depression in formerly abducted youth in Uganda. Front Psych. 2015;6:2.
187. Kelly JT, Branham L, Decker MR. Abducted children and youth in Lord's Resistance Army in Northeastern Democratic Republic of the Congo (DRC): mechanisms of indoctrination and control. Confl Heal. 2016;10:11.
188. Miles GM. Drawing together hope: 'listening' to militarised children. J Child Health Care. 2000;4(4):137–42.
189. Rowe C, Watson-Ormond R, English L, Rubesin H, Marshall A, Linton K, et al. Evaluating art therapy to heal the effects of trauma among refugee youth: the Burma art therapy program evaluation. Health Promot Pract. 2016. https://doi.org/10.1177/1524839915626413.

190. Schandorph Lokkegaard S, Ronholt S, Karsberg S, Elklit A. Validation of the PTSD screening cartoon test "Darryl" in a Danish clinical sample of children and adolescents. Int J Methods Psychiatr Res. 2017;26(1). https://doi.org/10.1002/mpr.1514.
191. Thakkar MJ, Jaffe AM, Vander Linden RS. Guidelines for conducting a victim-sensitive interview. J Child Sex Abus. 2015;24(7):717–30.
192. Sheehan DV, Lecrubier Y, Sheehan KH, Amorim P, Janavs J, Weiller E, et al. The Mini-International Neuropsychiatric Interview (M.I.N.I.): the development and validation of a structured diagnostic psychiatric interview for DSM-IV and ICD-10. J Clin Psychiatry. 1998;59(Suppl 20):22–33. quiz 4–57
193. Loughry M, Flouri E. The behavioral and emotional problems of former unaccompanied refugee children 3-4 years after their return to Vietnam. Child Abuse Negl. 2001;25(2):249–63.
194. Mollica RF, Poole C, Son L, Murray CC, Tor S. Effects of war trauma on Cambodian refugee adolescents' functional health and mental health status. J Am Acad Child Adolesc Psychiatry. 1997;36(8):1098–106.
195. Huemer J, Karnik N, Voelkl-Kernstock S, Granditsch E, Plattner B, Friedrich M, et al. Psychopathology in African unaccompanied refugee minors in Austria. Child Psychiatry Hum Dev. 2011;42(3):307–19.
196. Steinberg AM, Brymer MJ, Decker KB, Pynoos RS. The University of California at Los Angeles post-traumatic stress disorder reaction index. Curr Psychiatry Rep. 2004;6(2):96–100.
197. Elhai JD, Layne CM, Steinberg AM, Brymer MJ, Briggs EC, Ostrowski SA, et al. Psychometric properties of the UCLA PTSD reaction index. Part II: investigating factor structure findings in a national clinic-referred youth sample. J Trauma Stress. 2013;26(1):10–8.
198. Steinberg AM, Brymer MJ, Kim S, Briggs EC, Ippen CG, Ostrowski SA, et al. Psychometric properties of the UCLA PTSD reaction index: part I. J Trauma Stress. 2013;26(1):1–9.
199. Hafstad GS, Thoresen S, Wentzel-Larsen T, Maercker A, Dyb G. PTSD or not PTSD? Comparing the proposed ICD-11 and the DSM-5 PTSD criteria among young survivors of the 2011 Norway attacks and their parents. Psychol Med. 2017;47(7):1283–91.
200. Deeba F, Rapee RM, Prvan T. Psychometric properties of the children's revised impact of events scale (CRIES) with Bangladeshi children and adolescents. PeerJ. 2014;2:e536.
201. Salari R, Malekian C, Linck L, Kristiansson R, Sarkadi A. Screening for PTSD symptoms in unaccompanied refugee minors: a test of the CRIES-8 questionnaire in routine care. Scand J Public Health. 2017;45(6):605–11.
202. Meiser-Stedman R, Smith P, Bryant R, Salmon K, Yule W, Dalgleish T, et al. Development and validation of the child post-traumatic cognitions inventory (CPTCI). J Child Psychol Psychiatry. 2009;50(4):432–40.
203. Sourander A. Behavior problems and traumatic events of unaccompanied refugee minors. Child Abuse Negl. 1998;22(7):719–27.
204. Derluyn I, Broekaert E. Different perspectives on emotional and behavioural problems in unaccompanied refugee children and adolescents. Ethn Health. 2007;12(2):141–62.
205. Bronstein I, Montgomery P, Ott E. Emotional and behavioural problems amongst Afghan unaccompanied asylum-seeking children: results from a large-scale cross-sectional study. Eur Child Adolesc Psychiatry. 2013;22(5):285–94.
206. Goodman R, Meltzer H, Bailey V. The Strengths and difficulties questionnaire: a pilot study on the validity of the self-report version. Eur Child Adolesc Psychiatry. 1998;7(3):125–30.
207. Goodman R. Psychometric properties of the strengths and difficulties questionnaire. J Am Acad Child Adolesc Psychiatry. 2001;40(11):1337–45.

A Culture-Sensitive and Person-Centred Approach: Understanding and Evaluating Cultural Factors, Social Background and History When Working with Refugees

5

Hanna Kienzler, Cameron Spence, and Thomas Wenzel

Abstract

In recent years, research methods and data from cultural anthropology and transcultural psychiatry have highlighted the importance of paying attention to the ways in which culture shapes expressions of distress and help- and health-seeking. This chapter builds on these insights and offers an overview of selected major aspects of the role culture plays in refugee mental healthcare. It will also summarise concrete tools that can be used to explore the needs, expressions of distress and help-seeking behaviours among the diverse ethnic and religious groups. We suggest that these tools can be used to guide interventions and treatment models in practical but culture-sensitive ways.

5.1 Introduction

In contexts of forced migration and resulting displacement, affected persons tend to be less or ill-prepared to cope with a new and culturally different environment compared to those who were able to plan their migration well in advance. For the latter (i.e. migrant workers and their families), it is often possible to prepare their journey by learning the host country language and later maintain social ties and networks in both their home and host countries. However, in situations of forced migration and

H. Kienzler (✉) · C. Spence
Department of Global Health and Social Medicine, King's College London, London, UK
e-mail: hanna.kienzler@gmail.com; cameron.spence@kcl.ac.uk

T. Wenzel
World Psychiatric Association Scientific Section,
Psychological Aspects of Persecution and Torture, Geneva, Switzerland
e-mail: drthomaswenzel@web.de

T. Wenzel, B. Drožđek (eds.), *An Uncertain Safety*,
https://doi.org/10.1007/978-3-319-72914-5_5

displacement, individuals and groups are forced to leave their home country and their social environments are often fragile and disrupted. The insecurity related to not knowing about the fate of family members and friends can further exacerbate distress and decrease success in managing emergencies and integration into host societies. Besides social fragmentation and a lack of linguistic skills, refugees arriving in host countries might therefore lack access to support networks and have limited access to stabilising factors such as professional occupation, social and institutional support mechanisms (i.e. legal assistance, social institutions, healthcare and welfare) and religious and other social communities. Within such unstable and insecure environments, refugees seeking support for war-related emotional and physical health problems may be confronted with diagnostic and treatment procedures that pay little or no attention to the cultural and social determinants of their health, thus failing to provide adequate care. As such, in the following sections, we will highlight the important impact of culture on health and wellbeing and outline first attempts to provide culturally sensitive diagnoses and treatments especially in mental health.

5.2 The Importance of Cultural Sensitivity in the Context of Refugee HealthCare

Anthropological and psychiatric research has shown how contextual factors shape both the physical and mental health consequences of violence and insecurity among refugee populations [1] and impact on help- and health-seeking, interaction with health providers and the evaluation of services [2]. Such contextual or trans-cultural factors are (in the next chapter) defined as those "(…) shaping a person's identity and behaviour, including the specific expression of her background religion, ethnic, social, national and political background". Based on this definition, it is recommended that health providers become familiar with the ways in which culture influences their patients' expressions of distress, needs and health beliefs. Indeed, cultural sensitivity or competency [3] in health practice has been recommended for more effectively tailored services to refugee- or other marginal ethnic populations. It has also been shown that the incorporation of cultural health beliefs and practices into healthcare provision impacts positively on health and mental health outcomes [4].

At the same time, it is important to note that the concept of "cultural competency" has been criticised for stereotyping sufferers and for interpreting their behaviour through a generalising cultural lens, informed by a simplistic understanding of what "culture" is supposed to be. Castaneda [4] eloquently writes that cultural competency trainings that use a narrow definition of culture reduce the concept "to a static set of characteristics based on ethnicity, while ignoring the dynamic interplay between history and power as recognized in the anthropological culture concept" (p. 14). What is more, such an approach fails to recognise that health providers and their practice are also shaped by a culture that includes particular medical, social, ethical and religious belief and value systems. Overemphasising the cultural background of patients (while ignoring the cultural background of clinicians) has been shown to have negative consequences for health outcomes. Specifically, refugees can receive inadequate health information due to assumptions about the lack of particular competencies (i.e. reading and writing skills) or incorrect assumptions made about their worldviews. For instance, women from societies stereotyped as patriarchal sometimes receive inadequate information about sexuality and sexual health as it is assumed that they lack decision-making power over their own bodies. Moreover, cultural determinism deflects attention from structural factors such as racism, sexism, political violence, poverty and immigration politics, all of which have been directly and indirectly related to negative health outcomes [4, 5].

Culture, thus, must be viewed within this broader framework as one among other determinants, including social, economic and political ones that affect people's health and wellbeing. With this understanding in mind, we will now introduce various ways in which culture has found its way into diagnostic procedures in the field of mental health. We will do so by first introducing the concept of local idioms of distress, in order to then outline how such ideas have influenced diagnostic standards such as the DSM 5.

5.2.1 Culture-Specific Expressions of Distress and Diagnostic Categories

In the recent past, research on trauma-related mental health problems has focused mainly on post-traumatic stress disorder (PTSD), depression and anxiety. These have been considered universally represented. For instance, Marsella and colleagues concluded from a substantial body of research in 1996: "We are not aware of any ethno-cultural cohort in which PTSD could not be diagnosed" ([6], p. 531). Though such results seem to confirm PTSD as a "global" problem, such findings have led to controversial debates whereby many psychiatrists (notably Summerfield [7, 8]) and social scientists have questioned the syndrome's global validity and value (see also Chap. 11 in this book).

Over time, these debates have led to an increasing agreement concerning the fact that the mere identification of PTSD symptomatology does not reveal the extent to which the disorder has any local currency or therapeutic utility in specific situations. It has also been recognised that other distress reactions, such as local idioms of distress or grief reactions shaped by culture [9] might be more relevant in terms of understanding mental health problems within particular sociocultural groups. Kohrt and Hruschka [10] have noted, for instance that the "observation of PTSD symptoms does not, in and of itself, immediately reveal optional clinical care or other interventions" (p. 323). Instead, they highlight the importance of understanding personal and social meanings given to experiences of traumatic events and the culturally resonant ways in which people express their distress [11, 12].

In order to better understand how complaints, symptoms and syndromes are expressed in particular sociocultural contexts, anthropologists have developed the relatively open concept of local "idioms of distress". In fact, Mark Nichter coined the concept in the early 1980s to describe alternative modes of expressing distress, defining it more recently as a "(…) socially and culturally resonant means of experiencing and expressing distress in local worlds. They are evocative and index past traumatic memories as well as present stressors, such as anger, powerlessness, social marginalization and insecurity, and possible future sources of anxiety, loss and angst" [13]. He goes on to explain that when idioms of distress are experienced along with significant pathology, they express personal and interpersonal distress beyond that associated with universal disease processes.

Research has shown that such idioms are not static but are, instead, subject to change and must not be consistent over time as they flexibly adapt to changes in the social environment [14, 15]. Idioms of distress that have been explored in various sociocultural contexts and include, among others, experiences as diverse as nervios, susto, llaki, ñakary, ihahamuka, open mole and khyâl attacks ([16–18], see also Table 5.1). These categories vary greatly with regards to their symptomatology and related illness experience, attributions of causality, coping strategies and healing procedures. What makes them comparable is that they are both polysemic (multiple meanings) and idiosyncratic (peculiar to a particular group) phenomena that bridge and transcend somatic, psychic and social phenomena [19, 20]. For instance, Jenkins [21] analyses "nervios" suffered by Salvadoran women refugees living in exile in North America. The twenty-two women who participated in the study had fled El Salvador to escape large-scale political violence, regularised violence by male kin and impoverished economic conditions. Jenkins found that the cultural category of nervios indexes an array of dysphoric affects (anxiety, fear, anger), diverse somatic complaints (bodily pain, shaking, trembling) and often calor (heat). She concludes that the cultural lack of diagnostic specificity concerns more the social and moral status of the ill individual than the psychopathological manifestation of illness behaviour; and, therefore, the "examination of people's reactions to overwhelmingly horrific conditions will require that the parameters of the PTSD construct be expanded considerably to take into account gendered, socio-political, and ethno cultural dimensions of experience" (p. 178).

The clinical relevance of such local expressions of distress have also been highlighted, as they can help clinicians to understand "sufferers' views of the causes of their distress, constitute key therapeutic targets and help increase therapeutic empathy and treatment adherence" [17] but also to adapt treatment approaches [22–24]. However, in contexts of migration or displacement, the new host country environment might not adequately identify and respond to such idioms or messages, especially by host-country physicians without training in transcultural medicine [25]. The problem of recognising idioms in the clinical setting is confounded by a number of factors, which include translation problems (see Chap. 14 in this book) and lack of cultural competence [3], the dearth of data [10], the large number of cultures represented in a global context and a resulting lack of comprehensive databases. Another concern is that health professionals do not generally access anthropological data published in social science journals as they can appear far removed from clinical contexts and practical concerns. Consequently, medical research tends to be limited to standardised research instruments and questionnaires (see in Chap. 4 in

Table 5.1 Common expressions and idioms of distress in Syrian Arabic[a]

Arabic term or phrase	Transcription	Literal translations	Emotions, thoughts and physical symptoms that may be conveyed through these expressions
قياضتم – ةرتفلاه ريتك يلاح سساح – قياضتم جياض – يسفن – ةقونخم	– Meddayyek ketir hal fatra – Haassess haalii meddek – Dayej – Nafsi makhnouka	– I am very annoyed these days – I feel annoyed – To be cramped – My psyche is suffocating	– Rumination tiredness, physical aches, constriction in the chest, repeated sighing – Unpleasant feelings in the chest, hopelessness, boredom
– Hassess rouhi ’am tetla’	علطت مع يحور سساح	– I feel my soul is going out	– Dysphoric mood, sadness – Inability to cope, being fed up – Worry, being pessimistic
-يبلق – ضوبقم ىلع ىمعنا – يبلق	– Qalb maqboud – In’ama ’ala kalbi	– Squeezed heart – Blindness got to my heart	– Dysphoria – Sadness – Worry, being pessimistic
نابعتً – ايسفن يلاح سساح – نابعت يتلاح – ةنابعت سفن – هنابعت	– Taeban nafseyan – Hassess halii ta3ban – Halti taebaneh – Nafs ta’bana	– Fatigued self/soul	– Undifferentiated anxiety and depression symptoms, tiredness, fatigue
لمحتا رداق ام – يلع طغضلا – ريتك زكر رداق وم – تاطوغضلا نم	– Ma ader athammel – El daght ‘alayy ketiir – Mou kaader rakkezz men el doghoutaat	– Can’t bear it anymore – The pressure on me is too much – Can’t concentrate because of the pressure	– Feelings of being under extreme stress or extreme pressure – Helplessness
فرطت –	– Faratit	– I am in pieces	– General state of stress, sadness, extreme tiredness, inability to openup and to control oneself or to hold oneself together
وم هللا و – يمادق فياش	– Wallah mou shayef oddaamii	– By God, I can’t see in frontof me	– General state of stress, feelings of loss of options, loss of ability to project into the future – Confusion, hopelessness
ايندلا سساح – يشوب ةركسم مع يش يف ام – يعم طبزي	– Hases eddenia msakkra bwishi – Ma f shi ’am yizbat ma’i	– I feel the world is closing in front of my face – Nothing is working as planned with me	– Hopelessness, helplessness, state of despair

(continued)

Table 5.1 (continued)

Arabic term or phrase	Transcription	Literal translations	Emotions, thoughts and physical symptoms that may be conveyed through these expressions
– يدب وش – ىوكشلا...يكحإ ريغل – ذم هللا – – هلل دمحلا –	– Sho baddi 'ehki… el shakwa le gher allah mazalleh – Al hamdullillah	– What am I supposed to say… it is humiliating to complain to someone other than God – Praise be to God	– Reference to shame in asking for help – State of despair, surrender
– Maa ba'ref shou beddi a'mel be halii	– ام فرعب وش يدب لمعإ يلاحب	– I don't know what I am going to do with myself	– General state of distress – Feeling upset, edgy, helplessness – Hopelessness, lack of options
– Mitwatter	– رتوتم	– I feel tense	– Nervousness, tension
– نافيخ – – ساسح فوخلاب – بوعرم	– Khayfan – Hases bil khof Mar'oub	– I am afraid – I feel fear – Frightened, horrified	– Fear, anxiety – Worry – Extreme fear
– بّصَعْم –	– M3asseb	– I feel angry	– Anger, aggressiveness – Nervousness

Sources: This table is based on suggestions by Arabic-speaking mental health professionals, including: Alaa Bairoutieh, Tayseer Hassoon, Ghayda Hassan, Maysaa Hassan, Hussam Jefee-Bahloul, and Mohamed el Shazli

[a]From Hassan G., et al. in *Culture, Context and the Mental Health and Psychosocial Wellbeing of Syrians:A Review for Mental Health and Psychosocial Support staff working with Syrians Affected by Armed Conflict*. Geneva: UNHCR, 2015

this book) that might fail to integrate measures to assess refugee populations' varied traumatic experiences and related expressions of distress. Consequently, existing research data, as well as ongoing and future assessment, must be expected to miss indicators of distress that would require further exploration and response. To counteract this, Kohrt recommends the use of a combined diagnostic tool to assess, for example, symptoms of depression and idioms of distress [26] based on a study combining modules of the Composite International Diagnostic Interview (CIDI) with screening for local idioms of distress (Nepali, manko samasya) in Nepal. Nevertheless, it is important to acknowledge that much progress has already been made in integrating local expressions of distress into standardised diagnostic tools such as the new edition of the Diagnostic and Statistical Manual of Mental Disorders.

5.2.2 The Integration of Culture and Transcultural Psychiatry into DSM 5

Medical diagnostic models are increasingly influenced by cultural anthropology and transcultural psychiatry. This holds especially true for the recent revision of the American Psychiatric Associations Diagnostic and Statistical Manual of Mental Disorders (DSM 5) [27], the most common research and clinical standard in mental health. The recent revision has substantially extended the discussion, definitions and integration of cultural factors in regard to mental health and its treatment [28, 29].

The DSM 5 organises its description of the Cultural Formulation Model into three main categories, namely: (1) cultural syndrome defined as "clusters of symptoms and attributions that tend to co-occur among individuals in specific cultural groups, communities, or contexts (…) that are recognized locally as coherent patterns of experience"; (2) cultural idiom of distress which refers to a "linguistic term, phrase, or way of talking about suffering among individuals of a cultural group (e.g., similar ethnicity and religion) referring to shared concepts of pathology and ways of expressing, communicating, or naming essential features of distress"; and (3) cultural explanation or perceived cause which is described as "label, attribution, or feature of an explanatory model that provides a culturally conceived aetiology or cause for symptoms, illness, or distress". These categories are envisioned to be used as a guide for practitioners and researchers in order to enable them to derive culturally sensitive therapeutic interventions [30].

The DSM concept of cultural factors in health is similar to, though more narrow than, the models in cultural anthropology [31]. The concept of "cultural explanation or perceived cause" is partly identical with the term "Health Belief Models" (HBM) (that include "explanatory" or "attribution" models of illnesses) which can be seen as an important concept in understanding, assessing and planning interventions [32] in that it links physical, psychological and cultural aspects of illness and illness behaviour. Health belief models make assumptions about health and illness and, consequently, behaviour including help seeking, compliance and trust in treatment [33]. Culture-based health belief models are considered to be shared by a specific culture or ethnic group, but can differ between different sub-groups as defined by, for example, gender [34] or age [35, 36]. More concretely, depending on people's sociocultural background, they might classify their mental health problems as "metaphysical" (e.g. explaining illness as caused by "ghosts", "spirits" or "Djinn" [37]); as physical, psychological and ethical (e.g. social withdrawal in depression seen as "laziness"); or, in present "state-of-the-art" models, as "integrative" if they offer models combing somatic and psychological aspects [38]. Depending on the ways in which people understand and explain their illness causation, they will resort to different kinds of health-seeking. In the case of spirit possession, the afflicted will probably turn to a religious or traditional healer rather than to a psychiatrist or surgeon [39, 40]. Therefore, when people are confronted with alternative or conflicting explanatory models and treatment offers in a host-country context, these might, at least at first, be approached with suspicion or disbelief and, consequently, might lead to low compliance by the client.

Research findings and clinical experience have convincingly demonstrated that it can be of decisive importance for health organisations to plan their interventions by exploring such factors first [41]. The insights gained can then inform mental health as well as physical health (i.e. infection control or vaccination programmes tailored to specific populations) intervention strategies [42–44] by allowing alternative forms of treatment, such as prayer or other religious practices, to exist side by side or in dialogue with biomedicine [41]. When it comes to alternative or complementary herbal treatment, a word of caution is important as their medical effects can in some cases lead to complications when combined with "Western" medicine [45–48]. Therefore, uncertain composition and possible toxicity of herbal medicines that may form part of traditional healing practices and health belief systems [49] should be taken into consideration when delivering treatment [50–52] (see also Chap. 16 in this book).

5.3 Assessing Distress and Mental Health Problems in Culturally Resonant Ways

With an increased recognition of the impact of culture on mental health and its treatment, research and evaluation methods are currently developed to capture these complexities. Interestingly, there is a tendency to shift away from quantitative survey research toward qualitative or mixed-methods approaches that capture meanings, subjective evaluation and wider contextual factors that impact on people's health and wellbeing (see, e.g. [53–58]). It is important to note that qualitative research is not only an accepted standard in social sciences but also in public health and nursing sciences where researchers and interventionists work with relatively small samples to gain in-depth insights. Yet, care needs to be taken when choosing a qualitative research strategy as the methods can be time intensive when it comes to data collection, analysis and reporting. Software tools such as Atlas.ti™ [59, 60] or NVivo™ [61, 62] are used by many researchers to support the process of data entry and analysis.

The following approaches are recommended.

In situations when researchers are not sure about what the right questions may be to ask due to the novelty of the situation or patient group, *unstructured interviews* are recommended as a first step. Here, interviewers begin "with the assumptions that they do not know in advance what all the necessary questions are. Consequently, they cannot predetermine fully a list of questions to ask" [63]. Unstructured interviews are also useful for building rapport with refugees whose level of trust is low before moving into more formal interviews. Additionally, and most importantly, during conversations about sensitive topics (such as violence, powerlessness, sacred knowledge, corruption or political decision-making) the interviewees are granted control over what they find important to talk about, the phrasing of their responses, and when to shift the topic or quit the conversation altogether. On the other hand, *semi-structured interviews* (such as the McGill Illness Narrative Interview (MINI) described separately) allow researchers to elicit in-depth qualitative information on specific topics such as the flight experience, the situation in refugee camps, notions of self-perceived health and wellbeing, coping strategies and so on. *Focus group discussions*, in turn, may be defined as "a discussion in which a small number (usually six to twelve) respondents, under the guidance of a moderator, talk about topics that are believed to be of special importance to the investigation" [64]. Such focus groups are particularly useful as they facilitate the identification of common traits, beliefs and motives of culture, subculture, social class, etc. in addition to the disclosure or critical discussion of information study participants might not have revealed during an individual interview. To use Folch-Lyon and Trost's words, "[i]n group discussions, the internalized influence of cultural factors and the value structures of the social group to which participants belong and on which they have modelled their perceptions are reinforced and manifest themselves readily" (p. 444–445). Yet, there is a caveat when it comes to ensuring confidentiality. In certain, sensitive contexts, focus group discussions can be inappropriate as they may lead to public disclosure of attitudes, ethnic affiliations or religious views that could endanger individual participants. The same is true for other methods commonly used in community research such as testimony methods and photography (i.e. photovoice).

An increasingly popular approach in refugee research is *participatory action research* (PAR). PAR is based on data collection and action that aims to improve living conditions as well as health and reduce inequities by involving affected people as researchers rather than just as research subjects [65]. Data are collected and analysed together with study participants on an on-going basis. Methods used usually combine verbal and non-verbal data collection through story-telling circles, mapping and modelling exercises, Venn and flow diagrams, case studies, daily routine diagrams and "future possible" scenarios to elicit both individual and community views. Additionally, this method can include transect walks, which involves walking with refugees through an area and discussing different aspects related to community inclusion, barriers and resources. This is a good way to get a better understanding about the physical and social environment in which refugees live, locations where they feel safe or threatened and what it takes to navigate these locations on a daily basis. With this method, it is also important to discuss issues pertaining to anonymity, confidentiality and privacy beforehand as research participants may be co-authors on research outputs. The UNHCR model for Participatory Assessment with Children (see again Chap. 4 in this book) follows a similar approach. Where PAR is not practical or achievable, or where it has led to a specific need for deeper insight, semi-structured interview tools may provide a more direct approach.

5.3.1 Semi-structured Interview Tools

Interview tools have been developed to capture the ways in which culture affects illness experiences, causal explanations, health-seeking and treatment evaluations. Prominent among them are the McGill Illness Narrative interview (MINI) and the Cultural Formulation Interview which forms part of the DSM.

The McGill Illness Narrative Interview [66] is used to elicit illness narratives in various cultural contexts. It is a theoretically driven, semi-structured, qualitative interview protocol which is structured into three sections: (1) a basic temporal narrative of symptom and illness experience, organised in terms of the contiguity of events; (2) salient prototypes related to current health problems, based on the previous experience of the interviewee, family members or friends and mass media or other popular representations; and (3) any explanatory models, including labels, causal attributions, expectations for treatment, course and outcome. The supplementary sections of the MINI explore help seeking and pathways to care, treatment experience, adherence and impact of the illness on identity, self-perception and relationships with others. The MINI has been translated and applied in cross-cultural settings to diverse health problems including mental health (both severe and common mental disorders), breastfeeding, diabetes, medically unexplained symptoms, myocardial infarction, non-epileptic seizures and scleroderma (for the original English version, translated versions and publications, see[1]).

The Cultural Formulation Interview (CFI) is a tool that has been well established and tested in earlier research and is based on principles common in cultural anthropology [67] (see also Chap. 11 in this book). Data resulting from the application of this tool might be used to guide interaction and diagnostic and treatment models tailored to various ethnic or cultural groups. It has also fed into international handbooks such as the one developed by Kirmayer discussed later in this chapter. The CFI can be expected to be of special importance in practical work with refugees [68].

Specifically, the CFI is a publicly available, 16-question interview, in a core (client) version, but also in a CFI-informant version which is to be used with family and social network members, included in the DSM 5 and on the DSM 5 official website.[2] It evaluates four aspects of the cultural formulation (domains): cultural definition of the problem; cultural perceptions of cause, context and support (including cultural identity); cultural factors that affect self-coping and past help seeking; and cultural factors that affect current help seeking.

The interview tool is supported by 12 supplementary modules that are not included in the DSM 5 main handbook but are again available from the same website (Explanatory Model; Level of Functioning; Psychosocial Stressors; Social Network; Cultural Identity; Spirituality, Religion, and Moral Traditions; Coping and Help Seeking; Patient-Clinician Relationship; Immigrants and Refugees; School-Age Children and Adolescents; Older Adults; and Caregivers). A special tool has also been developed to measure the degree of physician fidelity to the interview protocol (Cultural Formulation Interview-Fidelity Instrument (CFI-FI)) [69].

Training should be considered when implementing the CFI, especially in clinical practice, as the tool follows a model not common in medical curricula [70, 71]. A number of supportive materials published by APA include a handbook[3] and an online movie[4] in a blended media approach to facilitate education in the new tool. Mills et al. have demonstrated improvement in cultural competence in a study with residents already after a one-hour training in the CFI, an effect that can be expected to improve with a more comprehensive training model [72]. Aggarval et al. have conducted a study to evaluate training models and teach the use of the interview in clinical practice with 75 clinicians from five continents as part of a major project on the CFI. They recommend a combination of reviewing written guidelines, video demonstration and behavioural simulations [73].

---

[1] https://www.mcgill.ca/tcpsych/research/cmhru/mini.

[2] http://www.dsm5.org.

[3] See also on http://www.dsm5.org for this and further materials.

[4] https://www.appi.org/Lewis-Fernandez. Accessed 30 May 2017.

Recently, a Dutch group has also reported on the development of an abbreviated version, particularly for the use in refugees [74], that could become an important tool if further data confirm the validity of the instrument. As with several similar instruments, the more general international application of the cultural formulation interview would require clarification of the process of granting translations and extended copyrights that at present are with the American Psychiatric Association (APA), which might complicate the situation.

5.3.2 Developing Tools Reflecting Specific Cultural Aspects

Providing questionnaires and assessment tools that are actually sensitive to differences, not only in language but also in culture, and follow the high standards common in psychological testing or research can be a challenging, time-consuming and resource-intensive process. Such tools should be based on revalidation and might require adaptation, such as the definition of new cut-off points, demonstrated by Ventevogel in Afghan groups [75]. This can rarely be done in emergencies, though a translation using validation by translation re- translation procedures [76] can at least be used as a preliminary tool in screening or basic assessment, but it may not be suitable for research (see also Chap. 14 in this book). A frequently neglected risk of such a simplified process is that important aspects are not properly identified and cultural expressions and idioms of distress remain undetected leading to what Bhui calls a “closed process” [77]. The MINI, CFI instruments, or qualitative research would be required to identify such important indicators of suffering.

5.4 Integrating Transcultural Models into Research and Clinical Practice

Solutions are currently being sought to address the necessary integration of the results of improved understanding of cultural factors into healthcare systems. Besides the increased use of research models taken from anthropology and the new instruments to support culture-based assessments, some institutions have begun to offer cultural *consultation services*—an approach developed earlier by the Division of Transcultural Psychiatry at McGill University [78]. These services include the assessment and evaluation of patients from different cultural backgrounds, including immigrants and refugees, and the re-evaluation of ongoing treatment if required through collaborative expertise derived from culture brokers, translators, health professionals and researchers.[5] An evaluation of this particular cultural consultation service has shown that it is an effective way to supplement existing services and improve diagnostic assessment and treatment for diverse populations. However, it was also noted that clinicians require more training in working with culture brokers

[5] See https://mcgill.ca/culturalconsultation/.

and interpreters, while culture brokers would benefit from formal training in mental health [78].

Training programmes to improve "transcultural literacy" or competence of the healthcare professional [79] including those mentioned in the context of the CFI are the next important step that should be embedded in both pre- and postgraduate training in health professions. Moreover, comprehensive *guidelines* should be developed that give access to the characteristic models and idioms of distress in different cultures to researchers and clinicians alike, in order to guide and improve their praxis. A helpful example of such integration would be the special handbook developed by Kirmayer and his group for UNHCR, focusing on Syrian refugees entitled *Culture, Context and the Mental Health and Psychosocial Wellbeing of Syrians*.[6] The handbook explores regional idioms of distress with Arabic, Kurdish (Kirmanji) and English listings (see also table 5.1), but also explanatory models, religious practices, and a chapter on Islam. The authors organise idioms in categories that could also be used as organising principles in other similar settings: (1) general distress, (2) fear and anticipated anxiety, (3) feeling nervous or tense, (4) sadness and difficulty in adjustment to an acute stressor, (5) depression, (6) lack of resources and helplessness, (7) cognitive symptoms, (8) madness and (9) suicidality. A final chapter explores the experience with the application of the MHPSS model in Syria.

The project can be recommended as an example of an integrated and thorough interdisciplinary approach, and it is to be hoped that UNHCR or other organisations will provide similar handbooks for other regions and major ethnic groups.

Conclusions

As this chapter made apparent, medicine in general and psychiatry in particular, increasingly draw on anthropological and transcultural insights as well as research methods in order to better understand the impact of culture on migrants' and refugees' mental health and wellbeing. Recognising and understanding how clients from various cultural backgrounds negotiate changing identities and identify and interpret psychological and/or physical illness has led to an engagement with concepts such as local idioms of distress or health belief models. Integrative models in healthcare, which are increasingly accepted when it comes to the therapeutic work with refugee and migrant populations, are actively being developed. The recognition of these aspects is also reflected in recent changes in standard diagnostic systems like the DSM 5,[7] which we consider an important step toward the improvement of medicine and mental healthcare for refugees.

---

[6] Hassan, G, Kirmayer, LJ, MekkiBerrada A., Quosh, C., el Chammay, R., Deville-Stoetzel, J.B., Youssef, A., Jefee-Bahloul, H., Barkeel-Oteo, A.: Coutts, A., Song, S. & Ventevogel, P. *Culture, Context and the Mental Health and Psychosocial Wellbeing of Syrians: A Review for Mental Health and Psychosocial Support staff working with Syrians Affected by Armed Conflict*. Geneva: UNHCR, 2015.

[7] www.dsm5.org/.

References

1. Tol WA, Kohrt BA, Jordans MJ, Thapa SB, Pettigrew J, Upadhaya N, et al. Political violence and mental health: a multi-disciplinary review of the literature on Nepal. Soc Sci Med. 2010;70(1):35–44.
2. Groen S. Recognizing cultural identity in mental health care: rethinking the cultural formulation of a somali patient. Transcult Psychiatry. 2009;46(3):451–62.
3. Kirmayer LJ. Cultural variations in the clinical presentation of depression and anxiety: implications for diagnosis and treatment. J Clin Psychiatry. 2001;62(Suppl 13):22–8. discussion 9–30
4. Castañeda H. Im/migration and health: conceptual, methodological, and theoretical propositions for applied anthropology. Napa Bull. 2010;34(1):21.
5. Miller KE, Rasmussen A. War exposure, daily stressors, and mental health in conflict and post-conflict settings: bridging the divide between trauma-focused and psychosocial frameworks. Soc Sci Med. 2010;70(1):7–16.
6. Marsella AJ, Friedman M, Spain H. Ethnocultural aspects of PTSD: some closing thoughts. In: Marsella AJ, Friedman MJ, Gerrity ET, Scurfield RM, editors. Ethnocultural aspects of posttraumatic stress disorder: issues, research, and clinical applications. Washington, DC: American Psychological Association; 1996. p. 529–38.
7. Summerfield D, Hume F. War and posttraumatic stress disorder: the question of social context. J Nerv Ment Dis. 1993;181(8):522.
8. Bracken PJ, Giller JE, Summerfield D. Psychological responses to war and atrocity: the limitations of current concepts. Soc Sci Med. 1995;40(8):1073–82.
9. Tay AK, Rees S, Chen J, Kareth M, Silove D. Factorial structure of complicated grief: associations with loss-related traumatic events and psychosocial impacts of mass conflict amongst West Papuan refugees. Soc Psychiatry Psychiatr Epidemiol. 2016;51(3):395–406.
10. Kohrt BA, Hruschka DJ. Nepali concepts of psychological trauma: the role of idioms of distress, ethnopsychology and ethnophysiology in alleviating suffering and preventing stigma. Cult Med Psychiatry. 2010;34(2):322–52.
11. Boasso AM, Steenkamp MM, Fox AB, Nash WP, Larson JL, Litz BT. The structure of PTSD in active-duty marines across the deployment cycle. Psychol Trauma. 2016;8(2):127–34.
12. Groleau D, Kirmayer LJ. Sociosomatic theory in Vietnamese immigrants' narratives of distress. Anthropol Med. 2004;11(2):117–33.
13. Nichter M. Idioms of distress revisited. Cult Med Psychiatry. 2010;34(2):401–16.
14. Sameer M, Menon V, Chandrasekaran R. Is 'Pure' Dhat syndrome a stable diagnostic entity? A naturalistic long term follow up study from a tertiary care centre. J Clin Diagn Res. 2015;9(8):VC1–3.
15. Ventriglio A, Ayonrinde O, Bhugra D. Relevance of culture-bound syndromes in the 21st century. Psychiatry Clin Neurosci. 2016;70(1):3–6.
16. Abramowitz SA. Trauma and humanitarian translation in Liberia: the tale of open mole. Cult Med Psychiatry. 2010;34(2):353–79.
17. Hinton DE, Lewis-Fernandez R. Idioms of distress among trauma survivors: subtypes and clinical utility. Cult Med Psychiatry. 2010;34(2):209–18.
18. Pedersen D, Kienzler H, Gamarra J. Llaki and nakary: idioms of distress and suffering among the highland Quechua in the Peruvian Andes. Cult Med Psychiatry. 2010;34(2):279–300.
19. Davis D, Joakimsen L. Nerves as status and nerves as stigma: idioms of distress and social action in Newfoundland and Northern Norway. Qual Health Res. 1997;7(3):20.
20. Kienzler HL, Locke P. The effects of societal violence in war and post-war contexts. In: White RG, Jain S, David MR, editors. The Palgrave handbook of global mental health: socio-cultural perspectives. Basingstoke: Palgrave Macmillan; 2017. p. 285–305.
21. Jenkins J. Culture, emotion, and PTSD. In: Marsella AJ, Friedman MJ, Gerrity ET, Scurfield RM, editors. Ethnocultural aspects of posttraumatic stress disorder: issues, research and clinical applications. Washington, D.C.: American Psychological Association; 1996.

22. Hinton DE, Hofmann SG, Rivera E, Otto MW, Pollack MH. Culturally adapted CBT (CA-CBT) for Latino women with treatment-resistant PTSD: a pilot study comparing CA-CBT to applied muscle relaxation. Behav Res Ther. 2011;49(4):275–80.
23. Hinton DE, Hofmann SG, Pollack MH, Otto MW. Mechanisms of efficacy of CBT for Cambodian refugees with PTSD: improvement in emotion regulation and orthostatic blood pressure response. CNS Neurosci Ther. 2009;15(3):255–63.
24. Otto MW, Hinton DE. Modifying exposure-based CBT for Cambodian refugees with post-traumatic stress disorder. Cogn Behav Pract. 2006;13(4):261–70.
25. Bhugra D. Cultural identities and cultural congruency: a new model for evaluating mental distress in immigrants. Acta Psychiatr Scand. 2005;111(2):84–93.
26. Kohrt BA, Luitel NP, Acharya P, Jordans MJ. Detection of depression in low resource settings: validation of the Patient Health Questionnaire (PHQ-9) and cultural concepts of distress in Nepal. BMC Psychiatry. 2016;16:58.
27. American Psychiatric Association, American Psychiatric Association, DSM-5 Task Force. Diagnostic and statistical manual of mental disorders: DSM-5, vol. xliv. 5th ed. Washington, D.C.: American Psychiatric Association; 2013. p. 947.
28. Lewis-Fernandez R, Aggarwal NK. Culture and psychiatric diagnosis. Adv Psychosom Med. 2013;33:15–30.
29. Stephenson C. The epistemological significance of possession entering the DSM. Hist Psychiatry. 2015;26(3):251–69.
30. Hinton DE, Kredlow MA, Bui E, Pollack MH, Hofmann SG. Treatment change of somatic symptoms and cultural syndromes among Cambodian refugees with PTSD. Depress Anxiety. 2012;29(2):147–54.
31. Wenzel T, Frewer A, Mirzaei S. The DSM 5 and the Istanbul Protocol: diagnosis of psychological sequels of torture. Torture. 2015;25(1):51–61.
32. Mikhail BI, Petro-Nustas WI. Transcultural adaptation of Champion's Health Belief Model Scales. J Nurs Scholarsh. 2001;33(2):159–65.
33. Tamez EG, Vacalis TD. Health beliefs, the significant other and compliance with therapeutic regimens among adult Mexican American diabetics. Health Educ. 1989;20(6):24–31.
34. Alidu L, Grunfeld EA. Gender differences in beliefs about health: a comparative qualitative study with Ghanaian and Indian migrants living in the United Kingdom. BMC Psychol. 2017;5(1):8.
35. Federman AD, Wolf M, Sofianou A, Wilson EA, Martynenko M, Halm EA, et al. The association of health literacy with illness and medication beliefs among older adults with asthma. Patient Educ Couns. 2013;92(2):273–8.
36. Smith A, MacEntee MI, Beattie BL, Brondani M, Bryant R, Graf P, et al. The influence of culture on the oral health-related beliefs and behaviours of elderly chinese immigrants: a meta-synthesis of the literature. J Cross Cult Gerontol. 2013;28(1):27–47.
37. Stefanovics EA, He H, Cavalcanti M, Neto H, Ofori-Atta A, Leddy M, et al. Witchcraft and biopsychosocial causes of mental illness: attitudes and beliefs about mental illness among health professionals in five countries. J Nerv Ment Dis. 2016;204(3):169–74.
38. Wenzel T, Kinigadner S. Auf der Flucht [To be fleeing]. Psychol Österreich. 2016;36(3):135–43.
39. Neuner F, Pfeiffer A, Schauer-Kaiser E, Odenwald M, Elbert T, Ertl V. Haunted by ghosts: prevalence, predictors and outcomes of spirit possession experiences among former child soldiers and war-affected civilians in Northern Uganda. Soc Sci Med. 2012;75(3):548–54.
40. van Duijl M, Kleijn W, de Jong J. Are symptoms of spirit possessed patients covered by the DSM-IV or DSM-5 criteria for possession trance disorder? A mixed-method explorative study in Uganda. Soc Psychiatry Psychiatr Epidemiol. 2013;48(9):1417–30.
41. Shoeb M, Weinstein HM, Halpern J. Living in religious time and space: Iraqi refugees in Dearborn, Michigan. J Refug Stud. 2007;20(3):29.
42. Kwong EW, Lam IO. Chinese older people in Hong Kong: health beliefs about influenza vaccination. Nurs Older People. 2008;20(7):29–33.

43. Nan X, Kim J. Predicting H1N1 vaccine uptake and H1N1-related health beliefs: the role of individual difference in consideration of future consequences. J Health Commun. 2014;19(3):376–88.
44. Alqahtani AS, Sheikh M, Wiley K, Heywood AE. Australian Hajj pilgrims' infection control beliefs and practices: insight with implications for public health approaches. Travel Med Infect Dis. 2015;13(4):329–34.
45. Smith RM, Nelsen LA. Hmong folk remedies: limited acetylation of opium by aspirin and acetaminophen. J Forensic Sci. 1991;36(1):280–7.
46. Carruth L. Camel milk, amoxicillin, and a prayer: medical pluralism and medical humanitarian aid in the Somali Region of Ethiopia. Soc Sci Med. 2014;120:405–12.
47. Volpato G, Kourkova P, Zeleny V. Healing war wounds and perfuming exile: the use of vegetal, animal, and mineral products for perfumes, cosmetics, and skin healing among Sahrawi refugees of Western Sahara. J Ethnobiol Ethnomed. 2012;8:49.
48. van Andel T, Westers P. Why Surinamese migrants in the Netherlands continue to use medicinal herbs from their home country. J Ethnopharmacol. 2010;127(3):694–701.
49. Villa-Torres L, Gonzalez-Vazquez T, Fleming PJ, Gonzalez-Gonzalez EL, Infante-Xibille C, Chavez R, et al. Transnationalism and health: a systematic literature review on the use of transnationalism in the study of the health practices and behaviors of migrants. Soc Sci Med. 2017;183:70–9.
50. Ramzan S, Soelberg J, Jager AK, Cantarero-Arevalo L. Traditional medicine among people of Pakistani descent in the capital region of Copenhagen. J Ethnopharmacol. 2017;196:267–80.
51. Mizzi C, Dalabira E, Kumuthini J, Dzimiri N, Balogh I, Basak N, et al. A European spectrum of pharmacogenomic biomarkers: implications for clinical pharmacogenomics. PLoS One. 2016;11(9):e0162866.
52. Straka RJ, Hansen SR, Walker PF. Comparison of the prevalence of the poor metabolizer phenotype for CYP2D6 between 203 Hmong subjects and 280 white subjects residing in Minnesota. Clin Pharmacol Ther. 1995;58(1):29–34.
53. Arriaza P, Nedjat-Haiem F, Lee HY, Martin SS. Guidelines for conducting rigorous health care psychosocial cross-cultural/language qualitative research. Soc Work Public Health. 2015;30(1):75–87.
54. Bellamy K, Ostini R, Martini N, Kairuz T. Erratum to: seeking to understand: using generic qualitative research to explore access to medicines and pharmacy services among resettled refugees. Int J Clin Pharm. 2016;38(2):469.
55. Saadi A, Bond BE, Percac-Lima S. Bosnian, Iraqi, and Somali refugee women speak: a comparative qualitative study of refugee health beliefs on preventive health and breast cancer screening. Womens Health Issues. 2015;25(5):501–8.
56. Szajna A, Ward J. Access to health care by refugees: a dimensional analysis. Nurs Forum. 2015;50(2):83–9.
57. Ingvarsson L, Egilson ST, Skaptadottir UD. I want a normal life like everyone else: daily life of asylum seekers in Iceland. Scand J Occup Ther. 2016;23(6):416–24.
58. Kay M, Wijayanayaka S, Cook H, Hollingworth S. Understanding quality use of medicines in refugee communities in Australian primary care: a qualitative study. Br J Gen Pract. 2016;66(647):e397–409.
59. Weine S, Muzurovic N, Kulauzovic Y, Besic S, Lezic A, Mujagic A, et al. Family consequences of refugee trauma. Fam Process. 2004;43(2):147–60.
60. Jirovsky E, Hoffmann K, Maier M, Kutalek R. "Why should I have come here?"--a qualitative investigation of migration reasons and experiences of health workers from sub-Saharan Africa in Austria. BMC Health Serv Res. 2015;15:74.
61. Kowal SP, Jardine CG, Bubela TM. If they tell me to get it, I'll get it. If they don't...: immunization decision-making processes of immigrant mothers. Can J Public Health. 2015;106(4):e230–5.
62. Bellamy K, Ostini R, Martini N, Kairuz T. Perspectives of resettled African refugees on accessing medicines and pharmacy services in Queensland, Australia. Int J Pharm Pract. 2016;25:358–64.

63. Berg B. Qualitative research methods for the social sciences. 6th ed. Boston: Pearson Allyn Bacon; 2007.
64. Folch-Lyon E, Trost JF. Conducting focus group sessions. Stud Fam Plan. 1981;12(1):7.
65. Baum F, MacDougall C, Smith D. Participatory action research. J Epidemiol Community Health. 2006;60(10):854–7.
66. Groleau D, Young A, Kirmayer LJ. The McGill illness narrative interview (MINI): an interview schedule to elicit meanings and modes of reasoning related to illness experience. Transcult Psychiatry. 2006;43(4):671–91.
67. Aggarwal NK, Desilva R, Nicasio AV, Boiler M, Lewis-Fernandez R. Does the cultural formulation interview for the fifth revision of the diagnostic and statistical manual of mental disorders (DSM-5) affect medical communication? A qualitative exploratory study from the New York site. Ethn Health. 2015;20(1):1–28.
68. Rohlof H, Knipscheer JW, Kleber RJ. Use of the cultural formulation with refugees. Transcult Psychiatry. 2009;46(3):487–505.
69. Aggarwal NK, Glass A, Tirado A, Boiler M, Nicasio A, Alegria M, et al. The development of the DSM-5 cultural formulation interview-fidelity instrument (CFI-FI): a pilot study. J Health Care Poor Underserved. 2014;25(3):1397–417.
70. Padilla A, Benjamin S, Lewis-Fernandez R. Assessing cultural psychiatry milestones through an objective structured clinical examination. Acad Psychiatry. 2016;40(4):600–3.
71. Luciano M, De Rosa C, Del Vecchio V, Sampogna G, Sbordone D, Atti AR, et al. Perceived insecurity, mental health and urbanization: results from a multicentric study. Int J Soc Psychiatry. 2016;62(3):252–61.
72. Mills S, Wolitzky-Taylor K, Xiao AQ, Bourque MC, Rojas SM, Bhattacharya D, et al. Training on the DSM-5 cultural formulation interview improves cultural competence in general psychiatry residents: a multi-site study. Acad Psychiatry. 2016;40(5):829–34.
73. Aggarwal NK, Lam P, Castillo EG, Weiss MG, Diaz E, Alarcon RD, et al. How do clinicians prefer cultural competence training? Findings from the DSM-5 cultural formulation interview field trial. Acad Psychiatry. 2016;40(4):584–91.
74. Groen SP, Richters A, Laban CJ, Deville WL. Implementation of the cultural formulation through a newly developed brief cultural interview: pilot data from the Netherlands. Transcult Psychiatry. 2017;54(1):3–22.
75. Ventevogel P, De Vries G, Scholte WF, Shinwari NR, Faiz H, Nassery R, et al. Properties of the Hopkins symptom checklist-25 (HSCL-25) and the self-reporting questionnaire (SRQ-20) as screening instruments used in primary care in Afghanistan. Soc Psychiatry Psychiatr Epidemiol. 2007;42(4):328–35.
76. Gautam S, Nijhawan M, Kamal P. Standardisation of hindi version of goldbergs general health questionnaire. Indian J Psychiatry. 1987;29(1):63–6.
77. Bhui K, Bhugra D. Transcultural psychiatry: some social and epidemiological research issues. Int J Soc Psychiatry. 2001;47(3):1–9.
78. Kirmayer LJ, Groleau D, Guzder J, Blake C, Jarvis E. Cultural consultation: a model of mental health service for multicultural societies. Can J Psychiatr. 2003;48(3):145–53.
79. Kirmayer LJ, Rousseau C, Guzder J, Jarvis GE. Training clinicians in cultural psychiatry: a Canadian perspective. Acad Psychiatry. 2008;32(4):313–9.

Integrative Mental Health and Psychosocial Support Interventions for Refugees in Humanitarian Crisis Settings

6

Inka Weissbecker, Fahmy Hanna, Mohamed El Shazly, James Gao, and Peter Ventevogel

Abstract

Refugees are often exposed to various interrelated stressors including the loss of resources and belongings, death of, or separation from, loved ones as well as direct exposure to armed conflict and violence. Psychological distress is common amongst refugees, with a substantial percentage developing mild to moderate mental disorders such as depression or anxiety disorders. A small percentage of people in refugee settings have severe mental disorders (often exacerbations of pre-existing disorders) and they are especially vulnerable.

This chapter outlines complex challenges in addressing the mental health and psychosocial support (MHPSS) needs of refugees and describes key global guidelines, programmatic elements and recommendations in the areas of MHPSS including situational assessments, coordination of services and functional integration of mental health interventions within existing health systems. Various

I. Weissbecker (✉)
Technical Unit, International Medical Corps, Washington, DC, USA
e-mail: iweissbecker@internationalmedicalcorps.org

F. Hanna
WHO Department of Mental Health and Substance Abuse, Geneva, Switzerland
e-mail: hannaf@who.int

M. El Shazly
Public Health Unit, United Nations High Commissioner for Refugees, Erbil, Kurdistan Region, Iraq
e-mail: ELSHAZLM@unhcr.org

J. Gao
Centre for Global Mental Health, London, UK

P. Ventevogel
Public Health Section, United Nations High Commissioner for Refugees, Geneva, Switzerland
e-mail: ventevog@unhcr.org

T. Wenzel, B. Drožđek (eds.), *An Uncertain Safety*,
https://doi.org/10.1007/978-3-319-72914-5_6

specific intervention modalities will be discussed, including psychological first aid, scalable psychological interventions, community-based psychosocial work and training of health workers in basic mental health care. This chapter has the potential to inform the planning, implementing or researching of MHPSS considerations for programmes in humanitarian refugee crises.

6.1 The Context of Refugee Mental Health in Humanitarian Crisis

6.1.1 Introduction

The world today is facing an unprecedented number of refugees and forcibly displaced persons: estimated at over 65 million people worldwide [1]. The effects of forced displacement and its subsequent stressors on mental health can be pervasive and profound. In the past, some donors, academics and humanitarian decision-makers assumed, mistakenly, that mental health problems were of less importance compared to other health problems and that populations outside highly developed industrial countries would not consider mental health and psychosocial wellbeing a priority. However, field experience and research have shown that people affected by humanitarian emergencies do view mental health as a significant issue of concern [2–4]. As a consequence, over the last decade, attention to mental health in humanitarian emergencies has been increasing, whilst programmes for mental health and psychosocial support have become routine elements of the humanitarian response to refugee crises [5, 6]. The field has evolved over the past several years and moved away from being overly focused on psychological trauma, posttraumatic stress disorder (PTSD) and on specialised interventions by mental health clinicians from high-income countries and has become a burgeoning field of research and interventions moving towards a more inclusive approach; one which recognises the scope and significance of different types of culturally shaped mental health problems and one which seeks to develop existing strengths and build capacities over time in order to integrate mental health care within already existing health, social and community systems [7–10].

Increasingly, humanitarian responses now include programming for mental health and psychosocial support (MHPSS). This often includes interventions in a wide range of sectors and thematic areas such as health, education, community-based protection, sexual and gender based violence, and child protection. There is growing awareness that all staff involved in the humanitarian response should know the basics of MHPSS and understand how their own actions can influence mental health and psychosocial wellbeing [11, 12]. All professionals working in humanitarian emergencies can contribute to alleviating the tremendous psychological suffering of the populations they serve.

Over the years, funding for mental health as part of development has slowly increased [13], and major stakeholders are starting to realise the importance of investing in mental health within refugee situations [14–16]. In practice, however, mental health is often not given a high priority, and inclusion of MHPSS within donor funding for humanitarian crises still often falls short of the total needs. In the 2016 Syrian Arab Republic Humanitarian Response Plan (SHARP), for example, MHPSS represented less than 0.1% of the overall budget of the humanitarian response [17].

This chapter intends to outline basic principles to inform the planning, implementing or researching of mental health and psychosocial support considerations for programmes in humanitarian crises, particularly in situations of forced displacement, with refugees and internally displaced persons (IDPs) in low- and middle-income countries.

6.1.2 Stressors and Mental Health Problems

Refugees and others affected by humanitarian crises frequently suffer various severe and interrelated stressors including the loss of homes, livelihoods, material belongings, communities and social support systems. They may also witness horrific events and atrocities, lose loved ones, become separated from family members. Many refugees are at a greatly increased risk of physical assault, gender-based violence and malnutrition [18]. Specific population groups such as children and youth are especially vulnerable as they are often dependent on caregivers and may become orphaned or separated in situations of crises.

Even when the acute emergency is over, the affected displaced populations continue to experience significant stress and hardships because of harsh living conditions, the erosion of mutual social support mechanisms, limited access to basic needs and services and lack of opportunities for maintaining livelihoods and education. Health and social services, which existed before the crisis, have often broken down whilst humanitarian aid attempts to fill the gaps. Poorly organised humanitarian services may contribute to making problems worse and increase tensions and stress in refugee populations [19]. It is often hugely challenging to create available and acceptable service of good quality for refugees and other displaced populations. Refugees may not be allowed to utilise local treatment services, which may also be expensive, or they may not have access to services outside refugee camps. Often, cultural and language barriers complicate the situation even further.

Many emotional, cognitive, physical and behavioural reactions are normal adaptive reactions to severe stressors; these are more likely to resolve if a supportive family or community environment is available. Unfortunately, in humanitarian settings, many of the protective informal community networks have deteriorated. Some people are at increased risk of developing prolonged mental health problems or disorders, especially those who already had difficulties in functioning before the emergency, those who have experienced cumulative stressors and those who have limited social support. People may develop negative behaviours to cope with stress such as the consumption of alcohol or drugs further putting them at risk [20]. People who have suffered mental health difficulties in the past, or are suffering from

Table 6.1 WHO projections of mental disorders and distress in adult populations affected by emergencies [22]

	Before emergency: 12-month prevalence	After emergency: 12-month prevalence
Severe disorder (e.g. psychosis, severe depression, severely disabling form of anxiety disorder)	2–3%	3–4%
Mild or moderate mental disorder (e.g. mild and moderate forms of depression and anxiety disorders, including mild and moderate PTSD)	10%	15–20%
Normal distress/other psychological reactions (no disorder)	No estimate	Large percentage

a pre-existing mental disorder, may find their symptoms relapsing or exacerbated. Humanitarian emergencies cause high rates of distress although precise estimates of prevalence are not known [21]. Nevertheless, only a minority of those suffering distress will develop frankmental disorders as shown in Table 6.1.

6.1.3 Global MHPSS Guidelines and Approaches

6.1.3.1 Key Definitions

Mental Health

Mental health is not just the absence of mental disorder. The World Health Organization (WHO) defines mental health as a state of wellbeing in which every individual realises his or her own potential, is able to cope with normal stresses of life, can work productively and fruitfully and is able to make a contribution to their community [23].

Mental Health and Psychosocial Support

Health agencies tend to speak of ‘mental health care’ to describe treatment interventions for people with mental disorders. However, outside of the health sector, the term ‘psychosocial support’ or ‘psychosocial intervention’ may cover a broader range of activities that support both the psychological and social wellbeing of families, groups and communities—not just those who suffer from mental disorders. This binary has led to confusion in the humanitarian sector, and so many organisations have agreed to use the composite term ‘mental health and psychosocial support’ to indicate ‘any type of local or outside support that aims to protect or promote psychosocial wellbeing and/or prevent or treat mental disorder’ [18].

Community-Based Approach

MHPSS places a large focus on the level of the community: a community-based approach implies working closely with affected populations, recognizing their individual and collective capacities and resources, and building on these to ensure wellbeing and protection [24].

Mental Health and Psychosocial Support Approach
The term 'MHPSS approach' is sometime used to promote the understanding that all actions and interventions in a humanitarian setting may have effects on mental health and psychosocial wellbeing, even if this is not the primary intention of the action [25]. For example, building shelters for refugees has as primary aim to provide a safe place to live, but *the way* in which such housing is realized can greatly affect psychological wellbeing. Consulting refugee communities and promoting active participation of refugees in the design and construction of their shelter, and ensuring that marginalized or vulnerable sections of the population feel safe and included, may create a sense of collective ownership and foster a sense of belonging.

Mental Health and Psychosocial Support Interventions
Whilst many interventions in a humanitarian setting may affect mental health and psychosocial wellbeing, a core MHPSS intervention has the specific aim to contribute to improved mental health and psychosocial wellbeing [25].

6.1.3.2 IASC Guidelines on Mental Health and Psychosocial Support in Emergency Settings

In 2007, the Inter-Agency Standing Committee (IASC), the primary mechanism for inter-agency coordination of humanitarian assistance, published the 'Guidelines on Mental Health and Psychosocial Support in Emergency Settings'. These guidelines represent a consensus framework that provides humanitarian actors with a set of minimum multisectoral responses to protect and improve people's mental health and psychosocial wellbeing in emergencies. The guidelines include a matrix with recommended key interventions spanning emergency preparedness, minimum responses during or after an emergency as well as comprehensive responses including potential additional responses for an emergency that becomes stabilised or is in the process of reconstruction. These responses work across domains of coordination, human resources, community mobilisation, community support, health, nutrition and water and sanitation. Furthermore, the guidelines emphasise collaboration between sectors and with non-health actors and core clusters such as child protection, sexual- and gender-based violence, community-based protection and education. They contain 25 action sheets placing an emphasis on multisectoral and coordinated action. Each action sheet contains the following information: background, key actions, selected sample process indicators, examples of good practice in previous emergencies and a list of further resource materials [18].

The guidelines are useful for the planning and coordination of activities and provide organisations from various backgrounds with a common conceptual framework for setting up services. IASC guidelines on MHPSS endorse six main principles: human rights and equity, participation, do no harm, building on available resources and capacities, integrated support systems and multilayered supports (see Fig. 6.1).

A 2014 review of the IASC guidelines found that they helped strengthening the role of MHPSS in emergencies, and the use of the 'MHPSS' term had improved understanding and linkage between mental health and psychosocial actors [5]. Furthermore, the intervention pyramid (Fig. 6.1) was found as a useful tool in training, coordination and discussions at the cluster level. Guidelines were found to be helpful in the communication between agencies and donors and were influential in developing and disseminating MHPSS policies.

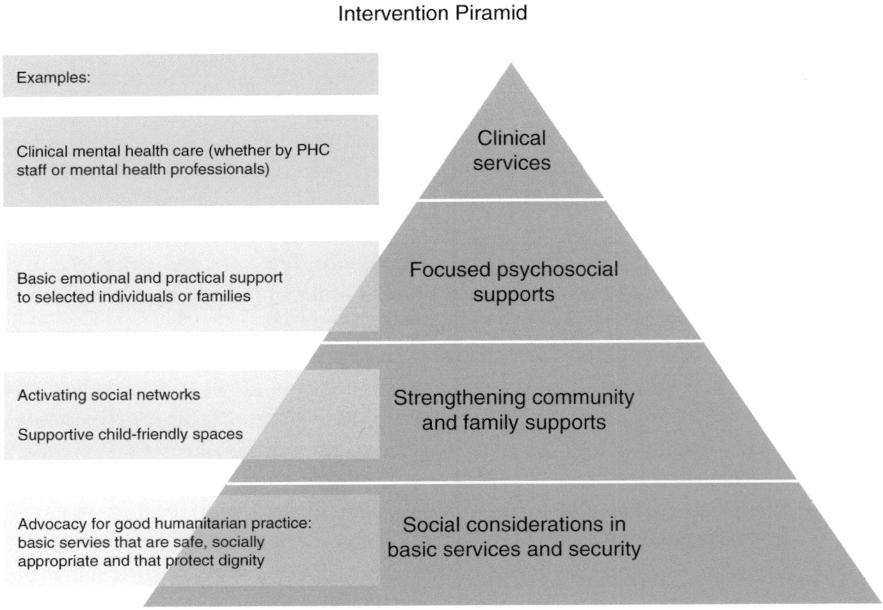

Fig. 6.1 The intervention pyramid for MHPSS in emergencies [18]

6.1.4 Cultural Considerations

Vignette: Cultural, Social and Contextual Factors

Khamis is a 35-year-old man in an East African country. He is married with five children. One year ago, he had to flee his native country due to ethnic and religious violence. He witnessed the pillaging of his village, and several family members were killed. One of his children died from illness during the flight. He and his family have been in a refugee camp in a foreign country for 4 months. Khamis, who used to be a farmer and carpenter, cannot use his skills because, as a refugee, he is not allowed to work. He and his wife argue much more than before, and he sometimes beats his wife but feels bad afterwards. He feels increasingly useless and has lost hope that his life will ever improve. His appetite is not good and he does not sleep well. He does not want to show his sadness, and in order to forget his problems he has started drinking excessively. He frequently visits the health centre and a local healer to complain of tiredness and stomach pains, but they have been unable to help him.

Discussion: This patient, who may suffer from depression and alcohol use disorder, does not self-identify as having a mental disorder and will be unlikely to seek help from a mental health professional. However, he makes numerous visits to the primary health-care provider for somatic complaints. Any adequate solution for Khamis needs to take the individual, family and environmental context into account and address both psychological and social problems.

The way in which refugees experience mental disorders is strongly influenced by factors such as semiotics and the cultural meaning and significance of concepts of mental illness. Describing any disorder is influenced by language and culture. In many languages, the terms 'mental disorder' and 'mental illness' may translate to 'craziness' or 'madness', carrying strongly negative connotations and stigma. Such terms are often only used for people with severe mental disorders. Causes for such disorders are often seen as spiritual which results in those affected seeking help from traditional healers and religious leaders. Mild and moderate forms of mental disorder—including depression, anxiety and substance use disorders—are not always identified as mental disorders but rather as social or moral issues or problems related to a person's character. Those affected usually seek help from trusted community members or leaders first. Consequently, the way people define 'mental disorder' has major implications for their health and help-seeking behaviour. Worldwide there are major variations in:

- How problems of thinking, feeling, perceiving or behaving are described and labelled
- Beliefs about the causes of mental disorders
- Coping mechanisms
- How mental distress is managed as part of formal services (e.g. health and social services)
- How mental distress is managed as part of informal services (e.g. community traditional or religious healers)
- How people with mental illness are perceived and treated within communities

People often use culturally patterned expressions to communicate that they 'do not feel well' and are having difficulty with the tasks and functions of daily living. Often these are not discrete diagnostic categories with a specific set of symptoms but are pragmatically applied concepts with fluid boundaries. These idioms of distress may be indicative of strong emotional or psychopathological states that undermine the wellbeing of a person but do not necessarily imply that the person has a mental disorder; in a lot of cases, these idioms are focused on a typical symptom or localised to one area of the body. Some examples include:

- Idioms related to thoughts, e.g. *kufungisisa* meaning 'thinking too much' in Shona in Zimbabwe and *yeyeesi* meaning 'many thoughts' in Kakwa in South Sudan [26–28]
- Idioms related to the heart, e.g. *poil-heart* meaning 'heavy hearted' in Krio in Sierra Leone, *qalbi-jab* meaning 'broken heart' in Somalia, *qalb maaboud* meaning 'squeezed heart' in Arabic (referring to dysphoria and sadness) and *houbout el qalb* meaning 'falling or crumbling of the heart' (referring to the somatic reaction of sudden fear) [29–31]
- Idioms related to the head, e.g. *amutwe alluhire* meaning 'my head is tired' in Nande in the Democratic Republic of Congo [28]
- Idioms related to the general body, e.g. *jiu sukera gayo* meaning 'drying of the body' used by Bhutanese refugee in Nepal to indicate a situation of loss and desperation [32] or *lashe mn grana* meaning 'my body is heavy' in the Kirmanji Kurdish dialect [30]

Health workers should make attempts to identify and understand salient local idioms in the settings where they work. This can help facilitate more effective communication with their patients through the identification of local coping methods which may, in some cases, be more appropriate than Western interventions. For example, *poil-heart* is described by an adolescent girl in Kailahun, Sierra Leone, as 'Someone who is *poil-heart* is in a group but she's withdrawn from it, she suffers from something and does not pay attention. If she has a baby she is confused and can neglect the baby. When she or he imagines what happened she cries all day and cannot sleep or eat. She tries to work but it is no good. When she is at school her concentration is poor' [31]. On a superficial level, the problem seems to resemble the psychiatric concept of 'major depressive disorder', but the people in Sierra Leone did not see it as a problem that required professional medical or traditional healing assistance. Thus the treatment for *poil-heart* was described as '... If my friend was *poil-heart* I would go to her and talk with her to encourage her. If there was a football game I would encourage her to go. If lonely I would ask her problems and exchange ideas. If she told me she could not sleep or was afraid I would take her to my bed and share it. One should hear the problem, explain it and solve it'. Western therapeutic efforts and interventions should identify and support such positive and constructive mechanisms which may already be in place, rather than assume that the toolkit of medical psychiatry will always have the best and only solution [33].

This requires that MHPSS workers develop 'cultural competence' which is the 'capacity of practitioners and health services to respond appropriately and effectively to patients' cultural backgrounds, identities and concerns' [34]. Guiding principles for cultural competence in disaster mental health programmes include recognising the importance of culture and respecting diversity, obtaining knowledge about the cultural composition of the community, recruiting MHPSS workers who are representatives of the community and providing training and guidance to MHPSS staff [35]. Besides, it is important to ensure that services are accessible, appropriate and equitable and involve existing support networks. A way to do this in refugee populations is to train and involve some of them as 'cultural brokers' or 'cultural mediators' as has been successfully introduced in new humanitarian settings with refugees and migrants in Europe [36]; this has had a long antecedent in humanitarian settings in low- and middle-income countries in which refugees or other conflict-affected people are often engaged as intermediaries between 'population' and 'services'.

6.1.5 Human Rights Considerations

Worldwide, people with severe mental disorders are at a higher risk for abuse and neglect, such as physical restraining, seclusion or isolation and being denied basic needs and human rights [37]. The widespread stigma and discrimination surrounding mental disorders prevent people from seeking and receiving care. In many emergencies, human rights violations are particularly common due to increased vulnerabilities such as displacement, breakdown of social structures, violence, absence of accountability and a lack of access to health services and resources such as psychotropic medication [38, 39]. It is important that MHPSS practitioners are aware of the human rights frameworks and are able to go beyond narrowly defined clinical approaches and collaborate with human rights advocates to address the range of rights violations that people with severe mental disorders face [40–42]. This may require using a more inclusive vocabulary that goes beyond medical terminology. Those using human rights-based approaches often avoid terms such as 'mental disorders' or 'psychiatric disease' and favour the terms 'psychosocial disabilities' and 'mental disabilities'. This emphasises that the problem is more than an impairment or disorder that resides in the individual but that disability is the result of an interaction between impairment and attitudinal or environmental barriers which hinders full and effective participation in society on an equal basis with others [41]. Using a human rights perspective will emphasise the barriers which prevent people with psychosocial or mental disabilities to enjoy full use of their rights including rights for self-determination and making treatment decisions, as well as rights to fully participate in society and to access key opportunities such as employment and education. Barriers to realising those rights may be legal, economic and social and can also be related to barriers within the health-care system. In humanitarian settings, MHPSS practitioners, together with affected persons and their families, can raise awareness and advocate for mental health policies and laws which promote the improvement of human rights conditions for people with mental health problems [43]. It is also important to involve people affected by mental illness and their families in making sure programmes are designed to meet their needs and to foster participation and leadership roles amongst mental health service users.

6.2 Key Aspects of the MHPSS Response

6.2.1 Assessment

Before planning activities in mental health and psychosocial support, an assessment should be conducted to gain a better understanding of the humanitarian situation, to identify the priority issues around mental health and psychosocial support which need attention and to evaluate the available resources. Such assessments should focus both on needs and on available resources and include both finding new information (through qualitative and quantitative means) and the systematic collection of information that already exist. This includes general humanitarian assessments and reports by non-governmental organisations [22] as well as a review of existing mental health system information including World Health Organization Assessment Instrument for Mental Health Systems (WHO-AIMS), WHO Mental Health Atlas and other relevant documents [22, 44–46]. MHPSS assessments in humanitarian emergencies are essential but also run the risk of causing harm by asking sensitive questions and not having trained data collectors who can respond supportively and link those with urgent needs to available services. Assessments which are not well planned and informed by existing tools and ethical guidelines may not result in useful knowledge leading to uninformed planning or inappropriate interventions. There are concerns that the preoccupation with individual psychopathological responses, which characterise many assessments, may ignore the sociopolitical contexts, the various cultural idioms of distress, priorities of the affected population and existing strengths and resources and do not translate into project planning [47–50]. It is therefore critical that assessments pay attention to aspects of coordination, selection of appropriate measures and inclusion of contextual information as well as adhering to key ethical considerations.

Coordination with other actors during an assessment is essential to maximise resources, identify gaps and avoid duplication and burdening affected communities with multiple questionnaires which may not result in appropriate services [47]. Assessments should be announced and planned with MHPSS coordination groups in order to coordinate efforts with other humanitarian actors and agencies. Additionally, assessments should coordinate with and engage existing stakeholders—such as governments, communities and national and international agencies—in initial discussions about needs and priorities. Lack of coordination during the assessment phase may cause 'assessment fatigue' amongst refugees who are sometimes multiple times being asked similar things whilst they do not see any visible improvements in their situation.

A set of key resources for assessment is readily available for MHPSS humanitarian actors [22, 51, 52]. It is important to remember to choose relevant questions and adapt them to the specific settings, avoid lengthily interviews and be aware of highly sensitive questions which might put people in danger. A diverse range of groups should also be considered and included in MHPSS assessments such as children, youth, women, men, older people and other minority groups. Commonly used and recommended global guidelines for MHPSS assessments in humanitarian settings have been frequently used for assessing the needs of refugees [22, 51]. Tools and questions cover the areas of:

- Relevant contextual information, e.g. culture-specific beliefs and practices, practices around death and mourning, vulnerable groups at risk and attitudes towards severe mental disorder
- Experience of the emergency, e.g. perceived causes and expected consequences
- Mental health and psychosocial problems, e.g. culture-specific idioms of distress, priority mental health-related problems and impairment of daily activities
- Existing sources of psychosocial wellbeing and mental health, e.g. coping methods and community sources of support and resources
- Available services (e.g. 4Ws mapping, mental health checklists for health facilities)

Desk reviews of existing resources can be important to synthesise what is already known about cultural concepts and local beliefs and practices [53–56]. In light of current humanitarian emergencies, several recent assessments highlighting cultural and contextual aspects refugees have been produced, including on Syrian refugees [30, 57], Somali refugees [29] and people displaced by the Nepal earthquake of 2015 [58]. The work of MHPSS actors can be synthesised using the 4W mapping tool: 'Who is doing What, Where and When' [59–61]. Mapping reviews of MHPSS actors and services have been regularly updated, for example, for refugees in Jordan [62, 63].

Assessment reports have also examined the perceived physical, social and psychological needs in refugee populations ranging from South Sudanese refugees in Uganda to displaced Syrians and their host communities in Jordan [64, 65]. Assessments of local perceptions of the causes for different mental health problems, and ways in which communities seek help, are also helpful for programme planning. Amongst the Somali refugee population in Ethiopia, for example, depression is thought to be caused by a loss of resources so community members try to help those affected by replacing their lost belongings and providing social support [29, 66]. On the other hand, psychotic disorders and epilepsy were seen to have spiritual causes, and families of those affected often sought care from traditional healers. Rapid MHPSS assessment reports combining review of existing documents, perceptions of community members and available mental health and psychosocial support services and capacities are also available [67–70].

Published assessments of mental health needs amongst refugees or other people in humanitarian emergencies often focus on or include surveys examining the prevalence of specific mental disorders such as depression or PTSD [71–74]. However, prevalence surveys are resource and cost intensive and often pose their own unique challenges; among humanitarian agencies there is consensus that such epidemiological surveys are not part of a routine assessment in emergencies [22]. In the past, prevalence surveys in humanitarian settings have been unable to distinguish between normal stress reactions and mental disorders leading to inflated estimates [75]. These surveys often use symptom checklists which have been validated only in Western settings and therefore may misclassify local expressions of mental disorders [76] or miss important information [77]. Such local idioms of distress—including concepts and experiences of mental health—may vary considerably from the Western diagnostic categories of the *Diagnostic and Statistical Manual of Mental Disorder* (DSM) or the *International Classification of Diseases* (ICD) [78–81]. Mental health symptom checklists have a large focus on psychopathology with little attention to positive factors which drive wellbeing such as hope, social functioning or social support [82]. Whilst surveys predominantly focus on psychiatric symptoms, which may help with advocacy for potential donors, they are of only limited usefulness for programme planning. Generic WHO estimates of prevalence already exist, as outlined earlier in this chapter (see Table 6.1), and these are often sufficient for the initial stages of programmatic planning.

Any assessment of mental health problems amongst emergency-affected populations needs to use instruments that are culturally validated for the local population and should include severe mental health problems (e.g. impaired functioning, bizarre behaviour, immediate danger to self or others) [18, 22]. Some researchers have developed culturally and methodologically sound methods of assessing mental health problems in varying contexts using mixed qualitative and quantitative methods of capturing local idioms and distress and can develop culturally relevant indicators of functioning and validation measures for use [18, 83, 84].

MHPSS research in humanitarian settings requires careful considerations of ethical issues given the population group under study. Guidance documents have been developed for mental health research in humanitarian settings which are also relevant for MHPSS assessments [47, 52, 85]. It has been recommended that research should:

- Benefit the affected population
- Use culturally valid assessment instruments and measures
- Consider power dynamics and the relative social statuses of researchers and beneficiaries
- Do no harm by protecting participants from potential negative effects of participation such as stigmatisation, discrimination and security threats
- Minimise psychological risks such as raised expectations and labelling whilst ensuring review of research by affected communities
- Protect confidentiality
- Involve affected communities in selection of research topics
- Obtain genuine informed consent (e.g. understandable explanations, avoiding inappropriate incentives, repeating consent as appropriate)
- Share findings with affected communities and make reports accessible to relevant stakeholders and others in the field

Too often, humanitarian or academic actors only use assessment findings internally or publish findings many months or years later. This can lead to duplication of efforts and a less coordinated and informed response. After the assessment is complete, it is therefore recommended to share it with other relevant agencies and stakeholders and to disseminate recommendations for action. Several MHPSS assessment reports using the tools discussed have been disseminated (e.g. via on dedicated Web platforms for MHPSS in humanitarian settings such as www.MHPSS.net) or have been published [64–66, 86].

6.2.2 Coordination

In humanitarian emergencies, coordination is essential between different actors to share information, avoid duplication, fill gaps and advocate for best practices [18]. Coordination can also help ensure that different aspects of the humanitarian response are implemented in a way which promotes mental health and psychosocial wellbeing, ensuring that specific mental health and psychosocial interventions and mechanisms are included in the humanitarian response [18]. National-level MHPSS coordination groups are often jointly led by a UN agency (e.g. UNHCR, WHO) and an international non-governmental organisation (INGO). They are closely linked and coordinate with other groups such as health, protection and education; these groups often take on important tasks such as producing brief inter-agency notes on MHPSS for other actors, which include key points about best practices and guidance tailored to a specific emergency based on global guidelines. Such guidance notes are the effort of multiple organisations and have in the past been developed in settings such as Jordan, for the Syrian and Iraqi refugee response, Haiti after the 2010 earthquake and Gaza [87–89].

Coordination groups can also serve as an important platform to discuss proposed MHPSS interventions from different actors in order to help ensure that global best practice guidelines are followed as well as to provide orientation seminars and information on these guidelines. In Jordan in 2012, for example, when Zaatari camp for Syrian refugees was first constructed, a foreign psychiatrist working at a field hospital proposed conducting a survey to assess the prevalence of mental illness in the camp. The idea was discussed in the coordination group which also included national actors from the Ministry of Health; it was agreed that such an assessment would not be appropriate and that organisations would collaborate in developing assessment methods and tools in line with the UNHCR and WHO MHPSS Assessment Toolkit [22].

Another important function of coordination groups is the creation of referral pathways and procedures between different local and international agencies. In response to the Syrian refugee crisis in Greece, for example, the local organisation Babel began a coordination group inviting different local and international mental health professionals to discuss common problems, needs and pathways to refer between different agencies. Gaps which were noted in referring refugees between camps and urban sites were subsequently addressed in a project which funded mental health outreach teams going from local urban-based organisations to camps. In Jordan, the MHPSS coordination group has developed a common referral form for mental health problems, including consent to refer and provide essential information, which was then used by many different agencies [89]. This common referral form together with a guidance note has more recently been further developed and adapted for global use by the MHPSS IASC Reference Group [90].

6.2.3 Psychological First Aid (PFA)

In the aftermath of disasters there may be a range of direct and indirect sequelae such as the loss of family members, loss of sense of control over one's own life or a lack of access to basic needs and social support; psychological consequences tend to manifest in different ways and with a broad range of reactions, impacting not only on the individual but also extending to wider layers of the general population. These reactions are not necessarily pathological in nature and should not be regarded as precursors to subsequent mental disorders. Adequate provision of support and access to services will result in normalcy, fostering the healing process and resilience of affected populations [91].

Large-scale disasters affecting large numbers of individuals necessitate the need for basic supportive interventions which go beyond the bounds of psychotherapy or professional counselling. Such basic support should not be provided only by specialised professionals but also by lay community members [91]. The need for such early interventions, combined with the lack of evidence and potential for harm for single-session individual debriefing, has led to the development of psychological first aid (PFA) [92]. The term PFA encompasses a brief set of supportive, non-clinical, response to a person who is suffering and who may require social or emotional support [93]. It is meant to elicit feelings of safety, connection and self-help in people recently exposed to serious crisis events to promote recovery. The action principles of PFA are look, listen and link. PFA can be provided by anyone who is in the position to help by:

- Providing nonintrusive, practical care and support
- Assessing needs and concerns
- Helping people to address basic needs (e.g. food and water, information)
- Listening to people but not pressuring them to talk
- Comforting people and helping them to feel calm
- Helping people connect to information, services and social supports
- Protecting people from further harm

It is important to realise that PFA is not akin to professional counselling or psychological debriefing. It is based on robust principles that are rooted in evidence, but until now there are not yet many quantitative data and a strong evidence base around PFA in the scientific literature, and it is difficult to generate direct results for the effectiveness of PFA [94, 95].

Because of its simplicity and utility, PFA has been recommended by many expert groups [18, 96], and it has become one of the most popular interventions in the acute phases of humanitarian crises [97, 98]. It has been translated in at least 20 different languages, and specific adaptations have been made to address distress in children and in the context of Ebola [99, 100].

6.2.4 Integrating with Existing Health Services

> "To address the mental health needs of large populations, we need definite strategies and plans. Ad hoc arrangements and improvisations in response to each emergency will no longer be acceptable. Specific management ability, strong field experiences and evidence-based approaches are required... WHO strongly recommends the establishment of community-based mental health care from emergency through reconstruction. Earliest integration of mental health within the public health care system available in refugee camps and national services is the most efficient, and cost-effective strategy. The concerned communities must be mobilized and actively involved to decrease psychiatric morbidity and increase sustainability." [101]

The above statement by a former director of the World Health Organization was made at an international consultation in Geneva focusing on the importance of involving communities. Since then, these words have lost nothing of their urgency. Since 2000, the number of refugees and displaced populations has soared, with many more and more protracted crises, and the recommendations remain highly relevant.

6.2.4.1 Staffing and Resource Shortage for Mental Health

In today's world, health systems, particularly in low- and middle-income countries with a high number of refugees, face an unprecedented increase in need for mental health and psychosocial support. According to the WHO Mental Health Atlas, more than 45% of the world population are living in countries where there is less than one mental health specialist for every 100,000 populations [45]. Huge inequalities in access to mental health services exist depending on where people live. On average, globally, there is less than one mental health worker per 10,000 people [102]. In low- and middle-income countries, rates fall below 1 per 100,000 people, whereas in high-income countries the rate is 1 per 2000 people. Worldwide nearly one in ten people have a mental health disorder, but only 1% of the global health workforce is working in mental health. Low- and middle-income countries spend less than US$ 2 per capita per year on mental health, whereas high-income countries spend more than US$ 50 [45]. The majority of spending for mental health is on psychiatric institutions which only serve a small proportion of those who need care. Task sharing of mental health care by non-specialised health professionals as well as providing mental health care integrated with community-based settings remains a key and cost-effective solution to bridge the gap in mental health services and resources [103, 104]. In countries with many refugees, mental health services require special considerations. Factors such as an increased prevalence of mental health problems, weakened or overwhelmed mental health infrastructure as well as challenges of coordinating agencies and actors contribute to the difficulties of providing support for refugees [105]. On the other hand, postemergency reconstruction presents significant possibilities to raise awareness of the major gaps, worldwide, in the realisation of comprehensive, community-based mental health care. This is especially true in low- and middle-income countries where resources are scant [106].

6.2.4.2 Common Challenges in Integrating Mental Health Care for Refugees

Refugee crises and other humanitarian emergencies create enormous challenges to ensure even a minimum level of services for mental health and psychosocial support. In their attempts to alleviate suffering as rapidly as possible, humanitarian programmes may inadvertently create problems on the long run such as (1) creating parallel systems that are not sustainable and cause inequities between refugees and non-affected local population or even undermine the existing mental health-care system, (2) being driven by 'outsiders' and ignoring what people already do themselves and thus silencing or marginalising local perspectives and local views and (3) providing insufficient supervision and follow-up training due to the short nature of much humanitarian programming [107]. Many of these risks are not unique for refugee settings, but they may become more pronounced and urgent in such situations. Common contextual challenges in providing integrated mental health care for refugees include various interrelated factors as outlined below:

Emergency contextual factors:

- Global political interest in an emergency usually attracts donors and brings more funding opportunities (e.g. Syria crisis). Yet in several countries in Africa, large emergencies with huge numbers of refugees (e.g. in Chad or Cameroon) remain unnoticed [108].
- Protracted crises will suffer from gradually decreasing funding even if needs remain large [109].
- Complex security situations which prevent access to certain geographical areas will have a negative impact on training and supervision activities [110].
- Geopolitics and the historical nature of relationships between host populations and refugee populations can contribute to conflict, tensions and additional stressors.

Refugee population-related factors:

- Access to services may be impacted by language barriers and limited command of the host population language. Even if interpretation is available, the lack of direct communication may complicate proper assessments and establishment of supportive client-provider relationships.
- Cultural expectations are also important to consider. Refugees may have different cultural beliefs about causes and treatment of mental disorder and their own views on what to expect from mental health care and on what kind of information they want to disclose. This may impact on whether they accept a mental health diagnosis and the consequent treatment.
- Cultural belief systems of help seeking and coping amongst refugees may differ from what is common in the host country. Different belief systems may hinder mental health assessments and conflict with the practitioners' understanding, such as the possible tendency to seek physical explanations for psychological problems and to seek out traditional healers for severe mental illness.
- Refugees may be particularly distrustful of services and authorities because of previous negative experiences in their country of origin or in the host country. Moreover, they may be unfamiliar with the health-care system in the host country, in particular with the way mental health care works.
- In urban areas, there may be other factors hindering access for refugees such as cost of treatment or medications and cost of transport (e.g. the nearest service provider may be in another city).

Host country-related factors:

- The quality of social services in host country can also have an impact. A study of refugees from the former Yugoslavia, conducted 9 years after the end of the Balkan war, showed the importance of the support provided in the host country. Lower mental disorder rates were linked to being in employment, having appropriate living arrangements and feeling accepted in the host country [111]. This would also be consistent with the finding that on the other hand continued daily stressors increase the risk for mental health problems amongst conflict-affected populations [112–114]. Many low- and middle-income countries, hosting the majority of the world's refugees, do not have effective mental health systems to absorb the increased needs.

6.2.4.3 Clinical Tools for Mental Health in Low-Resource Settings

Training of general health care staff in mental health is critical to building capacity for recognising and treating persons with both severe and common mental disorders. In 2010, the WHO launched the Mental Health Gap Action Programme Intervention Guide (mhGAP-IG) for mental, neurological and substance use disorders in non-specialised settings; its newest version was published recently [115]. The mhGAP-IG presents integrated management of priority conditions using protocols for clinical decision-making. The target audience of mhGAP-IG are non-specialised health-care providers working at first- and second-level health-care facilities in low- and middle-income countries. These include primary care doctors, general practitioners, nurses and other members of the health-care workforce who are not specialized in treating mental health problems. Currently mhGAP-IG is being used in more than 100 countries, and mhGAP materials have been translated into more than 20 languages. The WHO and UNHCR published a specific mhGAP module for the Assessment Management of Conditions Specifically Related to Stress [116]. This module was then incorporated into the mhGAP Humanitarian Intervention Guide to address specific challenges of humanitarian emergency settings [117]. This humanitarian version is even more succinct than the regular version of the mhGAP Intervention Guide and can be seen as stepping stone to the full mhGAP. The conditions and chapters included in mhGAP-HIG are shown in Table 6.2.

6.2.4.4 Principles of Integration Mental Health into General Health Care

The World Association for Family Doctors together with the World Health Organization has developed a report highlighting principles as well as case studies for mental health integration into primary health care. These ten principles are central for the successful integration into primary health care and bear special relevance to countries with a large number of refugees (Table 6.3).

Table 6.2 Modules in the mhGAP Humanitarian Intervention Guide [117]

• Acute stress
• Grief
• Moderate-severe depressive disorder
• Posttraumatic stress disorder (PTSD)
• Psychosis
• Epilepsy/seizures
• Intellectual disability
• Harmful use of alcohol and drugs
• Suicide
• Other significant mental health complaints

Table 6.3 Principles of mental health integration into primary care [118]

WHO/WONCA principles of mental health integration into primary health care	Relevance to the context of integration of mental health into primary health care in refugees contexts
Policy and plans need to incorporate primary care for mental health	National policy and plans need to consider universal access to health-care services to all persons in the country, including refugees, and must ensure the system is enabling access to refugees at equal or lower costs than the host population
Advocacy is required to shift attitudes and behaviour	Refugees with mental disorders may suffer from dual discrimination limiting access to health care, first as a refugee and second as a person living with mental disorder
Adequate training of primary care workers is required	Training of health workers on recognition of various cultural presentation of symptoms as well on the available range of services for the refugees in community
Primary care tasks must be limited and doable	Experts can use available tools (e.g. mhGAP-HIG) which focus on selected group of priority mental health conditions
Specialist mental health professionals and facilities must be available to support primary care	Involvement of specialists from the refugee population to support on the job training and management of complicated cases. Recruitment of health staff and community health workers (CHWs) amongst the refugee population and involvement of the refugee community leadership in coordination will ensure a health-care programme that is culturally appropriate, accessible and affordable [119]
Patients must have access to essential psychotropic medications in primary care	Mental health professionals should adapt pharmacological and psychological interventions to the culture and needs of the refugee population. Programmes should adhere to national and global guidelines on which psychotropic medications to include and work towards sustainability of medication supply. Professionals should also be aware of the substantial variation of psychopharmacological responses across cultures and ethnicities
Integration is a process, not an event	The integration process can take several years and requires advocacy targeting decision-makers as well as at donors. Public health programme planers and implementers can use demonstration pilot projects as proof of concept to attract further support and funds for mental health reform and scale-up of services for refugees as well as for host population [106]. Important is to take explicit actions against inadvertently favouring pharmacological solutions as a 'quick fix' above more appropriate psychological and social interventions [120]
A mental health service coordinator is crucial	Optimise the coordination of services. Research has shown that in almost all Western countries, experts identify the fragmentation of care systems as a major problem for marginalised groups, such as refugees [121]. Coordination should include specialised as well as generic services

(continued)

Table 6.3 (continued)

WHO/WONCA principles of mental health integration into primary health care	Relevance to the context of integration of mental health into primary health care in refugees contexts
Collaboration with other non-health sectors, non-governmental organisations, village and community health workers and volunteers is required	Refugees can present with complex medical and nonmedical needs. Medical needs can include infectious diseases, non-communicable diseases and complications from injuries due to trauma, including torture and violence. Reasons for the complexity of medical needs include the high burden of disease in the country of origin, the lack of access to health care and other pre- and post-migration stressors. Nonmedical needs can include housing, employment and education. The integration of services for refugees who have mental disorders typically requires collaboration amongst various sectors and stakeholders, both specialist and non-specialist health services providers, service users, family and friends, community leaders, education and employment services. Governmental health services (e.g. public health justice system, child welfare, disability, transportation) as well as non-governmental organisations (e.g. UN agencies, legal aid, protection services, gender-based violence programmes) also need to be involved
Financial and human resources are needed	Funding is required to establish and maintain care services for large number of refugees, to mainstream interpreting services and to provide and disseminate information to both refugee groups and professionals

6.2.4.5 Health Professionals Amongst the Refugee Population Supporting Other Refugees

In Turkey, during the Syrian Crisis, the Ministry of Health together with the International Humanitarian Community is building the capacity of Syrian doctors living in Turkey using mhGAP-IG to provide services at migrant health centres to Syrian refugees. Another strong example comes from Syria itself. In 2011, before the Syria conflict, UNHCR and the International Medical Corps in Syria were already in the area, operating comprehensive mental health and psychosocial support programmes for Iraqi refugees who were already in the country. When the crisis started, the Syrian population had increasing mental health needs. In 2012, programmes were expanded to support Syrians affected by conflict through a mixture of (mobile) individualised case management, family- and community-level supports provided by outreach volunteers and targeted assistance to displaced persons living in collective shelters [121].

6.2.4.6 Utilising Refugee Crises as an Opportunity to Foster Mental Health System Reforms

Whilst providing comprehensive and culturally appropriate and sustainable mental health services to refugees poses numerous challenges, refugee setting can also provide opportunities that, paradoxically, provide ingredients for structural improvement of mental health services such as increased funding opportunities, an influx of good human resources and an increased awareness of the importance of mental health and psychosocial wellbeing, sometimes generated through media attention on the topic [122, 123]. The availability of such factors, in otherwise disadvantaged or marginalised regions, can provide real opportunities to start new initiatives that boost mental health care, and the massive needs arising in acute refugee settings may prompt health authorities to accept piloting new initiatives for mental health-care provision, including the training of general health workers, the use of paramedical staff and working closely with communities which may provide the impetus to include mental health care in health sector reforms [124–129]. This can lead to real change as has been demonstrated by the case studies of ten emergency-affected populations collected in the WHO publication *Building Back Better: Sustainable mental health care after disasters* [106]. Enablers of integrating refugee services to health-care services include:

- Sufficient funding
- Refugee and host population champions
- Government buy-in and support for need of mental health services
- MH services integrated with existing systems that serve both refugee and host populations (rather than parallel mental health services only for refugees)
- Good service organisation
- Good rollout of both training and supervision [130–133]

The Middle East and North Africa region is one of the largest sources of refugees and IDPs due to the crises in Iraq, Syria, Yemen and Palestine; the region correspondingly also hosts most refugees. The mental health systems in this region are typically reliant on large psychiatric institutions centralised around major cities with limited community mental health services. The influx of large number of refugees in countries such as Jordan and Lebanon has brought several challenges as well as several opportunities [8]. If such opportunities are utilised, real change can happen as is illustrated in the following vignettes.

Vignette: Introducing Community-Based Mental Health Services in Jordan with Iraqi Refugees

Displaced Iraqi refugees in Jordan have received substantial support from several aid agencies. Within this context community-based mental health care was initiated, and a new mental health unit was established within the Ministry of Health to lead mental health governance. One of the challenges to mental health reform in Jordan—as in other countries—was the initial reluctance amongst many mental health specialists. Historically, psychiatrists were the sole professionals treating people with mental disorders, and their main approach was through a biological model. The reform has posed a challenge to this approach as it promoted comprehensive, biopsychosocial interventions emphasising the role of multidisciplinary teams; the reform also focused on the integration of mental health services at a primary health-care level for the first time and advocated for providing care for selected priority mental health conditions using general practitioners. This challenge was addressed through several means: involving all psychiatrists in the reform process, relying on supportive 'champions' to serve as change agents within their fields, harnessing the motivation and determination of other mental health professionals to support reform and benefiting from strong support at the highest political level [106].

Discussion: The Middle Eastern region represents the largest source of displaced people as well as the largest host of refugees. In each of the refugee-hosting countries, there are unique health systems; however mental health systems in the Middle East are typically reliant on psychiatric hospitals, centralised around major cities with limited community mental health services. An influx of refugees thus brings not only challenges but opportunities to develop these services and to 'build back better' [106].

Vignette: Reform of Mental Health Care of Lebanon Following Syrian Refugee Crisis

In Lebanon, with more than 1 million Syrian refugees (about one fourth of the population), the Ministry of Public Health has identified a wide gap in mental health services and decided to respond to the urgent need to strengthen the mental health system in the country [134, 135]. The National Mental Health Plan supported by organisations and agencies such as WHO, International Medical Corps and UNICEF was launched to reform the mental health system in the country [122]. Additionally, the Ministry of Public Health established a Mental Health and Psychosocial Support Task Force. This task force currently includes more than 60 organisations working on the Syrian crisis response in Lebanon with the aim of harmonising and mainstreaming mental health and psychosocial support in all sectors and improving access to care. One of the highlights of Lebanon's Mental Health Action Plan—which was unique in the Middle Eastern region—was the adoption of a human rights perspective as a cornerstone of the strategy. Equally the strategy highlighted not only the mental health of refugees but also of other vulnerable groups including other displaced populations (e.g. Palestinian refugees); persons in prisons; survivors of torture; families of those enforcedly disappeared; the lesbian, gay, bisexual and transgender community; and foreign domestic workers. Lebanon's Ministry of Public Health, together with international partners, is using mhGAP-IG to integrate mental health services into primary health-care facilities in order to provide services to both the host population and refugees.

Discussion: The importance of working with host communities has been a large part of the Middle Eastern refugee response. For example, before the Syrian conflict organisations such as UNHCR and International Medical

Corps were already working in the area operating a comprehensive mental health and psychosocial support programme for Iraqi refugees [136, 137]. When the crisis began and mental health needs were further increasing, an MHPSS programme was already well established through the resources and capacities of the Iraqi refugee population. Therefore in 2012, existing programmes were expanded to support displaced Syrians affected by conflict through a mixture of mobile, individualised case management and family- and community-level supports provided by outreach volunteers [138]. Equally, the resources and skills of the refugee population should not be underestimated: in Turkey, during the Syrian conflict, the Ministry of Health together with the international community built on the capacity of Syrian doctors living in Turkey to provide services at migrant health centres for Syrian refugees, using mhGAP-IG [139, 140].

6.2.5 Scalable Psychological Interventions

Existing specialised human resources, such as psychologists and psychiatrists, are often limited in refugee settings, and existing health systems, including mental health services, can be overwhelmed or unavailable for refugees (e.g. due to distance, cost). Nevertheless, the mental health needs are likely to be high in this population. One of the most effective and cost-efficient ways to make psychosocial interventions available and accessible to refugees is to train non-specialised staff in delivering basic interventions. Whilst several intervention studies targeting common metal health problems (e.g. anxiety, PTSD, depression) amongst refugees have been published, the intervention manuals used in these studies are rarely made public or shared with other agencies. There is a significant need to develop more evidence-based, culturally adapted and publicly available interventions which can be used by non-specialists. A number of evidence-based psychological therapies have been introduced into humanitarian settings in the last few years [141–145]. There is good evidence for their effectiveness in high-resource settings, whilst the evidence in crisis-affected settings is still limited but promising. These interventions can be adapted for use by trained and supervised non-specialists; however one major challenge is to ensure that such interventions are not used as ‘stand-alone therapies’ or to be seen as quick fixes for complex problems. Brief evidence-based psychotherapies can be used if they are contextually well adapted and functionally integrated within sustainable systems of care with appropriate training and supervision by more specialised professionals.

Problem-Solving Counselling or Therapy Problem-solving counselling or therapy is a psychological treatment involving the offering of direct and practical support. The service provider and person work together to identify and isolate key problem areas that might be contributing to the person’s mental health problems. This is done in order to break the problems into specific, manageable tasks and to problem-solve and develop better coping strategies overall. It can be used as an additional treatment option for depression and as a treatment option for alcohol use disorders or drug use disorders. WHO has recently developed Problem Management Plus (PM+) [146], a brief, non-specialist-delivered basic version of cognitive behavioural therapy (CBT) for adults in communities affected by adversity [146]. It is designed to address psychological and social problems through problem-solving counselling plus a range of interventions such as stress management, behavioural activation and strengthening social support systems. PM+ can be used with people experiencing a range of common mental health problems—such as depression, anxiety and stress—at different symptom severity levels. Initial research has found that PM+ is a promising intervention for reducing depression and anxiety symptoms in conflict-affected populations and there is potential for further developing and scaling up this intervention targeting refugee populations [147–150].

Interpersonal Psychotherapy (IPT) Interpersonal psychotherapy is a time-limited psychological treatment for depression, bipolar disorder, PTSD and other conditions [151]. It focuses on the links between the person's problems with functioning, mental health symptoms and interpersonal crises—such as loss, conflicts with others, social isolation and life changes. IPT can be conducted individually or in groups, and in community, clinical, primary care or other settings. In high-income countries, IPT is typically provided by clinicians. Evidence from low- and middle-income countries suggest that it is possible to train non-specialists, such as primary care staff, community health workers, community psychosocial workers and others, to successfully help people with depression in 8–16 session group IPT [150–153]. In Lebanon, IPT training has recently been provided to various non-specialised psychosocial workers and case managers addressing the needs of Syrian refugees and the vulnerable host community [154].

Interventions for Families There is a need for additional interventions to be developed including interventions focusing on families. Recent research on conflict-affected children found that important mediators for the relationship between armed conflict and a child's wellbeing include family variables such as harsh parenting, parental distress and the witnessing of intimate partner violence [155]. Furthermore, research has shown that parental mental health has consistently been found to predict child mental health in conflict-affected and refugee settings [155]. Therefore, efforts to improve child mental health should engage thoughtfully a consideration of mental health and psychosocial family wellbeing across generations. Most psychosocial interventions for children in conflict-affected settings have focused more narrowly on children rather than on their families and their broader environments [156]. Few case studies have described the use of family therapy in conflict-affected settings, and this is an area where more research is needed [157, 158].

Interventions for Harmful Use of Alcohol and Drugs Harmful use of alcohol and drugs is an often-neglected consequence of displacement given that those affected often seek to cope with the past and existing stressors using drugs or alcohol [159–162]. Factors that could drive people to abuse of alcohol and substance include higher levels of stress, unemployment and lack of livelihoods and problems in coping with a new environment and often a new culture [20]. Substance use problems can develop in the country of origin, in transit, in temporary refuge or in resettlement. Particularly at risk are men and those exposed to war trauma and people with coexisting mental health problems [163–165]. Much less is known about alcohol and drug use patterns amongst children, adolescents and women refugees. Adolescents and young adults could be specifically vulnerable considering the fact that these age groups are more vulnerable to drug use and disruption of social norms and family structure can add to this vulnerability.

Evidence-based approaches, such as screening followed by motivational interviewing or community self-help groups, show promise, but there is a need for a greater evidence base of interventions at the community level to address this problem in crisis-affected populations [160, 166, 167]. In practice, interventions for alcohol and substance disorders are often neglected in humanitarian settings [168]. Solutions likely require multilevelled interventions that include training health workers in identification and management of substance use problems accompanied by policy measures to restrict marketing and sales of drug and alcohol and with a strong involvement of communities [169, 170].

6.2.6 Community-Based Psychosocial Work

One of the main problems in societies affected by chronic adversity, including armed conflict and forced displacement, is the rupture of the 'social fabric'. As a result, people begin to lose trust in each other and mutual support systems which had existed before the crisis do not function anymore [4, 171]. Interventions to strengthen social support, mutual trust and solidarity are usually not seen as the unique responsibility of health actors, who tend to focus on the dysfunctional individual rather than the dysfunctional group or community. In many humanitarian emergencies, social and community interventions belong to the realm of specialists outside of the health sector such as in community-based protection, child protection or community mobilisation. It is, however, important for health workers to be aware of the social effects of humanitarian emergencies and to liaise with and connect people to agencies and groups involved in social interventions. Important elements include the use of participatory approaches and the promotion of community organisation, ownership and empowerment [172]. A key approach is to foster self-help within local communities as much as possible and to make use of internal support structures amongst displaced populations. With a greater involvement, people become more hopeful, more able to cope and more active in rebuilding their own lives and communities [173]. Community mobilisation and support are critical to care for people with mental distress or disorders. Key actions to include communities are listed below:

- Avoid doing what local people can do for themselves—and instead build on what local people are already doing to help themselves, including using internal community resources, knowledge, individual skills and talents.

- Support community initiatives and encourage additional ones to promote family and community support for all emergency-affected community members, including people at the greatest risk.
- Use multifunctional teams in UN agencies and NGOs in emergency settings.
- Use participatory and community-based approaches within a rights-based framework (e.g. if certain groups appear to be marginalised or excluded, find respectful ways to include them in decision-making processes, including people with mental disorders and their caregivers).
- When necessary, advocate within and beyond the community on behalf of marginalised and at-risk people such as people with severe mental disorders.
- Address human rights abuses in sensitive and culturally competent ways and address stigmatising or abusive practices [174].

Much of this can be achieved through community-based protection, a multi-leveled approach which may be used in refugee contexts. The approach works to provide services that are urgently required to prevent threats and abuses whilst also implementing programmes to enable people to improve their situation and restore dignity [173]. Finally, community-based protection action allows the changing of the underlying circumstances which obstructs a person's ability to realise their human rights. These levels are all strengthened via the active involvement and input of the community; the capacities, agency, rights and dignity of people are at the centre of programming [24]. Within the humanitarian response, such actions are not always explicitly labelled or framed as 'psychosocial', but they have, nevertheless, important effects on the psychosocial wellbeing of refugees and other forcible displaced populations. Some examples of this type of action are below.

Child-Friendly Spaces In the chaos of humanitarian emergencies, particularly in the early stage when comprehensive services are still being set up, the needs of children and young people can easily be overlooked. Displaced families and humanitarian workers have many competing priorities such as registration, providing food and shelter and ensuring access to other basic services including health care. Such contexts can constitute an unstable and stressful environment which negatively affects the emotional and social wellbeing of children who have already endured difficult events and hardships. Child wellbeing is often best fostered by the restoration of a sense of normalcy and safety in crises. For example, schools are often not yet established in the beginning of a refugee crisis and parents are often overwhelmed. A widely used intervention for children in emergencies is the establishment of child-friendly spaces. These are 'specific, identifiable spaces that protect children and young people from physical harm and psychosocial distress whilst assisting them to play and develop through participation in organised and supervised activities during emergencies' [175]. Child-friendly spaces are often hosted in temporary structures, such as a large tent or container, and provide a supportive environment in which children, under the supervision of trained facilitators, can be engaged in a range of activities including song, drama, dance, drawing, play, storytelling/reading, sports as well as learning basic literacy and numeracy. Child-friendly spaces have multiple goals that are not all strictly related to MHPSS in a narrow sense but also goals related to provision of physical protection and detection of children with specific needs, acting as a rallying point for community mobilisation or providing some emergency education activities. [176]. They are generally assumed to have a positive effect on the emotional wellbeing of children, but the evidence base for this is still rather limited [177]. Recent rigorous long-term evaluation of child-friendly spaces in various emergencies has shown positive effects, but not for all children in all settings.

Refugee Outreach Volunteers In many refugee operations, refugees are engaged as volunteers into a wide range of programmes in health, education and social services. Particularly in non-camp environments, where refugees would otherwise have difficulties in accessing services for themselves, the establishment of network of refugee outreach volunteers has proven to be of critical importance. Refugee outreach volunteers constitute a link between the professional humanitarian services and the refugee community. When programmes for refugee outreach volunteers are set up, psychosocial elements can be integrated in the training and supervision of the volunteers who can then be involved in information sharing, linking people to mental health services when needed and setting up support groups amongst other functions [138, 178, 179].

Community-Based Sociotherapy In Rwanda, a community-based group approach, community-based sociotherapy, was introduced in 2005 to address the social and psychological consequences of the 1994 Rwandan genocide [180]. Groups of community members, with different personal histories of adversity and suffering, share daily problems in weekly group meetings over 15 weeks. These problems can range from problems of family conflicts, fear, mistrust, gender-based violence, stigma and poverty. Through this process, the group functions as a therapeutic medium and facilitates the development of peer support structures. The groups are guided by trained facilitators who aim to create a safe environment where trust, care and respect can be built and rebuilt and where broken social relations can be restored [181]. The focus of sociotherapy is on the relationships between people rather than on individual symptoms, but there is some evidence to show positive effects on mental health symptoms as well [182, 183]. Whilst this approach was not initially developed for refugees, the method of community-based sociotherapy has been successfully adapted for use with Congolese refugees to Rwanda [184].

Narrative Theatre This approach uses community theatre to assist communities to identify and discuss common issues which are at stake in the community. The use of communal techniques creates a social space where people can exchange stories, discuss problems and share experiences from different perspectives. Participants both tell their stories and act them out in interactive theatre. Narrative theatre is usually done in environments characterised by poor resources, disrupted social networks and dependency on aid agencies and in areas of high psychosocial and physical problems, such as refugee camps or post-conflict settings [185–187]. More research is needed to investigate the effects of methods focused on collective healing on mental health and psychosocial wellbeing.

Working with Traditional Healers The involvement of community traditional healers can be important for providing culturally relevant mental health care. Healers can provide valuable insights on local beliefs, local terms used to describe symptoms and idioms of distress as well as information about identifying clients; in many cultures, people will go to these healers before instead of using Western medical approaches and seeking care at health centres. Involvement of traditional healers can be very successful but can also be marred with complexities [188, 189]. A collaborative system, with cross referrals, creates opportunities for mutual learning about beneficial treatments, addressing inappropriate and harmful practices, improving public health education (e.g. via conveying messages regarding misuse of alcohol or drugs) as well as getting support for follow-up of cases (e.g. administering and monitoring chronic treatment).

6.3 Future Directions and Recommendations

This chapter has outlined the complex challenges of addressing mental health amongst refugee populations including contextual factors (e.g. limited mental health systems in host countries, cultural barriers) and often limited donor funding and attention to mental health. We have also outlined key programmatic elements and recommendations in the areas of MHPSS assessments, coordination, psychological first aid, integration with existing health systems, scalable psychological interventions and community-based psychosocial work.

Past research on MHPSS in refugee settings has focused on establishing prevalence rates of disorders such as PTSD or has evaluated the effectiveness of specialised interventions delivered by professionals. It is now time to move on to broader and more operationally relevant research [144] and for researchers to engage with contemporary notions of resilience and social ecology [158, 190, 191]. For example, it is important to shed more light on question about how changes in the social environment can influence individual wellbeing and to investigate the effectiveness of interventions such as training parents of distressed refugee children and of other family- and community-focused interventions.

There is also especially a need for innovative and methodologically sound research on scalable low-cost mental health interventions that can be delivered by non-specialists (e.g. health staff, teachers, community health workers and other community workers) [192]. It has, by now, been well established that incorporating basic psychiatric services into general health care within humanitarian emergencies is possible, but little is known about if and how such interventions can be brought to scale and be incorporated in sustainable routine systems of care without unacceptable loss of quality [193, 194]. Similarly, there is now solid evidence that brief psychological interventions delivered by trained non-specialists yield remarkable results in research trials [195]. However, it remains a challenge to scale up and integrate such interventions without losing quality. Implementation research is needed that addresses questions around scale-up, supervision, staff retention and quality control [196].

Key features of effective MHPSS interventions include community engagement, partnership with government and/or local actors, delivery by trained providers, socially and/or culturally meaningful programme activities, being group based and programme providers who build trusting and supportive relationship with programme recipients [197].

Lastly, it is essential to make research findings accessible to implementing organisations such as international and local NGOs through open-access journals and to foster collaborative research involving national actors and including refugees [198, 199].

The field of mental health and psychosocial support for refugees has gained in strength, but the danger of losing momentum continues. We feel that real opportunities exist to include quality interventions within the humanitarian response for refugees in resource-constrained settings. This will require concerted efforts by researchers, practitioners and policymakers.

References

1. UNHCR. Global Trends Forced Displacement in 2015 [Internet]. 2016. https://s3.amazonaws.com/unhcrsharedmedia/2016-2016-06-20-global-trends/2016-06-14-Global-Trends-2015.pdf.
2. Baron N. Community based psychosocial and mental health services for southern Sudanese refugees in long term exile in Uganda. In: De Jong J, editor. Trauma, war, and violence: public mental health in socio-cultural context. New York: Kluwer/Plenum; 2002. p. 158–203.
3. Rasmussen A, Katoni B, Keller A, Wilkinson J. Posttraumatic idioms of distress among Darfur refugees: Hozun and Majnun. Transcult Psychiatry. 2011;48(4):392–415.
4. Ventevogel P. The effects of war: local views and priorities concerning psychosocial and mental health problems as a result of collective violence in Burundi. Intervention. 2015;13(3):216–34.
5. IASC Reference Group for Mental Health and Psychosocial Support. Review of the implementation of the IASC guidelines on Mental Health and Psychosocial Support in emergency settings [Internet]. 2014. https://interagencystandingcommittee.org/system/files/1_iasc_guidelines_on_mhpss_review-2014-final_2_0.pdf.
6. Weissbecker I, Jones L. International response to natural and manmade disasters. In: Okpaku S, editor. Essentials of global mental health. Cambridge: Cambridge University Press; 2014. p. 326–35.
7. Tol W, Purgato M, Bass J, Galappatti A, Eaton W. Mental health and psychosocial support in humanitarian settings: a public mental health perspective. Epidemiol Psychiatr Sci. 2015;24(6):484–94.
8. van Ommeren M, Hanna F, Weissbecker I, Ventevogel P. Mental health and psychosocial support in humanitarian emergencies. East Mediterr Health J. 2015;21(7):498–502.
9. Van Ommeren M, Saxena S, Saraceno B. Mental and social health during and after acute emergencies: emerging consensus? Bull World Health Organ. 2005;83(1):71–6.
10. Wessells M. A reflection on the strengths and limits of a public health approach to mental health in humanitarian settings. Epidemiol Psychiatr Sci. 2015;24(6):495–7.

11. IASC Reference Group for Mental Health and Psychosocial Support. Mental health and psychosocial support in humanitarian emergencies: what should camp coordination and camp management actors know? 2012.
12. Inter-Agency Standing Committee (IASC) Global Protection Cluster Working Group, & IASC Reference Group for Mental Health and Psychosocial Support in Emergency Settings. Mental Health and Psychosocial Support in Humanitarian Emergencies: What should Protection Programme Managers Know? Geneva; 2010.
13. Mackenzie J, Kesner C. Mental health funding and the SDGs: What now and who pays? [Internet]. 2016. https://www.odi.org/sites/odi.org.uk/files/resource-documents/10573.pdf.
14. Baingana F, Bannon I, Thomas R. Mental health and conflicts. Washington, DC: World Bank; 2005.
15. Marquez P. Mental health among displaced people and refugees: making the case for action at the World Bank Group. Washington: World Bank Group; 2017.
16. Meyer S. UNHCR's mental health and psychosocial support for persons of concern. Geneva; 2013.
17. UNOCHA. 2016 Humanitarian response plan Syrian Arab Republic. 2015.
18. IASC. IASC guidelines on mental health and psychosocial support in emergency settings [Internet]. Geneva: IASC. 2007. https://interagencystandingcommittee.org/system/files/legacy_files/guidelines_iasc_mental_health_psychosocial_june_2007.pdf.
19. Wessells M, van Ommeren M. Developing inter-agency guidelines on mental health and psychosocial support in emergency settings. Intervention. 2008;6(3):199–218.
20. Hanna F. Alcohol and substance use in humanitarian and postconflict situations. East Mediterr Health J. 2017;23(3):231–5.
21. Silove D, Ventevogel P, Rees S. The contemporary refugee crisis: an overview of mental health challenges. World Psychiatry. 2017;16(2):130–9.
22. World Health Organization, United Nations High Commissioner for Refugees. Assessing mental health and psychosocial needs and resources: toolkit for major humanitarian settings [Internet]. 2012. http://apps.who.int/iris/bitstream/10665/76796/1/9789241548533_eng.pdf?ua=1.
23. World Health Organization. Mental health: a state of well-being [Internet]. 2014. http://www.who.int/features/factfiles/mental_health/en/.
24. UNHCR. A community-based approach in UNHCR operations [Internet]. 2008. http://www.unhcr.org/47f0a0232.pdf.
25. United Nations High Commissioner for Refugees. Operational guidance for mental health and psychosocial support programming in refugee operations. Geneva; 2013.
26. Kaiser B, Haroz E, Bolton P, Bass J, Hinton D. "Thinking too much": a systematic review of a common idiom of distress. Soc Sci Med. 2015;147:170–83.
27. Patel V, Simunyu E, Gwanzura F. Kufungisisa (thinking too much): a Shona idiom for non-psychotic mental illness. Cent Afr J Med. 1995;41(7):209–15.
28. Ventevogel P, Jordans M, Reis R, de Jong J. Madness or sadness? Local concepts of mental illness in four conflict-affected African communities. Confl Health. 2013;7(1):3.
29. Cavallera V, Reggi M, Abdi S, Jinnah Z, Kivelenge J, Warsame A, et al. Culture, context and mental health of Somali refugees: a primer for staff working in mental health and psychosocial support programmes. Geneva: UNHCR; 2016.
30. Hassan G, Kirmayer L, Quosh C, el Chammay R, Deville-Stoetzel J, Ventevogel P. Culture, context and the mental health and psychosocial wellbeing of Syrians: a review for mental health and psychosocial support staff working with Syrians affected by armed conflict. [Internet]. Geneva. 2015. http://www.unhcr.org/55f6b90f9.pdf.
31. Jones L. Responding to the needs of children in crisis. Int Rev Psychiatry. 2008;20(3):291–303.
32. Sharma B, van Ommeren M. Preventing torture and rehabilitating survivors in Nepal. Transcult Psychiatry. 1998;35(1):85–97.
33. Kirmayer L, Pedersen D. Toward a new architecture for global mental health. Transcult Psychiatry. 2014;51(6):759–76.

34. Kirmayer L. Cultural competence and evidence-based practice in mental health: epistemic communities and the politics of pluralism. Soc Sci Med. 2012;75(2):249–56.
35. U.S. Department of Health and Human Services. Developing cultural competence in disaster mental health programs: guiding principles and recommendations. Rockville: Center for Mental Health Services, Substance Abuse and Mental Health Services Administration; 2003.
36. Crepet A, Rita F, Reid A, Van den Boogaard W, Deiana P, Quaranta G, et al. Mental health and trauma in asylum seekers landing in Sicily in 2015: a descriptive study of neglected invisible wounds. Confl Heal. 2017;11:1.
37. Dudley M, Silove D, Gale F. Mental health and human rights: vision, praxis, and courage. Oxford: Oxford University Press; 2012.
38. Human Rights Watch. "Chained like Prisoners" abuses against people with psychosocial disabilities in Somaliland. 2015.
39. Silove D, Ekblad S, Mollica R. The rights of the severely mentally ill in post-conflict societies. Lancet. 2000;355(9214):1548–9.
40. Handicap International. Disability in humanitarian contexts: views from affected people and field organizations. Lyon: Handicap International; 2015.
41. United Nations. Convention on the rights of persons with disabilities. New York: United Nations; 2006.
42. United Nations. International covenant on economic. New York: Social and Cultural Rights; 2006.
43. World Health Organization. WHO quality rights tool kit to assess and improve quality and human rights in mental health and social care facilities. Geneva: WHO; 2012.
44. World Health Organization. WHO-AIMS: mental health systems in selected low-and middle-income countries: a WHO-AIMS cross-national analysis [Internet]. 2009. http://www.who.int/mental_health/evidence/who_aims_report_final.pdf.
45. World Health Organization. Mental health atlas 2014 [Internet]. 2009. http://apps.who.int/iris/bitstream/10665/178879/1/9789241565011_eng.pdf?ua=1&ua=1.
46. World Health Organization. WHO MiNDbank: more inclusiveness needed in disability and development [Internet]. World Health Organization. 2017. http://www.mindbank.info.
47. Allden K, Jones L, Weissbecker I, Wessells M, Bolton P, Betancourt T, et al. Mental health and psychosocial support in crisis and conflict: report of the mental health working group. Prehosp Disaster Med. 2009;24(S2):s217–27.
48. Miller K, Omidian P, Quraishy A, Quraishy N, Nasiry M, Nasiry S, et al. The Afghan symptom checklist: a culturally grounded approach to mental health assessment in a conflict zone. Am J Orthopsychiatry. 2006;76(4):423–33.
49. Summerfield D. A critique of seven assumptions behind psychological trauma programmes in war-affected areas. Soc Sci Med. 1999;48(10):1449–62.
50. White R, Jain S, Orr D, Read U. The Palgrave handbook of sociocultural perspectives on global mental health. 2017.
51. IASC Reference Group for Mental Health and Psychosocial Support. IASC reference group mental health and psychosocial support assessment guide [Internet]. 2012. http://www.who.int/mental_health/publications/IASC_reference_group_psychosocial_support_assessme.
52. IASC Reference Group for Mental Health and Psychosocial Support. Recommendations for conducting ethical mental health and psychosocial research in emergency settings [Internet]. 2014. https://interagencystandingcommittee.org/system/files/1._iasc_recommendations_for_ethical_mhpss_research_in_emergency_settings_0.pdf.
53. Greene M, Jordans M, Kohrt B, Ventevogel P, Kirmayer L, Hassan G, et al. Addressing culture and context in humanitarian response: preparing desk reviews to inform mental health and psychosocial support. Confl Heal. 2017;11:21.
54. IASC Reference Group for Mental Health and Psychosocial Support. Nepal Earthquake 2015: Desk review of existing information with relevance to mental health and psychosocial support. Kathmandu; 2015.
55. Medeiros E, Orr D, Deventer J. Mental health and psychosocial support in Guinea-Conakry/Santé mentale et soutien psychosocial en Guinée-Conakry. 2015.

56. World Health Organization & Pan American Health Organization. Culture and Mental Health in Haiti: a literature review. Geneva; 2010.
57. Hassan G, Ventevogel P, Jefee-Bahloul H, Barkil-Oteo A, Kirmayer L. Mental health and psychosocial wellbeing of Syrians affected by armed conflict. Epidemiol Psychiatr Sci. 2016;25(2):129–41.
58. Kane J, Luitel N, Jordans M, Kohrt B, Weissbecker I, Tol W. Mental health and psychosocial problems in the aftermath of the Nepal earthquakes: findings from a representative cluster sample survey. Epidemiol Psychiatr Sci. 2017;2017:1–10.
59. Fitzgerald C, Elkaied A, Weissbecker I. Mapping of mental health and psychosocial support in post conflict Libya. Intervention. 2012;10(2):188–200.
60. IASC Reference Group for Mental Health and Psychosocial Support. Who is where, when, doing what (4Ws) in mental health and psychosocial support: manual with activity codes. 2012.
61. O'Connell R, Poudyal B, Streel E, Bahgat F, Tol W, Ventevogel P. Who is where, when, doing what: mapping services for mental health and psychosocial support in emergencies. Intervention. 2012;10(2):171–6.
62. Baca M, Fayyad K, Marini A, Weissbecker I. The development of a comprehensive mapping service for mental health and psychosocial support in Jordan. Intervention. 2012;10(2): 177–87.
63. Mental Health and Psychosocial Support Working Group. Who is doing what, where and when (4Ws) in Mental Health Psychosocial Support in Jordan [Internet]. 2016. https://data.unhcr.org/syrianrefugees/download.php?id=10531.
64. Adaku A, Okello J, Lowry B, Kane J, Alderman S, Musisi S, et al. Mental health and psychosocial support for South Sudanese refugees in northern Uganda: a needs and resource assessment. Confl Heal. 2016;10:18.
65. International Medical Corps, & Sisterhood is Global Institute. Mental Health and Psychosocial Support (MHPSS) Needs Assessment of Displaced Syrians and Host Communities in Jordan [Internet]. 2015. http://www.data.unhcr.org/syrianrefugees/download.php?id=10165.
66. International Medical Corps. Baseline Mental Health Situational Analysis Dollo Ado Somali Refugee Camps [Internet]. 2013. http://www.mhinnovation.net/sites/default/files/files/IMC%20Ethiopia%20MHPSS%20Situational%20Analysis%20Jan%2010%202013.pdf.
67. International Medical Corps. IMC Libya Mental Health and Psychosocial Support Assessment Report [Internet]. 2011. http://internationalmedicalcorps.org/document.doc?id=239.
68. International Medical Corps. Rapid mental health and psychosocial support situational assessment services, identified needs, and recommendations following the April and May 2015 earthquakes in Nepal [Internet]. 2015. http://internationalmedicalcorps.org/document.doc?id=672.
69. International Medical Corps. Syria Crisis addressing regional mental health needs and gaps in the context of the Syria crisis [Internet]. 2015. http://internationalmedicalcorps.org/document.doc?id=526.
70. International Medical Corps South Sudan & UNHCR. Maban refugee camps rapid mental health situational analysis: Mental health priority conditions, community practices and available services and supports [Internet]. 2017. http://www.mhinnovation.net/sites/default/files/files/IMC%20South%20Sudan%20Maban%20MH%20Assessment%20Apr2013-Final.pdf.
71. Cardozo B, Talley L, Burton A, Crawford C. Karenni refugees living in Thai–Burmese border camps: traumatic experiences, mental health outcomes, and social functioning. Soc Sci Med. 2004;58(12):2637–44.
72. Mollica R, Cardozo B, Osofsky H, Raphael B, Ager A, Salama P. Mental health in complex emergencies. Lancet. 2004;364(9450):2058–67.
73. Roberts B, Damundu E, Lomoro O, Sondorp E. Post-conflict mental health needs: a cross-sectional survey of trauma, depression and associated factors in Juba, Southern Sudan. BMC Psychiatry. 2009;9(1):7.
74. Scholte WF, Olff M, Ventevogel P, de Vries GSJ, Jansveld E, Cardozo BL, Crawford CAG. Mental health symptoms following war and repression in Eastern Afghanistan. JAMA. 2004;292(5):585.

75. Rodin D, van Ommeren M. Commentary: explaining enormous variations in rates of disorder in trauma-focused psychiatric epidemiology after major emergencies. Int J Epidemiol. 2009;38(4):1045–8.
76. Ventevogel P. Psychiatric epidemiological studies in Afghanistan. A critical review of literature and future directions. J Pak Psychiatr Assoc. 2005;2(1):9–12.
77. Rasmussen A, Ventevogel P, Sancilio A, Eggerman M, Panter-Brick C. Comparing the validity of the self reporting questionnaire and the Afghan symptom checklist: dysphoria, aggression, and gender in transcultural assessment of mental health. BMC Psychiatry. 2014;14(1):206.
78. Kleinman A. Writing at the margin. 1st ed. Berkeley: University of California Press; 1997.
79. Kohrt B, Rasmussen A, Kaiser B, Haroz E, Maharjan S, Mutamba B, et al. Cultural concepts of distress and psychiatric disorders: literature review and research recommendations for global mental health epidemiology. Int J Epidemiol. 2013;43(2):365–406.
80. Haroz E, Ritchey M, Bass J, Kohrt B, Augustinavicius J, Michalopoulos L, et al. How is depression experienced around the world? A systematic review of qualitative literature. Soc Sci Med. 2017;183:151–62.
81. Kirmayer L, Gomez-Carrillo A, Veissière S. Culture and depression in global mental health: An ecosocial approach to the phenomenology of psychiatric disorders. Soc Sci Med. 2017;183:163–8.
82. Tol W, Komproe I, Susanty D, Jordans M, Macy R, De Jong J. School-based mental health intervention for children affected by political violence in Indonesia. JAMA. 2008;300(6):655.
83. Bolton P, Bass J, Betancourt T, Speelman L, Onyango G, Clougherty K, et al. Interventions for depression symptoms among adolescent survivors of war and displacement in Northern Uganda. JAMA. 2007;298(5):519.
84. Eisenbruch M, de Jong J, van de Put W. Bringing order out of chaos: A culturally competent approach to managing the problems of refugees and victims of organized violence. J Trauma Stress. 2004;17(2):123–31.
85. Chiumento A, Rahman A, Frith L, Snider L, Tol W. Ethical standards for mental health and psychosocial support research in emergencies: review of literature and current debates. Glob Health. 2017;13(1):8.
86. International Medical Corps. Rapid Mental Health and Psychosocial Support Assessment: needs, services, and recommendations for support to refugees, asylum seekers, and migrants in Northern and Central Greece [Internet]. 2016. https://data.unhcr.org/mediterranean/download.php?id=1814.
87. IASC. Interagency Statement on Mental Health and Psychosocial Support in Gaza in 2009: principles and response [Internet]. 2009. http://internationalmedicalcorps.org/document.doc?id=2.
88. IASC. Guidance Note for Mental Health and Psychosocial Support Haiti Earthquake Emergency Response [Internet]. 2010. https://www.apa.org/international/resources/info/haiti-guidelines.pdf.
89. IASC. Inter-Agency Guidance Note for Mental Health and Psychosocial Support Jordan Response to Displaced Syrians [Internet]. 2017. https://data.unhcr.org/syrian refugees/download.php?id=4079.
90. IASC Reference Group for Mental Health and Psychosocial Support. Inter-agency referral form and guidance note. Geneva; 2017.
91. Hobfoll S, Watson P, Bell C, Bryant R, Brymer M, Friedman M, et al. Five essential elements of immediate and mid-term mass trauma intervention: empirical evidence. Focus. 2009;7(2):221–42.
92. Rose S, Bisson J, Churchill R, Wessely S. Psychological debriefing for preventing post traumatic stress disorder (PTSD). Cochrane Database Syst Rev. 2002;2:CD000560.
93. World Health Organization, War Trauma Foundation & World Vision International. Psychological first aid: guide for field workers. Geneva: WHO; 2011.
94. Bisson J, Lewis C. Systematic review of psychological first aid [Internet]. 2009. https://mhpss.net/?get=178/1350270188-PFASystematicReviewBissonCatrin.pdf.

95. Dieltjens T, Moonens I, Van Praet K, De Buck E, Vandekerckhove P. A systematic literature search on psychological first aid: lack of evidence to develop guidelines. PLoS ONE. 2014;9(12):e114714.
96. Sphere Project. Sphere handbook: humanitarian charter and minimum standards in disaster response, 2011 [Internet]. 1st ed. 2011 [cited 12 June 2017]. http://www.ifrc.org/PageFiles/95530/The-Sphere-Project-Handbook-20111.pdf.
97. Gkionakis N. The refugee crisis in Greece. Intervention. 2016;14(1):73–9.
98. Schafer A, Snider L, van Ommeren M. Psychological first aid pilot: Haiti emergency response. Intervention. 2010;8(3):245–54.
99. Save the children. Save the children psychological first aid training manual for child practitioners. Copenhagen. 2013.
100. World Health Organization, CBM, World Vision International & UNICEF. Psychological first aid during Ebola virus disease outbreaks [Internet]. Geneva. 2014. http://apps.who.int/iris/bitstream/10665/131682/1/9789241548847_eng.pdf?ua=1.
101. Brundtland G. Presentation presented at 2000 Mental Health of Refugees and Displaced Populations in Conflict and Post-Conflict Situations from Crisis Through Reconstruction, Geneva.
102. Kakuma R, Minas H, van Ginneken N, Dal Poz M, Desiraju K, Morris J, et al. Human resources for mental health care: current situation and strategies for action. Lancet. 2011;378(9803):1654–63.
103. Rebello T, Marques A, Gureje O, Pike K. Innovative strategies for closing the mental health treatment gap globally. Curr Opin Psychiatry. 2014;27(4):308–14.
104. Sørensen C, Bæk O, Kallestrup P, Carlsson J. Integrating mental health in primary healthcare in low-income countries: changing the future for people with mental disorders. Nord J Psychiatry. 2016;71(2):151–7.
105. World Health Organization. Rapid Assessment of Mental Health Needs of Refugees, displaced and other populations affected by conflict and post-conflict situations [Internet]. 2001. http://www.who.int/hac/techguidance/pht/7405.pdf.
106. World Health Organization. Building back better: sustainable mental health care after disaster. Geneva. 2013.
107. Ventevogel P, Perez-Sales P, Fernandez Liria A, Baingana F. Integration of mental health into existing systems of care during and after complex humanitarian emergencies: an introduction to a special issue. Intervention. 2011;9(3):195–210.
108. Goldberg M. The world's top 12 most neglected humanitarian emergencies [Internet]. 2013. http://www.undispatch.com/the-worlds-top-12-most-neglected-humanitarian-emergencies/.
109. UN News Centre. Between protracted and emergency crises - a case study of the humanitarian funding conundrum in Sudan. 2016.
110. Gavlak D. Healing invisible wounds of the Syrian conflict. Bull World Health Organ. 2016;94(1):6–7.
111. Bogic M, Ajdukovic D, Bremner S, Franciskovic T, Galeazzi G, Kucukalic A, et al. Factors associated with mental disorders in long-settled war refugees: refugees from the former Yugoslavia in Germany, Italy and the UK. Br J Psychiatry. 2012;200(3):216–23.
112. Miller K, Rasmussen A. War experiences, daily stressors and mental health five years on. Intervention. 2014;12:33–42.
113. Riley A, Varner A, Ventevogel P, Taimur Hasan M, Welton-Mitchell C. Daily stressors, trauma exposure, and mental health among stateless Rohingya refugees in Bangladesh. Transcult Psychiatry. 2017;54(3):304–31.
114. Jordans M, Semrau M, Thornicroft G, van Ommeren M. Role of current perceived needs in explaining the association between past trauma exposure and distress in humanitarian settings in Jordan and Nepal. Br J Psychiatry. 2012;201(4):276–81.
115. World Health Organization. mhGAP intervention guide for mental, neurological and substance use disorders in non-specialised health settings [Internet]. 2016. http://apps.who.int/iris/bitstream/10665/250239/1/9789241549790-eng.pdf?ua=1.

116. World Health Organization & United Nations High Commissioner for Refugees. Assessment and management of conditions specifically related to stress [Internet]. 2013. http://apps.who.int/iris/bitstream/10665/85623/1/9789241505932_eng.pdf.
117. World Health Organization & United Nations High Commissioner for Refugees. mhGAP Humanitarian Intervention Guide (mhGAP-HIG): clinical management of mental, neurological and substance use conditions in humanitarian emergencies [Internet]. 2017. http://apps.who.int/iris/bitstream/10665/162960/1/9789241548922_eng.pdf.
118. World Organization of Family Doctors & World Health Organization. Integrating mental health into primary care: a global perspective [Internet]. 2008. http://www.who.int/mental_health/resources/mentalhealth_PHC_2008.pdf.
119. UNHCR. Refugee health [Internet]. 1995. http://www.unhcr.org/uk/excom/scaf/3ae68bf424/refugee-health.html.
120. Ventevogel P. Integration of mental health into primary healthcare in low-income countries: Avoiding medicalization. Int Rev Psychiatry. 2014;26(6):669–79.
121. Giacco D, Priebe S. WHO Europe policy brief on migration and health: mental health care for refugees. World Health Organization Europe; 2015.
122. El Chammay R, Ammar W. Syrian crisis and mental health system reform in Lebanon. Lancet. 2014;384(9942):494.
123. Epping-Jordan J, van Ommeren M, Ashour H, Maramis A, Marini A, Mohanraj A, et al. Beyond the crisis: building back better mental health care in 10 emergency-affected areas using a longer-term perspective. Int J Ment Heal Syst. 2015;9(1):15.
124. Baingana F, Mangen P. Scaling up of mental health and trauma support among war affected communities in northern Uganda: lessons learned. Intervention. 2011;9:291–303.
125. Budosan B. Mental health training of primary health care workers. Intervention. 2011;9(2):125–36.
126. Budosan B, Bruno R. Strategy for providing integrated mental health/psychosocial support in post earthquake Haiti. Intervention. 2011;9:223.
127. Eisenman D, Weine S, Green B, Jong J, Rayburn N, Ventevogel P, et al. The ISTSS/rand guidelines on mental health training of primary healthcare providers for trauma-exposed populations in conflict-affected countries. J Trauma Stress. 2006;19(1):5–17.
128. Perez-Sales P, Fernandez-Liria A, Baingana F, Ventevogel P. Integrating mental health into existing systems of care during and after complex humanitarian emergencies: rethinking the experience. Intervention. 2017;9(3):345–58.
129. Sadik S, Abdulrahman S, Bradley M, Jenkins R. Integrating mental health into primary health care in Iraq. Ment Health Fam Med. 2011;8(1):39–49.
130. Bhugra D, Gupta S, Bhui K, Craig T, Dogra N, Ingleby J, et al. WPA guidance on mental health and mental health care in migrants. World Psychiatry. 2011;10(1):2–10.
131. Kane J, Ventevogel P, Spiegel P, Bass J, van Ommeren M, Tol W. Mental, neurological, and substance use problems among refugees in primary health care: analysis of the Health Information System in 90 refugee camps. BMC Med. 2014;12(1):228.
132. UNHCR. Ensuring access to health care operational guidance on refugee protection and solutions in urban areas [Internet]. Geneva. 2011. http://www.unhcr.org/uk/protection/health/4e26c9c69/ensuring-access-health-care-operational-guidance-refugee-protection-solutions.html.
133. Watters C. Emerging paradigms in the mental health care of refugees. Soc Sci Med. 2001;52(11):1709–18.
134. El Chammay R, Kheir W, Alaouie H. Assessment of mental health and psychosocial support services for Syrian refugees in Lebanon [Internet]. Beirut, Lebanon: United Nations High Commissioner for Refugees (UNHCR). 2013. http://www.alnap.org/resource/19540.
135. Ministry of Public Health. Mental health and substance use prevention promotion and treatment, situation analysis and strategy for Lebanon 2015-2020 [Internet]. Beirut. 2015. http://www.mhinnovation.net/sites/default/files/downloads/resource/MH%20strategy%20LEBANON%20ENG.pdf.

136. Harrison S, Dahman R, Ismail M, Saada E, Hassan M, Hassan R, et al. Against all odds. Intervention. 2013;11(2):190–4.
137. Hijazi Z, Weissbecker I, Chammay R. The integration of mental health into primary health care in Lebanon. Intervention. 2011;9(3):265–78.
138. Quosh C. Mental health, forced displacement and recovery: integrated mental health & psychosocial support programme for urban refugees in Syria. Intervention. 2013;11(3):295–320.
139. World Health Organization Europe. Training Syrian doctors in Turkey to boost health services [Internet]. World Health Organization. 2014. http://www.euro.who.int/en/countries/turkey/news/news/2014/12/training-syrian-doctors-in-turkey-to-boost-health-services.
140. World Health Organization Europe. Psychological first aid: first-line support in emergency situations [Internet]. World Health Organization. 2017. http://www.euro.who.int/en/countries/turkey/news/news/2016/11/psychological-first-aid-first-line-support-in-emergency-situations.
141. Bass J, Annan J, McIvor Murray S, Kaysen D, Griffiths S, Cetinoglu T, et al. Controlled trial of psychotherapy for congolese survivors of sexual violence. N Engl J Med. 2014;370(26):2547.
142. Neuner F, Schauer M, Klaschik C, Karunakara U, Elbert T. A comparison of narrative exposure therapy, supportive counseling, and psychoeducation for treating posttraumatic stress disorder in an african refugee settlement. J Consult Clin Psychol. 2004;72(4):579–87.
143. Patel V, Chowdhary N, Rahman A, Verdeli H. Improving access to psychological treatments: lessons from developing countries. Behav Res Ther. 2011;49(9):523–8.
144. Purgato M, Gastaldon C, Papola D, van Ommeren M, Barbui C, Tol W. Psychological therapies for the treatment of mental disorders in low- and middle-income countries affected by humanitarian crises (protocol) [Internet]. Cochrane Database Syst Rev. 2015. http://onlinelibrary.wiley.com/doi/10.1002/14651858.CD011849/abstract.
145. World Health Organization. Thinking healthy: a manual for psychosocial management of perinatal depression [Internet]. 2015. http://apps.who.int/iris/handle/10665/152936.
146. World Health Organization. Problem management plus (PM+) Individual psychological help for adults impaired by distress in communities exposed to adversity [Internet]. 2016. http://apps.who.int/iris/bitstream/10665/206417/1/WHO_MSD_MER_16.2_eng.pdf?ua=1.
147. Dawson K, Bryant R, Harper M, Kuowei Tay A, Rahman A, Schafer A, et al. Problem Management Plus (PM+): a WHO transdiagnostic psychological intervention for common mental health problems. World Psychiatry. 2015;14(3):354–7.
148. Rahman A, Hamdani S, Awan N, Bryant R, Dawson K, Khan M, et al. Effect of a multicomponent behavioral intervention in adults impaired by psychological distress in a conflict-affected area of Pakistan. JAMA. 2016;316(24):2609.
149. Sijbrandij M, Bryant R, Schafer A, Dawson K, Anjuri D, Ndogoni L, et al. Problem Management Plus (PM+) in the treatment of common mental disorders in women affected by gender-based violence and urban adversity in Kenya; study protocol for a randomized controlled trial. Int J Ment Heal Syst. 2016;10(1):44.
150. Sijbrandij M, Acarturk C, Aktas M, Bryant R, Burchert S, Carswell K, et al. Strengthening mental health care systems for Syrian refugees in Europe and the Middle East: Integrating scalable psychological interventions in 8 countries. Eur J Psychotraumatol. 2017;8:1388102.
151. World Health Organization & Columbia University. Group Interpersonal Therapy (IPT) for depression [Internet]. 2017. http://apps.who.int/iris/bitstream/10665/250219/1/WHO-MSD-MER-16.4-eng.pdf?ua=1.
152. Lewandowski R, Bolton P, Feighery A, Bass J, Hamba C, Haroz E, et al. Local perceptions of the impact of group interpersonal psychotherapy in rural Uganda. Global Mental Health. 2016;3:e23.
153. Meffert S, Abdo A, Alla O, Elmakki Y, Omer A, Yousif S, et al. A pilot randomized controlled trial of interpersonal psychotherapy for Sudanese refugees in Cairo, Egypt. Psychol Trauma. 2014;6(3):240–9.

154. Verdeli H, Clougherty K, Onyango G, Lewandowski E, Speelman L, Betancourt T, et al. Group interpersonal psychotherapy for depressed youth in IDP camps in Northern Uganda: adaptation and training. Child Adolesc Psychiatr Clin N Am. 2008;17(3):605–24.
155. Verdeli H, Clougherty K, Sonmez N. Training in Interpersonal Psychotherapy (IPT) in Lebanon. Amman/New York; 2016.
156. Panter-Brick C, Grimon M, Eggerman M. Caregiver-child mental health: a prospective study in conflict and refugee settings. J Child Psychol Psychiatry. 2013;55(4):313–27.
157. Miller K, Jordans M. Determinants of children's mental health in war-torn settings: translating research into action. Curr Psychiatry Rep. 2016;18(6):58.
158. Charlés L. Scaling up family therapy in fragile, conflict-affected states. Fam Process. 2014;54(3):545–58.
159. Jordans M, Pigott H, Tol W. Interventions for children affected by armed conflict: a systematic review of mental health and psychosocial support in low- and middle-income countries. Curr Psychiatry Rep. 2016;18(1):9.
160. Ezard N. Substance use among populations displaced by conflict: a literature review. Disasters. 2011;36(3):533–57.
161. Lai L. Treating substance abuse as a consequence of conflict and displacement: a call for a more inclusive global mental health. Med Confl Surviv. 2014;30(3):182–9.
162. Roberts B, Murphy A, Chikovani I, Makhashvili N, Patel V, McKee M. Individual and community level risk-factors for alcohol use disorder among conflict-affected persons in Georgia. PLoS ONE. 2014;9(5):e98299.
163. Weaver H, Roberts B. Drinking and displacement: a systematic review of the influence of forced displacement on harmful alcohol use. Subst Use Misuse. 2010;45(13):2340–55.
164. Clejan P. Alcohol and substance abuse: A quantitative and qualitative field study among the Chin community in Malaysia. 2011.
165. Ezard N, Oppenheimer E, Burton A, Schilperoord M, Macdonald D, Adelekan M, et al. Six rapid assessments of alcohol and other substance use in populations displaced by conflict. Confl Heal. 2011;5(1):1.
166. Luitel N, Jordans M, Murphy A, Roberts B, McCambridge J. Prevalence and patterns of hazardous and harmful alcohol consumption assessed using the AUDIT among Bhutanese Refugees in Nepal. Alcohol Alcohol. 2013;48(3):349–55.
167. Chen A, Smart Y, Morris-Patterson A, Katz C. Piloting self-help groups for alcohol use disorders in Saint Vincent/Grenadines. Ann Glob Health. 2014;80(2):83–8.
168. Ezard N, Debakre A, Catillon R. Screening and brief intervention for high-risk alcohol use in Mae La refugee camp, Thailand: a pilot project on the feasibility of training and implementation. Intervention. 2010;8(3):223–32.
169. Roberts B, Ezard N. Why are we not doing more for alcohol use disorder among conflict-affected populations? Addiction. 2015;110(6):889–90.
170. Benegal V, Chand P, Obot I. Packages of care for alcohol use disorders in low- and middle-income countries. PLoS Med. 2009;6(10):e1000170.
171. Streel E, Schilperoord M. Perspectives on alcohol and substance abuse in refugee settings: lessons from the field. Intervention. 2010;8(3):268–75.
172. Somasundaram D. Scarred communities. Psychosocial impact of man-made and natural disasters on Sri Lankan society. New Delhi: Sage; 2014.
173. UNHCR. Participatory assessment in operations [Internet]. 2006. http://www.refworld.org/pdfid/462df4232.pdf.
174. UNHCR. Protection policy paper understanding community-based protection [Internet]. 2014. http://www.refworld.org/pdfid/5209f0b64.pdf.
175. UNHCR. Community-based protection and mental health & psychosocial support. Geneva. 2017.
176. Davie S, Stuart M, Erwin E. Child friendly spaces: protecting and supporting children in emergency response and recovery. Aust J Emerg Manage. 2014;29(1):25–30.
177. Global Education Cluster, Global Protection Cluster, Interagency Network for Education in Emergencies & Interagency Standing Committee. Guidelines for child friendly spaces in emergencies. Field-testing version [Internet]. 2011. https://www.unicef.org/protection/Child_Friendly_Spaces_Guidelines_for_Field_Testing.pdf.

178. Ager A, Metzler J, Vojta M, Savage K. Child friendly spaces. Intervention. 2013;11(2): 133–47.
179. Hassan M. Personal reflections on a psychosocial community outreach programme and centre in Damascus, Syria. Intervention. 2013;11(3):330–5.
180. Mirghani Z. Healing through sharing. Intervention. 2013;11(3):321–9.
181. Richters A, Dekker C, Scholte W. Community based sociotherapy in Byumba, Rwanda. Intervention. 2008;6(2):100–16.
182. Richters A. Suffering and healing in the aftermath of war and genocide in Rwanda: Mediations through community-based sociotherapy. In: Kapteijns L, Richters A, editors. Mediations of violence in Africa: fashioning new futures from contested pasts. 1st ed. Leiden: Brill; 2010. p. 173–210.
183. Scholte W, Verduin F, Kamperman A, Rutayisire T, Zwinderman A, Stronks K. The effect on mental health of a large scale psychosocial intervention for survivors of mass violence: a quasi-experimental study in Rwanda. PLoS ONE. 2011;6(8):e21819.
184. Verduin F, Smid G, Wind T, Scholte W. In search of links between social capital, mental health and sociotherapy: a longitudinal study in Rwanda. Soc Sci Med. 2014;121:1–9.
185. Duhumurizanye Iwacu Rwanda. Community based sociotherapy pilot project Kiziba-Nyabiheke refugee camps. Kigali Rwanda. 2015.
186. Sliep Y. Healing communities by strengthening social capital: a narrative theatre approach. Diemen: War Trauma Foundation; 2009.
187. Sliep Y, Meyer-Weitz A. Strengthening social fabric through narrative theatre. Intervention. 2003;1(3):45–56.
188. Sliep Y, Weingarten K, Gilbert A. Narrative theatre as an interactive community approach to mobilizing collective action in Northern Uganda. Fam Syst Health. 2004;22(3):306–20.
189. Le Roy J. How can participation of the community and traditional healers improve primary health care in Kinshasa. In: De Jong J, editor. Trauma, war, and violence: public mental health in socio-cultural context. 1st ed. New York: Kluwer Academic/Plenum; 2002. p. 405–40.
190. West H. Working the borders to beneficial effect: the not-so-indigenous knowledge of not-so-traditional healers in Northern Mozambique. In: Luedke T, West H, editors. Borders and healers: brokering therapeutic resources in Southeast Africa. 1st ed. Bloomington: Indiana University Press; 2017. p. 21–42.
191. Jordans M, Tol W. Mental health in humanitarian settings: shifting focus to care systems. Int Health. 2012;5(1):9–10.
192. Vindevogel S. Resilience in the context of war: a critical analysis of contemporary conceptions and interventions to promote resilience among war-affected children and their surroundings. Peace Conflict: J Peace Psychol. 2017;23(1):76–84.
193. Patel V, Saxena S. Transforming lives, enhancing communities—innovations in Global Mental Health. N Engl J Med. 2014;370(6):498–501.
194. Eaton J, McCay L, Semrau M, Chatterjee S, Baingana F, Araya R, et al. Scale up of services for mental health in low-income and middle-income countries. Lancet. 2011;378(9802):1592–603.
195. Ventevogel P. Borderlands of mental health, Explorations in medical anthropology, psychiatric epidemiology and health systems research in Afghanistan and Burundi. Ph.D. Dissertation, University of Amsterdam; 2016.
196. Singla D, Kohrt B, Murray L, Anand A, Chorpita B, Patel V. Psychological treatments for the world: lessons from low- and middle-income countries. Annu Rev Clin Psychol. 2017;13(1):149–81.
197. Murray L, Tol W, Jordans M, Sabir G, Amin A, Bolton P, et al. Dissemination and implementation of evidence based, mental health interventions in post conflict, low resource settings. Intervention. 2014;12:94–112.
198. Bangpan M, Dickson K, Felix L, Chiumento A. The impact of mental health and psychosocial support interventions on people affected by humanitarian emergencies: a systematic review. Oxford: Oxfam GB; 2017.
199. Kohrt B, Upadhaya N, Luitel N, Maharjan S, Kaiser B, MacFarlane E, et al. Authorship in global mental health research: recommendations for collaborative approaches to writing and publishing. Ann Glob Health. 2014;80(2):134–42.

The Mantra of 'Do No Harm' in International Healthcare Responses to Refugee People

7

Nimisha Patel

Abstract
In the context of refugee movements as a result of a proliferation of armed conflicts and humanitarian crises, the role of international organisations in responding to healthcare needs is crucial. The ethical principle of 'do no harm' is oft-repeated but begs an examination of how power and interest may manifest in the attempts to develop and provide appropriate healthcare for refugee people and potentially lead to harm. This chapter examines these issues and identifies key tasks for those responsible for funding, developing and delivering healthcare for refugee people, to ensure the principle of 'do no harm' is not an empty mantra.

7.1 Introduction

At a time of protracted armed conflicts, a proliferation of humanitarian crises and related unprecedented refugee movements, the role of international organisations and civil society has arguably never been as critical as now. International organisations can play a vital role in developing and disseminating good practice and facilitating cooperation with and supporting states. There are a plethora of international organisations and non-governmental organisations working within and across regions to address the healthcare needs of refugee people, including life-saving healthcare and other mental health and psychosocial services. Yet, they seem to be increasingly bureaucratised, engaged in complex funding structures within a context of shrinking humanitarian budgets; many embroiled in competitiveness largely over funding and faced with a general lack of a coordinated response, entrenched conceptual debates and exigent challenges in implementing services for mental health and psychosocial well-being.

N. Patel
Clinical Psychology, University of East London, London, UK
e-mail: n.patel@uel.ac.uk

T. Wenzel, B. Droždek (eds.), *An Uncertain Safety*,
https://doi.org/10.1007/978-3-319-72914-5_7

The impact of violence in armed conflicts and the upheavals, multiple losses and traumas related to humanitarian crises can be devastating, wide-ranging and enduring, impacting on individual children and adults, families and whole communities. In addition, sexual and gender-based violence in these conflicts and crises can lead to life-threatening outcomes, including homicide, suicide, maternal and infant mortality and mortality related to AIDs, as well as many other health problems such as psychological distress, trauma responses and physical pain. The isolation of survivors, exacerbated by social stigma, shame and fear, can contribute to further health problems, as well as poverty and social exclusion as well as heightening vulnerability to exploitation and further harm. Those with pre-existing mental health problems and others with special needs can be particularly vulnerable to many risks and a deterioration in health, compounded by a lack of access to health services and specialist interventions.

Inevitably, healthcare, including psychological healthcare, is one essential component of an international response to refugee movements. Despite many innovations, initiatives and developments in the field of refugee health, where psychological health is concerned, globally we are still some way away from delivering evidence-based, culturally relevant, context-appropriate, prompt and quality services. In recognising that inappropriately designed interventions in humanitarian work can undermine local coping methods and reinforce unequal power dynamics and thus contribute to harm [1], there is increasing consensus across international organisations that any healthcare responses to refugees must do no harm, although what this means in practice remains unclear. This chapter outlines some of the key international organisations active in refugee mass movements and their contributions to mental and psychosocial healthcare. It discusses how we may first understand the mantra of 'do no harm' and, second, examine using the lens of power and interest, some of the shortcomings in the approaches of international organisations and traps which may compromise the delivery and quality of psychosocial care for refugee people. The chapter concludes by offering reflections on how the ambition to do no harm can be realised, beyond a mantra without teeth.

7.2 International Agencies and Healthcare for Refugee People

A number of international organisations have remits which encompass healthcare development, yet few exist primarily or exclusively for the delivery of refugee healthcare. International organisations include multilateral agencies, bilateral agencies and non-governmental organisations.

7.2.1 Multilateral Agencies

Multilateral agencies are intergovernmental agencies dependent on funding from multiple governments and NGOs, some taking voluntary donations too, and distributed worldwide depending on their strategic priorities. Examples of multilateral agencies which contribute to healthcare of refugee people include those outlined below.

The Office of the United Nations High Commissioner for Refugees (UNHCR) provides international protection and aid to refugee people and facilitates resettlement in other countries for those eligible. It provides aid to refugee people directly, as well as relies on extensive partnerships with other international and local NGOs, including by directly funding them to carry out activities to provide protection, assistance and support to refugees. In complex refugee situations and humanitarian crises, UNHCR operates the Refugee Coordination Model, in collaboration with partners, leading a strategic response to providing protection and life-saving assistance (including emergency shelter kits, basic needs support and other assistance covering legal services, detention monitoring and resettlement activities) by developing/using comprehensive interagency refugee response plans. UNHCR's emergency preparedness and response plan includes a strategy for the deployment of swift assistance, depending on the classification of the emergency, including the provision of health, alongside its stand-by partners.

The United Nations Works and Relief Agency (UNWRA) provides assistance and protection to registered Palestinian refugees in the West Bank, Gaza, Lebanon, Jordan and Syria. Operational since 1950, it is the oldest agency working with refugees. Its services are extensive, addressing immediate crises and long-term needs and spanning emergency responses, education, relief and social services, healthcare, psychosocial support, microfinance and protection and refugee camp improvement. Funding is from voluntary contributions and member states.

United Nations International Children's Emergency Fund (UNICEF) focuses on healthcare of the most vulnerable children globally, particularly those under age of 5 and mothers in developing countries. UNICEF works alongside WHO, and it also contributes to sanitation and water supply, child nutrition and emergency relief. It is funded by voluntary contributions of governments, non-governmental organisations, private sector and private individuals.

The United Nations Population Fund (UNFPA) focuses on family planning and poverty reduction.

The United Nations Development Programme (UNDP) focuses on health (maternal and child nutrition, maternal mortality and AIDs), education and employment.

World Health Organization (WHO) is an intergovernmental agency related to the United Nations, working autonomously but with the UN, within coordination mechanisms of the UN Economic and Social Council. Its central goal is the 'attainment by all peoples of the highest possible level of health', which includes mental health. The WHO provides direction, public information and education for health, technical assistance, training, health systems development and monitoring and evaluation systems for health programmes; it promotes research and develops standards and coordinates international health activities in different countries. Funding is from member states, voluntary contributions and non-state funders.

International Organisation for Migration (IOM) is an intergovernmental organisation whose mandate is to provide humanitarian assistance and services to migrants, including refugees and internally displaced persons, as well as advice to governments regarding migration. Its work includes the provision of training and support for psychosocial support programmes for migrants, including internally displaced persons and those affected by conflict.

7.2.2 Bilateral Agencies

Bilateral organisations are essentially government agencies from one country but where aid is distributed to developing countries. United States Agency for International Development (USAID) is one of the largest bilateral agencies. Other examples include the Danish International Development Agency (DANIDA), the international development cooperation for the Danish government; the British ministerial Department for International Development (Dfid); and Deutsche Gesellschaft für Internationale Zusammenarbeit GmbH or 'German Corporation for International Cooperation' (GIZ), the international development cooperation of the German government. Their contributions to humanitarian assistance, including healthcare, vary and depend on historical and political priorities, including foreign policy of the respective donor government. International healthcare agencies or NGOs funded by these bilateral agencies may then develop healthcare, sometimes offering basic healthcare, others investing in longer-term healthcare, in those countries prioritised by the funding bilateral agency.

7.2.3 Non-governmental Organisations

Non-governmental organisations (NGOs) may have a mandate only within a country or across a region or internationally. NGOs tend to be diverse in size, remit and reach, varying in terms of their contribution to healthcare, some offering more systematic services than state health services. The largest non-governmental humanitarian organisation is the International Red Cross and Red Crescent Movement, which comprises the International Committee of the Red Cross (ICRC) (under the Geneva Conventions, it provides protection and medical assistance to prisoners of war and civilians in international armed conflicts), the International Federation of Red Cross and Red Crescent Societies and the national Red Cross and Red Crescent Societies which offer a range of services, including disaster relief and emergency support. Medecins Sans Frontieres (MSF) is also an NGO providing health aid across many countries to victims of war and natural disasters, which may include refugee people. War Child provides assistance and psychosocial support to children in areas of conflict and in the aftermath of conflict. International Medical Corps also works across many countries providing emergency relief and health services, including mental health and psychosocial support to those affected by war and disaster, and helps rebuild devastated health systems. In addition, there are numerous national NGOs which operate within the country in which they are based, contributing to or specialising in providing health and social care and other services, such as legal, educational and vocational support to refugee people.

Overall, the healthcare response of international agencies is substantial, though with the exceptions of UNHCR, UNWRA and IOM, the healthcare response is not specifically for refugee people (including asylum seekers and internally displaced people). Most healthcare responses for refugee people are limited to medical emergency care (e.g. after sexual violence, injuries sustained midst armed conflict) and basic healthcare, whilst mental healthcare is largely neglected and psychosocial healthcare is limited to basic psychosocial support offered primarily via community workers and counsellors.

7.3 Mantra of 'Do No Harm'

Amongst international organisations, one dominant principle is to 'do no harm', in other words to not cause further physical or psychological harm or create further risks for refugee people. Whilst organisational mission statements, strategies and guidance may all avow the principle of do no harm, rarely is this principle unpacked beyond considering protection responses to a range of refugee protection concerns, such as child labour, exploitation, neglect or abuse, gender-based violence and the protection of others considered vulnerable (e.g. those with mental health problems, special needs, disabilities).

In professional healthcare, the principle of do no harm is derived from the Hippocratic oath in medicine and more widely incorporated in other health professional ethics. The principle is two-pronged in that it refers to both refraining from engaging in any activity which can cause harm and preventing harm by taking necessary action. Yet, harm is constructed largely in individualist terms—harm to individuals and the professional obligation in the dyadic professional relationship to protect the individual client or patient from harm in the course of healthcare. This individualised construction of 'do no harm' is limited in the context of refugee healthcare, for a number of reasons.

First, in refugee crises and mass movements of people, the risk of harm is not only to individuals but to families and whole communities, as well as to staff working with them. Individuals may be at risk of economic or sexual exploitation; physical, sexual or emotional abuse from others; trafficking; neglect; and self-harm or suicide. Families may also be at risk of destitution, exploitation and violence, whilst entire communities may be at risk of intercommunal violence, ongoing security threats, widespread destitution, illness, disease and malnutrition. International organisations have a positive obligation to do no harm to individual refugee children and adults, to refugee families and to refugee communities. Whist many international organisations have protection strategies and protocols, they rarely extend to considering the overlap between protection activities and the provision of physical, mental and psychosocial healthcare or the risk of harm within the actual delivery of physical, mental and psychosocial healthcare services. The risk of harm, then, is constructed as being 'out there', whilst neglecting the potential for harm embedded *within* the organisational structures, policies and practices—in other words, institutionalised harm.

Second, the individualised construction of the ethical obligation to do no harm also obscures the positive obligation of international organisations to do no harm to staff required to work with refugee individuals, families and communities. This positive obligation requires preventive action to ensure the security, safety, emotional and physical well-being of all staff, not just frontline staff since the experience of working with refugee people who are faced with threats, destitution, violence and insecurity can reverberate at every level of an organisation and staff from administration, communications, finance, fundraising and management can also be exposed to horrific and distressing stories and images of refugee people they seek to support and be left with feelings of helplessness, anger, guilt, exhaustion and distress. Again, whilst many international organisations have begun to address staff care, it is recognised as 'good practice', implying choice, rather than as a manifestation of the organisational obligation to do no harm.

Third, the imperative to 'do no harm' is rarely applied in international organisations as a matter of governance and ensuring due diligence in all its activities. Herein lie fundamental challenges for international organisations and those who work for and with them, since the negative obligation to do no harm requires a sustained and honest scrutiny of the complex and interrelated dynamics of and impresses of power and interest at *every level* and *every type* of healthcare responses for refugee people.

7.4 Challenges to Providing Mental and Psychosocial Healthcare for Refugee People

There are numerous challenges which arise in developing and delivering mental and psychosocial healthcare for refugee people. Some of these challenges are general and others may be specific to where these services are, for example, in resettlement countries (e.g. high-income countries such as in Europe, North America, Australia) or in particular regions (e.g. Middle East, Great Lakes) where the countries are in the low- and middle-income bracket. In focussing on the provision of mental and psychosocial healthcare for refugee people in low- and middle-income countries, some of the constraints and challenges international organisations face in implementing the 'do no harm' obligation are discussed, using the lens of power and interest.

7.4.1 Power and Interest

Power in relation to understanding distress and the work of international organisations with refugee people is considered here as both social materialist [2], including the adverse impact of the vast array of social, economic and material factors in the everyday lives and experiences of refugee people which impact on their distress (e.g. poverty, food insecurity, inadequate housing, lack of safety, sexual violence), and as discursive [3, 4], constructed in language and producing dominant social discourses, with particular social consequences. For example, the dominant discourses of psychological trauma and biomedical mental disorders in refugee people can be seen as biopolitical power manifest in the proliferation of the machinery and methods of 'trauma psychology' (research, tools, measures, interventions, etc.) which governs the practice of practitioners (individualising the distress of refugee people and 'treating' them by focussing on symptom alleviation). One consequence of such dominant discourses is the particular types of psychological and mental health services they determine, services which ignore or distance themselves from the social and material causation of refugee people's distress and suffering, thereby rendering the individualistic trauma discourse unquestioned and privileged over other subjugated discourses, for example, collective suffering, and subjugating and devaluing local and different cultural ways of understanding and working with the social and material realities of refugee individuals, families and communities.

Any exploration of power demands attention to the various parallel and related interests. These interests are not necessarily or intentionally malign or coercive, but may have negative consequences for refugee people. Interests can include macro-level economic and political interests of governments, funders, global corporations, international organisations, pharmaceutical companies and the 'psy' professions (e.g. psychaitry, psychology, psychotherapy etc.). Interests can also include everyday and micro-level human interests we all have [5], including our own motivations, influenced also by social and environmental actors [2], professional and personal status, preoccupations, beliefs and values, with which also come our own blind spots or hypervigilance related to culture (manifest in cultural hegemony in healthcare and counter-resistance to the dominance of Eurocentrism), 'race' (manifest often in the dominance of Whiteness) and gender (manifest in the dominance of patriarchal worldviews and practices).

Inevitably, many of the challenges international organisations and other service providers face are extremely complex, highly interrelated and shaped by economic, geopolitical, historical and cultural factors. Some of these common issues of power and interest are explored, by looking at four interconnected areas: (a) refugee communities, (b) international organisations, (c) staff within international organisations and other service providers they fund and (d) concepts, models and methods used in refugee healthcare.

7.4.1.1 Refugee Communities and Power

Refugee communities in refugee camps or those seeking asylum or resettled within particular countries may have numerous and differing challenges and concerns. Three of these key concerns which explicate the dynamics of power and interest are presented here: safety and security, health and well-being and justice, reparation and rehabilitation.

The primary concern for refugee communities, particularly those in refugee camps, though also a concern for those resettled, is almost invariably safety and security against harm as a result of armed conflict, persecution, torture and other grave human rights violations, in other words safety from the abuse of power in discriminatory and violent actions of the state and/or other non-state and private actors. For those who may be particularly vulnerable (such as children, single parents, women, those with mental health problems, disabilities or special needs), safety becomes paramount and protection a legal, human rights and a humanitarian obligation.

Another key concern is that of health and well-being, also a matter of power, since the experience of being a refugee can mean a profound sense of powerlessness, partly as a consequence of multiple traumas, multiple losses and extreme hardship and lack of control over the circumstances in which refugeedom becomes necessary and where survival is thwarted by bureaucracy, a breakdown and absence of effective social support networks, lack of material and emotional resources, an overwhelming sense of uncertainty and lack of access to prompt, appropriate and accessible healthcare. That being said, refugee people also demonstrate phenomenal resilience and creativity in their survival, a riposte to the impresses of power and a robust expression of constructive and transformative resistance. Decidedly not passive victims of their circumstances, many refugee people can and do exercise power, in whatever way they can, active and creative in their survival. Yet, many of their attempts at survival are distorted by states, the public and media alike, mired in political debates which centre on whether refugee people are legal, truthful, manipulative, exploitative, criminal or terrorists in our midst. For many, surviving the battle to seek refuge is an ongoing threat to their safety, well-being and dignity. The threats posed by the external environment, hostility and violence from border guards, police and the public, combined with ongoing destitution may render many refugee people feeling they have no choice but to accept whatever help they are offered, by local NGOs or international organisations, however humiliating, enraging and disempowering that may feel or even where some of that 'help' is experienced as culturally inappropriate. Not being able to exercise the choice to refuse 'help', when desperate, is itself another manifestation of powerlessness. How indeed can refugee people say 'thank you for offering this accommodation, but no thank you it's not enough or adequate'; or 'thank you for offering us support, but no thank you to counselling'?

A third main concern for refugee people is how to access justice mechanisms and reparation for human rights violations, including torture, sexual violence, extrajudicial killings, arbitrary detention, disappearances, loss or confiscation of land, destruction of their homes and livelihood—all manifestations of the abuses of power by states and non-state actors. Whilst some international organisations have extensive protection mechanisms, not all those who work with refugee communities have the specialist knowledge, skills or mechanisms to ensure the identification and documentation of torture and other grave human rights violations, nor the means to offer or refer them to specialist rehabilitation services, nor the means to offer legal support to access justice mechanisms, if available. The lack of reparation and justice, with continued impunity and uncertainty, is also often a result of corruption, power and political interests. The continued material conditions of economic deprivation, temporary or no adequate housing, crowding, poor sanitation, limited food and inadequate clothing, compounded with impunity, prolonged uncertainty and ongoing lack of security, all create a vast arena of disempowerment, impacting adversely on health and well-being.

For refugee communities, these conditions and injustices can be experienced as a continued injury, exacerbating psychological health problems, for which healthcare services are inadequate or, worse, simply unavailable. Healthcare responses, where present, may be little more than short-term psychosocial support, and for many, with no options for other and more specialised psychosocial healthcare services, such support can be a lifeline in a vortex of suffering, yet insufficient to address the enormity of their distress and health problems and almost inconsequential in their impact on the root causes in their material and political realities. Essentially, the potential for harm lies in any diversion of the gaze of international organisations from these root causes, whilst offering psychosocial support which may be seen as a 'fix'. Nevertheless, such support is vital and an imperative as a humanitarian response, but cannot be said to fulfil conceptions of 'psychosocial healthcare' for refugee people or what would constitute 'rehabilitation' (United Nations Convention Against Torture and other cruel, inhuman or degrading treatment or punishment, Article 14) as a form of reparation for human rights violations such as torture [6] experienced by refugee people.

7.4.1.2 International Organisations and Power

As noted earlier, multilateral and bilateral agencies may provide healthcare services directly or fund others to do so, yet they operate within a politicised context of humanitarianism, beset with dynamics of power and interest: historical, political and economic. Their own funding may be from member states (e.g. UN multilateral organisations) and from private donors making voluntary contributions (including pharmaceutical companies), and United Nations member states or NGOs may be funded by multilateral or bilateral organisations, alongside other funders. The nature of funding and donors for international organisations may shape their funding policies and priorities. Similarly, decisions about where funding is directed is heavily influenced, particularly for bilateral agencies, by historical relationships, for example, former colonial relationships, between donor countries and recipient countries hosting refugee populations. Political interests, including foreign policies of donor countries, or of regions, also weigh significantly in decisions about which refugee communities in which humanitarian crises are prioritised and for how long, thereby shaping the strategic objectives of funding programmes, international organisations and, subsequently, the services offered to refugee people and their quality, reach and sustainability.

Many psychosocial support services funded or offered by international organisations may appear to be extensive (at least in creative calculations of the numbers of 'beneficiaries'—refugee people, reached), but remain relatively superficial in scope and short-lived in the face of enormous and enduring need. The country context, for example, a context of intransigent armed conflict, political and economic instability, lack of security and the sheer vastness and geography of a country, can also make the provision of comprehensive and quality healthcare services an elusive goal, particularly where some refugee communities may be dispersed and geographically inaccessible. Pragmatics and the availability of economic and staff resources inevitably determine what can be offered, by whom, in which areas and for how long.

Many international organisations have their bases in developed countries, where many of the healthcare strategies, training materials, manuals and guidance are developed and 'expert technical advice' is almost exclusively drawn from those developed countries with 'international consultants' (e.g. clinical psychologists, psychiatrists, psychotherapists) who are used to train local staff. Often international organisations use multiple 'experts'—international consultants, sometimes simultaneously and other times sequentially, none working in communication or coordination with each other, and sometimes with differing theoretical orientations and approaches, dependent on their own professional and academic training and their own country contexts. Few international consultants collaborate with local experts even where they exist, since international organisations most often privilege (and fund) Western expertise and knowledge, over and above local understandings and approaches. The control exerted via psychosocial and mental health programming has been described as international therapeutic governance, a form of control exercised by humanitarian actors acting on behalf of Western interests in order to manage global social risk [7] by using mental and psychosocial care to apparently promote development, human rights and peace; whilst programme funding is returned to Western economies [8], and geopolitical power is maintained.

Whilst the reasons for this are extremely complex and riddled with ethical and funding dilemmas and the policies and political interests of international organisations, it is an example of the impresses of power—how the politicisation of funding can determine the way in which psychosocial healthcare services evolve and related international programmes implemented for refugee communities. Since some refugee communities are transient, these services and their outcomes may be short-lived. New international consultants are often used for subsequent refugee crises and different refugee communities or sometimes even with the same refugee community, with each new consultant introducing new approaches and sometimes reinventing or reversing the wheel set in motion by previous consultants.

The consequences of the dominant or sole reliance of international organisations on multiple, external, predominantly 'international' (Western) staff and consultants are potentially manifold. Consequences can include (a) absence of a clear organisational strategy for the design, implementation, monitoring, evaluation and ongoing development of mental and psychosocial healthcare services; (b) absence of an integrated system and methodology embedded within the organisation to ensure periodic and routine needs assessment of mental and psychosocial health needs of the refugee communities in question; (c) absence of consensus on what is the most culturally and context-appropriate way to conceptualise the needs of heterogenous refugee communities and what are the most appropriate interventions for the relevant refugee communit(ies); (d) an absence of a systematic programme for the development of skills and knowledge for staff working with mental and psychosocial health needs; (e) absence of regular and meaningful monitoring and evaluation of mental and psychosocial healthcare services offered; (f) lack of integration of mental and psychosocial healthcare considerations across different departments and services offered by international organisations (e.g. education, social services, protection and advocacy services, vocational services, community activities); and (g) fragmentation and marginalisation of mental health and psychosocial healthcare services within international organisations. Together, many of these consequences serve to inhibit progress and the development of high-quality and sustainable mental health and psychosocial healthcare responses to refugee people.

In some cases of chronic refugee situations, for example, as seen in the Middle East currently, the absence of an effective state health and social care services and infrastructure in the host country (which may also be in a state of economic and political turbulence) can mean that neither the host population nor refugee communities they host can access appropriate services. The lack of services, trained personnel and effective referral pathways and mechanisms can further serve to maintain stagnation, if not chaos, in any mental and psychosocial healthcare services. Notwithstanding these immense challenges, protracted refugee situations provide an opportunity and make absolutely imperative the establishment of more longer-term strategies and sustainable mental and psychosocial healthcare services.

Arguably, external 'international' consultants may have a role, but mental and psychosocial healthcare services can only be effective and sustainable if they engage local staff, local experts and local NGOs and state healthcare services, working with international organisations, in developing a coordinated, integrated and coherent national and regional strategy and approach to service delivery. The issue of power however remains critical—which body should be responsible for the coordination of such an approach, and should the leadership be provided by the state or local consortiums comprising state bodies, local NGOs and experts or driven by the interests of international organisations and international external consultants with invariably relatively far less knowledge of and expertise in the local context? There are some, though scarce, examples of extensive partnerships and collaboration between international multilateral organisations and local NGOs, such as UNHCR's organisational strategy and practices; consortiums including international organisations as well as local NGOs and service providers, yet coordinated and led by state ministry of health (e.g. Lebanon); and innovations and extensive service development from local staff and experts, working alongside 'international' experts who maintain longer-term relationships with services, supporting the implementation and development of psychosocial healthcare services, as exemplified by UNWRA (e.g. in Gaza, Lebanon, Jordan).

Nonetheless, the operations of power are pervasive and transparent in what are designed as healthcare solutions for refugee people, by whom, for whom and to which (or whose) end. Competition for funding provided by donors and multilateral and bilateral international organisations also adds to these dynamics of power, fuelling bitter competition which can sometimes lead to the sacrifice of ethics and quality of healthcare or 'support' services provided, in exchange for funding for local and international NGOs desperate for survival, recognition and stake. For some NGOs, such competition can lead to opportunism and reaching beyond their organisational remit, mission and expertise—with adverse consequences for refugee people offered substandard services, which they do not have the power to question, nor the privilege to refuse, in the absence of other support.

The funding competition, financial and risk management conditions imposed by donors [9], financial instability and limited collaboration between agencies, often in the same arena, working for the same refugee communities, and in the same countries or regions, have been without doubt some of the most significant obstacles to developing effective and sustainable healthcare responses for refugee communities. This is despite a crucial advancement in multi-agency collaboration, illustrated by the work of the Inter-Agency Standing Committee (IASC) established in 1992 in response to General Assembly Resolution 46/182. The IASC's function is to be the primary mechanism for interagency coordination in relation to humanitarian assistance in response to complex and major emergencies, with many of its standing members including UNHCR, UNICEF, UNDP, UNFPA, WHO as well as invitees such as IOM, ICRC and the International Federation of Red Cross and Red Crescent Societies.

7.4.1.3 Staff Working with Refugee Communities and Power

Services offered by international organisations vary in the extent to which they recruit and rely on local staff. Where local staff are employed by international organisations, typically community workers and counsellors, their training or capacity-building, is increasingly seen as essential to ensuring a quality psychosocial service. How the need for such training is decided, who the training is delivered to and by whom also highlight various power dynamics.

Sometimes, extensive service delivery programmes are designed by international organisations, intended to be delivered by local staff, once provided with what is deemed by international advisors or consultants to be necessary training. Where local staff are trained to be trainers to build local capacity, often the training is dictated by Eurocentric models and interventions. The capacity-building of local staff is often shaped by needs assessments (if at all conducted) by external, international consultants, not local experts. The justification is often that local experts are insufficiently trained or expert or few and far between, though a careful mapping by international organisations of local experts is rarely to be found. Utilitarian arguments abound, but serve to obscure power dynamics and can lead to a culture of resignation and helplessness within international organisations and within local NGOs and health service providers, whilst also alienating local experts who could be crucial to ensuring cultural and context-appropriateness and sustainability of services.

Some international organisations employ 'psychosocial advisors' as staff. The role of psychosocial advisors can include contributing to the analysis of what is needed within the international organisation and on the ground in different country contexts. In addition, they may also contribute to the organisation or provision of training to staff within the organisation and developing relevant models and materials on mental health and psychosocial support. Few international organisations may employ regional psychosocial advisors who have an expertise relevant to the region. However, rarely do international organisations employ psychosocial advisors who are local and qualified health professionals, who speak the commonly spoken language in the region and who come with experience of designing professional psychosocial healthcare services and/or with clinical or field experience of working directly and specifically with the psychosocial needs of refugee communities. Yet, the influence of psychosocial advisors employed as staff of international organisations on what is funded by the international organisation or what is offered as services can have a profound impact on the ground. Whilst they may rely on advice from external (often also not local) clinicians with relevant expertise, the selection and prioritisation of any such advice is made by nonspecialist staff within the organisation, with guidance from the psychosocial advisors.

Where services are offered by an international organisation, or by local NGOs funded by the international organisation, the quality, breadth and standard of these services can depend on the number of available local staff who already have the necessary basic qualifications (such as in counselling, clinical psychology, social work, prior to any 'specialist international' training), to benefit from such additional training and to then offer psychosocial healthcare specifically for refugee adults, children and families and psychosocial support to communities. This in turn can be a result of educational and professional training opportunities locally and their accessibility and affordability—a matter of power and social inequalities, with privilege or disadvantage determining which staff have been able to access relevant opportunities in order to acquire the necessary prerequisite qualifications, locally in private institutions, or abroad, for those who can afford to seek such training abroad.

Some international organisations offer salaries to local staff which far exceed those which can be offered by local NGOs providing services to refugee people with local staff. This can mean that those with more qualifications are more likely to seek employment by international organisations, leaving local NGOs struggling to provide services to refugee communities, depleted of their most qualified and experienced staff and unable to financially compete with international organisations. International organisations are often then criticised for poaching or deliberate 'brain-drain', seen as undermining the sustainability of healthcare services for refugee people provided locally, either in local NGOs or the national health system.

Where training is offered by international organisations to local staff, it is almost exclusively provided by 'international experts'. Inevitably, the expertise of local staff, which includes their lived experience (sometimes as refugees themselves) and their intimate knowledge of the local and regional context, the local host population and the refugee communities and the nuances of the tensions and challenges which exist between these communities, is effectively not valued. Moreover, the 'expertise' of international staff is valued as better, unfortunately reinforcing the axiom 'West is best'. This is harmful to effective and respectful collaboration between international organisations and local staff, to the potential detriment to services for refugee people. The damage to the morale and trust of local staff employed by international organisations is also not uncommon, with few being able to openly voice their discomfort, for fear of adversely affecting their employment or future prospects. Where paid work is difficult to find and families depend on the salaries of local staff employed by international organisations, the scope to be critical or raise questions regarding these issues is constrained.

Another area where there is potential for harm to staff is paradoxically in situations where the safety and well-being of staff are of concern. The interest in embedding 'self-care' or 'help for helpers' has gained momentum in recent years within international organisations. Yet, self-care is typically constructed as an individual activity, in other words what individual staff must do to ensure their own 'self-care', or well-being, with the implication that 'help' for 'helpers' is actually individual staff's own individual responsibility. Self-care is one dimension of ensuring safety and well-being. The corollary is staff care, which specifically points to the organisational responsibility of international organisations (and the organisations they fund to carry our psychosocial healthcare for refugee people) to take necessary actions for the protection and well-being of all staff so as to ensure their own safety and to ensure they are able to carry out their work safely and do no harm to others. The tensions between these individual and organisational responsibilities lie at the heart of the mantra of do no harm. Where staff are concerned, who must do what in order to do no harm?

Harm in this context may also include exploitation or bullying of local staff and refugee people. Exploitation of local staff may take the form of differential salaries and working conditions for local and international staff conducting the same work, working the same hours and, in the same context, facing the same occupational hazards. Harm may also include sexual or other exploitation and the imposition of Western priorities and approaches in training, whilst ignoring or belittling and dismissing, if not eradicating, any pre-existing practices and models of service delivery as primitive, unsophisticated and incorrect. Harm may also constitute not valuing local staff and their knowledge and skills and their own expertise and lived experiences and understanding of local and refugee communities. Harm may also follow in the continuation of training and short-term initiatives in the same vein, by international organisations, failing to recognise that sometimes the positive feedback provided on training funded by international organisations is subject to a political economy where the end goal for local staff is not just improved skills and services but increasing the likelihood that there will be continued funding and salaries. Harm may also include the insistence and imposition of research agendas of the international organisation (or consultants or international experts they recruit) on local NGOs and service providers, in exchange for providing 'specialist training', but ostensibly to further the interests of the international organisation. Whilst it can be argued that local NGOs and service providers can benefit from such activities by the international organisations, the issue of power cannot be evaded—the extent to which local NGOs and service providers can turn away such offers linked to funding is extremely limited, particularly in a context of dwindling resources and fierce competition amidst service providers and local NGOs for funding and survival.

Harm can also lie in the potential to impose Western, gendered norms and Western values, when training local staff, for example, by ignoring local norms such as the need to allow appropriate breaks for prayer times; ridiculing (amongst trainers) the dress codes of women trainees wearing the niqab in the presence of men; minimising the need for professional interpreters by using lay persons (including staff who are not professional interpreters) to translate or not funding the professional translation of training materials; and dismissing requests or comments by staff during training for culturally or religiously appropriate material, or methods of intervention, such as Islamic counselling, as fundamentalist, amusing or absurdly unrealistic, etc.

The dynamics of power with respect to staff working with psychosocial healthcare for refugee people are not only pervasive at every level of services but often mirror the very experiences of the refugee people themselves. For example, feeling powerless, marginalised and voiceless, subject to economic and political interests of states and the interests of international organisations, feeling that one has to be grateful for any support or opportunity offered, even if it not one of their choosing, the feeling of constant insecurity, financial and in terms of their own safety and ongoing uncertainty—not knowing what may happen next, if and for how long their current state of relative stability will continue. These institutional group processes can be observed in many organisations providing healthcare, where the stresses, threats, fragile and temporary stability and uncertainties experienced by those who receive services are mirrored in the anxieties and defences staff and institutions use. Common social defences may paradoxically serve to bind together staff facing common anxiety and threats [10]. They can be seen in institutional practices displaying rigidity, authoritarianism, building of ever more bureaucratic structures and protocols, splitting, mutual suspiciousness, secrets and scapegoating. They can also be manifest in the overt dissatisfaction, frustration and anger misdirected at clients where staff feel unable to express their anxiety to management or the leadership within the organisations, who may be experienced by staff as oppressing debate, criticism, healthy conflict or open reflection on distress arising from the work itself. Unfortunately, failure to address these group processes, which include dynamics of power and the experience of powerlessness, can lead to organisations losing sight of their primary goals and functions [11], with risks to the sustainability and quality of any mental or psychosocial healthcare services offered to refugee people.

7.4.1.4 Concepts, Models, Methods and Power

An overarching impress of power in the field of refugee psychosocial healthcare is evident in the language and construction of 'mental health and psychosocial support', otherwise known as 'MHPSS'. MHPSS is a relatively new acronym, emerging in the last decade within the humanitarian field (though unfamiliar in the wider field of mental and psychological healthcare and social care). Used often as an umbrella term, MHPSS constructs mental health and psychosocial support as separate interventions, without articulating theoretically why and how they are separate or without demonstrating how and justifying why they should be separate in practice (see also the chapter by Wenzel et al. and other chapters in this book). In contrast, decades of advancement in the field of mental health and psychosocial healthcare globally points to a continuum and complexity of human suffering and distress, rather than as distinct categories of distress as *either* 'psychosocial' or as 'mental disorders', as the term MHPSS implies. Further, there is burgeoning literature which highlights the relevance of social factors to distress, including to enduring, complex mental health problems (e.g. [12–16]), thereby questioning the construction of only so-called 'psychosocial' problems as warranting a distinct and separate type of 'psychosocial support'.

To date, there is no agreed definition of MHPSS, and the now commonly used term 'psychosocial' is not easily directly translated into other languages [17], or culturally meaningful or familiar across different refugee communities. Yet, interventions for mental healthcare and for psychosocial support are rolled out, often as separate, silo programmes, by international organisations. These programmes commonly include one or more interventions, including the use of international psychiatrists and researchers on a time-limited basis, the provision of basic supportive counselling or trauma-focussed counselling, community awareness and development activities and the provision of safe spaces and activities for children.

In the World Health Organization's Pyramid for Optimal Services in Mental Health [18], mental health is defined primarily as a specialist area requiring specialist services (such as those provided by psychiatrists and psychologists), as well as what is referred to as 'informal support'. Informal support, according to the WHO can include community support, self-care and services which can be provided by 'non-specialists' (such as community workers, counsellors) in the community, in schools or religious organisations, predominantly identified as low-cost services. Specialist services in ascending order of specialism, and at higher cost, can be provided in primary family health centres, community mental health services and psychiatric services within general hospitals and, lastly, specialist and long-stay mental health hospitals. One difficulty of the WHO's pyramid model is the lack of any specific mention of psychosocial interventions (though the model may imply that it is included in the community and schools), which renders it invisible, or relegated to 'informal support', in contrast to what are considered 'specialist' interventions. Interestingly, whilst the WHO, amongst others (e.g. [19]), has established the importance of social determinants, specifically in mental health [16], its model of interventions does not address how those social determinants may be addressed. Further, this model for optimal services in mental health is not specific to refugee people, including those in crisis and conflict situations.

The Inter-Agency Standing Committee proposes an 'intervention pyramid for mental health and psychosocial support' specifically in emergencies (including natural disasters and armed conflict) [20]. This pyramid and guidance are not specific to refugee people but include mass movements of refugee and internally displaced people. The IASC guidelines, seen as representing best and current practice amongst UN and other humanitarian actors, use the term MHPSS to 'describe any type of local or outside support that aims to protect or promote psychosocial well-being and/or prevent or treat mental disorder' [21], p. 1. Whilst useful in its very broad definition of MHPSS and in acknowledging that support may be from local or 'outside' (presumably international) staff, this conceptualisation still makes a distinction between 'psychosocial well-being' and 'mental disorder'. Whilst acknowledging the importance of heterogeneity of recipients of services, in still distinguishing 'psychosocial well-being' from 'mental disorder', it too fails, like the WHO's pyramid for services in mental health, to address the nature, complexity, multifaceted nature and multiplicity of difficulties and distress that refugee individuals, families and communities experience—which do not fit into apparently neat and discrete categories of psychosocial distress or mental disorders—but which constitute physical, material, psychological and social distress and suffering.

Both the WHO's and IASC's pyramids of intervention are problematic in relation to refugee people in a number of ways. They do not address the scale, ubiquity and severity of distress and the abundance of social, economic, political and other factors which influence the well-being of all refugee people and internally displaced persons. Both pyramids of intervention do not acknowledge the wide range of interventions aimed at addressing the agglomeration of complex needs of not just refugee individuals but entire families and diverse refugee communities, including the needs of those who are subjected to human rights violations such as torture and sexual violence, where interventions require a range of interdisciplinary skills and methods, not easily or meaningfully discernable as 'specialist mental health interventions' or as 'psychosocial support'. Both risk the homogenisation and pathologisation of the experiences and the needs [7] of refugee communities.

In current practice, many interventions for refugee communities, families and individuals are not 'disorder'-specific, but address the very wide-ranging, interconnected and labyrinthine physical health, psychological health, social, welfare and legal difficulties which many refugee people experience simultaneously. These include lack of basic needs and impact of economic and food insecurity; malnutrition, illness and diseases as a result of the conditions in which they are forced to live; injuries and disabilities related to war; profound and ongoing grief for multiple losses, chronic fearfulness and anxiety related to ongoing food and economic insecurity, threats and uncertainty; individual and collective trauma reactions related to war, exile, torture and other human rights violations and abuses; lack of safety and security with ongoing risks of harm, violence and exploitation; physical and sexual abuse, violence, exploitation and neglect within families, within communities and in schools and refugee camps; and legal complexities and chronic uncertainty about legal status and the consequences for the rights to work, education and healthcare and whether they can ever build a life and home again. In the case of refugee torture survivors which constitute a significant proportion of refugee communities, interventions need to be specialised and interdisciplinary, providing psychological, physical, social, welfare, legal, educational and vocational support, sometimes simultaneously or sequentially, as needs dictate [22]. Such support is specialised and long-term, not a short-term, emergency response common in humanitarian healthcare, whether it is provided to individuals, in groups or to families; and it explicitly integrates the social or 'psychosocial' *within* specialist interventions.

As such, 'psychosocial support' interventions in humanitarian situations, relevant to all the aforementioned difficulties experienced by refugee people, are anything but 'soft' or 'basic' or 'informal' and can address a range and multiplicity of difficulties with consequences for overall psychosocial health as well as promote and build resiliency for refugee individuals, families and communities. Such interventions for refugee people may be more accurately described as 'psychosocial healthcare', to refer to a range of interventions of differing complexity, offered at every level of the 'intervention pyramid', by a range of staff. 'Specialists' may include psychiatrists, clinical psychologists, mental health and general nurses, physicians, social workers, counsellors and indigenous healers. Additional and complementary emotional support and 'specialist' social care for emotional and social well-being can be offered by all those working with refugee people, including teachers, community support staff, vocational support staff, legal advisors, protection and welfare staff, traditional healers and faith leaders within the local or refugee communities.

Such broad and interdisciplinary care can be and is delivered by some local NGOs whose core work is to address needs of refugee communities. Rarely do international organisations have the access to resources, expertise or experience to offer such care directly, given their remit is often to work in emergencies, providing immediate to short-term humanitarian support. The absence of adequate resources to offer such holistic healthcare is undoubtedly one of the greatest challenges faced by international and local organisations, though where resources are available, priorities and funding decisions are influenced by this conceptual blurring and artificial distinctions by international organisations between 'specialist' interventions for 'mental disorders' and apparently basic or informal support for 'psychosocial problems'. These practices in the field of 'MHPSS' also exemplify the dynamics of power.

First, power is manifest in the continued and unquestioned dominance of Eurocentric conceptualisations of well-being, based on Cartesian dualism in health paradigms, whereby the mind is seen as independent from, though related to, the physical brain, or as a function of it, and mental illness understood as disease categories. There is growing body of literature since the 1960s which refutes the medicalisation of distress and suffering, the location of pathology in individual biology and the neglect of social and cultural understandings of psychological distress (e.g. [23–31]) and the drift into drug-based psychiatry [32].

Current conceptualisations also highlight the predominance of the biomedical model of health, evidenced in the proliferation of the psychiatric diagnosis-driven approach promoted by the World Health Organization in its mhGAP programme [33] and applied widely, increasingly and unquestioningly to refugee communities in resource-poor settings. Ironically, the early definition of health in the constitution of the WHO adopted a broad social and holistic vision, defining health as 'a state of complete physical, mental and social well-being, and not merely the absence of disease or infirmity' [34] (p. 1). Latterly this definition has been criticised in its wording of 'complete', for unintentionally medicalising society, supporting tendencies of drug industries and professional bodies to redefine diseases and lower thresholds for new conditions not previously seen as health problems and requiring new drugs [35].

The WHO defines mental health as 'a state of well-being in which every individual realizes his or her own potential, can cope with the normal stresses of life, can work productively and fruitfully, and is able to make a contribution to her or his community' [36]. Yet in describing mental disorders (not mental health), the WHO [37] states that there 'are many different mental disorders, with different presentations. They are generally characterized by a combination of abnormal thoughts, perceptions, emotions, behaviour and relationships with others'. It acknowledges that 'access to health care and social services capable of providing treatment and social support is key'. Treatment is described as including medication and, in addition, for depression and talking therapies and family involvement for developmental disorders. No mention is made of specific psychosocial interventions for those with complex, enduring mental health problems, only medication and support to access education, housing and employment. These Eurocentric, medicalised constructions of mental distress as 'disorders' ignore social context, social material factors and social determinants of health, culture and gendered norms of differing refugee communities, and they dismiss alternative (and local) understandings of health and well-being which include the interrelationships between social context, the environment and the physical, psychological, spiritual and interpersonal (social) well-being.

Second, in constructing some interventions as specialist (invariably medicalised) and others as informal psychosocial support, there is an implication that the former are for more serious 'mental disorders' (effectively disease categories) and the latter less so, thus warranting lower-level support. This artificial split and underlying assumptions ignore the fundamental, lived reality of many refugee people—many may suffer severely and have needs which fall anywhere along the continuum of distress, whilst at the same time demonstrate immense survival and coping abilities, without crossing the diagnostic thresholds that may apparently indicate that they need specialist interventions in the form of 'treatment', including medication. The diversity, breadth and totality of their suffering is largely neglected; their needs homogenised and pathologised in trauma paradigms utilised by humanitarian agencies in psychosocial programmes [38, 39]; their suffering is fragmented by international organisations and other service providers and channelled towards separate activities and one-off or short-term interventions aimed at protection or general support or recreational and social activities or problem-solving and relaxation activities or counselling or medication, where resources permit. For those refugee people with pre-existing complex and enduring mental health difficulties, their suffering may be amplified by their experiences of becoming a refugee and the related stresses of social stigma, discrimination, abandonment or separation from family members and former carers. Interventions for them also warrant an interdisciplinary response which addresses their social and material reality and social determinants of poor mental health, isolation, marginalisation and psychological distress.

Psychosocial healthcare responses for refugee people should hence address the diverse and interconnected needs and lived realities of refugee people and involve a range of multidisciplinary, contextually relevant interventions aimed at the individual, group, family and community levels, which adopt a holistic and contextualised approach to a range of welfare; legal, social, physical, mental and psychological health; and interpersonal, familial and other difficulties. Such an approach is not biological, though recognises the biological aspects of distress. It does not rely on diagnosing 'mental disorders' which warrant only diagnosis-specific interventions (rather than those which address the maze of interconnected problems faced by refugee people), nor does it rely on expensive and potentially harmful medication [40–42] in the service of pharmaceutical conglomerates [43, 44] and their partners, which refugee people or local service providers are unable to afford or access.

There are several advantages of a contextualised, interdisciplinary, psychosocial healthcare response. One advantage of course is its focus on understanding and addressing the continuum of distress in an integrative way. Another related advantage is that it could go some way to address power asymmetries, by engaging and genuinely addressing a range of culturally, contextually and gender-appropriate interventions, integrating approaches deemed locally more meaningful, acceptable and appropriate. However, calls for 'evidence-based practice' [45] often ignore the absolute centrality of context in what might be considered 'evidence', for whom and where. 'Evidence-based practice' and, in particular, evidence-based medicine [46] have been intensely critiqued in recent years and questioned on the basis of ethical dimensions [47] and on grounds of being selective and ignoring questions of scientific validity in transferring from one region to another and 'scaling up' mental health interventions [48]. Power is also evident in the prioritisation and funding of so-called evidence-based interventions designed originally within high-income countries, predominantly for European and North American populations, based on studies often excluding those deemed 'different' (linguistically, ethnically, culturally) and then transferred and imposed on those for whom the original interventions and measurement tools were not designed.

In the humanitarian context of supporting refugee people, evidence-based practice should mean that there are (a) genuine efforts to establish the *evidence of such a range of individual, group-based, family-based and community-based interventions* for refugee people; (b) interventions assessed by *context-appropriate methods* and only using Eurocentric tools where strictly necessary, alongside other culturally meaningful and acceptable methods, and with tools which have cultural and construct validity and which are not merely linguistically translated and asserted as 'culturally valid' [49, 50]; (c) interventions which are *acceptable to and appropriate* for those with whom they are utilised; and (d) interventions which genuinely engage with concepts of health and well-being and *outcomes as defined by local refugee populations*—not imposing dominant Eurocentric constructs, tools and empirical methods privileged by international researchers, donors and service providers as 'scientific' and apparently as superior.

The third advantage of a contextualised approach is that services can more effectively integrate legal support and provide this in a way which attends to the psychosocial difficulties refugee people experience in attempting to seek safety and to rebuild their lives. Legal support and related activities can enable refugee people to exercise their rights and be empowered to seek and access justice and reparation for violations to which they were subjected. Together, such advocacy and legal support activities can be integrated as part of a range of simultaneous or sequential interventions to facilitate individual and social well-being, individual and collective agency and reparation.

Such service models for refugee people can be found in local NGOs in different high- and low- and low- and middle-income countries, including those hosting significant numbers of refugee and internally displaced people; and some international agencies, such as UNRWA, have also developed more integrative and contextualised services for refugee individuals, families and communities. Costs, unstable funding and lack of appropriately trained staff remain an ongoing challenge though, resulting in difficult funding decisions for international organisations in terms of where their interventions and funding are best placed to ensure effective psychosocial healthcare for large populations of internally displaced and refugee people. Some have argued that the state health ministries can take specific actions, for 'MHPSS' in emergency settings, by establishing health and emergency preparedness plans; providing national guidelines, standards and tools in responding to emergencies; training health professionals to identify and manage 'priority mental disorders'; and using opportunities to develop sustainable mental health services

[51]. Whilst laudable in the recommendations to states to ensure more long-term, sustainable mental health services, the need for contextualised and integrative services for both long-term and specifically for refugee crises situations is obscured; and criticisms of global mental health as the medicalisation of distress, or 'medical imperialism' [52] and a colonial discourse [53], remain unaddressed.

In the absence of stable and robust national health and social care systems, international organisations often fill a gap, effectively providing in the stead of statutory services, whilst funded by humanitarian aid, not state financing. In such circumstances, the scope of international organisations to impose critically unexamined 'international' standards, invariably constructed as universal, 'evidence-based' (yet Eurocentric) interventions supported by pharmaceutical industries, is enormous. In the context of mass refugee movements, the scale of the need is often used to argue that humanitarian activities (services) should reach as many people as possible and, by implication, that regardless of these dynamics of power and the shortcomings and potential harm of Eurocentric models and interventions, they are 'better than nothing'. Undoubtedly, human distress in individuals, families and communities warrants a humane healthcare response. In the absence of local, state-provided services, international organisations can offer an invaluable source of support, and such support may also contribute to preventing further harm within families and communities, prevent future crises and provide the basis of possible reconciliation and reconstruction of societies—as apparent in many post-conflict and transitional justice country situations. However, services for refugee people which rely largely on international organisations can rarely be anything other than relatively short-term fixes and relatively superficial in their reach and impact, yet devastating in their long-term impact of denigrating and eradicating local, culturally meaningful and appropriate ways of understanding and coping with suffering and distress.

The issues of power are discernible in (a) the dominance of Eurocentric models and methods; (b) the mantra of evidence-based interventions where evidence is defined within the narrow confines of positivist epistemologies, using Eurocentric, medicalised constructs and measures lacking cultural validity; (c) the artificial distinctions made between 'more serious' mental health problems and those apparently less serious psychosocial problems, requiring informal or basic support—leaving many in great need unable to access specialist and multidisciplinary and integrative care; and (d) local, culturally and gender-appropriate methods being rejected by international organisations as not meeting so-called international standards, thereby excluding local and regional experiences and understandings, which, if included, may point to more context-appropriate standards. The impact of these dynamics may be seen in the absence of coherent strategies and implementation of integrative psychosocial and mental healthcare services for refugee people by international organisations which in turn are also ill-equipped and inadequately resourced to establish such comprehensive healthcare systems. An additional consequence is the continued reinforcement of divisions between various programmes, such as mhGAP, focussing on 'mental disorders' and psychosocial support services. Where international organisations provide other healthcare, this too is often ill-defined, and typical activities such as emergency medical aid, food relief and providing water and sanitation are almost never seen as also including or necessitating psychosocial healthcare.

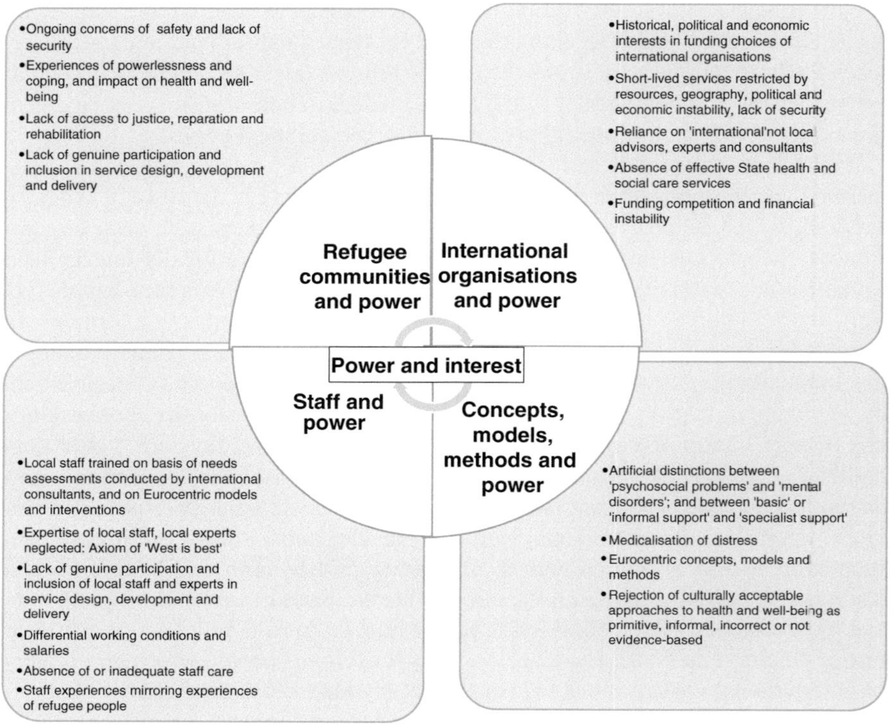

Fig. 7.1 Power and interest: psychological, mental health and social care for refugee people

In summary, the genesis of harm in the form of incoherent and predominantly Eurocentric models and methods arguably lies in the poor conceptualisation of what MHPSS actually means and, specifically, what it means for the suffering of refugee individuals, families and whole communities. The absence of any meaningful collaboration with local experts and any genuine respect and integration of culturally acceptable and appropriate interventions, which address local cultural and gender norms, adds to the potential for harm. Not only does this unquestioning propagation of Western standards and interventions as the 'gold standard' risk dismiss alternative understandings and interventions, but it precludes any real dialogue, genuine participation and inclusion of refugee communities themselves, local NGOs and local experts from similar or the same refugee communities in deciding what is best and most appropriate for refugee people in their society. Essentially, these are all issues of power, privilege and interest (summarised in Fig. 7.1).

7.5 Realising the Mantra of 'Do No Harm'

In examining some of the power dynamics and impresses of power in the healthcare responses of international organisations and other service providers they fund, for refugee people, one key question which arises is: What would be an appropriate and less disempowering way for international organisations to address mass psychological, social, welfare, physical, legal and other needs of large numbers of refugee people (children, adults, families, communities) affected by war, human rights abuses, displacement and related injustices, deprivation and ongoing insecurity?

The response to this question is dependent on many factors, such as the refugee community in question, the geopolitical and economic context, the cultural context of the relevant communities as well as the nature of the persecution, conflict, injustices and human rights violations that refugee children, adults and families have suffered historically, including in near history, and continue to suffer in the current context. Nonetheless, there are broad steps which may help to ensure that the dynamics of power are not harmful to refugee people.

The first step towards 'do no harm', it seems, may be to reformulate the concept of 'MHPSS' as 'psychological, mental health and social care for refugee people' (Box 7.1)—in a way that both honours the continuum of distress and explicitly acknowledges the role of social context and range of social, economic, political and cultural factors and experiences impacting on the continuum of suffering, distress and mental health difficulties which refugee people experience. The term 'psychological, mental health and social care' also does not make a distinction between 'psychosocial' and mental health—rather it acknowledges that psychological and mental healthcare and social care are inextricably bound.

Box 7.1 Conceptualising Psychological, Mental Health and Social Care for Refugee People

Psychological, mental health and social care for refugee people as

- Addressing the psychological and social care needs of
  - Refugee individuals (children and adults), couples, families and multiple refugee communities
  - Refugee people suffering from psychosocial health difficulties, including distress related to their social, housing and welfare conditions; food insecurity; legal status or uncertainty; lack of safety; multiple losses (of home, family and friends killed, separated, died during exile or disappeared); multiple traumatic experiences; torture; sexual violence; lack of employment, education or livelihood-building opportunities; social stigma and marginalisation; threat of ongoing violence, abuse, exploitation or neglect; etc.
- Addressing mental health needs which may be pre-existing, including those refugee people with
  - Severe, enduring and complex mental health problems, perhaps previously living at home, in hospitals or in long-stay institutions
  - Severe, enduring and complex mental health problems who may be particularly vulnerable during war or emergencies, not least because of their difficulties in social functioning, not having access to appropriate protection and appropriate healthcare and not having access to family support where family members have become separated, killed, displaced or disappeared, etc.

- Addressing mental health problems which arise during conflict and ongoing crises including refugee people who
  - May not have had a previous history of such difficulties or
  - Had no previous history of impaired social functioning as a result of complex mental health and psychosocial health problems
  - As a result of events and experiences during conflict, displacement and subsequent and ongoing crises develop severe mental health problems which also impair their social functioning and ability to care for themselves or others (e.g. their children)
- Ensuring psychological, mental health and social care services which embed the core principles of being
  - Holistic in the care and support provided for ALL refugee people, in a way that addresses the breadth of needs, strengths and coping methods
  - Interdisciplinary and which draw on the range of knowledge and skills of local staff
  - Available and accessible for children, adults, families and communities
  - Seamless, coherent and having transparent referral pathways between community-based services and hospital-based services
  - Preventive and aimed at raising awareness, building resiliency of refugee communities, and enabling early identification of those most vulnerable and in need of health protection, welfare protection and legal protection
  - Targeted to also address needs of those particularly vulnerable (including torture survivors; children; women; those with disabilities, special needs and complex and enduring mental health difficulties; and older adults) and in need of more intensive, longer-term healthcare and possibly legal support services and protection
  - Attentive to the dangers, stresses and other risks faced by staff and proactive in providing formal support structures and supervision mechanisms for caregivers, frontline and other staff
  - Sustainable in that they (a) provide support which is ongoing, not just short-term or emergency support provided during or post-emergencies, and (b) embed an approach which builds individual, family and community resiliency, resources and social connectedness—to cope with future crises and to support social reconstruction and peace-building
  - Relevant to the particularities of multiple refugee communities they serve and their needs
  - Culturally, gender and context-appropriate
  - Ethical and inclusive in that they (a) engage, respect and honour diverse local understandings, knowledge, skills, priorities and (b) uphold the human rights of those they serve

The second step towards doing 'no harm' may be for international organisations and other service providers to conduct an honest and sustained analysis of power and interest in their own organisation (e.g. by using Fig. 7.1). This would facilitate the third step of reconfiguring healthcare responses as integrated 'care services' (psychological, mental, physical and social care) for refugee people in a way that better tries to implement the mantra of 'do no harm'.

This presents donors, international organisations, service providers and practitioners with challenges but more than that key tasks (Box 7.2).

Box 7.2 Key Tasks in Addressing Power and Interest in Care Services for Refugee People

1. Non-oppressive and nonexploitative care	• Identify power asymmetries at all levels, and acknowledge these in a transparent way • Acknowledge the limitations and biases of 'international' (Eurocentric) standards • Address the distal and proximal impresses of power: recognise and name the distal impresses of power (including the wider societal dominant discourses and the social, cultural, political, economic, legal and structural influences) and the proximal impresses of power (family conflicts, abuse and violence in interpersonal relationships, etc.) on the suffering and distress of refugee people and on their capacity to cope and survive adversity • Ensure that care-providing services are non-pathologising in that they do not medicalise or pathologise (as psychiatric disorders) human suffering related to the experiences of becoming and being a refugee, without explicitly naming the context and reasons of that suffering • Address the expresses of power: Recognise and facilitate the different and creative ways in which individuals, families and communities express their individual and collective agency, their strengths and personal, social and other resources in coping with and surviving adverse circumstances and extreme distress
2. Meaningful participation	• Include local experts and other colleagues at every level of decision-making about what is needed and what would be considered seen as culturally and gender-appropriate as well as practical, affordable, realistic and effective at the local level • Include local experts and colleagues (including refugee staff members) in genuine consultations with the relevant refugee communities • Include refugee communities (individuals, families, children, adults) in all consultations to decide what is needed; what are priorities for them; and what would be culturally, gender and contextually appropriate, meaningful and relevant to them
3. Respect for local knowledge, expertise and experience	• Acknowledge that local power structures may differ and be at odds with the interests and goals of international organisations, manifesting in different, competing and contradictory values and methods or even mutually exclusive approaches with the same identified 'problems' • Recognise local experts and local colleagues, including refugee staff, as equal and as having their own unique expertise, and lived experience within the socioeconomic, cultural and political context and realities on the ground • Recognise the role that local experts, colleagues and refugee staff can play in developing realistic and appropriate services and including them in relevant decision-making • Recognise that knowledge, models, methods and interventions are inevitably context-bound (and therefore prone to bias and to causing harm when unquestioningly transferred or imposed in other contexts) • Recognise that expertise is not the prerogative of 'international' professionals, consultants, scholars or organisations and guard against approaches to service delivery which ignore context and different and changing cultural norms and which adopt a colonising and oppressive 'West is best' approach

4. Meaningful partnerships and collaboration	• Recognise the need for meaningful, not tokenistic, collaborative working which is an interagency, interdisciplinary, holistic and inclusive of refugee people and local experts, local colleagues and refugee staff • Recognise that collaboration requires a process of ongoing mutual learning with international organisations, other service providers and practitioners having the primary responsibility to learn from refugee communities and local experts • Ensure commitment in actual practice to developing reciprocal trust—which depends on consistent transparency, mutual respect and openness to learning from each other
5. Independence from coercion and affirmation of self-determination	• Ensure that there is no coercion or deliberate denial of autonomy of refugee people and their right to choose whether they refuse or accept whatever services, interventions or research activities presented by international organisations and service providers funded by them, without punishment or withdrawal of other support provided to them by the international organisation or service provider • Be alert to guard against the unquestioning use of hegemonic psychological discourses, methods and practices which have the potential to harm and to ignore cultural, gendered and local understandings and ways of coping • Ensure that services and practitioners do not engage in cultural homogenisation, leading to harmful generalisations which are demeaning, disrespectful and racist towards refugee people
6. Focus on process	• Ensure that international organisations do not focus on targets for service delivery (e.g. number of 'beneficiaries') at the expense of process. Specifically, • Attend to questions such as – How are refugee people engaged; how are dialogue, mutual understanding, collaboration and participation facilitated? – How is dialogue and mediation between competing institutions (e.g. state and other non-state service providers, universities) facilitated? – How is the building of social capital and tolerance between local communities and refugee communities facilitated? – How are local staff and refugee staff engaged, included and facilitated to participate in decision-making related to services? – How are services adapted to meet changing local needs and priorities?
7. Critical reflexivity adopting lens of power and interest	• Ensure critical reflexivity by all staff and managers, examining the part they play and their assumptions, prejudices, biases, values, language and actions which sustain the negative impresses of power on refugee people • Ensure there is critical appraisal and evaluation of all psychosocial and mental healthcare projects and all care services and their sustainability, which adopts the lens of power and interest • Ensure this critical reflection is a responsibility of all international organisations, their internal advisors and external consultants, trainers, all partners and staff

Conclusions

The mantra of do no harm extends beyond the narrow confines of the dyadic relationship between a staff member and a client and demands attention to the collective harm international organisations, their donors and partners can do to refugee people and communities, in the development of healthcare responses. Addressing and preventing such harm are the ethical duties of all staff, external consultants, and advisors and a matter of due diligence in organisational governance for all international organisations and their donors, to be rigorous and transparent in scrutinising the impresses of power and interest which question the core values and undermine the very endeavour of what we all call 'humanitarianism'.

References

1. Wessells M. Do no harm: toward contextually appropriate psychosocial support in international emergencies. Am Psychol. 2009;64(8):842–54.
2. Smail D. Power, interest and psychology: elements of a social materialist understanding of distress. Ross-on-Wye: PCCS; 2005.
3. Foucault M. Discipline and punish. Harmondsworth: Penguin; 1979.
4. Foucault M. In: Gorden C, editor. Power/knowledge: selected interviews and other writings 1972-1977. New York: Pantheon; 1980.
5. Habermas J. Knowledge and human interests. London: Heinemann; 1978.
6. Smith E, Patel N, MacMillan L. A remedy for torture survivors in international law: Interpreting rehabilitation. Discussion paper. London: Medical Foundation; 2010.
7. Pupavac V. Therapeutic governance: psycho-social intervention and trauma risk management. Disasters. 2001;25(4):358–72.
8. van Ommeren M, Saxena S, Saraceno B. Mental and social health during and after acute emergencies: emerging consensus? Bull World Health Organ. 2005;83:71–5.
9. IASC. Donor conditions and their implications for humanitarian response. IASC; 2016.
10. Jaques E. Social systems as a defence against persecutory and depressive anxiety. In: Klein M, Heimann P, Money-Kyrle R, editors. New directions in psychoanalysis. London: Tavistock; 1955.
11. Bion WR. Experiences in groups. London: Tavistock; 1968.
12. Mirowsky J, Ross C. The social causes of distress. 2nd ed. Hawthorne: Aldine de Gruyter; 2003.
13. Pilgrim D. Mental health and inequality. London: Palgrave; 2002.
14. Rogers A, Pilgrim D. Mental health and inequality. Basingstoke: Palgrave Macmillan; 2003.
15. Rogers A, Pilgrim D. A sociology of mental health and mental illness. 4th ed. Berkshire: OUP; 2010.
16. World Health Organization, Calouste Gulbenkian Foundation. Social determinants of mental health. Geneva: WHO; 2014.
17. Aggarwal N. Defining mental health and psychosocial in the Inter-Agency Standing Committee Guidelines: constructive criticisms from psychiatry and anthropology. Intervention J. 2011;9(1):21–5.
18. World Health Organization. The optimal mix of services for mental health, mental health policy, planning and service development, information fact sheet No. 2 (Geneva); 2007. http://www.who.int/mental_health/policy/services/2_Optimal%20Mix%20of%20Services_Infosheet.pdf. Accessed 3 Mar 2017.

19. Wilkinson R, Pickett K. The spirit level. London: Allen Lane; 2010.
20. IASC. Guidelines on mental health and psychosocial support in emergency settings. Geneva: IASC; 2007.
21. IASC. Mental health and psychosocial support in humanitarian emergencies: what should humanitarian health actors know? Geneva: IASC; 2010.
22. Patel N, Rytter T, Søndergaard E. Good practices and current challenges in the rehabilitation of torture survivors. Discussion paper. Geneva: CTI & Copenhagen: DIGNITY; 2016.
23. Szasz TS. The myth of mental illness. London: Secker and Warburg; 1962.
24. Scheff TJ. Being mentally ill: a sociological theory. Chicago: Aldine; 1966.
25. Bentall RP. Doctoring the mind. Why psychiatric treatments fail. London: Penguin; 2010.
26. Schizophrenia BM. A scientific delusion? 2nd ed. London: Routledge; 2002.
27. Read J, Dillon J. Models of madness: psychological, social and biological approaches to psychosis. London: Routledge; 2013.
28. Tew J. Social approaches to mental distress. Basingstoke: Palgrave Macmillan; 2011.
29. Rapley M, Moncrieff J, Dillon J. Demedicalising misery. Psychiatry, psychology and the human condition. Basingstoke: Palgrave Macmillan; 2011.
30. Johnstone L. Users and abusers of psychiatry: a critical look at psychiatric practice. London: Routledge; 2009.
31. Fernando S. Cultural diversity, mental health and psychiatry. Hove: Brunner-Routledge; 2003.
32. Fernando S. Mental health worldwide. Culture, globalization and development. London: Palgrave Macmillan; 2014.
33. World Health Organisation. mhGAP intervention guide for mental, neurological and substance use disorders in non-specialized health setting. Geneva: WHO; 2010.
34. World Health Organization. Constitution of the World Health Organization; 1948. Available from: www.who.int/governance/eb/who_constitution_en.pdf. Accessed 3 Mar 2017.
35. Huber M, Knotterus JA, Green L, van der Horst H, Jadad A, Krombout D, Leeonard B, Lorig K, Loureiro M, van der Meer JW, Schnabel P, Smith R, van Weel C, Smid H. How should we define health? Br Med J. 2011;343:d4163. https://doi.org/10.1136/bmj.d4163.
36. World Health Organization. What is mental health? Geneva: WHO; 2013. Available from: http://www.who.int/mental_health/action_plan_2013/en/. Accessed 3 March 2017.
37. World Health Organisation. Mental disorders. Geneva: WHO; 2016. Available from: http://www.who.int/mediacentre/factsheets/fs396/en/. Accessed 3 March 2017.
38. Pupavac V. Pathologizing populations and colonizing minds: International Psychosocial Programs in Kosovo. Alternatives. 2002;27(3):489–511.
39. Pupavac V. Humanitarian politics and the rise of international disaster psychology. In: Reyes G, Jacobs A, editors. Handbook of international disaster psychology. Connecticut: Praeger; 2006.
40. Moncrieff J. The myth of the chemical cure. A critique of psychiatric drug treatment. Basingstoke: Palgrave Macmillan; 2009.
41. Kirsch I. The emperor's new drugs: exploding the antidepressant myth. London: Bodley Head; 2009.
42. Carlat D. Unhinged: the trouble with psychiatry – a doctor's revelation about a profession in crisis. New York: Free Press; 2010.
43. Moncrieff J, Hopker S, Thomas P. Psychiatry and the pharmaceutical industry: who pays the piper? A perspective from the critical psychiatry network. Psychiatr Bull. 2005;29:84–5.
44. Goldacre B. Bad pharma. How drug companies mislead doctors and harm patients. London: Fourth Estate; 2012.
45. Cochrane AL. Effectiveness and efficiency. Random reflections on health services. London: Nuffield Provincial Hospitals Trust; 1972.
46. Sackett DL, Rosenberg WM, Gray JA, Haynes RB, Richardson WS. Evidence based medicine: what it is and what it isn't. Br Med J. 1996;312(7023):71–2.
47. Gannon K. Evidence-based practice - the ethical dimension. In: Tribe R, Morrissey J, editors. The handbook of professional and ethical practice for psychologists, counsellors and psychotherapists. 2nd ed. London: Routledge; 2015.

48. Ingleby D. How 'evidence-based' is the movement for global mental health? Disability Global South. 2014;1(2):203–26.
49. Hollifield M, Warner T, Lian N, Krakow B, Jenkins JH, Kesler J, Stevenson J, Westermeyer J. Measuring trauma and health status in refugees: a critical review. J Am Med Assoc. 2002;288: 611–21.
50. Patel N, de C Williams A, Kellezi B. Reviewing outcomes of psychological interventions with torture survivors: conceptual, methodological and ethical issues. Torture. 2016;26(1):2–16.
51. van Ommeren M, Hanna F, Weissbecker I, Ventevogel P. Mental health and psychosocial support in humanitarian emergencies. East Mediterr Health J. 2015;21(7):498–502.
52. Summerfield D. Afterword: against 'global mental health. Transcult Psychiatry. 2012;49(3): 519–30.
53. Mills C. Decolonizing global mental health: the psychiatrization of the majority world. Abingdon: Routledge; 2014.

Part II

Psychological and Psychosocial Health in Host Countries

Refugees in Host Countries: Psychosocial Aspects and Mental Health

8

Branka Agic, Lisa Andermann, Kwame McKenzie, and Andrew Tuck

Abstract

In the last few years, the number of refugees worldwide has increased significantly, reaching the highest levels ever recorded. As described in the literature, the mental health of refugees is affected by their pre-migration, migration, and post-migration experiences. It is well documented that the circumstances that refugees go through can impact both their physical and mental health. While the pre-migration and migration factors cannot be altered, host countries can make the greatest impact on the mental health trajectories for refugees by addressing the post-migration psychosocial factors. This chapter discusses how certain social factors and policies can affect the psychological well-being and mental health of refugees and asylum seekers in Canada and other developed countries.

B. Agic (✉)
Centre for Addiction and Mental Health (CAMH), Toronto, ON, Canada

University of Toronto, Toronto, ON, Canada
e-mail: Branka.Agic@camh.ca

L. Andermann
University of Toronto, Toronto, ON, Canada

Mount Sinai Hospital, Toronto, ON, Canada
e-mail: lisa.andermann@utoronto.ca

K. McKenzie
Centre for Addiction and Mental Health (CAMH), Toronto, ON, Canada

University of Toronto, Toronto, ON, Canada

Wellesley Institute, Toronto, ON, Canada
e-mail: Kwame.McKenzie@camh.ca

A. Tuck
Centre for Addiction and Mental Health (CAMH), Toronto, ON, Canada
e-mail: Andrew.Tuck@camh.ca

T. Wenzel, B. Drožđek (eds.), *An Uncertain Safety*,
https://doi.org/10.1007/978-3-319-72914-5_8

We will focus on the impact of the seven Ds: detention, denial of employment, dispersal, denial of health care, destitution, delayed decisions on applications, and discrimination. While these are often interrelated issues, they each play a role in the integration of refugees and influence their short- and long-term mental health and well-being. Restricting access to employment or health care and forcing refugees to live in certain areas or in impoverished circumstances without any certainty of their acceptance all have negative effects on mental health while reducing the likelihood of integrating and developing strong social bonds.

8.1 Introduction

Political violence and turmoil, internal conflicts, and wars have led to a large number of people who have been displaced from their homes and forced to seek refuge in other countries. In the last few years, the number of displaced people has increased significantly, reaching the total highest levels ever recorded in 2015 [1]. The UNHCR reports that there are currently 65 million people displaced worldwide. The majority of these individuals have been internally displaced within their own countries; however, about 24 million people are currently living as refugees or seeking asylum in other countries [1]. The number of refugees has consistently been increasing for years but seems to have slowed in 2015 [1, 2]. Yet, the number of refugees able to return to their country of origin has been trending downward [2]. This puts added strain on host countries, and they in turn need to consider how their policies, strategies, and requirements around entering the country, living and working in the country, and socialization can have an impact on the mental health of refugees within their country in both the short and long term.

"Refugee" is the term commonly used to describe people fleeing their home due to armed conflict or persecution. However, in international law, "refugee" is a very specific term that refers to individuals who are outside of their country of origin due to a well-founded fear of persecution based on their race, religion, nationality, membership of a particular social group, or political opinion. Refugees are protected by international law [3]. Asylum seekers or refugee claimants are people who are seeking asylum within a host country and whose request for sanctuary has yet to be determined [4]. These two terms are sometimes used interchangeably, but refugee claimant is the term used primarily within the Canadian context. Resettled refugees are people who have been granted permanent settlement in another country [5]. They are commonly all called refugees, and the different terms are often used interchangeably.

Most refugees seek protection in countries that border their original home. This is reasonable as these countries are easier to get to due to their proximity to the refugees' home country. Often, although it is not always the case, these host countries are fairly similar to the original country. They are likely to have similar cultures, religions, politics, and histories. While a vast majority of refugees stay in neighboring countries, others take greater risks and attempt a longer journey for a multitude of reasons to developed countries or apply for resettlement to potential host countries to be accepted as a refugee. While some countries like Turkey, Pakistan, or

Lebanon have hosted millions of refugees in the past few years [1], other countries, for example, Mexico, that are much further away from the region where most people are currently fleeing also receive asylum seekers and accept refugees annually, just in lower numbers [1]. Recent turmoil in Central America has seen a fivefold spike, from 2012 to 2015, in the number of people from Guatemala, El Salvador, and Honduras seeking refuge in Mexico and the United States [1]. The numbers of refugees and asylum seekers coming to North America as compared to countries in Africa, Asia, and even Europe are less abundant due to the complexity and danger of trying to reach the North American countries from Asia or Africa.

In 2014, there were nearly 900,000 new asylum applications to the "44 industrialized countries"; 30 of these countries reported a rise in asylum applicants during the year [5]. Germany received the largest number of asylum seekers in 2014, an increase by 58% from the previous years, and the seventh consecutive annual increase. The United States, Turkey, and Sweden were the countries that received the second through fourth highest number of asylum seekers with all four countries seeing large increases over recent years [6]. Most asylum seekers in 2014 to these 44 industrialized countries were from the Syrian Arab Republic. Other countries of note with high levels of people seeking asylum were Iraq, Afghanistan, Serbia, and Kosovo [6]. While industrialized nations have seen increases in refugee applications, refugees, and asylum seekers, the nations hosting the most refugees are in developing regions. The top five countries with the most refugees in 2015 were Turkey, Pakistan, Lebanon, Islamic Republic of Iran, and Ethiopia [1].

While legislation is specific about which refugee groups the international and national laws and rules apply to, this does not necessarily translate into other areas. In the public realm, the different groups are often lumped together as refugees, and the distinctions are not always clear in the academic literature either. Some research clearly defines the group that they are researching; others use generic terms such as migrant or refugee to define different classifications of refugees. In some cases, immigrants are also included in the refugee classification. In recognition of these methodological challenges, we try to be as specific as possible when providing evidence about the effects of the refugee experience on mental health.

Refugee mental health is affected by pre-migration, migration, and post-migration experiences. The difficult circumstances that refugees go through can impact both their physical and mental health. While refugees are more likely to experience some mental health problems than either immigrants or host country residents, overall, most problems will occur in refugee populations at similar levels to host populations [7–9]. It is important to note that only a small portion of refugees with mental health problems require specialized treatment (e.g., from a psychiatrist) and only a few will develop chronic problems. The estimated rate of mental illness in refugee populations is wide ranging and likely higher among war-affected refugees [7, 9]; these differences are in part linked to the varying social responses [7, 8].

Post-migration experiences can exert enormous influence on the mental health of refugees [10]. Mental health problems limit the potential of the individual both economically and socially and may place greater burdens onto the host country's social institutions [10]. Stresses such as unemployment, poverty, and lack of access to services have an adverse effect on everyone, but migration and resettlement increase the probability of experiencing these stresses [10]. Precarious status, detention, and prolonged status insecurity put additional stress on asylum seekers. Post-migration stressors experienced by refugees, in particular those exposed to pre-migration trauma, have been positively associated with mental disorders [9].

While the pre-migration and migration factors cannot be altered, host countries can make the greatest impact on the mental health trajectories for refugees by addressing the post-migration psychosocial factors. Considering the policies that directly affect how refugees are received and the resources and system in place to respond to refugees can directly affect the long-term mental health of refugees. The way groups are welcomed into a country, the opportunity for sustainable high-quality employment, access to education and training, and initiatives to foster their social inclusion within their community and the larger society are fundamental aspects in reducing social isolation, reducing hopelessness, and producing good mental health.

This chapter discusses how certain social factors and policies affect the psychological well-being and mental health of refugees and asylum seekers in Canada and mainly other developed countries. We will focus on the impact of the seven Ds [11, 12]: detention, denial of employment, dispersal, denial of health care, destitution, delayed decisions on applications, and discrimination.

8.2 The Seven Ds

8.2.1 Detention

Different countries have different policies and procedures on whom to accept, the process of acceptance, and how refugees or asylum seekers are treated once they've arrived within the country based on a set of criteria which includes security of the nation and human rights. Many developed and developing nations currently have policies or guidelines relating to the detention of asylum seekers at a port of entry or after arrival. These regulations, as well as the treatment of asylum seekers, also differ from country to country.

As examples we outline the regulations in Canada and Australia to emphasize differences and similarities across nations. Detention of asylum seekers, in particular those who have undergone traumatic experiences, can be detrimental to their mental health [13–20] (see also the chapter by den Otter et al. in this book).

8.2.1.1 Canada

In Canada, the Immigration and Refugee Protection Act (IRPA) [4] governs the admission of foreign nationals into the country. Under the IRPA, the Canada Border Services Agency (CBSA) agents may arrest and detain asylum seekers designated as part of an "irregular arrival" if they have reasonable grounds to believe the individual is inadmissible under the IRPA and poses a danger to the public; is unlikely to appear for an examination, an admissibility hearing, or a removal from Canada; cannot prove their identity; or is part of an irregular arrival as designated by the Minister of Public Safety and Emergency Preparedness. Detained asylum seekers are held in either Immigration Holding Centers (IHCs) or provincial jails. According to the IRPA [4], anyone 16 or older who is detained is held until their case for refugee protection is acknowledged, or the Immigration Division or the Minister orders their release. They do have to receive a review within 48 h of being detained, and this must be reviewed at least once a month. However, there is no defined maximum length of stay, so that essentially a refugee claimant who is detained under the Act can be detained indefinitely [4]. The IRPA specifically states that no attempt be made to detain any minor under the age of 16, except under extraordinary circumstances. Children of detained asylum seekers who are under 16 are either taken away from parents and handed over to provincial child protection services or unofficially detained with their mother in an immigration holding center [21]. In Canada, the UNHCR has full access to all detention centers where asylum seekers are detained.

8.2.1.2 Australia

In Australia, under the Migration Reform Act introduced in 1992, all "unlawful" non-citizens to Australia are required to be detained [22, 23]. The Act ensures that anyone who arrives without "lawful authority" is not allowed to enter Australia until they have satisfactorily completed health, character, and security checks and been granted a visa, or they are removed from the country. Mandatory detention was introduced as a temporary and exceptional measure in response to the wave of "boat people" coming from Indo-China. The maximum time someone can be detained is indefinite and some cases of years-long detention have been documented [23]. The Australian Migration Reform Act has a few notable differences from the Canadian Immigration and Protection Act: in Australia a detainee is liable to pay the Commonwealth for their detention or removal, and dependent children can also be detained [22].

The Effects of Detention on Mental Health

While the conditions of detention vary considerably within and across countries, often these centers are like prisons (or are actual prisons), with surveillance cameras, guards, controlled locks, and fences, and sometimes the centers are located on islands off the mainland of the country [13, 16, 19, 23, 24]. Detention of asylum seekers has been shown to be associated with increased risk of mental health problems and disorders including anxiety, depression, and post-traumatic stress disorder [18, 19, 25]. Exposure to detention can provoke intense fear and anxiety, sleep disturbances, and depressed mood in individuals who have previously experienced torture [18]. Detention often leads to feelings of hopelessness and powerlessness, which can lead to increased substance use [15], worsening mental health, and suicidal ideation and attempts [14–16, 18]. Detention seems to adversely affect the mental health of men and boys more than women and girls [15, 17, 19]. Detention, even short term, has a detrimental impact on the psychosocial well-being of children including developmental delays, diagnosed mental health problems, and suicidal behaviors [26, 27].

Length of stay in detention is directly linked to poor mental health. Nielsen and colleagues [17] studied asylum-seeking children in Denmark. They found that children aged 11–16 who had lived in asylum centers for more than 1 year had a relative risk for mental difficulties 30 times higher than those children who had lived in asylum centers less than a year [17]. Keller et al. [13] followed a number of asylum seekers in the United States over a number of years and found that 70% of participants perceived their mental health worsening during detention; subsequent analysis correlated this with an association between length of detention and levels of anxiety, depression, and post-traumatic stress disorder which improved for those who were eventually released. Similarly, prolonged detention in Australia [28] has been shown to exert long-term impact on psychosocial well-being in refugees, with the mental health problems persisting after release. Furthermore, the Commonwealth and Immigration Ombudsman found a strong correlation between the rise in the average time in detention and the increase in self-harming behavior [29].

Cleveland and Rousseau [19] examined differences between asylum seekers in detention in Canada and those never detained. They found that the proportion of asylum seekers in detention above clinical cutoffs were significantly higher for post-traumatic stress, depression, and anxiety symptoms than the non-detained group. Symptom levels and the number of cases of mental health problems were found to be significantly higher in the detained group after a relatively short stay in detention, 17.5 median days [19].

Moving Forward

Policies of detention are brought into effect for a number of reasons, including but not limited to security and deterrence of irregular migrants. However, even the most stringent detention policies have been shown not to deter people [30], and as the research shows, detention clearly affects mental health both in the short and long term. In light of the increased interest in detention policies and the increased displacement around the world, the UNHCR has been striving to reduce, if not eliminate, the use of detention. In June 2014, UNHCR launched its Global Strategy—Beyond Detention 2014–2019, which aims to support governments to end the detention of asylum seekers and refugees. The strategy lays out three main goals:

> to "end the detention of children;
>
> to ensure that alternatives to detention are available in law and implemented in practice;
>
> [and] to ensure that conditions of detention, where detention is necessary and unavoidable, meet international standards by, inter alia, securing access to places of immigration detention for UNHCR and/or its partners and carrying out regular monitoring" [30], p. 7.

The strategy calls for a select group of 12 focus countries to develop national action plans in the first 2 years. As of December 2015, there had been action plans developed for the following countries: the United States, the United Kingdom, Thailand, Lithuania, Israel, Malaysia, Canada, Indonesia, Mexico, Malta, Zambia, and Hungary. The country-specific action plans differ depending on which goal(s) they choose to pursue, the specific objectives and actions to success [30]. For example, ending the detention of children is a key priority of the Canada's NAP with several actions listed under four subgoals: (a) legal and policy framework are in place to ensure that children are not detained, (b) best interests of the child prevail, (c) appropriate alternative reception and care arrangements are available, and (d) child-sensitive screening and referral procedures are in place to refer them to relevant child protection institutions or organizations [31]. In the case of Malta and the United Kingdom, for example, the UNHCR has outlined slightly different routes for ending the detention of children. In Malta in 2014 the government specifically created legislative provisions, and the Prime Minister publicly stated that children should not be in detention, so the UNHCR plans to support the implementation of the policy [32]. The United Kingdom has made progress already toward ending detention of children, but focus is to be placed on short-term holding facilities. Where there are no specific rules in place, the UNHCR will support the government to address this gap [33]. These global strategy and national action plans are only the start of a long process in addressing the issue of negative impacts of detention.

8.2.2 Denial of Employment

Individuals need productive tasks to give them meaning, to create purpose, and to find constructive uses of their time. Employment is one avenue that if meaningful, worthwhile, and challenging can help to reduce the chance for mental illnesses to develop and alleviate present symptoms. Getting and keeping a job is never an easy task, but it is often made more difficult for refugees based on their status (legal or not) within the host country, recognition of education, and professional degrees from their home country and fluency in the host country's language.

Refugees may at first experience downward employment mobility within a host country. A refugee who is not successful in acquiring work in their field and proving adequately their ability to work within the host country may end up underemployed. Underemployment is employment which is of inferior quality than could be expected given a person's education, skills, and/or experience [34]. This can include temporary, casual, contract, and part-time employment even within the person's field of expertise [34]. Refugee populations, in particular recent arrivals, are less likely to be employed or are underemployed in many host countries. In Canada, for example, some research suggests that refugees are less likely to be in steady employment at a level appropriate to their educational attainment [35]. Overemployment occurs when workers in full-time jobs experience increased pressure, increased workload, longer shifts and hours, as well as demands for high organizational performance with and without increases in compensation for these expectations and demands [36].

8.2.2.1 The "Right to Work"

Being granted the right to work and having the capacity to find employment are important in restoring psychological well-being. While the ability to work is a given right under international law [37], denial to work for refugees, especially asylum seekers, still occurs for certain designations of refugees in some countries. The

International Covenant on Economic, Social, and Cultural Rights (ICESCR) recognizes a set of rights that includes the right of everyone to make a living by work that is freely chosen or accepted with fair wages and equal remuneration for work of equal value and under safe and healthy work conditions [37]. Despite recognition of this law, refugees and asylum seekers sometimes fall into a gray area as their employment rights within a host country are dependent on the policies and legislations that confer certain classifications to different classification of refugees within each country. If they are allowed to work, the policies may also specify how many hours (or weeks) and sometimes where (in the country and/or only in certain industries) they may work. They may be required to prove their ability to speak the host country language, have a set number of hours of experience within the country, and/or may have difficulty proving their qualifications because of loss of documentation. As examples, we outline the rights to work for refugees and asylum seekers in Canada, Germany, and the United Kingdom.

Canada

Refugees with permanent resident status are allowed to work anywhere in Canada. However, asylum seekers (refugee claimants) may not work in Canada unless authorized to do so [4]. Asylum seekers have to apply for a work permit from Immigration, Refugees and Citizenship Canada (IRCC) and prove they need to work to support themselves. Resettled refugees are provided assistance for up to 12 months from the federal government, or through private sponsors. This support is to help them get established and settled until they can find employment. Refugee claimants have access to social assistance. In their first 4 years in Canada, it has been found that as a group the rate of employment among refugees goes up and the rate of unemployment drops [38]. However, the unemployment rate for those refugees was 29% [38] which was much higher than the unemployment rate in Canada of 6.6% at the same time [39]. Similarly, the percentage of refugee claimants receiving social assistance declines significantly with time in Canada [40].

Germany

In Germany, refugees fall under one of three possible immigration statuses, and these confer different rights and access to the labor market [41]. The permissions and rights to work are laid out in three acts: the Asylum Act, the Residence Act, and the Employment Ordinance [41]. Persons with a residence permit may work without restrictions. Applicants who are still in the asylum proceedings (permission to reside) and those with temporary suspension of deportation must obtain work permission from their immigration authority and the local employment agency. They can be given permission to work 3 months after the formal asylum application has been filed. However, individuals obliged to live in reception facilities are not allowed to work while living in the facility, which could last for up to 6 months. Asylum seekers from designated safe countries within Member States of the European Union who file for asylum are required to live within the reception facility for the entire asylum process and therefore are not eligible to work [41].

United Kingdom

In the United Kingdom (UK), similar to Canada and Germany, individuals granted convention refugee status are permitted to work, [42]. In contrast asylum seekers generally are not allowed to work. They can apply for permission if they have waited over 12 months for an initial decision on their asylum claim or they have been refused asylum but not received a response to further submissions submitted over 12 months ago and they are not considered responsible for the delays [43]. If granted permission to work, asylum seekers are only eligible to take jobs from the official shortage occupation lists of the United Kingdom and Scotland [43]. However, they may not be self-employed or start their own business [43, 44].

8.2.2.2 Mental Health and the Relationship to Various States of "Employment"

Employment status has been clearly linked to mental health. Being unemployed is associated with higher levels of anxiety and depression in general populations [45–47], and high unemployment rates have been associated with suicide patterns [45]. Both underemployment and overemployment have also been linked to levels of stress and depression [36, 48]. In general, individuals who are adequately employed report significantly lower rates of depression than either the unemployed or the underemployed [46]. The relationship between employment and depression is complex as people who are depressed are less likely to be employed. However, longitudinal research has shown that the direction of causation from unemployment to illness is greater than illness causing unemployment [45, 46]. Transitioning from employed to either underemployed or unemployment, when controlling for depression at baseline, has been linked to increased depression as compared to staying employed [46].

The effect of employment status on mental health may be greater for some subgroups of refugees than others. Women and lower-educated individuals are more likely to be unemployed or underemployed [46, 49], and the adverse effects of being unemployed have been noted to be greater in the highly educated refugees [46].

Similar trends around employment and mental health problems from general population studies have been found within refugee groups [50–59]. Having employment (any employment) is better than being unemployed for the mental health of refugees [52, 55]. A study comparing Somali refugees living in London (UK) and Minneapolis (USA) found much higher rates of depression among refugees in London where participants were more likely to be unemployed; employment status had the highest impact on reducing the odds of major depression [58]. Longitudinal studies conducted with Southeast Asian refugees in Canada found that refugees who were stably employed and people who found jobs between baseline and second follow-up had the best mental health outcomes [50]. On the other hand, refugees who were chronically unemployed or newly unemployed had the worst mental health [50]. Unlike general population studies, this work suggests that depression levels at baseline increased the probability of unemployment at second follow-up [50, 52]. Temporary, part-time, and low-paid work is linked to poorer mental health in refugee populations [9, 57].

8.2.3 Dispersal

Over time numerous countries have implemented policies of dispersion with regard to refugee and/or asylum populations [60–62]. The premise for implementing these policies is usually stated as one of or a combination of the following: spreading the costs across a number of local authorities, achieving better integration, avoiding pressure on housing and social services, deterrence and control, and reducing spatial concentrations of minority ethnic populations [60, 61, 63, 64]. These policies sometimes target asylum seekers and in some cases resettled refugees, and they provide different supports depending on the conceptual framework of the country. Some countries view the welfare responsibility largely as a familial one where services are provided by volunteer organizations, and other countries provide a welfare safety net to ensure access to services for all refugees [63].

8.2.3.1 Dispersal in Canada and the United Kingdom

Canada

Canada takes a safety net approach, but it does not have designated legislation around dispersal of asylum seekers or refugees. Instead Immigration, Refugees and Citizenship Canada (IRCC) has in place a practice for dispersing government-assisted refugees (GARs), but not refugee claimants or privately sponsored refugees (PSRs) [65]. Refugee claimants in Canada must find their own accommodations until there is a determination on their claim for refugee protection. The sponsoring organization or family is responsible for helping PSRs find accommodations. The main reason for dispersion of GARs in Canada is to share resources. Canada sends refugees to a location within the country where community resources and services will best support their resettlement and integration needs [65]. Officials attempt whenever possible to resettle refugees in communities where relatives or close friends live, if disclosed by potential resettled refugees [65].

Government-assisted refugees (GARS) are met at the airport upon arrival by someone from one of the federally funded service provider organizations (SPOs). These agents of the SPO have already obtained temporary accommodation for the refugees; they also provide basic orientation to Canada and assist them in finding other settlement services and permanent accommodations [66–69]. Success of this program has been mixed [68]. The support offered by SPO agents is often critical to the integration of refugees in Canada; however, the allotted destinations do not always take into account the requests of refugees. Research suggests that the destination preference of refugees has previously been ignored [66]. The government of Canada attempts to refer GARs to communities that they've requested or as close to their request; however, the process is complicated in that regions and CIC offices are involved in the normal process and SPOs are located primarily in larger metropolitan cities [65].

The United Kingdom

The United Kingdom introduced legislation in 1999 that created a centralized system of housing and welfare support for asylum seekers [42]. The system was created for the purpose of dispersing asylum seekers to reduce the demand and pressure on housing and resources in London and spreading it throughout the nation [42, 63]. The dispersal system is on a no-choice basis; asylum seekers are not entitled to permanent housing but instead are sent to state-provided housing wherever the government deems and they can be moved multiple times (between about ten major centers) [11, 42, 61–63, 70]. Asylum seekers can refuse dispersal and then they would have to give up the financial support offered by the government, so dispersal may not be compulsory, but it is mandatory for those who cannot support themselves nor have a support system already in place [61]. Individuals granted refugee status who are not dispersed instead can apply for social housing and claim benefits [42].

It has been suggested that this dispersal policy was put in place to accomplish two tasks: (1) deter and control the flow of refugees and (2) disperse the financial burden of asylum seekers across multiple cities and agencies [42, 61, 63]. The dispersal system in the United Kingdom has not been viewed as a successful endeavor for integration of asylum seekers or refugees [42, 61–63, 70]. The condition of the housing situation is often poor, overcrowded, and considered substandard [42, 62]. Once asylum seekers have been given refugee status, they must leave the state-sponsored housing within 28 days, and those who are not priority refugees must find their own housing, with one exception being those dispersed to Scotland [62, 70]. Asylum seekers granted refugee status in Scotland can move freely to another part of Scotland or the rest of the United Kingdom and still qualify for local authority housing [70].

The Effects of Dispersing on Well-Being

Dispersal practices and policies often result in refugees and asylum seekers experiencing reduced social support, increasing feelings of hopelessness, and increasing isolation. Migrant networks play a critical role in providing support, and advice [60]. Dispersal away from support networks can lead to feelings of powerlessness, fear, and isolation [71]. The instability of housing available through the dispersal program in the United Kingdom for asylum seekers and after receiving refugee status in the United Kingdom has been shown to force them to move frequently, leading them to feel isolated, and they often face harassment and discrimination all of which reduce their likelihood of integration and decrease psychological well-being [42, 62]. Some research also suggests that refugees who were dispersed as asylum seekers in the United Kingdom have higher levels of secondary migration than other refugees [72].

Refugees who are sent to smaller communities in Canada have reported a marked sense of isolation and often have difficulty finding employment for which they are qualified [66, 73]. There seems to be large secondary migration as a means to be closer to family and friends and find employment [66, 67]. Family and friends provide forms of support that the government sources available in Canada cannot adequately provide, such as transportation, childcare, and help in times of illness [66]. While refugees often tend not to stay in small communities, one Canadian study reported that some refugees may decide to stay. Key reasons are the welcoming nature of the community, partnering refugees with a local family as social hosts, and the low ethnic diversity mean that newcomers are not likely to socialize exclusively with others from their country thereby widening their social ties to the larger community [74].

The UK dispersal policy may contribute directly to increased emotional problems in asylum seekers [72]. However, the link between dispersal practices and diagnosed mental health problems has not been fully explored. The dispersal literature does establish a link between how dispersal reduces social support and increases isolation. Mental health research has clearly shown that there is a detrimental relationship between low social support and mental health problems in refugee populations [9, 75, 76]. Less social support has been associated with more symptoms of Posttraumatic Stress Disorder (PTSD), anxiety [75], and depression [9, 75, 76].

8.2.4 Denied Access to Health Care

Denial of health care for refugees and asylum seekers may depend on changes in government, but legal rights to health care do not always guarantee actual rights and understanding the situation is complex. In some countries, governments provide access to the health-care system for refugees and asylum seekers at multiple levels. In countries such as Canada, the United Kingdom, and Australia where health care is funded by the government, convention refugees often have similar access to citizens; however, not all refugees and asylum seekers are afforded the same rights. Sometimes countries provide limited access for some groups (e.g., vulnerable populations) or to emergency health care, but this multi-tiered system can create uncertainty as both health-care providers and refugees are not sure if they are eligible or for what services they are eligible.

Canada has recently seen its policy around health-care access for refugees change for the better [77]. However, in 2012 changes to the Canadian Interim Federal Health Program essentially removed access to medication coverage, dental care, and vision care for all refugees (except GARs) and refugee claimants from countries that the government deemed safe (i.e., should not be producing refugees) such that they no longer received any health coverage [78, 79]. These changes created a high level of confusion among health-care providers around the coverage available to refugees and refugee claimants [79, 80]. This confusion likely led to refusals and the foregoing of necessary health-care treatment for refugees and claimants [78, 80]. The changes also caused some refugees and claimants to incur significant bills from accessing health care which they were unlikely able to pay [78]. These changes to the Interim Federal Health Program were reversed in 2016 so that refugee claimants in Canada can now access basic health-care services and have access to a set of supplemental services during their period of ineligibility for provincial or territorial health-care coverage [77]. These changes make it easier, theoretically, to access health care in coverage. However, because of differences in access and understanding that existed before the 2012 changes, they are still likely to continue as refugees and asylum seekers in Canada still face many challenges in accessing health care [81, 82].

Germany restricts access to health care for asylum seekers and refugees [83, 84]. The regulation of the eligibility for and the level of coverage is regulated by the Asylum Seekers' Benefits Act [AsylibLG] [84]. Which services are covered, the process for accessing those services, and the restrictions on refugees and asylum seekers are laid out in the AsylibLG [84]; the health care they receive in Germany has been declared as third class [83]. This exclusion from health care was found to result in higher incident health expenditures than from granting regular access to the needed services in Germany and could not be explained completely by differences in need [84]. Bozorgmehr and Razum [84] found that per capita health expenditures were 40% higher among refugees and asylum seekers with restricted access compared to the expenditures in the group of refugees and asylum seekers with regular access in Germany.

Denying access to health care can reduce health-care supports and increase stress and is likely to increase long-term health impacts while leading to the use of costlier health services for refugees. Limiting access to publicly funded health care increases the costs incurred by refugees, the health-care system, and other social institutions [80, 84, 85]. Policies that limit access to health care also places health-care providers in situations where they have to make a moral decision about providing necessary health care to individuals who cannot afford it [80].

8.2.5 Destitution

Refugees and refugee claimants are vulnerable to destitution as they have been forced to flee their country and arrive in host countries with nothing; therefore they are dependent on the host country for their essential living needs [86–88]. It has been suggested that the threat of destitution has been used as a deterrent against asylum seeking and that countries that provide generous provisions are rendered too attractive to seekers [86, 88]. Many forced migrants are in poverty in a monetary sense and therefore often face disadvantages subjectively in terms of housing quality and residential facilities and are socially excluded [87].

Destitution affects many things in the lives of refugees, for example, educational opportunities, language acquisition, and housing which can affect the well-being of refugees and their ability to integrate with the host society. Individuals who are financially unstable have to make decisions, such as—do I first acquire English or find a job to pay for rent? Poverty often affects where we can live and the state of our environment. This includes the physical structure and environment of our home as well as the social environment such as access to a similar community, family, and friends. Refugees are vulnerable and face exploitation because of destitution [87, 88]. Exploitation and poverty reduce opportunities and reduce availability and accessibility of resources leading to experiences of low mood and sadness, frustration, and discontent [88, 89]. More chronic deprivation can lead to a sense of learned helplessness and antisocial behavior [89]. Poverty is considered a risk factor for mental illness [87, 89, 90]. Poverty is an intricate concept because of its interrelatedness with many other factors [89, 90]. One important factor that is often a result of destitution is poor housing. In Canada, sponsored refugees have reported far lower income levels 4 years after arriving than other immigrants [91]. They are less likely to own a home and more likely to still be living in crowded conditions compared to immigrants [91]. This need to share housing leads to a loss of privacy and additional stressors; poor housing conditions can intensify previous traumas and leave refugees open to abuse from other residents [71, 91].

8.2.5.1 The Effects of Poor Housing and the Built Environment on Mental Health

A review of the literature points to a number of associations between housing, the environment, psychosocial factors, and mental well-being [92]. For example, living in high-rise, multiple-unit dwellings has been linked to increased psychological distress in mothers with young children due to increased isolation, reduced chance for children to play, and reduced social networks [92]. Homes in need of repair or with unresponsive landlords are associated with worse mental health [92]. Evans [92] identified three processes (personal control, social support, and restoration) through which the built environment might indirectly affect mental health. When people can control their environment, they feel better; however, when they are thwarted in this, helplessness can occur. The physical environment is directly linked to recovery from cognitive fatigue and stress. Being exposed to nature has positive outcomes and has been shown to replenish cognitive energy [92].

Factors such as poor-quality housing, lack of control, and lack of social support can help contribute to unstable housing, and hence frequent movement, something which has been noted in refugees and asylum seekers in Canada and the United Kingdom [42, 66, 67, 70, 93]. The constant movement can destabilize social networks and disrupt the continuity of care [12, 42, 93]. The links between housing, the built environment, and mental health problems for refugees specifically have not been studied extensively. Warfa and colleagues [93] report that residential instability among Somali refugees living in London, England, is seen as stressful and that it compromised the refugees' mental health. Their preoccupation and worry about instability and their limited control were believed to contribute to psychological distress in the Somali refugees [93].

8.2.6 Delayed Decisions

The government of Canada, at the time of writing of this chapter, estimates that the length of time to a final decision on a refugee claimant application already in Canada is 10 months [94]. The current processing times for Offshore Humanitarian Refugees to be accepted as a refugee in Australia (convention refugees and special humanitarian program refugees that are not in Australia) will take 12 months from when the application is submitted until a decision is made [95]. For asylum seekers who are already in Australia to receive Onshore Protection Visas, the Australian government estimates that the time frame to a decision is the same 12 months [95].

These timelines provided by the Australian and Canadian governments are only estimates of the time to process applications. It is important to note that the manner to determine eligibility for refugee status is complex and difficult and will differ from country to country. This stems from the need for decision-makers to have sufficient knowledge of the cultural, social, and political environment of the country of origin, capacity to bear the psychological weight of hearings and the consequent decisions, and an ability to deal with legal issues, both international and local [96].

The government of Germany has previously published statistics on the asylum procedure through the Federal Office for Migration and Refugees [97]. They report that in 2013 nearly 60% of applications for asylum were processed with a decision delivered within 6 months. For those applications in 2012 that were decided beyond appeal, the total duration of the procedure occurred on average within 12.1 months, with nearly half being determined within 6 months and three-quarters were determined within 2 years at that time [97].

The Canadian government also provides estimate times for the process of applications for convention refugees. For individuals applying as a GAR to Canada, the processing time for their application differs depending on where they are applying from. For the majority of countries, the time to application completion is 15 months; however, there is not enough data to determine times for many countries [94]. The shortest processing times for GARS are for those currently in Jordan (1 month) and Lebanon (7 months), while the longest are for applications from individual currently in Ethiopia (46 months) and Kenya (32 months) [94]. For PSRs, the time for processing is about 50 months for applicants from many countries; the pattern for shorter and longer times is similar as it is for GARs with applicants from Jordan taking about 10 months, Lebanon about 8 months, while Ethiopia and Kenya about 73 months and 68 months, respectively [94]. These differences likely result from a prioritization of caseloads that has taken place because of recent conflicts in Syria.

8.2.6.1 Delayed Decision and Well-Being

A review of international studies of the asylum procedure concluded that the process itself is inherently damaging to mental health [98]. Not knowing whether they will be given refugee status, or how long they will wait, can take a toll on individuals. Claimants may fear the decision—that they may be turned down and hence deported back to their country of origin—and this leads to poorer mental health. Uncertainty and temporary protection in Australia has contributed to the risk of ongoing depression, PTSD, and disability related to mental health problems in refugees [28]. Legal status is an important factor in mental health; asylum seekers are more likely to report PTSD and depression/anxiety than recognized refugees in the Netherlands [75]. In both community and clinical samples of asylum seekers, the literature points to high rates of depression, anxiety, and PTSD [98]. The literature also suggests that mental health may deteriorate over time as asylum seekers wait for the outcome of their application [98]. One study of Iraqi asylum seekers in the Netherlands reported that those asylum seekers who had been in the country longer without a decision (more than 2 years) report more worries over the asylum procedure than asylum seekers who have been in the country for less than 6 months [54].

This study found a twofold chance of an anxiety disorder among those asylum seekers who had been waiting for a decision longer (over 2 years) compared to those with a shorter delay in their decision, less than 6 months [54].

8.2.7 Discrimination

Discrimination refers to inequitable or unjust treatment of individuals or groups based on their socially stratified classification, such as race/ethnicity, class, gender, sexuality, ability, age, and/or health status which results in social inequalities. The concept of discrimination focuses on behavior. The definition of discrimination includes "treatment" or "action" that is different for groups of people based on their socially constructed status, which may cause harm or disadvantage. Discrimination is defined on a number of dimensions including direct versus indirect and acute versus chronic [99–105]. A prominent dimension is the level at which discrimination occurs: individual or structural.

Structural discrimination is highly complex. Current conceptualization is not consistent and due to the magnitude of domains, types of discrimination, and the confusing binaries is far from simple to define or measure. If individual discrimination is considered to be an action, then structural discrimination would be in the operation of the system [99]. This does not mean that a government or institution is aiming to discriminate; though the structure may facilitate discrimination, it is the execution of policies and practices that may produce discrimination [99, 100]. It has been suggested that structural discrimination [100, 101] is (1) the practices of institutions rather than the actions of individuals; (2) the results (rather than intent) of indirect practices or direct actions; (3) the outcome of the connected system of practices, policies, and institutions; (4) innately made up of the interconnectedness of institutions and systems; (5) intersecting types and domains of oppression; (6) in part historically and socially constructed; (7) a fluid process that changes over time and space; and (8) justified and maintained, in part, by beliefs that are shared collectively.

8.2.8 Government Policy and Discrimination

Governments often do not specifically set an agenda of discrimination; however, policies have often been identified, by various parties (the media, professionals, advocates of equality and equity, and political opposition), as being discriminatory or discriminate against specific groups (for examples, see [106, 107]). These policies are usually enacted under the auspices of protection, protection of the country's citizenry and its culture. This seems to be in line with public perception in some countries that immigration and asylum policies are not enough and that refugees are taking all of the jobs and reducing the quality of life of the country's citizens [51, 108–110]. There is a culture of "us versus them" (see also the chapter by Vamik Volkan in this book), a fear of the "other," and links to terrorism within the discrimination literature [109–111]. Discrimination is a complex, multilevel phenomenon that is usually only addressed at the individual (perceived discrimination) level in the academic literature.

8.2.9 Discrimination and Mental Health

Government policies on protectionism and deterrence can produce outcomes that result in indirect practices and direct actions that are discriminatory to refugees and asylum seekers [108]. Media depictions also help to shape public perception [61, 109]. These result in oppression, segregation, and hostility (hate crimes) toward newcomers [109, 112]. It has been noted that hate crimes against asylum seekers are justified by the same arguments as other forms of discrimination and are the result of misinformation, frustration, and fear but may be more socially accepted [109]. While structural and institutional discrimination are difficult to measure and assess, individual racism, individual discrimination, and perceived discrimination have been shown to result in a significant psychological toll [54, 113–116].

Many refugees report having experienced everyday discrimination from host country residents and institutions around the world. Common forms of this are employment practices (e.g., not hiring them or firing them because of their race or status), feelings of exploitation, attitudes of a country's residents (e.g., that they are better than you or stereotyping and negative attitudes), and lack of recognition of identity and ability and in health-care settings [51, 93, 114–116]. These everyday discriminations have been associated with symptoms of PTSD and common mental disorders in refugee groups [114–116]. In their study of older Somali refugees living in Finland [116], depressive symptoms were most common among refugees exposed to everyday discrimination. Mölsä and colleagues [116] concluded that experiences of discrimination and racism formed a substantial risk for mental health problems among Somali refugees living in Finland. These everyday occurrences of discrimination have a psychosocial impact on the well-being of refugees especially adolescents. Continued exposure to discrimination may result in low feelings of self-worth and development of severe mental health problems in adolescent refugees [112, 114]. Adolescent boys and girls may be differentially affected; in a study of Somali refugees in America adolescent boys who adopted more of an American identity were less likely to experience depressive symptoms, and the association between discrimination and depression was weaker [114]. However, for adolescent girls maintaining a strong association with their Somali culture resulted in a similar effect, while they still experienced high levels of discrimination, the effects on depression were less but those who tried to adopt a greater American identity tended to experience discrimination from within their own culture [114].

Individuals who have previously experienced discrimination can provoke emotional responses which may result in heightened stress reaction, mistrust, chronic worry, and rumination [116, 117]. In the long term, this may result in cognitive changes with increased vigilance, anticipation of discrimination, and adaptations in personal development to avoid opportunities, situations, and places where they may be vulnerable [116, 117]. Discrimination impacts mental health in a number of ways: through socially inflicted trauma (indirect or witnessed), economic and social inequality, decreased mobility (lack of education, or employment opportunities), and inadequate, inappropriate, or degrading medical care [117]. Not all refugees experience discrimination, and not all of those that do will develop mental health problems but discrimination greatly impacts the social and emotional well-being of individuals.

8.3 Potential Avenues for Change: Educating Professionals to Support Refugees

When a country chooses to open its home to accept refugees fleeing from war and conflict, they have often to consider a balance between the humanity of the act and the security and prosperity of their current citizens. They do not strive to worsen or cause mental illness, but sometimes their policies and practices can detrimentally affect the refugees' lives and hence produce mental health problems for them. It is important to recognize that there is a lot that host country governments can do to support refugees, but the responsibility for integration, support, and reduction of mental health problems does not lie solely with governments. Industries, agencies, and individuals within a host country have an obligation to provide a welcoming environment and to provide opportunities and support to refugees. In recognition of this and to bestow the necessary knowledge and expertise to health and settlement professionals, the Refugee Mental Health Project (RMHP) was developed in Ontario, Canada. The RMHP was developed at the Center for Addiction and Mental Health (CAMH) to build settlement, social and health service providers' knowledge, and skills for supporting and promoting refugee mental health and to promote inter-sectoral and inter-professional collaboration.

This project was developed as a follow-up to a national Refugee Mental Health Practices study that identified needs and promising practices in refugee mental health in Canada. This study included an environmental scan, literature review, and in-depth interviews and focus groups with 150 participants in nine provinces across Canada, including refugee clients, settlement workers, program managers, policy-makers, and clinicians [118]. One of the key findings of the study was that building knowledge, skills, and partnerships among service providers is essential to better support complex and changing refugee mental health needs during resettlement. A comprehensive network of service provision would help refugees' access appropriate services when they need them. Health care, social service, and settlement professionals, by being knowledgeable and skilled in this area, can help build the foundation for an effective and sustainable network of service providers promoting refugee mental health during refugees' resettlement in Canada [118].

The findings of the national study were used to develop a guide on promising practices and partnership-building resources for refugee mental health [118] and to inform the refugee mental health capacity-building project. This project includes a self-directed online course on refugee mental health for settlement workers and a version of the same course targeted to health-care providers, a community of practice and a toolkit of resources (www.porticonetwork.ca/web/rmhp). The course covers a wide range of topics including information on refugees in Canada, mental health problems around refugees' experience, information on vulnerable populations, and how to work with interpreters in settlement and health-care settings. This project has met with a high level of success, providing training to over 3500 service providers from 2012 to 2016, and has now expanded nationally. Demand from the settlement sector across Canada consistently exceeds the projects' capacity to offer training. Project evaluations show improvements in learning, and participants regularly express their gratitude for the opportunity to acquire skills and a stronger appreciation of refugee mental health issues.

8.4 Summary

The seven Ds is a useful framework to review the psychosocial impacts of post-migration stressors on the mental health of refugees. These seven factors can lead to social isolation of refugees, leading to feelings of low self-worth and being unwanted by the host society, increasing hopelessness, and potentially re-traumatizing individuals. In contrast, when social support and positive opportunities are made available in resettlement countries, outcomes can include thriving in the new setting, growth, and resilience.

We recognize that the various classifications of refugees (e.g., convention refugee, asylum seeker) make it difficult to specify differences among the research internationally, also noting that refugees are dealt with differently in different political systems in countries around the world. Refugees who are deemed to be deserving of protection and rights should be treated as such, and exposing them to conditions that cause or worsen social isolation, hopelessness, trauma, and stress increases the chances of mental health problems including suicidal ideation. The evidence presented above points overwhelmingly to the need to improve the post-migration experience for newcomers, as this can mitigate mental health outcomes and offer opportunities for a new life.

References

1. United Nations High Commissioner for Refugees [UNHCR]. Global trends: forced displacement in 2015. Geneva: UNHCR; 2016.
2. United Nations High Commissioner for Refugees [UNHCR]. Mid-year trends 2015. Geneva: UNHCR; 2015.
3. United Nations (UN) General Assembly. Convention relating to the status of refugees. 1951. http://www.unhcr.org/3b66c2aa10.html. Accessed 30 Sept 2016.
4. Government of Canada. Immigration and Refugee Protection Act (S.C. 2001, c.27). Ottawa, Canada; 2001.
5. United Nations High Commissioner for Refugees [UNHCR]. UNHCR refugee resettlement trends 2015. Geneva: UNHCR; 2015.
6. United Nations High Commissioner for Refugees [UNHCR]. Asylum trends 2014: levels and trends in industrialized countries. Geneva: UNHCR; 2015.

7. Fazel M, Wheeler J, Danesh J. Prevalence of serious mental disorder in 7000 refugees resettled in western countries: a systematic review. Lancet. 2005;365(9467):1309–14.
8. Porter M, Haslam N. Predisplacement and postdisplacement factors associated with mental health of refugees and internally displaced persons. A meta-analysis. JAMA. 2005;294:602–12.
9. Bogic M, Njoku A, Priebe S. Long-term mental health of war-refugees: a systematic literature review. BMC Int Health Hum Rights. 2015;15:29.
10. Beiser M. The health of immigrants and refugees in Canada. Can J Public Health. 2005;96(Suppl 2):S30–44.
11. McColl H, McKenzie K, Bhui K. Mental healthcare of asylum-seekers and refugees. Adv Psychiatr Treat. 2008;14:452–9.
12. McKenzie K, Tuck A, Agic B. Mental healthcare policy for refugees in Canada. In: Simich L, Andermann L, editors. Refugee and resilience: promoting resilience and mental health among resettled refugees and forced migrants. New York: Springer; 2014. p. 181–94.
13. Keller AS, Rosenfeld B, Trinh-Shevrin C, Meserve C, Sachs E, Leviss JA, Singer SH, Wilkinson J, Kim G, Allden K, Ford D. Mental health of detained asylum seekers. Lancet. 2003;362:1721–3.
14. Koopowitz LF, Abhary S. Psychiatric aspects of detention: illustrative case studies. Aust N Z J Psychiatry. 2004;38:495–500.
15. Dupont HJBHM, Kaplan CD, Verbraeck HT, Braam RV, van de Wijngaart GF. Killing time: drug and alcohol problems among asylum seekers in the Netherlands. Int J Drug Policy. 2005;16:27–36.
16. Silove D, Austin P, Steel Z. No refuge from terror: the impact of detention on the mental health of trauma-affected refugees seeking asylum in Australia. Transcult Psychiatry. 2007;44(3):359–93.
17. Nielsen SS, Norredam M, Christiansen KL, Obel C, Hilden J, Krasnik A. Mental health among children seeking asylum in Denmark—the effect of length of stay and number of relocations: a cross-sectional study. BMC Public Health. 2008;8:293. https://doi.org/10.1186/1471-2458-8-293.
18. Robjant K, Hassan R, Katona C. Mental health implications of detaining asylum seekers: systematic review. Br J Psychiatry. 2009;194:306–12. https://doi.org/10.1192/bjp.108.053223.
19. Cleveland J, Rousseau C. Psychiatric symptoms associated with brief detention of adult asylum seekers in Canada. Can J Psychiatr. 2013;58(7):409–16.
20. Filges T, Montgomery E, Kastrup M. The impact of detention on the health of asylum seekers: a systematic review. Res Soc Work Pract. 2016. https://doi.org/10.1177/1049731516630384.
21. Cleveland J, Rousseau C, Kronick R. The harmful effects of detention on family separation on asylum seekers' mental health in the context of Bill-C31, Brief submitted to the House of Commons Standing Committee on Citizenship and Immigration concerning Bill-C31, the Protecting Canada's Immigration System Act. 2012. https://www.csssdelamontagne.qc.ca/fileadmin/csss_dlm/Publications/Publications_CRF/brief_c31_final.pdf. Accessed 30 Sept 2016.
22. Australian Government. Migration Reform Act 1992 no. 184, 1992. Canberra, Australia; 1992.
23. Phillips J, Spinks H. Immigration detention in Australia. Department of Parliamentary Services, Parliament of Australia. 2013. http://www.aph.gov.au/About_Parliament/Parliamentary_Departments/Parliamentary_Library/pubs/BN/2012-2013/Detention. Accessed 30 Sept 2016.
24. Dawson C. Refugee hotels: the discourse of hospitality and the rise of immigration detention in Canada. Univ Tor Q. 2014;83(4):826–46.
25. Gros H, van Groll P. "We have no rights" arbitrary imprisonment and cruel treatment of migrants with mental health issues in Canada. International Human Rights Program, University of Toronto Faculty of Law. 2015. http://www.law.utoronto.ca/utfl_file/count/media/ihrp_we_have_no_rights_report_web_version_final_170615.pdf. Accessed 30 Sept 2016.

26. Human Rights and Equal Opportunity Commission [HREOC]. A last resort? National inquiry into children in immigration detention. 2004. http://www.humanrights.gov.au/sites/default/files/content/human_rights/children_detention_report/report/PDF/alr_complete.pdf. Accessed 30 Sept 2016.
27. Steel Z, Momartin S, Bateman C, Hafshejani A, Silove DM, Everson N, Roy K, Dudley M, Newman L, Blick B, Mares S. Psychiatric status of asylum seeker families held for protracted period in a remote detention centre in Australia. Aust N Z J Public Health. 2004;28(6):527–36.
28. Steel Z, Silove D, Brooks R, Momartin S, Alzuhairi B, Susljik N. Impact of immigration detention and temporary protection on the mental health of refugees. Br J Psychiatry. 2006;188(1):58–64.
29. Commonwealth of Australia. Suicide and Self-harm in the immigration detention network. Canberra, Australia. 2013. http://www.ombudsman.gov.au/__data/assets/pdf_file/0022/30298/December-2013-Suicide-and-self-harm-in-the-Immigration-Detention-Network.pdf. Accessed 20 Nov 2016.
30. United Nations High Commissioner for Refugees [UNHCR]. Beyond detention 2014-2019: a global strategy to support governments to end the detention of asylum-seekers and refugees. Geneva: UNHCR; 2014.
31. United Nations High Commissioner for Refugees [UNHCR]. Beyond detention 2014-2019: a global strategy to support governments to end the detention of asylum-seekers and refugees - National Action Plan—Canada. Geneva: UNHCR; 2015.
32. United Nations High Commissioner for Refugees [UNHCR]. Beyond detention 2014-2019: a global strategy to support governments to end the detention of asylum-seekers and refugees - National Action Plan—the republic of Malta. Geneva: UNHCR; 2015.
33. United Nations High Commissioner for Refugees [UNHCR]. Beyond Detention 2014–2019: a global strategy to support governments to end the detention of asylum-seekers and refugees - National Action Plan—United Kingdom of Great Britain and Northern Ireland. Geneva: UNHCR; 2015.
34. Feldman DC. The nature, antecedents and consequences of underemployment. J Manag. 1996;22(1):385–407.
35. Krahn H, Derwing T, Mulder M, Wilkinson L. Educated and underemployed: refugee integration into the Canadian labour market. J Int Migr Integr. 2000;1(1):59–84.
36. Dollard MF, Winefield AH. Mental health: overemployment, underemployment, unemployment and healthy jobs. Australian e-Journal for the Advancement of Mental Health. 2002;1(3):170–95.
37. United Nations. International covenant on economic, social and cultural rights. Geneva: Office of the United Nations High Commissioner for Human Rights [OHCHR]; 1966.
38. Xue L. Initial labour market outcomes: a comprehensive look at the employment experience of recent immigrants during the first four years in Canada. Ottawa: Citizenship and Immigration Canada; 2008.
39. Statistics Canada. Labour force indicators by age group and sex for Canada, provinces and territories. Labour Highlight Tables, 2006 Census. Statistics Canada Catalogue no. 97–559-XWE2006002. 2008. http://www12.statcan.ca/census-recensement/2006/dp-pd/hlt/97-559/Index-eng.cfm. Accessed 30 Sept 2016.
40. Lu Y, Frenette M, Schellenberg G. Social assistance receipt among refugee claimants in Canada. Econ Inst. 2015;51:1–7. Statistics Canada Catalogue no. 11–626-X
41. Federal Office for Migration and Refugees. Access to the labour market for refugees. Nuremburg, Germany. 2016. http://www.bamf.de/EN/Infothek/FragenAntworten/ZugangArbeitFluechtlinge/zugang-arbeit-fluechtlinge-node.html. Accessed 30 Sept 2016.
42. Phillips D. Moving towards integration: the housing of asylum seekers and refugees in Britain. Hous Stud. 2006;21(4):539–53.
43. Gower M. Should asylum seekers have unrestricted rights to work in the UK? Briefing Paper No. 1908. House of Commons Library, London; 2016.
44. Home Office. Asylum policy instruction: permission to work. London: Home Office; 2014. https://www.gov.uk/government/publications/handling-applications-for-permission-to-take-employment-instruction. Accessed 30 Sept 2016.

45. Jin RL, Shah CP, Svoboda TJ. The impact of unemployment on health: a review of the evidence. Can Med Assoc J. 1995;153(5):529–40.
46. Dooley D, Prause J, Ham-Rowbottom KA. Underemployment and depression: longitudinal relationships. J Health Soc Behav. 2000;41:421–36.
47. Breslin FC, Mustard C. Factors influencing the impact of unemployment on mental health among young and older adults in a longitudinal, population-based survey. Scand J Work Environ Health. 2003;29(1):5–14.
48. Angrave D, Charlwood A. What is the relationship between long working hours, over-employment, under-employment and the subjective well-being of workers? Longitudinal evidence from the UK. Hum Relat. 2015;68(9):1491–515.
49. Bloch A. Refugees in the UK labour market: the conflict between economic integration and policy-led labour market restriction. J Soc Policy. 2007;37(1):21–36.
50. Beiser M, Johnson PJ, Turner RJ. Unemployment, underemployment and depressive affect among southeast Asian refugees. Psychol Med. 1993;23:731–43.
51. Pernice R, Brook J. Refugees' and immigrants' mental health: association of demographic and post-immigration factors. J Soc Psychol. 1996;136(4):511–9.
52. Beiser M, Hou F. Language acquisition, unemployment and depressive disorder among southeast Asian refugees: a 10-year study. Soc Sci Med. 2001;53:1321–34.
53. Papadopoulos I, Lees S, Lay M, Gebrehiwot A. Ethiopian refugees in the UK: migration, adaptation and settlement experiences and their relevance to health. Ethn Health. 2004;9(1):55–73.
54. Laban CF, Gernaat HPBE, Komproe IH, van der Tweel I, de Jong JTVM. Postmigration living problems and common psychiatric disorders in Iraqi asylum seekers in the Netherlands. J Nerv Ment Dis. 2005;193(12):825–32.
55. Bhui K, Craig T, Mohamud S, Warfa N, Stansfeld SA, Thornicroft G, Curtis S, McCrone P. Mental disorders among Somali refugees: developing culturally appropriate measures and assessing socio-cultural risk factors. Soc Psychiatry Psychiatr Epidemiol. 2006;41:400–8.
56. Davidson GR, Murray KE, Schweitzer R. Review of refugee mental health and wellbeing: Australian perspectives. Aust Psychol. 2008;43(3):160–74.
57. Bogic M, Ajdukovic D, Bremner S, Franciskovic T, Galeazzi GM, Kucukalic A, Lecic-Tosevski D, Morina N, Popovski M, Schützwohl M, Wang D, Priebe S. Factors associated with mental disorders in long-settled war refugees: refugees from the former Yugoslavia in Germany, Italy and the UK. Br J Psychiatry. 2012;200:216–23.
58. Warfa N, Curtis S, Watters C, Carswell K, Ingleby D, Bhui K. Migration experiences, employment status and psychological distress among Somali immigrants: a mixed-method international study. BMC Public Health. 2012;12:749.
59. Hagaman AK, Sivilli TI, Ao T, Blanton C, Ellis H, Cardozo BL, Shetty S. An investigation into suicides among Bhutanese refugees resettled in the United States between 2008 and 2011. J Immigr Minor Health. 2016;18(4):819–27.
60. Boswell C. Spreading the costs of asylum seekers: a critical assessment of dispersal policies in Germany and the UK. London: Anglo-German Foundation for the Study of Industrial Society; 2001.
61. Andersson R. Settlement dispersal of immigrants and refugees in Europe: policy and outcomes. Research on Immigration and Integration in the Metropolis Working Paper Series No. 03–08; 2003.
62. Bakker L, Cheung SY, Phillimore J. The asylum-integration paradox: comparing asylum support systems and refugee integration in The Netherlands and the UK. Int Migr. 2016;54(4):118–32.
63. Wren K. Supporting asylum seekers and refugees in Glasgow: the role of multi-agency networks. J Refug Stud. 2008;20(3):391–413.
64. Netto G. Strangers in the city: addressing challenges to the protection, housing and settlement of refugees. International Journal of Housing Policy. 2011;11(3):285–303.
65. Citizenship and Immigration Canada. In Canada processing of convention refugees abroad and members of the humanitarian protected persons abroad classes—part 1 (general)

[Resettlement Assistance Program (RAP)]. Ottawa, Canada. 2011. http://www.cic.gc.ca/english/resources/manuals/ip/ip03-part1-eng.pdf. Accessed 30 Sept 2016.
66. Simich L, Beiser M, Mawani F. Paved with good intentions: Canada's refugee destining policy and paths of secondary migration. Can Public Policy. 2002;28(4):597–607.
67. Simich L. Negotiating boundaries of refugee resettlement: a study of settlement patterns and social support. Can Rev Sociol. 2003;40(5):575–91.
68. Hyndman J, McLean J. Settling like a state: Acehnese refugees in Vancouver. J Refug Stud. 2006;19(3):345–60.
69. Citizenship and Immigration Canada. In Canada processing of convention refugees abroad and members of the humanitarian protected persons abroad classes—part 2 [Resettlement Assistance Program (RAP)]. Ottawa, Canada. 2015. http://www.cic.gc.ca/english/resources/manuals/ip/ip03-part2-eng.pdf. Accessed 30 Sept 2016.
70. Stewart ES. UK dispersal policy and onward migration: mapping the current state of knowledge. J Refug Stud. 2011;25(1):25–49.
71. Kissoon P. From persecution to destitution: a snapshot of asylum seekers' housing and settlement experiences in Canada and the United Kingdom. J Immigr Refug Stud. 2010;8:4–31.
72. Stewart E, Shaffer M. Moving on? Dispersal policy, onward migration and integration of refugees in the UK. 2015. http://www.onwardmigration.com/files/2012/12/Moving_On_Final_Report_2015.pdf. Accessed 30 Sept 2016.
73. Sherrell K, Hyndman J, Preniqi F. Sharing the wealth, spreading the "burden"? The settlement of Kosovar refugees in smaller British Columbia cities. J Can Ethn Stud. 2005;73(3):76–96.
74. El-Bialy R, Mulay S. Two sides of the same coin: factors that support and challenge the wellbeing of refugees settled in a small urban center. Health Place. 2015;35:52–9.
75. Gerritsen AAM, Bramsen I, Devillé W, van Willigen LHM, Hovens JE, van der Ploeg HM. Physical and mental health of Afghan, Iranian and Somali asylum seekers and refugees living in the Netherlands. Soc Psychiatry Psychiatr Epidemiol. 2006;41(1):18–26.
76. Fazel M, Reed RV, Panter-Brick C, Stein A. Mental health of displaced and refugee children resettled in high-income countries: risk and protective factors. Lancet. 2012;379(9812):266–82.
77. Government of Canada. Interim Federal Health Program Policy. Citizenship and Immigration Canada. Ottawa, Canada. 2016. http://www.cic.gc.ca/english/department/laws-policy/ifhp.asp. Accessed 30 Sept 2016.
78. Barnes S. The real cost of cutting refugee health benefits. Policy Paper, Wellesley Institute, Toronto, Ontario 2013.
79. Ruiz-Casares M, Cleveland J, Oulhote Y, Dunkley-Hickin C, Rousseau C. Knowledge of healthcare coverage for refugee claimants: results from a survey of health service providers in Montreal. PLoS One. 2016;11(1):e0146798. https://doi.org/10.1371/journal.pone.0146798.
80. Marwah S. Refugee health care cuts in Canada: system level costs, risks and responses. Toronto: Wellesley Institute; 2014.
81. McKeary M, Newbold B. Barriers to care: the challenges for Canadian refugees and their health care providers. J Refug Stud. 2010;23(4):523–45.
82. Campbell R, Klei AG, Hodges BD, Fisman D, Kitto S. A comparison of health access between permanent residents, undocumented immigrants and refugee claimants in Toronto, Canada. J Immigr Minor Health. 2014;16(1):165–76.
83. Pross C. Third class medicine: health care for refugees in Germany. Health Hum Rights. 1998;3(2):40–53.
84. Bozorgmehr K, Razum O. Effect of restricting access to health care on health expenditures among asylum-seekers and refugees: a quasi-experimental study in Germany, 1994–2013. PLoS One. 2015;10(7):e0131483. https://doi.org/10.1371/journal.pone.0131483.
85. Yates T, Crane R, Burnett A. Rights and the reality of healthcare charging in the United Kingdom. Med Confl Surviv. 2007;23(4):297–304.
86. Da Lomba S. The threat of destitution as a deterrent against asylum seeking in the European Union. Refuge. 2006;23(1):81–92.

87. Davidson GR, Carr SC. Forced migration, social exclusion and poverty: introduction. J Pacific Rim Psychology. 2010;4(1):1–6.
88. Mayblin L. Asylum, welfare and work: reflections on research in asylum and refugee studies. Int J Sociol Soc Policy. 2014;34(5/6):375–91.
89. Kuruvilla A, Jacob KS. Poverty, social stress and mental health. Indian J Med Res. 2007;126:273–8.
90. Lepièce B, Reynaert C, Jacques D, Zdanowicz N. Poverty and mental health: what should we know as mental health professionals? Psychiatr Danub. 2015;27(Suppl 1):92–6.
91. Murdie R. Precarious beginnings: The housing situation of Canada's refugees. In Canadian Issues. New York, NY, USA: ACS; 2010. pp. 47–51.
92. Evans GW. The built environment and mental health. J Urban Health. 2003;80(4):539–55.
93. Warfa N, Bhui K, Craig T, Curtis S, Mohamud S, Stansfeld S, McCrone P, Thornicroft G. Post-migration geographical mobility, mental health and health service utilisation among Somali refugees in the UK: a qualitative study. Health Place. 2006;12:503–15.
94. Government of Canada. Check application processing times. Ottawa: Citizenship and Immigration Canada. 2016. http://www.cic.gc.ca/english/information/times/index.asp. Accessed 30 Sept 2016.
95. Australian Government. Refugee or humanitarian programme visa processing times. Canberra: Department of Immigration and Boarder Protection; 2016. https://www.border.gov.au/about/access-accountability/service-standards/refugee-or-humanitarian-program-visa-processing-times. Accessed 30 Sept 2016.
96. Rousseau C, Crépeau F, Foxen P, Houle F. The complexity of determining refugeehood: a multidisciplinary analysis of the decision-making process of the Canadian immigration and refugee board. J Refug Stud. 2002;15(1):62–75.
97. Federal Office for Migration and Refugees. Germany's asylum procedure—in detail: responsibilities, procedures, statistics, legal consequences. 2015. http://www.bamf.de/SharedDocs/Anlagen/EN/Publikationen/Broschueren/das-deutsche-asylverfahren.html?nn=1451252. Accessed 30 Sept 2016.
98. Ryan DA, Kelly FE, Kelly BD. Mental health among persons awaiting an asylum outcome in western countries. Int J Ment Health. 2009;38(3):88–111.
99. King G. Institutional racism and the medical/health complex: a conceptualization analysis. Ethn Dis. 1996;6(1–2):30–46.
100. Pincus FL. Discrimination comes in many forms: individual, institutional, and structural. Am Behav Sci. 1996;40(2):186–94.
101. McKenzie K. Something borrowed from the blues? We can use Lawrence inquiry findings to help eradicate racial discrimination from the NHS. BMJ. 1999;318:616–7.
102. Henkel KE, Dovidio JF, Gaertner SL. Institutional discrimination, individual racism, and hurricane Katrina. Anal Soc Issues Public Policy. 2006;6(1):99–124.
103. McKenzie K, Bhui K. Institutional racism in mental health care: services have some way to go before they meet the challenges of a multicultural society. BMJ. 2007;334:649–50.
104. Pager D, Shepherd H. The sociology of discrimination: racial discrimination in employment, housing, credit, and consumer markets. Ann Rev Sociol. 2008;34:181–209.
105. Gee GC, Ro A, Shariff-Marco S, Chae D. Racial discrimination and health among Asian Americans: evidence, assessment, and directions for future research. Epidemiol Rev. 2009;31:130–51.
106. Black D. Immigration experts say bill C-24 discriminatory and weakens citizenship. The Toronto Star. 2014. https://www.thestar.com/news/immigration/2014/06/27/immigration_experts_say_bill_c24_discriminatory_and_weakens_citizenship.html. Accessed 30 Sept 2016.
107. Levitz S. Conservatives' refugee system overhaul dealt another blow by federal court: federal court ruling means refugees from 42 countries have the right to appeal. Toronto: The Canadian Press; 2015. http://www.cbc.ca/news/politics/conservatives-refugee-system-overhaul-dealt-another-blow-by-federal-court-1.3165544. Accessed 30 Sept 2016.

108. Lloyd C. Anti-racism, racism and asylum-seekers in France. Patterns Prejudice. 2003;37(3):323–39.
109. O'Nions H. What lies beneath: exploring links between asylum policy and hate crime in the UK. Liverp Law Rev. 2010;31:233–57.
110. Masocha S. Construction of the 'other' in social workers' discourses of asylum seekers. J Soc Work. 2015;15(6):569–85.
111. United Nations High Commissioner for Refugees [UNHCR]. Victims of intolerance. Refugees. 2006;142(1):1–30.
112. Stark L, DeCormier Plosky W, Horn R, Canavera M. 'He always thinks he is nothing': the psychosocial impact of discrimination on adolescent refugees in urban Uganda. Soc Sci Med. 2015;146:173–81.
113. Karlsen S, Nazroo JY, McKenzie K, Bhui K, Weich S. Racism, psychosis and common mental disorder among ethnic minority groups in England. Psychol Med. 2005;35:1795–803.
114. Ellis BH, MacDonald HZ, Klunk-Gillis J, Lincoln A, Strunin L, Cabral HJ. Discrimination and mental health among Somali refugee adolescents: the role of acculturation and gender. Am J Orthopsychiatry. 2010;80(4):564–75.
115. Hatch SL, Gazard B, Williams DR, Frissa S, Goodwin L. SELCoH study team, Hotopf M. Discrimination and common mental disorder among immigrant and ethnic groups: findings from a south East London community sample. Soc Psychiatry Psychiatr Epidemiol. 2016;51:689–701.
116. Mölsä M, Kuittinen S, Tiilikainen M, Honkasalo M-L, Punamäki R-L. Mental health among older refugees: the role of trauma, discrimination, and religiousness. Aging Ment Health. 2016. https://doi.org/10.1080/13607863.2016.1165183.
117. McKenzie K. Racial discrimination and mental health. Psychiatry. 2006;5(11):383–7.
118. Vasilevska B, Madan A, Simich L. Refugee mental health: promising practices and partnership building resources. Toronto: Centre for Addiction and Mental Health. 2010. https://www.porticonetwork.ca/documents/51609/273390/refugee_mental_health_prompractices.pdf/8b5f3b0d-19e0-4816-966b-3bf818eb279a. Accessed 30 Sept 2016.

Psychosocial Wellbeing of 'Vulnerable' Refugee Groups in (Post-)Conflict Contexts: An Intriguing Juxtaposition of Vulnerability and Resilience

9

Ilse Derluyn, Elisa van Ee, and Sofie Vindevogel

Abstract

Refugees often find themselves in a precarious situation, characterised by multiple vulnerabilities. The label 'vulnerable', as specifically applied to certain categories of refugees like unaccompanied minors, child soldiers or elderly, may ensure due attention to their specific needs at various stages of conflict and in post-conflict situations, yet it risks masking specific support needs at the individual level. Therefore, the allocation of support should always be based on needs assessment at the individual level rather than the categorical level. A complex constellation of factors at the individual as well as contextual level appears to play a part in determining the impact of traumatic events and the post-traumatic reactions. At the contextual level, support oriented towards addressing vulnerability and fostering resilience can help individuals to gain control over their life and life context and to deal with psychological challenges in a way that reduces their impact. This chapter concludes that a systemic, strengths-based, culturally-sensitive, relational framework should guide the design and implementation of future interventions for refugees. This would ensure that they are context-sensitive, based on the capacities and strengths of the target population, and designed to enhance support that a given context offers to its most affected and vulnerable members.

I. Derluyn (✉)
Department of Social Work and Social Pedagogy, Ghent University, Ghent, Belgium

Centre for Children in Vulnerable Situations, Ghent University, Ghent, Belgium
e-mail: Ilse.Derluyn@UGent.be

E. van Ee
Psychotraumacentrum, 's-Hertogenbosch, The Netherlands

The Radboud University, Nijmegen, The Netherlands
e-mail: elisavanee@gmail.com

S. Vindevogel
Department of Orthopedagogy, Expertise Centre on Quality of Life (E-QUAL), University College Ghent, Ghent, Belgium
e-mail: sofie.vindevogel@hogent.be

T. Wenzel, B. Drožđek (eds.), *An Uncertain Safety*,
https://doi.org/10.1007/978-3-319-72914-5_9

9.1 Introduction

James was born and raised in the eastern Ituri region of the Democratic Republic of Congo. He was only 12 years old when he was abducted and press-ganged into the Union of Congolese Patriots (UCP). As a child soldier, he was forced to kill his own parents and fight in a brutal Congolese militia. He remained captive for years, but managed to flee to a refugee camp in the border area. Despite his escape, he still feels trapped. He lives in constant fear both because he re-experiences his traumas night and day and because the UCP remains an active political force in Ituri. As a former child soldier, he feels stigmatised and rejected by the camp community. His greatest desire is to go to school and learn about new farming technology so that he can contribute to rebuilding of the community. At the same time, he does not dare to return to his community. He desperately wants to focus on the future, but is constantly reminded of the past.

In response to the unprecedented forced displacement of millions of people, the former High Commissioner for Refugees António Guterres said: 'Forced displacement is now profoundly affecting our times. It touches the lives of millions of our fellow human beings–both those forced to flee and those who provide them with shelter and protection. Never has there been a greater need for tolerance, compassion and solidarity with people who have lost everything' [1].

Refugees and internally displaced persons may have multiple vulnerabilities. It is accepted that certain groups, such as children (in particular unaccompanied minors), pregnant women, sexual minorities, individuals with disabilities and elderly persons, are 'vulnerable'. Children face serious risks; children who are unaccompanied or separated from their families are especially at risk of neglect, abuse, violence and exploitation. Women and girls are at risk of experiencing discrimination, exploitation, violence (in particular sexual violence) and intimidation. People may also be subjected to violence or threats of violence because of their sexual orientation or gender identity. According to the United Nations (UN) Special Rapporteur on torture, members of sexual minorities are disproportionately likely to be subjected to torture [2]. People with disabilities (intellectual disability, psychosocial, sensory or physical impairments) are at risk of isolation, neglect, abuse and undignified treatment and are often excluded from participation in the community. Although, as a group, elderly people are usually defined in terms of age, their vulnerability is, as with most vulnerable groups, depending on the specific country context where they live and the living standards and life expectancy here. In elderly people psychological distress may occur against a background of pre-existing age-related neurological or psychiatric disorders, such as dementia, depression, and a general reduction in mental capacity. Frailty can create dependence and make access to support difficult [3, 4].

Quantitative data on different 'categories' of vulnerable people are very limited, but it is apparent that the size of the current population of vulnerable persons is unprecedented. For example, more than half of the refugee populations are children under 18 years of age, and a considerable proportion of them have been separated from their parents or previous caregivers [1]. The latest global report on child soldiering estimated that roughly a quarter of a million children worldwide are currently serving as conscripts in armed conflicts, in roles such as soldier, spy, cook, porter or sexual slave [5–7].

There is often a marked increase in gender-based violence in crisis situations [8]. In the Democratic Republic of Congo, for example, it has been estimated that 12% of women have experienced sexual violence and that 6–17% of survivors fall pregnant as a result of sexual violence [9, 10]. In 2000, the World Health Organisation (WHO) released a report [11] in which children born of rape were described as being at risk of neglect, stigmatisation and racism, abandonment and infanticide. Despite these concerns, little is known about the fate of children born of sexual violence and their mothers [12].

Although to some extent vulnerability of these groups can be defined in terms of personal factors—in particular age, gender, sexual orientation and disability, it involves several additional, interrelated dimensions, including contextual factors. Contextual vulnerability is based on societal factors such as living environment, social and economic status, neighbourhood and community resources and intimate and instrumental support [13, 14]. For example, children can be forced to join an armed group or may join 'voluntarily', but in either case being inducted into an armed faction as a 'child soldier' places children at huge risk of experiencing a range of difficulties [15–18]. Children born of sexual violence are at heightened risk, because a pregnancy resulting from sexual violence is considered to add to the trauma of sexual violence itself, and the mother and/or her community may perceive a child born from such a pregnancy as a living reminder of rape and the rapist (enemy) [12, 19].

Vulnerabilities can be multiple and may intersect and change over time. Health and welfare problems such as destitution may multiply vulnerability, as they put individuals at risk of homelessness, inadequate nutrition, poor physical and mental health, isolation, exploitation, abuse and high-risk behaviour, thereby increasing the overall risk of harm. Victims of torture, other forms of trauma and human trafficking, may be in need of protection because of the trauma they have experienced and because of being at risk of further abuse. Adverse effects of early life difficulties may influence psychosocial development, enhance later vulnerabilities and substantially increase probability of poor outcomes [13]. Vulnerability is also depending from circumstances, for example, the availability of education, health services or food. In other words, vulnerability is shaped by both personal and environmental factors and changes over time and according to circumstances [3].

Further, we will elaborate specific psychosocial and mental health risks that have been documented in various groups of 'vulnerable refugees', in particular in conflict and post-conflict contexts. We will also look in detail at the 'resilience' that many refugees demonstrate. In addition we will explore factors at various levels of the socioecological system that may be associated with increased risk of mental health problems. Finally, we will discuss approaches to support and intervention for vulnerable groups of refugees. But first, we would like to reflect on the meaning of the 'vulnerability' label.

9.2 Labelled as 'Vulnerable'

Although being labelled as 'vulnerable' may ensure that a group receives particular attention or that its specific needs are met at different times and stages of conflict and post-conflict situations, using this label also carries important caveats. First, designations of 'vulnerability' are often based on the so-called 'objective' characteristics, such as age (e.g. children, elderly), gender (women) or a presence of clearly identifiable physical problems (e.g. disability, illness). Although it is clear that these 'objective' characteristics may indicate greater vulnerability to detrimental effects of war, displacement, armed conflict and collective violence, there is no absolute or direct causal relationship between such characteristics and risk or need for support and protection at individual level. Individual members of 'vulnerable' groups may not be in need of additional support and/or protection, and, even more importantly, individuals who are not belonging to a designated 'vulnerable group' may be in need of extra support and/or protection. Labelling certain groups as 'vulnerable' may thus mask the fact that individuals who are not members of a recognised vulnerable group may have huge needs and therefore need to be supported accordingly.

A related point is that governments are increasingly using group-level vulnerability classifications to determine allocation of resources. Furthermore, based on 'objective characteristics' and the related 'vulnerability' label, they create subcategories within categories or groups that are already entitled to receive extra support. A good example of this strategy can be seen in what happens to the group of 'unaccompanied minors': whilst this group as a whole is recognised as 'vulnerable', government increasingly indicates 'extra-vulnerable groups' within this group, such as those under the age of 14 or girls. This 'additional' label is then used to allocate 'scarce' resources to the 'extra-vulnerable' groups. This process can mean that individuals who are not members of an 'extra-vulnerable' group do not receive the support to which they are entitled, as per definition a 17-year-old Afghan boy would be in less need of support than a 14-year-old Angolan girl.

This attempt to make allocation of resources and support more 'objective' contrasts with the approach used in most care and support systems. In these systems support is 'needs-based' and an 'individualised care trajectory' is put forward: needs assessment is then always carried out at individual level (not at group level), and support is allocated according to specific, context-dependent needs of an individual, *not* assumptions about the needs of a group or category which he or she belongs to. Although it is important to pay particular attention to the needs of certain groups, it is thus equally important that attention is paid to possible side-effects of creating categories and subcategories based on an 'objective' approach to vulnerability.

9.3 Mental Health, Culture and Vulnerability

Poor mental health can be both a cause and a consequence of vulnerability [14]. There is evidence for a strong association between multiple and chronic extreme experiences in refugees and the diagnosis of post-traumatic stress disorder (PTSD), which has been defined as the presence of intrusive memories, avoidance, negative alterations in cognitions and mood and alterations in arousal and reactivity as a consequence of a single or a series of traumatic experiences. PTSD often co-occurs with other mental health conditions such as depression, anxiety disorders [20–22], complicated, persistent grief following violent loss [23–25] and other forms of psychological distress [26].

Deleterious effects of traumatic events on mental health and functioning in refugee populations have been well documented. Almost all systematic studies in conflict and post-conflict regions and across diverse cultural settings have reported rates of PTSD and depression that by far exceed those found in communities not affected by conflict. Reported prevalence of PTSD varies widely, ranging from 0% in a conflict-affected region of Iran [27] to 99% in Sierra Leone [28]. Weighted prevalence estimates from a subset of methodologically robust surveys included in a systematic review of Steel and colleagues [29] range between 13% and 25% and may be the most accurate indicator of PTSD rates, which is considerably higher than the prevalence rates found in Western countries.

In post-conflict populations, poor general psychological health has been associated with female gender, young or old age, low social status, bad living conditions and insecurity and violent and traumatic events, including forced displacement and child soldiering [30]. It has been consistently reported that the prevalence of PTSD, depression and anxiety in post-conflict populations is higher in females than in males [31–33]. In Sri Lanka, the prevalence of depression and associated factors increases with age in adult primary care patients, ranging from 0.3% in the youngest group to 11.6% in the oldest group [33]. Prevalence of depression reached 31% in a sample of elderly people in a Palestinian refugee camp [34]. There is, however, a dearth of studies on the impact of forced migration on mental health of elderly people. Equally, in post-conflict settings, deficits in mobility, cognition, self-care, seeing and hearing are associated with poor mental health, with a higher prevalence of PTSD and depression symptoms and worse social functioning [31, 33, 35]. A study of adolescents in the conflict regions of eastern Democratic Republic of Congo showed that displacement has placed them at increased risk for developing several mental health problems [36]. Furthermore, unaccompanied minor refugees are clearly at much greater risk than children fleeing with their parents; studies in resettlement contexts indicate that they are at up to a fivefold higher risk of developing symptoms of anxiety, depression and PTSD [37–39]. Psychological distress is also prevalent in former child soldiers [16, 40–43], although the reported prevalence varies between contexts and according to the specific measurement methods and study timeframes [44]. Symptoms of psychological distress that may occur in the aftermath of child soldiering include a range of internalising and externalising problems, such as stress, flashbacks and nightmares, feelings of guilt and shame, sleep disturbances, social isolation, aggressive behaviour and hyper-arousal, as well as a range of psychosomatic complaints such as headache, stomach ache and decreased appetite [7, 45, 46]. War-affected populations, particularly groups of adolescents, may exhibit 'internalising problems' such as symptoms of depression, anxiety and post-traumatic stress, as well as 'externalising behaviours', such as conduct disorders, substance use and high-risk sexual behaviour. Often several symptoms co-occur, for example, externalising behaviours may be associated with or even mediated by internalising problems, such as depressive symptoms [47].

Mental disorders such as PTSD are by definition characterised by a specific combination of symptoms affecting thinking, mood and behaviour and are associated with personal distress and/or impaired functioning. It is generally agreed, however, that good mental health amounts to more than a lack of symptoms of mental disorder. According to the WHO [48], 'concepts of mental health include subjective wellbeing, perceived self-efficacy, autonomy, competence, intergenerational dependence, and self-actualisation of one's intellectual and emotional potential, among others'. Mental illness is mainly defined in terms of symptoms, whereas mental health is mainly defined in terms of successful functioning manifested in productive activities, fulfilling relationships and resilience, i.e. the ability to adapt to change and cope with adversity [49]. Vulnerability in particular can limit the potential to function successfully. Trauma can severely disrupt child development, in particular psychosocial development which includes development of the ability to form fulfilling relationships. Relational aspects of adjustment after war and violence may be particularly salient in young children, because of their relatively greater dependence on caregivers [50]. In addition, caregivers who have been submitted to torture may present with parenting and family relationship problems [51, 52].

There is an ongoing debate, however, about whether Western psychological concepts of traumatic stress are relevant to populations in culturally diverse conflict and post-conflict regions [53]. Culture has been described as 'an acquired 'lens', through which individuals perceive and understand the world that they inhabit, and through which they learn how to live within it' [54]. All persons are influenced by—and in turn influence—their context and culture they identify with. Conceptions of the self and the other are shaped by culture and influence perspectives on normal and psychopathological phenomena [55]. Thus trauma and post-traumatic reactions can be viewed as products of a continuous, dynamic interaction between an individual and his or her context. Silove [56] argued that in post-conflict regions, core individual and societal adaptation systems are disrupted. 'In each society, historical and cultural factors will determine the specific way in which these adaptive systems are expressed, what constitutes a threat to each one and how the community reacts to repair the adaptive systems after periods of mass conflict and chaos' [57]. Derluyn and colleagues [15] and Kevers and colleagues [58] have also emphasised social impact of collective violence, war and armed conflict: collective violence affects not just individuals but also social fabric, destroying social relations and social networks, as well as social support structures. Individual trauma should, therefore, always be considered in a relational framework and its broader social context [58]. As such, although there is a large body of evidence showing that war, displacement and collective violence have a negative impact on mental health and psychosocial functioning of vulnerable groups, there are also accounts for high resilience and strength in these populations, and the resilience perspective is often emphasised by those who criticise over-pathologisation of vulnerable groups. We will further elaborate on this perspective in the next paragraph.

9.4 Resilience

The concept of resilience is critical to accounts of positive adaptation in the context of significant adversity. Resilience has been operationalised in various ways, but it is generally regarded as the capacity to withstand, adapt to or rebound from challenging or threatening circumstances. Demonstration of resilience is a dynamic process involving the interplay of multiple risk and protective processes over time and encompassing individual, family and wider sociocultural influences [59]. Multiple biological and psychological variables, internal and external to the person, inform and constrain other domains almost always bidirectionally. Resilience depends on continuously interacting and transforming complex adaptive systems [60, 61]. Ungar [62] drew attention to the role of culture and context in this process, specifically their role in facilitating culturally meaningful ways of coping, which necessitates reflections on the need for a stronger cultural conceptualisation of 'resilience' [63].

Turning once again to the example of children as a vulnerable group, systemic factors (e.g. the quality of a child's family, school or community) typically account for more of the variance in child outcomes than the cumulative impact of individual traits, particularly in highly adverse contexts [64]. Anna Freud's famous observations during World War II drew attention to the importance of the presence of parents and parental reactions as a buffer against the impact of war on children [65]. Parenting can not only mitigate effects of war and violence but can also enhance processes by which children become resilient despite an adverse context. It has been shown that during war loving and non-punitive parenting are associated with positive child outcomes, namely, high creativity and cognitive competence, which could in turn have a protective effect on mental health [66, 67].

Resilience can take diverse forms, and there are many ways of coping with adversity, war and collective violence embedded in different levels of the socioecological system [46, 68]. Neblett and colleagues [69], for example, found that amongst African American young adults, spirituality, positive affect and communalism are sources of resilience which promote adaptive outcomes to stressful situations and other negative circumstances. However, certain experiences, such as child soldiering, may affect resources to which children have access or which they perceive as valuable in their search for a way of coping with difficult experiences and challenges they face [46, 70, 71].

Vulnerability and resilience can be seen as two sides of the same coin as their existence derives from the context of stress. Affirming one's resilience and addressing one's vulnerability help one to gain control over his/her life and deal with psychological challenges. In all populations forced to deal with challenging situations, high levels of psychological distress alongside remarkable agency and resilience are observed: people seem to continue with their lives and invest in life and relationships despite psychological suffering [72]. Alongside great suffering people may show great strength and agency, but equally, individuals who appear to function well may nevertheless be experiencing deep psychological pain and distress.

9.5 Risk Factors for Psychosocial Wellbeing

High prevalence of mental health problems in refugee populations encompasses considerable variation, and therefore scholars have tried to identify factors that increase a risk for development of psychological problems in refugees. The most important risk factors will be further presented and discussed.

9.5.1 War-Related Traumatic Events

There is a large body of evidence that in all categories of refugees, including the 'vulnerable' groups discussed in this chapter, exposure to war-related traumatic events has a very high impact on the presence and persistence of mental health problems [73, 74], even years after a conflict has ended or upon resettlement [72].

Several studies, for example, have documented a high impact of past traumatic events on child soldiers [16, 18, 46]. Some studies have compared the prevalence of psychological problems in former child soldiers and their peers who were not recruited and have shown that child soldiering has a detrimental impact on mental health, beyond to that of exposure to war only [41, 75]. Although comparative studies are scarce and inconsistent, there is strong support for the added role of aversive child soldiering events, as studies indicate that child soldiers who experience the greatest quantity and severity of war events are often the ones who experience the most severe psychological distress afterwards [41, 76]. In other words, there seems to be a 'dose-effect' relationship between adversity-related factors and psychological wellbeing in this population [77].

There is also evidence that sexual violence has a large impact on victims' mental health, both in adult refugee populations [78, 79] and in adolescent war-affected groups [80]. Various studies have documented fairly high levels of symptoms across a wide range of problem areas in victims of sexual violence. Breslau and colleagues [81] estimated the lifetime prevalence of exposure to rape at 5.4% and the probability of PTSD after rape at 49%.

A study by Okello and colleagues [82] in Uganda documented the high impact of both war-related traumatic experiences and childhood adversities, whilst Mels and colleagues [36] noted that displaced, war-affected adolescents in eastern Democratic Republic of Congo report more mental health problems than their non-displaced, war-affected peers. A recent study by Shehadeh and colleagues [83] in the Palestinian occupied territories documented that imprisonment of a family member, especially the father, is associated with an increase in children's mental health problems. This evidence is in line with the considerable impact of past traumatic experiences in populations of child refugees separated from their parents [84, 85]. Similarly, elderly people having experienced a greater number of adverse events carry a higher risk of developing mental health problems [86]. Indeed, both the type of trauma and the number of difficult experiences are of high relevance to their meaning and the likelihood of vulnerabilities.

9.5.2 Current Daily Stressors in Conflict and Post-Conflict Contexts

Large attention that has been paid for long to the impact of war-related traumatic events has been submitted to critique [87]. In particular, an influential study by Miller and Rasmussen [77] highlighted the massive impact of 'daily stressors' on the psychological wellbeing of war-affected populations, and the role 'daily stressors' play in *mediating* the impact of traumatic events on mental health. This study led to increased interest in how post-conflict living conditions—daily material and social stressors—influence refugees' psychological wellbeing.

In the specific case of refugee children, a range of factors that may affect mental health have been identified, including daily material stressors (e.g. poor housing, lack of financial resources), daily social stressors (e.g. limited social network, exposure to racism and discrimination, acculturation) and lack of access to professional support, in particular psychological care [74, 88].

In the case of unaccompanied minor refugees, quantitative studies in resettlement contexts have illustrated a huge emotional impact of several daily (material and social) stressors [74, 85, 89], whilst qualitative research has highlighted the psychological burden imposed by certain stressors, including lack of (permanent) residence documents, poor housing and limited access to schooling [72, 78, 90].

It has also been reported that in adolescent victims of war-related sexual violence and in former child soldiers, social stressors, particularly stigma and social exclusion, are one of the main risk variables for development of mental health problems [80, 91]. Former child soldiers tend to have a very ambiguous position in society, oscillating between being seen as a victim and as a perpetrator [45, 76, 92]. Children born of sexual violence are perceived as objects of shame and humiliation [51]. For example, the Acholi culture (northern Uganda) condemns illegitimacy, with some tribes discriminating against illegitimate children [93]. This means that children born to mothers captured by the Lord's Resistance Army have the lowest possible social status as they are double stigmatised by association with the rebels and by illegitimacy [93]. It has been extensively documented that former child soldiers who are victims of (war-related) sexual violence and their children are both subjected to stigmatisation, discrimination, hostility and ostracism and that this is often a source of psychological distress [42, 51, 94–96]. Collective violence destroys social bonds and social networks, thus removing one of the most important protections against mental health risks associated with adversity and adding to other risks which war-affected populations face [15, 97].

The protracted refugee conditions of many refugee populations worldwide, whereby most of them live in very detrimental circumstances, clearly add to a mental health burden they already face as a result of past traumatic experiences, being uprooted and dealing with multiple losses. One could argue that these refugees experience the so-called condición migrante [98], a combination of post-migration stressors such as loss of family relationships, loss of social support and a loss of identity. Yet, living in a protracted refugee situation is even more complicated because of, amongst other things, a total lack of control upon immediate and longer-term future and high level of uncertainty over whether needs will ever be met. The result is often a 'life in limbo' that may feel temporary, but can become permanent [51].

9.6 Interventions for Refugee Populations in Conflict and Post-Conflict Settings

From the material presented earlier in this chapter, it seems obvious that interventions to support vulnerable groups should focus on reducing the main causes of their suffering. Considerable political effort is required to put an end to collective violence and destitution that compels these groups to leave their homelands in search for safety and a better living. Additionally, stress of post-conflict contexts should be minimised by rebuilding every aspect of a society (economy, infrastructure, education, health services, etc.) as soon as possible. Furthermore, specific interventions should be applied to address psychosocial wellbeing. Rather than presenting an overview of a variety of possible interventions, here we aim at setting out a broader framework for interventions in line with our argument that mental health problems should be considered in the broader context of problems an individual faces, strengths and resilience he or she presents with and relational and social context he/she is nested in. Although for a long time interventions focused on traumas which individuals had experienced stood central [7, 77], the increasing emphasis on the impact of daily material and social stressors on mental health and wellbeing is producing a gradual shift in focus. We therefore call for interventions to be based on a systemic, strengths-based, culturally sensitive, relational framework.

A *systemic approach* in interventions is necessary because psychological impact of collective violence is embedded in a spectrum of other factors that impinge individuals and their surroundings. This spectrum of challenges constitutes the context in which psychological wellbeing is shaped [45, 77]. This perspective implies that healing psychological wounds of war and collective violence at individual level also entails repairing the damage done to all areas of people's lives and to the context in which they exist, as such damage tends to multiply problems caused by war and collective violence [99, 100].

James's family lost most of their belongings during the devastating war in Eastern Congo. His sudden abduction by the UCP compounded that loss, depriving him of what remained of his possessions and of his family and the ancestral land on which the family had built their homes. When he escaped from the UCP and arrived in the refugee camp, James found there was little left to return to. A consortium of humanitarian organisations for war-affected young people heard about his situation and intervened to support his transition to society. He now benefits from basic services (e.g. food programme, basic health care) provided to all people in the camp and is further assisted by a support team who is trying to trace his relatives, assess the state of affairs in his former community, negotiate the return of his family's ancestral land and prepare James and his former community for reunification and reconciliation. This will require lengthy, delicate and extensive mediation at community level, but it is likely to make a huge difference to individuals like James. For instance, if the complex land disputes are resolved and James is able to reclaim his ancestral land through community-supported mechanisms, he might be able to start farming, start building a new home and settle down.

Our plea for a more *strengths-based approach* follows from the evidence of high levels of resilience in vulnerable populations, together with problems stemming from the pathologisation of the refugee experience and the objectivation of refugees' vulnerability. We need to look at interventions that support a range of intra- and interpersonal factors and processes and can strengthen capacities of individuals, families and communities to deal with aversive situations [101]. Paying more attention to people's resources and support mechanisms does justice to a complex reality of refugees' adaptability and functionality and recognises complexity of the interplay between challenges and resources [15, 46].

James's greatest desire is to go to school and learn about new farming technology. He believes that education will give him a better chance of finding a paid job and making a better future for himself. He also sees education and a paid job as the route to a better position in the community, because they would enable him to contribute to the development of the community development and thus earn him respect. James has missed several years of schooling because he was press-ganged into the UCP and at the moment there is no school operating in the camp. However, a group of parents and former teachers have got together to educate the camp's young people, and this means James can gradually catch up on his secondary education. Moreover, one of the elders in the camp, who took care of James when he arrived, has used his network of connections in the camp to introduce James to someone who used to work with new farm technology and is willing to share his experience and the lessons he has learned, to give James some familiarity with the job. This makes James focus more on the future and bolsters his hope that there is a better life ahead of him, which is crucial to his ability to cope with the stress and other psychological sequelae of his experience as a child soldier and the restrictions which camp life imposes on his development.

A *culturally sensitive approach* to interventions should address criticisms based on the cultural specificity of responses to stressful events. Interventions should be designed and organised collaboratively, with external agencies drawing on local partners' knowledge of a community's main psychosocial needs and resources and their understanding of the local relevance of particular psychosocial wellbeing indicators and ways of promoting wellbeing [100]. This should ensure that interventions are sensitive to a local context and cultural particularities.

Like many young people in the camp, James receives counselling from an international NGO that provides psychosocial support to war-affected young people. During one of the sessions, James told the counsellor that he is haunted by spirits. He often wakes up at night and sees the people he killed during his time with UCP in his room. He tells the counsellor that the spirits of these people wander around his room and threaten him. James also discloses that this arouses strong emotions in him, that it takes a long time for the fear and anxiety to dissipate and that even in the daytime he is haunted by vivid memories of the night. The counsellor discussed James's case during a meeting of the international team, and it elicited a discussion about the framing and interpretation of mental health symptoms. In line with his Western biomedical training, James's counsellor clearly interpreted James's re-experiencing as a symptom of post-traumatic stress for which he would suggest psychological therapy. His Congolese colleagues were able to offer insight into James's understanding of the concept of spiritual possession and explain that in their cosmological frame of reference, spiritual possession can best be treated by performing cultural ceremonies. The open discussion of cultural differences in this meeting stimulated the team to work towards an approach that aligned with the cultural framework of James's experiences and guaranteed that he received the support needed to alleviate his suffering and improve his mental health. His counsellor was thereby empowered to explore nonlinguistic and ceremonial approaches to processing traumatic events.

Finally, we call for a *relational approach* to support and humanitarian interventions. Healing and support interventions should recognise the importance of social contexts. Emphasis should be placed on interventions designed to repair local social contexts and social support networks, for example, through community-oriented therapeutic groups. Furthermore, when individuals and groups return home, a lot of resources should be directed towards family- and community-oriented programmes to help returnees reintegrate. There needs to be an acknowledgement that displacement and separation inevitably lead to changes in both the displaced and those left behind and hence that rather than trying to recover the old way of living, being and interacting, a new equilibrium must be constructed [95, 102]. In case of former child soldiers, particular attention must be paid to reconciliation processes as many of them have caused great harm to their own communities. Calls for active 'reconciliation' are often set against the dominant view amongst humanitarian intervention organisations (not amongst the affected communities, however) that child soldiers should be seen as 'victims' rather than 'perpetrators' [92]. Last, given the prevalence of social stressors and stigma, particularly amongst victims of war-related sexual violence and former child soldiers, and their huge impact on individual wellbeing, we should be wary of humanitarian interventions based on assigning people to categories. Indeed, providing certain groups, such as former child soldiers, with extra support may exacerbate feelings of hatred and revenge in a community, especially when a community itself suffers from numerous problems. Categorical approaches to humanitarian interventions are often derived from policies (at government level and in non-governmental and funding agencies) which see targeting 'the most vulnerable groups' as more 'attractive' in many ways (prospect of helpful media coverage, accessibility of the group, attraction of funding, etc.). It is important to remember that categorical approaches are at the expense of the noncategorical, 'holistic' approach which is increasingly advocated. Continuous tension between policy-driven interventions and programmes based on an assessment of needs taking into account complex circumstances of people's lives calls for intensive cooperation and networking between all actors in the field, including governmental and non-governmental, local, national and international agencies [95]. This kind of noncategorical approach would not only acknowledge that armed conflict affects all children and adolescents living in a conflict area, directly or indirectly [75], but also avoid the risk of stigmatisation caused by singling out particular (and often already contested) groups. A noncategorical approach also addresses our concerns regarding possible side-effects of labelling particular groups as 'vulnerable' purely on a basis of 'objective' characteristics, such as age, gender, disability or past experiences.

James has been stigmatised and rejected by other people in the camp ever since he arrived there after serving as a child soldier in the UCP. Although he tries to fit in, both he and his community have changed considerably since he was recruited by the UCP. He grew up listening to stories around the communal campfire. These stories taught him cultural norms and practices. Because there is no storytelling of this kind in the camp, he is missing out on an important source of guidance about how to behave respectfully towards fellow community members. Some of the things he does and some of his behaviour are frowned upon, feared and considered rebellious and result in his stigmatisation and rejection. To help tackle this kind of problem, a community-based organisation is trying to revive the storytelling tradition, by organising meetings amongst community members in the camp and encouraging them to discuss the everyday issues that bother them under the guidance of the community's leader. This leader is also being supported in the role of negotiator and in attempts to initiate dialogue between, for example, former child soldiers like James and fellow community members. Such meetings and attempts at conflict mediation may lead to an enhanced understanding of different frames of reference and shared expectations of community life, as well as to a more nuanced understanding of former child soldiers. Over time, these things are to reduce conflict, stigma and rejection within the community.

To conclude with, we call for holistic interventions and initiatives that address psychological distress as a part of a comprehensive package of support encompassing many life domains that have a bearing on psychosocial wellbeing rather than in isolation. Furthermore, interventions should not just be translated from one culture to another; they should be designed in a culturally sensitive manner, taking account local frames of reference and culturally specific responses to psychological distress. Interventions should not focus exclusively on psychopathology and difficulties, but acknowledge and make use of strengths and resources of survivors. The comprehensive approach we propose needs to consist of an integrated, multilayered pyramid of support, including basic services and security (e.g. basic health care), community and family support interventions (e.g. family tracing and reunification), focused non-specialist support (e.g. livelihood programmes) and specialist services (e.g. psychological counselling) [103]. Support should draw on and reinforce capacities and strengths available in a given context, with the aim of increasing the contextual and social support that is already present to all community members and in particular to those with specific needs [46].

References

1. UNHCR. Press release; 2015. http://www.unhcr.org/myt15/.
2. United Nations General Assembly. Annual report of the UN high commissioner for human rights: discriminatory laws and practices and acts of violence against individuals based on their sexual orientation and gender identity. Geneva: UN; 2011.
3. UNHCR. Vulnerability screening tool, identifying and addressing vulnerability: a tool for asylum and migration system. Geneva: UNHCR; 2016.
4. Virgincar A, Doherty S, Siriwardhana C. The impact of forced migration on the mental health of the elderly: a scoping review. Int Psychogeriatr. 2016;28:889–96.

5. Coalition to Stop the Use of Child Soldiers. Child soldiers. Global Report 2008. London: Coalition to Stop the Use of Child Soldiers; 2008.
6. Machel G. The impact of war on children. London: Hurst & Company; 2001.
7. Wessells M. Child soldiers. From violence to protection. Cambridge: Harvard University Press; 2006.
8. Stark L, Ager A. A systematic review of prevalence studies of gender-based violence in complex emergencies. Trauma Violence Abuse. 2011;12:127–34.
9. Peterman A, Palermo T, Bredenkamp C. Estimates and determinants of sexual violence against women in the Democratic Republic of Congo. Am J Public Health. 2011;101:1060–7.
10. Scott JS, Rouhani A, Greiner K, Allbutt P, Kuwert MR, Hacker M, van Roouen P, Bartels S. Respondent-driven sampling to assess mental health outcomes, stigma, and acceptance among women raising children born from sexual violence-related pregnancies in eastern Democratic Republic of Congo. BMJ Open. 2015;5:e007057.
11. World Health Organisation. Reproductive health during conflict and displacement: a guide for program managers. Geneva: World Health Organisation; 2000.
12. Van Ee E, Kleber RJ. Growing up under a shadow, key issues in research on and treatment of children born of rape. Child Abuse Rev. 2013;22(6):386–97.
13. Mechanic D, Tanner J. Vulnerable people, groups, and populations: societal ties. Health Aff. 2007;26:1220–30.
14. World Health Organisation. Mental health and development: targeting people with mental health conditions as a vulnerable group. Geneva: World Health Organisation; 2010.
15. Derluyn I, Vindevogel S, De Haene L. Toward a relational understanding of rehabilitation and reintegration processes of former child soldiers. J Aggress Maltreat Trauma. 2013;22:869–86.
16. Vindevogel S, Coppens K, Derluyn I, Loots G, Broekaert E. Forced conscription of children during armed conflict: experiences of former child soldiers in northern Uganda. Child Abuse Negl. 2011;35:551–62.
17. Vindevogel S, De Schryver M, Broekaert E, Derluyn I. Challenges faced by former child soldiers in the aftermath of war in Uganda. J Adolesc Health. 2013;52:757–64.
18. Vindevogel S, De Schryver M, Broekaert E, Derluyn I. War-related experiences of former child soldiers in northern Uganda: comparison with non-recruited youths. Paediatrics Int Child Health. 2013;33:281–91.
19. Van Ee E, Kleber RJ. Child in the shadowlands. Lancet. 2012;380(9842):642–3.
20. Fazel M, Wheeler J, Danesh J. Prevalence of serious mental disorder in 7000 refugees resettled in western countries: a systematic review. Lancet. 2005;365:1309–14.
21. Lindert J, Ehrenstein OS, Priebe S, Mielck A, Brähler E. Depression and anxiety in labor migrants and refugees–a systematic review and meta-analysis. Soc Sci Med. 2009;69:246–57.
22. Momartin S, Silove D, Manicavasagar V, Steel Z. Complicated grief in Bosnian refugees: associations with posttraumatic stress disorder and depression. Compr Psychiatry. 2004;45:475–82.
23. Craig CD, Sossou M, Schnak M, Essex H. Complicated grief and its relationship to mental health and wellbeing among Bosnian refugees after resettlement in the united states: implications for practice, policy, and research. Traumatology. 2008;14:103–15.
24. Schaal S, Jacob N, Dusingizemungu J, Elbert T. Rates and risks for prolonged grief disorder in a sample of orphaned and widowed genocide survivors. BMC Psychiatry. 2010;10:55.
25. Schaal S, Elbert T, Neuner F. Prolonged grief disorder and depression in widows due to the Rwandan genocide. J Death Dying. 2009;59:203–19.
26. Van Ommeren M, Saxena S, Saraceno B. Aid after disasters. BMJ. 2015;330:1160–1.
27. Hashemian F, Khoshnood K, Desai MM, et al. Anxiety, depression, and posttraumatic stress in Iranian survivors of chemical warfare. JAMA. 2006;296:560–6.
28. De Jong K, Mulhem M, Ford N, van der Kam S, Kleber R. The trauma of war in Sierra Leone. Lancet. 2000;355:2067–8.
29. Steel Z, Chey T, Silove D, Marnane C, Bryant RA, van Ommeren M. Association of torture and other potentially traumatic events with mental health outcomes among populations

exposed to mass conflict and displacement, a systematic review and meta-analysis. JAMA. 2009;302:537–49.
30. Roberts B, Browne J. A systematic review of factors influencing the psychological health of conflict-affected populations in low-and middle-income countries. Glob Public Health. 2011;6:814–29.
31. Cardozo BL, Bilukha OO, Crawford CAG. Mental health, social functioning, and disability in postwar Afghanistan. JAMA. 2004;292:575–84.
32. Ghumman U, McCord CE, Chang JE. Posttraumatic stress disorder in Syrian refugees: a review. Can Psychol. 2016;57:246–53.
33. Senarath U, Wickramage K, Peiris SL. Prevalence of depression and its associated factors among patients attending primary care settings in the post-conflict Northern Province in Sri Lanka: a cross-sectional study. BMC Psychiatry. 2015;14:85.
34. Chaaya M, Sibai AM, Fayad R, El-Roueiheb Z. Religiosity and depression in older people: evidence from underprivileged refugee and non-refugee communities in Lebanon. Aging Ment Health. 2007;11:37–44.
35. Rivera WH, Mari JDJ, Andreoli SB. Prevalence of mental disorder and associated factors in civilian Guatemalans with disabilities caused by the internal armed conflict. Int J Soc Psychiatry. 2008;54:414–24.
36. Mels C, Derluyn I, Broekaert E, Rosseel Y. The psychological impact of forced displacement: comparing risk factors in internally displaced, returned and non-displaced eastern Congolese adolescents affected by war. J Child Psychol Psychiatry. 2010;51:1096–104.
37. Bean T, Derluyn I, Eurelings-Bontekoe E, Broekaert E, Spinhoven P. Comparing psychological distress, traumatic stress reactions and experiences of unaccompanied refugee minors with experiences of adolescents accompanied by parents. J Nerv Ment Dis. 2007;195:288–97.
38. Derluyn I, Mels C, Broekaert E. Mental health problems in separated refugee adolescents. J Adolesc Health. 2009;44:291–7.
39. Mels C, Derluyn I, Broekaert E. Screening for traumatic exposure and post-traumatic stress symptoms in adolescents in war-affected eastern Democratic Republic of Congo. Arch Pediatr Adolesc Med. 2009;63:525–30.
40. Betancourt TS, Borisova I, Rubin-Smith J, Gingerich T, Williams T, Agnew-Blais J. Psychosocial adjustment and social reintegration of children associated with armed forces and armed groups: the state of the field and future directions. Psychology Beyond Borders: Austin; 2008.
41. Betancourt TS, Brennan RT, Rubin-Smith J, Fitzmaurice GM, Gilman SE. Sierra Leone's former child soldiers: a longitudinal study of risk, protective factors, and mental health. J Am Acad Child Adolesc Psychiatry. 2010;49(6):606–15.
42. Derluyn I, Broekaert E, Schuyten G, De Temmerman E. Post-traumatic stress in former Ugandan child soldiers. Lancet. 2004;363(9412):861–3.
43. Klasen F, Oettingen G, Daniels J, Adam H. Multiple trauma and mental health in former Ugandan child soldiers. J Trauma Stress. 2010;23(5):573–81.
44. Rodin D, van Ommeren M. Commentary: explaining enormous variations in rates of disorder in trauma-focused psychiatric epidemiology after major emergencies. Int J Epidemiol. 2009;38(4):1045–8.
45. Derluyn I, Broekaert E. Child soldiers. In: Brown J, Campbell E, editors. The Cambridge handbook of forensic psychology. Cambridge: University Press; 2010.
46. Vindevogel S, Broekaert E, Derluyn I. A global perspective on child soldiering. In: Conte JR, editor. Child abuse & neglect worldwide, Global responses, vol. 2. Santa Barbara: Praeger; 2014.
47. Okello J, Nakimuli-Mpungu E, Klasen F, Voss C, Musisi S, Broekaert E, Derluyn I. The impact of attachment and depression symptoms on multiple risk behaviors in post-war adolescents in northern Uganda. J Affect Disord. 2015;180:62–7.
48. World Health Organisation. The world health report 2001: mental health: new understanding, new hope. Geneva: World Health Organisation; 2001.

49. Surgeon General for Mental Health: A report of the Surgeon General; 1999. http://www.surgeongeneral.gov/library/mentalhealth/home.html.
50. Scheeringa MS, Zeanah CH. A relational perspective on PTSD in early childhood. J Trauma Stress. 2001;14:799–815.
51. Van Ee E. A new generation: how refugee trauma affects parenting and child development. Diemen: Arq; 2013.
52. Van Ee E, Kleber RJ, Jongmans MJ. Relational patterns between traumatized parents and their non-traumatized children, a review. Trauma Violence Abuse. 2015;17:186–203.
53. Summerfield D. The impact of war and atrocity on civilian populations: basic principles for NGO interventions and a critique of psychosocial trauma projects. London: Overseas Development Institute; 1996.
54. Kleber RJ, Figley CR, Gersons BPR. Introduction. In: Kleber RJ, Figley CR, Gersons BPR, editors. Beyond trauma: cultural and societal dimensions. New York: Plenum; 1995.
55. De Jong JT. Public mental health and culture: disasters as a challenge to western mental health care models, the self, and PTSD. In: Wilson JP, Drozdek B, editors. Broken spirits, the treatment of traumatized asylum seekers, refugees, war and torture victims. New York: Brunner-Routledge; 2004.
56. Silove D. The psychosocial effects of torture, mass human rights violations and refugee trauma: towards an integrated conceptual framework. J Nerv Ment Dis. 1999;187:200–7.
57. Silove D. The global challenge of asylum. In: Wilson JP, Drozdek B, editors. Broken spirits, the treatment of traumatized asylum seekers, refugees, war and torture victims. New York: Brunner-Routledge; 2004.
58. Kevers R, Rober P, Derluyn I, De Haene L. Remembering collective violence: broadening the notion of traumatic memory in post-conflict rehabilitation. Cult Med Psychiatry. 2016;40(4):620–40.
59. Walsh F. Family resilience: a framework for clinical practice. Fam Process. 2003;42:1–18.
60. Cicchetti D. Resilience under conditions of extreme stress: a multilevel perspective. World Psychiatry. 2010;9:145–54.
61. Masten AS. Global perspectives on resilience in children and youth. Child Dev. 2014;85:6–20.
62. Ungar M. Resilience, trauma, context and culture. Trauma Violence Abuse. 2013;14(3):255–66.
63. Vindevogel S, Ager A, Schiltz J, Broekaert E, Derluyn I. Toward a culturally sensitive conceptualization of resilience: participatory research with war-affected communities in northern Uganda. Transcult Psychiatry. 2015;52:396–416.
64. Ungar M. Practitioner review: diagnosing childhood resilience: a systemic approach to the diagnosis of adaptation in adverse social ecologies. J Child Psychol Psychiatry. 2015;56(1):4–17.
65. Freud A, Burlingham DT. War and children. New York: Medical War Books; 1943.
66. Punamäki RL. Resiliency in conditions of war and military violence: preconditions and developmental processes. In: Garralda ME, Flament M, editors. Working with children and adolescents, an evidence-based approach to risk and resilience. Oxford: Lanham; 2006.
67. Punamäki RL, Wouta S, El Sarraj E. Models of traumatic experiences and children's psychological adjustment: the role of perceived parenting, children's resources and activity. Child Dev. 1997;68:718–28.
68. Mels C, Derluyn I, Broekaert E, Garcia-Pérez C. Coping behaviours and post-traumatic stress in war-affected eastern Congolese adolescents. Stress Health. 2014;31:83–8.
69. Neblett EW Jr, Hammond WP, Seaton EK, Townsend TG. Underlying mechanisms in the relationship between Africentric worldview and depressive symptoms. J Couns Psychol. 2010;57(1):105.
70. Vindevogel S, Broekaert E, Derluyn I. "It helps me transform in my life from the past to the new". The meaning of resources for former child soldiers. J Interpers Violence. 2013;28:1–24.
71. Vindevogel S, Wessells M, Broekaert E, Derluyn I. Dealing with the consequences of war: resources of formerly recruited and non-recruited youth in northern Uganda. J Adolesc Health. 2014;55:134–40.

72. Vervliet M, De Mol J, Broekaert E, Derluyn I. "That I live, that's because of her". Intersectionality as framework for unaccompanied refugee mothers' experiences. Br J Soc Work. 2014;44:2023–41.
73. Betancourt TS, Williams WT. Building an evidence base on mental health interventions for children affected by armed conflict. Intervention. 2008;6:39–56.
74. Fazel M, Reed RV, Panter-Brick C, Stein A. Mental health of displaced and refugee children resettled in high-income countries: risk and protective factors. Lancet. 2012;379:266–82.
75. Annan J, Aryemo F, Blattman C, Green E, Brier M. Promoting recovery after war in northern Uganda: reducing daily stressors by building human capacity. J Child Adolesc Trauma. 2012;22:849–68.
76. Blattman C, Annan J. The consequences of child soldiering. Rev Econ Stat. 2010;92(4):882–98.
77. Miller KE, Rasmussen A. War exposure, daily stressors, and mental health in conflict and post-conflict settings: bridging the divide between trauma-focused and psychosocial frameworks. Soc Sci Med. 2010;70(1):7–16.
78. Keygnaert I, Vettenburg N, Temmerman M. Hidden violence is silent rape: sexual and gender-based violence in refugees, asylum seekers and undocumented migrants in Belgium and the Netherlands. Cult Health Sex. 2012;14:505–20.
79. Keygnaert I, Dialmy A, Manço A, Keygnaert J, Vettenburg N, Roelens K, Temmerman M. Sexual violence and sub-Saharan migrants in Morocco: a participatory assessment using respondent driven sampling. Glob Health. 2014;10:32.
80. Verelst A, De Schryver M, Broekaert E, Derluyn I. Mental health of victims of sexual violence in eastern Congo: associations with daily stressors, stigma, and labeling. BMC Womens Health. 2014;14:106.
81. Breslau N, Kessler RC, Chilcoat HD, Schultz LR, Davis GC, Andreski P. Trauma and post-traumatic stress disorder in the community. The 1996 Detroit area survey of trauma. Arch Gen Psychiatry. 1998;55:626–32.
82. Okello J, De Schryver M, Musisi S, Broekaert E, Derluyn I. Differential roles of childhood adversities and stressful war experiences in the development of mental health symptoms in post-war adolescents in northern Uganda. BMC Psychiatry. 2014;14:260.
83. Shehadeh AS, Vanderfaeillie J, Loots G, Derluyn I. The impact of parental detention on the psychological wellbeing of Palestinian children. PLoS One. 2015;10(7):e0133347.
84. Hodes M, Jagdev D, Chandra N, Cunniff A. Risk and resilience for psychological distress amongst unaccompanied asylum seeking adolescents. J Child Psychol Psychiatry. 2008;49:723–32.
85. Vervliet M, Lammertyn J, Broekaert E, Derluyn I. Longitudinal follow-up of the mental health of unaccompanied refugee minors. Eur Child Adolesc Psychiatry. 2014;23:337–46.
86. Chee YK, Levkoff SE. Culture and dementia: accounts by family caregivers and health professionals for dementia-affected elders in South Korea. J Cross Cult Gerontol. 2011;16:111–25.
87. Wessells M, Monteiro C. Psychosocial assistance for youth: toward reconstruction for peace in Angola. J Soc Issues. 2006;62:121–39.
88. Montgomery E, Foldspang A. Discrimination, mental problems and social adaptation in young refugees. Eur J Pub Health. 2008;18:156–61.
89. Montgomery E. Trauma and resilience in young refugees: a 9-year follow-up study. Dev Psychopathol. 2010;22:477–89.
90. Thommessen SAO, Corcoran P, Todd BK. Experiences of arriving to Sweden as an unaccompanied asylum-seeking minor from Afghanistan: an interpretative phenomenological analysis. Psychol Violence. 2015;5:374–83.
91. Verelst A, De Schryver M, De Haene L, Broekaert E, Derluyn I. The mediating role of stigmatization in the mental health of adolescent victims of sexual violence in eastern Congo. Child Abuse Negl. 2014;38:1139–46.
92. Derluyn I, Vandenhole W, Parmentier S, Mels C. Victims and/or perpetrators? Towards an interdisciplinary dialogue on child soldiers. BMC Int Health Hum Rights. 2015;15:a28.
93. Apio E. Bearing the burden of blame—the children of the Lord's resistance army, northern Uganda. Coalit Stop Use Child Soldiers. 2008;11:2–13.

94. Denov M. Child soldiers: Sierra Leone's revolutionary united front. Cambridge: Cambridge University Press; 2010.
95. Derluyn I. Towards a new agenda for rehabilitation and reintegration processes for child soldiers. J Adolesc Health. 2011;49(1):3–4.
96. Vindevogel S, Coppens K, De Schryver M, Loots G, Broekaert E, Derluyn I. Beyond child soldiering: the interference of daily living conditions in former child soldiers' longer term psychosocial well-being in northern Uganda. Glob Public Health. 2013;8:485–503.
97. Schiltz J, Vindevogel S, Derluyn I, Broekaert E. Dealing with relational and social challenges after child soldiering: perspectives of formerly recruited youth and their communities in northern Uganda. J Community Appl Soc Psychol. 2016;26:307–22.
98. Graafsma T, Tieken J. Leven in een 'condición migrante'. In: Lamers PA, editor. Hulpverlening aan migranten: De confrontatie van culturen in de geestelijke gezondheidszorg. Brussel: Samson Stafleu; 1987.
99. Ager A, Boothby N, Bremer M. Using the 'protective environment' framework to analyse children's protection needs in Darfur. Disasters. 2009;33(4):548–73.
100. Miller KE, Rasco LM. An ecological framework for addressing the mental health needs of refugee communities. In: Miller KE, Rasco LM, editors. The mental health of refugees: ecological approaches to healing and adaptation. Mahwah: Erlbaum; 2004.
101. Wessells M. Supporting the mental health and psychosocial well-being of former child soldiers. J Am Acad Child Adolesc Psychiatry. 2009;48(6):587–90.
102. Derluyn I, Mels C, Parmentier S, Vandenhole W. Re-member. Rehabilitation, reintegration and reconciliation of war-affected children, Series on transitional justice, vol. 11. Intersentia: Antwerp; 2012.
103. Inter-Agency Standing Committee. IASC guidelines on mental health and psychosocial support in emergency settings. Geneva: IASC; 2007.

War, Persecution, and Dual Transition: A Developmental Perspective of Care for Refugee Adolescents in Host Countries

10

Trudy Mooren, Julia Bala, and Marieke Sleijpen

Abstract

Most refugee adolescents arrive in Western industrialized countries with at least one caregiver, who is usually a parent. A growing number, however, apply for asylum as an unaccompanied minor. What are the consequences of these social changes due to flight, migration, and resettlement on the opportunities for development and well-being? In this chapter, we elaborate on backgrounds related to developmental stages, interrelationships, traumatic exposure, migration and acculturation experiences, and mental health consequences. We emphasize resilience and describe factors that contribute to it. Current prevention and intervention methods will be discussed as well.

10.1 Introduction

The number of refugee adolescents and children has never been as large as it is currently [1] (see Box 10.1). According to international conventions and laws, children are entitled to safety. Although they may seem a homogeneous group, there are many differences among the youth who have fled their homes to escape from threat, violence, and suppression. Most displaced children are in the company of one or both parents or another caretaking adult; however, an increasing number of teenagers are leaving their homes unaccompanied by a caregiver. For some, the flight takes

T. Mooren (✉) · J. Bala
Foundation Centrum'45, Arq Psychotrauma Expert Group, Diemen, The Netherlands
e-mail: t.mooren@centrum45.nl; bala.julia@gmail.com

M. Sleijpen
Foundation Centrum'45, Arq Psychotrauma Expert Group, Diemen, The Netherlands

Department of Clinical Psychology, Utrecht University, Utrecht, The Netherlands
e-mail: m.sleijpen@centrum45.nl

T. Wenzel, B. Droždek (eds.), *An Uncertain Safety*,
https://doi.org/10.1007/978-3-319-72914-5_10

years. For others, it is a direct and brief journey. For decades already, children are also used as soldiers. After their escape or the end of conflict, these former child soldiers have to adjust to their civil societies again. When we consider refugee youth in this chapter, we cannot do justice to the complexity of individual varieties in background and experiences.

In this chapter, we describe the consequences of forced migration on refugee adolescents. We focus on this age group because of its significance for further development. Not only are refugee teenagers in transition due to migration and flight; they also face transition from childhood to adulthood. What are the consequences of violence and disruption of social life and community for the development and well-being of this age group? Adolescents are on the edge between childhood and adulthood. They seek a balance between autonomy and dependency and between carelessness and risk taking versus responsibility.

We emphasize resilience or the ability to bounce back when under strain. Resilience is the multifaceted process of adjustment in response to severe turmoil. We will focus on the inter-relational challenges and resources that adolescent refugees show in particular. This interplay between strengths and strains is, among others, dependent upon the protection and support received. All children younger than 18 years are entitled to receive this protection (see Box 10.2). However, national governments develop different operationalization of legal and protective measures, partly in response to public discourse about immigration (see for a discussion [2, 3]). This chapter focuses on (a) the experiences of refugee adolescents, (b) developmental changes, (c) consequences of violence and forced migration on (mental) health, and (d) mental health interventions, at an individual, family, or community level (e.g., school). We will end the chapter with concluding remarks, including clinical and research implications. We start by presenting two case examples, first of an adolescent refugee living together with his mother and second of an unaccompanied refugee minor resettling in Western Europe.

Box 10.1: Figures of Refugees, Worldwide

Number of:

- Forcibly displaced people worldwide: 65.3 million.
- Refugees: 21.3 million.
- Asylum seekers: 3.2 million.
- Top recipients of asylum applications: Germany (441,900), the United States of America (172,700), Sweden (156,400), and Russian Federation (152,500).
- Stateless people: 10 million.
- Top host countries: Turkey (2.5 million), Pakistan (1.6 million), Lebanon (1.1 million), Islamic Republic of Iran (979,400), Ethiopia (736,100), and Jordan (664,100).
- Refugees under the age of 18: >50%.

- Unaccompanied children in 78 countries, mainly Afghans (50,300), Syrians (14,800) Eritreans (7300), Iraqis (5500), and Somalis (4100), lodged a total of 98,400 asylum applications in 2015.
- In the EU, the majority of unaccompanied minors are male (91%).
- In total in the EU, unaccompanied minors accounted for almost a quarter (23%) of all asylum applicants younger than 18 years in 2015.
- In the EU over half were aged 16–17 years (57%, 50,500 persons), 29% 15–15 years (25,800), and 13% less than 14 years (11,800).

Sources: Centraal Orgaan opvang asielzoekers (COA) [4]; United Nations High Commissioner for Refugees (UNHCR) [5, 6]; United Nations International Children's Emergency Fund (UNICEF) [1]

Note: The number of unaccompanied minors seeking asylum has increased in recent years, from 24,300 in 2013 and 34,300 in 2014 to 98,400 in 2015. This constitutes nearly 5% of all asylum requests. Particularly in Sweden, but also in Germany, there has been a significant increase of asylum requests by unaccompanied minors from Afghanistan, Syria, Somalia, Eritrea, and Iraq. These figures are based on provisional data; not all countries supply the specific numbers. Eurostat, for instance, reports a slightly higher number of asylum requests by unaccompanied minors in the EU in 2015 alone: 88,300, predominantly by Afghans (51%).

Box 10.2: Legal Definitions and Arrangements for Refugees, Including Adolescents

The distinction between refugees and asylum seekers is a legal definition. According to the UNHCR [7]:

- Refugees include individuals recognized under the 1951 Convention relating to the Status of Refugees, its 1967 Protocol, the 1969 OAU Convention Governing the Specific Aspects of Refugee Problems in Africa, those recognized in accordance with the UNHCR Statute, individuals granted complementary forms of protection, or those enjoying temporary protection.
- Asylum seekers are individuals who have sought international protection and whose claims for refugee status have not yet been determined, irrespective of when they may have been lodged.
- Internally displaced persons (IDPs) are people or groups of individuals who have been forced to leave their homes or places of habitual residence, in particular as a result of, or in order to avoid, the effects of armed conflict, situations of generalized violence, violations of human rights, or natural or man-made disasters, and who have not crossed an international border.

With regard to the protection of children and adolescents, the following regulations have been agreed upon by the United Nations:

- Convention on the Rights of the Child (CRC) expresses the protection of all children under the age of 18:
  - *Article 1*
    For the purposes of the present Convention, a child means every human being below the age of 18 years unless under the law applicable to the child, majority is attained earlier.
  - *Article 2*
    Parties shall respect and ensure the rights set forth in the present Convention to each child within their jurisdiction without discrimination of any kind, irrespective of the child's or his or her parent's or legal guardian's race, color, sex, language, religion, political, or other opinion, national, ethnic or social origin, property, disability, birth, or other status.
    Parties shall take all appropriate measures to ensure that the child is protected against all forms of discrimination or punishment on the basis of the status, activities, expressed opinions, or beliefs of the child's parents, legal guardians, or family members.

Source: United Nations (UN) [8].

10.2 Two Case Examples

10.2.1 Rakim

After a long imprisonment, Rakim, a 17 year old adolescent from South Asia, was continuously in fear. Upon release, he had been warned to never talk about what had happened. He felt as if he was still in danger and was petrified. During daytime he tried to stay alert to notice if someone was following him or if there was a police officer around the corner who might send him back. Or maybe people from his country would come here to capture him again. Rakim is convinced that if he returns to his home country, he won't escape death.

His mother, a tender woman, will bring Rakim a glass of water at night when he wakes up screaming from a nightmare. Her own suffering has diminished her capacity to offer her son more support than bringing him food daily and water at night. Overwhelmed with sadness and worry, she spends most of the day in bed crying. In moments of intensive hopelessness, she believes death is the only escape. Rakim worries a lot about his mother and tries to be with her as much as possible. In the moments when his worries about his mother and fear of being deported increase, he can hardly follow the lessons at school. After school Rakim goes home quickly to care for his mother. Some days he takes her to some appointments and will translate for her.

Rakim has given up intentions to seek contact with his peers. He believes that his experiences and daily reality are so different from his schoolmates that no common understanding can be found. Sometimes he wishes his father was alive to tell him how he should go on with his troubled life. He has often been insecure about which decisions to take. But, he knows he has to study hard. The schoolwork has become his goal, his relief, and his escape.

10.2.2 Karim

Karim, an 18-year-old, shy, unaccompanied adolescent from South Asia as well, hardly ever thinks about the painful and humiliating experiences he had during his imprisonment. He considers it as being over and belonging to the past. The torture he experienced has been far less upsetting for him than the loss of his parents who were killed during bombardments. Most of the time, Karim sits in his tiny room, asking himself again and again why it all has happened to him. Stunned by the losses and overwhelmed with sadness, he cannot generate enough interest for learning the language. He gave it a try, but gave up due to his difficulties concentrating. He can't remember new words, and this makes him feel deeply ashamed for not knowing an answer in the classroom.

Life without parents seems meaningless to Karim. He believes that "without a family you are no one. How do you restart your disrupted life in a strange country without your family, without friends, without a role, without a goal?" Sometimes Karim thinks he has to start something, but he is not sure what and does not know what would be a starting point in a limbo. Some weekends he manages to visit the church, which is a remaining pillar for him. Church is the only place he believes he belongs to—it is a source of strength to go on.

Both adolescents are from the same country, and although they have similar adverse experiences, the developmental pathways of these two adolescents were impacted differently. Similar adverse events can lead to different outcomes. Multiple, bidirectional, and interdependent interactions between the child and his or her environment contribute to adjustment [9]. In which ways do war, persecution, and dual, normative, and cultural transitions alter the biological and psychological developmental trajectories of refugee adolescents? Which factors and processes facilitate and hinder the developmental transformations and reorganization for adolescents confronted with long-lasting cumulative stress? The dynamic interplay of biological, psychological, family, and socio-contextual influences [10] provides broad, multiple perspectives for understanding the pathways to psychopathology and resilience.

10.3 Refugee Experience

Generally, three phases are distinguished among the experiences that refugees go through: (1) preflight circumstances, (2) migration, and (3) post-migration or resettlement phase. (1) It is usually during the period before flight when there is a high risk of being subjected to or becoming a witness of violence and death. Traumatic experiences, such as bombardments, personal losses, and (witnessing) experiences of violence and abuse affect individual members, multiple family subsystems [11], and the family as a whole [12]. Also, the threat of being drafted into the army or military service may cause young people to go into hiding or to seek safety elsewhere.

In addition to experiencing threat and violence in their country of origin, refugees face loss and separation due to death, imprisonment, combat, kidnapping, or flight. The worries about family members left behind or who have disappeared, along with the grief for lost ones, are often intertwined with anxieties and feelings of uncertainty due to the unpredictable outcomes of asylum procedures.

During the (2) next episode, the migration phase, or flight, there is a high risk of confrontation with violence or submersion as well. People pay enormous amounts of money to human traffickers. Young people, sometimes just children, leave their possessions and social networks and close relatives behind often without informing them about their whereabouts because of the perceived danger. Some young adolescents, for instance, from Eritrea, are known for their long and risky flight routes through the desert and across the sea [13]. They hope to be able to fulfill their own and their families' hopes for a better future in a Western society.

In the (3) post-migration, acculturation, or resettlement phase, young refugees need to readjust to new circumstances. They need to learn a new language, get accustomed to local rules, and bear the uncertainties of new and temporary life (e.g., for asylum seekers). They await legal procedures, for a permit to stay, and for family reunification. These procedures are hardly easy. In addition to dealing with many losses, adolescents often have to take on responsibilities that are beyond their developmental abilities and/or became confronted with impossible missions to bring family members to the host country or to financially support family left behind, all while having limited material resources [14]. Moreover, they may be worrying about their future and struggling to find their place in the new unfamiliar environment. Among the Syrian and Eritrean unaccompanied refugees, high pressure is being placed on them to organize family reunions. Hazardous legal and administrative procedures cause frustration and high levels of stress [15]. In Western European countries, asylum-seeking refugees under 18 years old go to school. Once they are 18 they often no longer have rights to education. Children usually adapt faster to their new surroundings than their parents, causing a feeling of dependency in adults. Many refugees miss the support of extended family members. Most live in harsh circumstances with poverty and societal hardships to endure.

On the one hand, there are many risks and challenges, but on the other hand, many adolescent refugees also see new opportunities in a host country, e.g., related to schooling and prospects of work.

10.3.1 Loss, Bereavement, and Grief

Refugee adolescents who have lost parents or siblings by violent death or separation during the journey, or under other circumstances, are at risk of prolonged and/or traumatic grief. Despite dual exposure to trauma and loss, there is little research focused on identifying different psychosocial consequences related to bereavement by refugees [16]. Grief can be experienced and expressed differently depending on the kind of death, the relation to the deceased, and cultural differences [17]. Morgos, Worden, and Gupta [18] connect high levels of traumatic grief by displaced children to stress and dangerous situations, disruptions, and lack of possibilities for mourning practices. Unaccompanied minors are especially at risk for traumatic grief, since they are missing support from family members and friends, as well as the usual rituals after a violent death of parents and/or siblings.

Scared of the unknown, outside world, and tormented by painful memories, Karim lived a withdrawn life. Lying on his bed, he longed for his parents, searching without success for answers to questions such as: "Why has all this happened?" "Why did my parents become victims of bombardments?" Despite his strong intention avoiding to talk about it, he managed slowly to describe the circumstances of his parents' death, give words to his thoughts and feelings, and construct a narrative. He could define what he was missing the most from his parents and how to preserve nice recollections of them. Encouraged by thoughts of what his parents would expect from him now, he started seeking support in church, attending Dutch lessons, learning step by step how he "can be someone, without a family," and building new friendships as a starting point in the limbo.

10.4 Adolescents' Developmental "Tasks"

During wartime in Sarajevo in 1991–1995, youngsters would wander around the graveyards during curfew. They would take the risk to gather. In the sheltered city, closed from the outside world, they needed the company of other people of their own age. They said that they did so not only to share their understanding of what was going on but also to have a sense of being alive. There was little opportunity for them to go to pubs, parties, or sports, which, during normal times, were regular activities for most of them.

Accomplishing several age- and stage-related developmental tasks is extra challenging for refugees, due to traumatic experiences, ongoing stressors, and cultural transition, especially if the support of parents is missing. This may occur because they are unaccompanied or as a consequence of psychological problems of the parents themselves. In addition to the usual developmental challenges, refugee adolescents face several extra developmental tasks. Some of these responsibilities weigh heavily, considering current age developmental stage, such as expectations to provide financial support to family members left behind or taking care of their traumatized parents in the host country. Some young refugees, who have had prolonged traumatic experiences, who have been kept imprisoned or sexually abused, or who became child solders, may have altered trajectories in their socio-emotional state, identity, sexual, or moral development.

Adolescents are on the bridge between childhood and adulthood. While time, duration, and form of transition may be similar in various cultures, there will also be differences in adolescents related to their specific social circumstances. Van der Veer [19] pointed out that adolescent refugees face not only general developmental tasks linked to their age but also additional developmental tasks related to their specific circumstances—such as dealing with the values of two cultures, coping with losses, adapting to a new society, and handling stress symptoms. Besides, general developmental tasks can be more challenging for young refugees–for example, reshaping family relationships. Van der Veer [19] mentioned three developmental themes: integration of impulses (aggressive and sexual), separation from parents, and building an independent future. We discuss these under the headings of (a) biological transition, (b) independency and autonomy, and (c) identity formation.

10.4.1 Biological Transition

Increasing autonomy in adolescence goes hand in hand with biological and physical changes. Adolescence is one of the periods of development when most of the changes in the body, e.g., the hormonal system, occurs. Between the ages of 10 and 16, children grow dramatically. Hormonal changes also impact the social relationships among youngsters; they may start to date and have their first sexual experiences.

Brain development continues, and this goes on into adulthood. Research has demonstrated that the control or inhibition of impulses is relatively difficult, specifically for adolescents [20]. A tendency to seek adventures and curiosity for new experiences may also be related to alcohol and/or drug abuse at this age. The roles of parents change from being central and pedagogically crucial to them becoming supportive coaches ("sitting in the passenger's seat"). This is frequently associated with an increase of conflicts in the house.

10.4.2 Independency and Autonomy

Many adolescents stretch but keep the elastic tie with their family members, in particular their parents; in times of trouble they need to be able to rely on parental support. For some refugee adolescents, the ties are prematurely broken. Unaccompanied minors miss the support of their families when they need them the most. Parents who are preoccupied with traumatic memories or grief are often limited in their abilities to protect and stimulate the development of their children.

Adolescents can demonstrate negative or aggressive behavior in response to their parents who attempt to communicate their authority. Both parties want to feel respected, but at the same time they have to become accustomed to their changed relationship. These processes take place within culturally varied contexts. These contexts are influential on how socialization occurs. In some societies, after they get married, girls move to live in the house of their husbands' family. The social ties may be stronger because they live closer than in Western industrialized cultures where there is an emphasis on individual independency. Adolescence, therefore, is a cultural and societal phenomenon that bridges childhood and adulthood, although the years of age when these changes take place may differ across cultures.

10.4.3 Identity Formation

Adolescents need their friends to discover or seek reinforcement of their own identity. The process of identity construction, which occurs through belonging to various groups, may become challenging for refugee adolescents who are in a cultural transition. Unaccompanied adolescents are often forced to take over adult responsibilities earlier than they may be ready for. In some refugee families, adolescents need to take over adult obligations when one or both parents' capacities are undermined by post-traumatic reactions or acculturation tempo [21].

Box 10.3
Adolescence and young adulthood constitute particularly challenging and interesting periods during which:

- Biological and physical changes are prominent.
- Peer groups and social relationships outside of the family contribute to defining a sense of identity. The extent to which friends have an impact on the significant choices in their lives may be different for refugees from different backgrounds.
- Parents change position: they move to the "passenger or back seat"; they are needed more as coaches who offer guidance than as caretakers. Again, various cultural backgrounds will use different codes for parental behavior in relation to young people.
- There may still be a strong (masked) need for guidance and support.

The developmental pathway of refugee adolescents can be challenged by the accumulation of stress. In order to examine consequences of the disruptive events in the lives of refugee adolescents on their development and well-being, we will now focus on their flight-related experiences and coping strategies.

10.5 The Impact of Cumulative Stress

10.5.1 Individual

Refugee children exposed to cumulative stress due to organized violence, forced migration, and long-lasting asylum procedures have a significant risk of suffering from a number of serious complaints [22–25]. Post-traumatic stress disorder (PTSD) and comorbidity of, in particular, anxiety and affective symptoms and disorders are the most familiar consequences of the interplay between accumulation of traumatic and ongoing stressors, internal vulnerabilities, lack of resources, and dysfunctional family coping and adaptation. Rates for PTSD or other symptoms vary tremendously across studies [22, 24]. Overall, elevated rates of mental disorders have been observed for asylum-seeking children [24].

10.5.2 Family

For many refugee families, it takes tremendous effort to deal with the losses and adjust to new social surroundings in a country of arrival, especially while lacking supportive relationships when they are most needed. Stress symptoms experienced by one or more family members impair family functioning and disrupt family routines and interactional patterns [26, 27]. Using a multilevel path analysis, Nickerson and colleagues [28] found that loss and trauma significantly impacted the psychological outcomes at both the individual and family levels. Trauma-related distress and symptoms are associated with insensitive caregiving behavior, lack of empathy, hostility [29], diminished emotional availability, and negative perception of the child's behavior [30]. While the literature and clinical practice demonstrate that an accumulation of stresses affect parent-child relations and family functioning, research findings also suggest that family processes are pivotal in influencing post-traumatic adjustment [28, 31]. Interpersonal relationships with family members improved psychosocial functioning and post-traumatic growth [32].

Unfortunately, there are only few prospective studies on refugee youth available, which make it hazardous to draw firm conclusions about the significance of predicting factors for adjustment, recovery, and healthy development. Based on studies so far, traumatic experiences are regarded as a risk factor for mental health problems. Refugees are particularly at risk once they have reached the host country [24, 33, 34]. While low education, higher age, and negative experiences in the host country (e.g., discrimination) jeopardize positive adjustment, education and social support from family members and friends foster decrease of symptoms [24, 33, 34]. It seems that in the (perceived) absence of support, traumatic experiences gain more significance in relation to coping and health over time.

10.5.3 Intergenerational Consequences

Traumatized refugee families need to "make peace with the past" [35] in order to reorganize the relations within the fragmented family, redefine the roles and relations within the changed family structure, adjust to a new environment, and reset the future perspectives [36]. Many families accomplish these tasks successfully and move on; others stay captured by the painful past, the frozen grief, and an inability to generate future perspectives. Assessment of systems and subsystems is needed to explore in which way cumulative stress influences family members and the family as a whole. It will help to identify factors and processes that contribute to positive adaptation and the individual, family, and community resources.

Traumatic experiences and loss can shatter the family cohesion, leading to isolation of family members who are unsupported in their grief [37]. Unshared memories and experiences and memories that result in silence due to the belief that it helps forgetting or that it protects other family members or cultural beliefs cause distancing among family members. Avoiding communication about the death of a child or parent in the family limits the possibility for exchanging thoughts and feelings, which would help construct a shared meaning and narrative and facilitate the grieving process. Factors that inhibit shared meaning include family secrets, fragile family ties, divergent beliefs, and certain family rules [38]. A blocked grieving process may lead to the internalization of problems, withdrawal of adolescents, and/or engagement in risky behavior [37]. Through individual trauma- or grief-focused therapy, the encouragement of mutual support, reestablishment of parental protective capacities, and creation of shared meanings and rituals can be achieved.

Lanida, an isolated, depressed 13-year-old girl from a post-Soviet Union country became withdrawn after the traumatic events she experienced. Her mother suffers from post -traumatic and depressive symptoms and stays in her own room most of the time. She believes that all the odds in her life, including the lasting uncertainty about the asylum procedure, are to blame for the political engagement of her husband. The escalating conflicts between Lanida's parents along with their anger and irritability lead to verbal hostility toward Lanida. This strengthens her withdrawal and refusal to communicate with her parents. Neither her mother, who is imprisoned in the past and struggling with painful memories, nor her father, who is unsuccessfully trying to control his emotions, is emotionally available for Lanida. They don't see her age-specific needs and they are incapable of supporting her. Lanida, confronting a wall of silence, tries without success to make sense of her experiences. Only when she said that she does not want to live any longer did her parents become worried.

Still, feelings of greater closeness with family members are described by refugees as well. Also, positive changes as a result of experiencing adverse circumstances or trauma may take place within the family unit.

10.5.4 School

For many refugee adolescents, school constitutes an important resource. School provides the opportunity to learn and obtain various activities that facilitate self-development, meet other peers, be a way-out from home, and a place just to be a normal kid, although there may be a flip side to school as well. For instance, attending school may induce stress when a refugee has overly high ambitions for achievement. Successful adjustment depends on the perceived quality and support by the adolescent and family [21].

10.5.5 Religion

For some adolescents, religious activities, including the attendance of ceremonies, may be beneficial. Religion can provide a framework for understanding and coping with adversity, social support, and sense of belonging to a community [39]. However, it can also hamper effective coping strategies by closing off alternative ways for communication and seeking help. Eritrean unaccompanied minors, for instance, maintain a strong reliance on God, church, and priests. Their private rooms are fully decorated with religious objects. Professionals working with them (e.g., their legal guardians or social workers) are worried about their emphasis on religion as a resource.

10.6 Mental Health Interventions

In the next sections of this chapter, we discuss mental health interventions at different levels: individual, family, and community. We have taken the stand that multimodal interventions work best: due to the complexities and comorbidity of symptoms, different approaches may be best combined in treatment. Cooperation between representatives of different levels of the ecological circles (e.g., with school or family) has beneficial outcomes. A good case conceptualization is needed in order to maintain an overview and transparency of interventions.

10.6.1 Contextual Assessment: Developing a Case Conceptualization

One of the essential tasks of the mental health professional is to explore the consequences of political violence, forced migration, cultural transition, and the asylum policies for the refugee adolescent and his family. The consequences of traumatic experiences are examined in the context of other stressors in the pre- and post-migration period within the sociopolitical and cultural context of the country of origin and arrival [40]. The risk and protective factors during different phases of migration, including pre-existing vulnerabilities and strengths, as well as their effects, need to be carefully explored [41, 42], individually, as well as within a family context whenever possible. Moreover, an understanding of suffering and coping within the adolescents' own cultural framework and idiom of distress needs to be acquired. Questions derived from DSM's cultural formulation [43] may be helpful.

Despite differences in traumatic experiences, life circumstances, and cultural diversity, refugee adolescents are comforted by questions such as: How can I make sense of what has happened? How can I reorganize my life in an unfamiliar world? How do I restart a meaningful life? The challenge for mental health professionals is to support adolescents in finding some answers to these questions.

Several therapeutic approaches are described within the limited literature on therapeutic approaches with refugee adolescents [14]. In general, there are still insufficient empirically supported treatments that fulfill the standards for evidence-based practices with refugee youth living in Western countries. Isakson, Legerski, and Layne [44] therefore propose the implementation of the APA guidelines for evidence-based practice, taking into account:

- The best available clinical evidence regarding interventions for trauma
- Youth and family culture, preferences, and experiences
- Professional expertise and wisdom

An integrated multisystemic approach [45] creates flexibility to meet young refugees' diverse needs. The complex problems of refugee adolescents require multimodal interventions that integrate individual, family, and community approaches [41, 46–49]. A flexible implementation and integration of psychosocial and therapeutic techniques need to be modified according to clients' traumatic experiences, developmental needs, cultural diversity, and phase of migration. Below we describe interventions that are oriented subsequently at the individual, family, and community. As already noted, they are not mutually exclusive.

10.7 Individual Intervention

Despite a high rate of psychopathology in refugee adolescents, many of them fail to access mental health services, often due to fear of stigma [50]. Bean and colleagues [51], for instance, showed that nearly 60% of refugees reported the need for mental health services due to emotional distress, while only 13% received help. Insufficient information about treatment possibilities, lack of trust or cultural beliefs about mental health institutes, or not being used to talking about problems outside the family constitute barriers to professional psychosocial services. Linguistic and cultural barriers to appropriate services may play a role as well [52]. Another reason may be related to the conceptualization of psychological functioning and treatment. A parent may be concerned with behaviors at home or in school, while they may not understand the psychological sequelae of these behaviors. This possibly reflects different cultural understandings of mental health issues [53]. Alternatively, these symptoms might be seen as less important relative to other stress factors they have been through or are still facing, such as post-migration stressors. Finally, Sullivan and Simonson [54] suggest that refugees often experience internalizing symptoms. This may be associated with a lower rate of treatment use. Maybe, their symptoms are less noticeable to others, and therefore it is less likely that they will be referred to mental health care. In addition to being provided with extended information about mental health institutions, treatment process, and expected outcomes, refugee adolescents need to be encouraged to express their doubts and hesitations. Even when adolescents do enter mental health institutions, many of them are hesitant, ambivalent, and distrustful.

Building up a trusting relationship and motivation requires an open attitude and acceptance of lack of trust, anxieties, and ambivalent thoughts on the part of the mental health practitioner. Including family members, a legal custodian, or other supportive adults in the treatment can facilitate the process of building up trust and help refugee adolescents feel more at ease. Understanding how adolescents and family members perceive and define their problems, how they make sense of experience, and what matters to them is helpful for co-creating shared meanings of the problems and clarifying expectations. Therapeutic interventions that can initiate minimal positive changes such as relaxation techniques, problem-solving skills, and emotional regulation facilitating maintenance of the "window of tolerance" [55] can increase motivation and positive expectations in the early stages of therapy.

10.7.1 Trauma-Focused Treatment: The Applicability of Evidence-Based Methods

Although studies evaluating PTSD treatments for young refugees are scarce, and tend to suffer from methodological problems [41, 56], there is growing evidence that a specific trauma-focused approach can be effective in reducing PTSD in young refugees. Promising treatments for reducing symptoms of war-related PTSD include cognitive behavioral treatment (CBT), narrative exposure therapy ((KID) NET) [44, 57], and eye movement desensitization and reprocessing (EMDR) [58, 59].

Preferably, the therapist should be prepared to offer more than one promising treatment option as a best choice for tailored interventions, depending on the nature and frequency of traumatic experiences, language fluency, cultural influences, and preference of the adolescent. Cultural adaptations may include detailed and transparent information for adolescent and family members as well as length and number of sessions and modules. Sufficient adult support needs to be created for unaccompanied adolescents during treatment. TF-CBT, KIDNET, and EMDR for adolescents are briefly described here.

Cognitive behavioral therapy (TF-CBT) with exposure and/or cognitive restructuring as core elements has emerged as one of the most successful evidence-based, culturally sensitive treatments of trauma-related symptoms in adults, and also in children and adolescents, both trauma and/or grief focused [60–62]. For application of TF-CBT in refugee adolescents, modifications are suggested, for instance, to include more sessions for modulating feelings and psycho-education [63]. In particular, the recommended flexibility in implementing the modules of TF-CBT and the inclusion of parents and focus on enhancement of parental skills makes it very adjustable to refugee youth.

There is some evidence that *narrative exposure therapy (NET),* a short-term effective treatment for PTSD in individuals who have been traumatized by conflict and organized violence [64], can work for refugee adolescents. Based on the neurocognitive theory of traumatic memory, this approach has been developed in refugee camps combining exposure with creating a testimonial record, using a lifeline along with stones and flowers that resemble negative and positive life events, respectively [65]. The testimony method, also integrated in the NET procedure, covers both the private and public domain. A written transcript of NET is given to the client, allowing him/her to decide whether to keep it, send it to a human rights organization, or use it for judicial processes. Small-scale studies employing NET with Somalian adolescent refugees yielded promising results [66, 67].

Eye movement desensitization and reprocessing (EMDR) is a promising choice in treatment for refugee youth, even though there is still scant literature and insufficient empirical evidence for its use in this group. An image of the most upsetting as a starting point is helpful for many adolescents to process and desensitize traumatic memories, without the need to talk in detail about painful events. Oras, de Ezpeleta, and Ahmad [68] studied the use of EMDR in only 13 young refugees. Clearly, more and better controlled studies are needed.

10.8 Family Interventions

A multimodal, integrative treatment of refugee adolescents includes, in addition to individual trauma and grief therapy, a family-centered, strengths-based, culturally sensitive intervention. The objective of family-oriented interventions is to facilitate functional family coping.

When meeting families from various cultures, an open attitude is required in order to create possibilities for sharing many potentially different perspectives and interpretations relating to "how problems are perceived, understood and responded to" [69]. Creating a space where mutual understanding and negotiation of various meanings is possible can be seen as the precondition for co-constructing definitions of the problems and establishing therapeutic goals [40].

Box 10.4: Questions that Guide Assessment of Family Consequences

- What has happened and to whom?
- What are (un)shared memories held between family members?
- What separations and losses have occurred?
- What are ongoing stressors?
- Who is left behind or missing?
- How have the family dynamics, the relationships, and the roles changed?
- How do family members support each other and are they isolated, consumed with their own memories and sorrows?
- How do family members make sense of their experiences?
- Do different cultural values between family members lead to conflicts?

The therapeutic interventions target the family consequences of traumatic experiences and cumulative stress in the pre- and post-migration period aiming to (a) increase mutual understanding, (b) improve communication between family members, (c) reestablish competent parenting and improve parent-child relations, (d) reorganizing roles and obligations, and (e) strengthen coping, family and external resources.

10.8.1 Increasing Mutual Understanding

The better family members understand each other's changed reactions, behavior, and needs, the more they can increase their mutual support. Stimulating mentalization (the capacity to understand other's intentions, thoughts, and feelings), which is often reduced by trauma and stress, helps parents to understand the developmental and specific needs of their children in changed circumstances. Information may be given by a professional about traumatic and grief reactions especially when given with openness to possible different cultural interpretations.

10.8.2 Facilitating Family Communication

Communication patterns can facilitate or hinder the process of post-traumatic family adaptation. How families assign meaning and construct a family narrative depends upon the manner in which the parents and children communicate [70]. Avoidance of sharing painful memories or feelings may serve a purpose for the family, such as protecting oneself or other family members, adhering to cultural traditions and beliefs, or anxieties about the consequences. When the unspoken blocks the mourning process or the process of "making peace with the past" [35], the therapist can explore the ways that these unspoken issues influence the daily lives of the family. The importance of the timing of disclosure and the manner in which it takes place are more important than the effects of open communication or silencing strategies [71]. Disclosure should not, of course, be imposed on the family.

10.8.3 Improving Parenting and Parent-Child Relations

There is increasing evidence that cumulative and chronic (traumatic) stress, as well as trauma-related symptoms and comorbidity, undermine parental functioning and parent-child interactions [11, 26, 30, 72]. For many refugee parents, it is a challenge to become good parents while struggling with consequences of their own traumatic experiences, cultural transition, and ongoing stress. Interventions that focus on improvement of mentalization and emotional regulation are efficient for increasing functional parenting and improving parent-child relations.

10.8.4 Reorganizing Roles and Obligations

Tasks and roles or functions in the family change often during resettlement. In families with missing or traumatized parents or a parent hindered by acculturation issues, children often take over many parental tasks. It takes a careful estimation to assess whether this facilitates the functional adaptation of the family or endangers the development of children. Cultural factors need to be taken in consideration. When a parentified position interferes with the developmental tasks of adolescents, parents can be helped to understand and get sufficient external help to take over various roles from their children.

10.8.5 Strengthening Coping, Family, and External Resources

Even though many refugee families believe that their resources have been depleted and that the coping strategies on which they have relied in the past are no longer effective [36], each family has a range of coping abilities, strengths, and resource reserves [35]. It is up to the therapist to explore, support, and assist in activating these dormant resources and coping, mapping what family members find helpful, how they support each other, and how they use external resources. The therapist can discuss which rituals the family uses to facilitate the mourning process and how, despite cultural transitions, they could use these old traditions or invent new traditions that could help. Religious beliefs that were effective before or that are helpful now can be discussed. Parents are encouraged to tell their children what they learned from their own parents and other important individuals that they relied on in difficult times.

Unfortunately, so far there is little evidence for the efficacy of family-oriented interventions in the field of psychotrauma for refugees in particular. However, Weine and colleagues [31, 73] have reported positive effects of strengthening family adjustment and coping in Bosnian and Kosovar refugees through using a group format. Communication within families was improved in families where one of its members was suffering from PTSD.

Separate psychotherapy for Rakim and his mother was combined with family sessions, helping his mother to understand what her wish to die meant to her son. When his mother became able to reassure Rakim that she would stay alive and could be motivated to accept external practical help, Rakim regained a feeling of safety. His parentified role diminished. By strengthening the mutual support between the mother and her son and involving external support, sufficient holding was created to start the trauma-focused therapy. Several months after receiving a residence permit, Rakim could slowly find his way to build friendships and engage in pleasurable activities.

10.9 Community-Oriented Interventions: Working with School

There are various programs that foster empowerment, coping competencies, and resilience in refugee youth. Preventive programs generally have a broad scope, directing at creative expression, identity development, and social support. School may be particularly supportive for strengthening an adolescent's ability to cope with stress and adversity. However, psychological distress may impact a person's ability to concentrate, and it can hinder his or her executive functioning, which also interferes with the building of social relationships [74]. And vice versa, poor academic performance and inconsistent attendance are early signs of emerging mental health problems [75]. A sense of hopelessness in asylum-seeking youth in the Netherlands, for instance, caused difficulties in holding on to the belief that they want to perform well at school [15].

School participation in general is associated with resilience in refugee youth [24]. Many adolescent refugees see education as the key to a higher status or better future and as a way of gaining control over their lives [21]. A greater sense of school belonging is associated with lower depression and higher self-efficacy in adolescent refugees [76]. Besides, positive relationships with other students can help young refugees to integrate into their new society [15].

School could be the ideal place to offer extra support for refugee children [77]. At the same time, mental health interests cannot dominate the priorities of teaching and learning in school. Teachers working with refugees and immigrant children are usually faced with extra demands in the classroom already. While school is an ideal place to meet young people, meeting their mental health needs entails a collaboration of educational and mental health professionals.

10.9.1 School-Based Mental Health Interventions

School-based mental health services vary tremendously; they vary in terms of focusing on prevention versus more acute intervention and also in terms of who provides these services (e.g., teachers or clinicians with special training) and what are targeted domains, dosage, and more. A recent review by Sullivan and Simonson [54] included 13 studies of school-based interventions with young refugee, asylum-seeking, or war-traumatized immigrants. They distilled three different types of school-based interventions: (1) creative expression therapy (including music, drama, writing, and drawing activities), (2) cognitive behavioral therapeutic interventions, and (3) multimodal interventions. Most of the school-based intervention programs that were offered to refugee, asylum-seeking, or war-traumatized immigrant children and youth were previously developed for other populations who have experienced trauma. Although the effects varied, the findings suggested that school-based interventions can be effective in reducing young refugees' trauma-related symptoms (see also [78]). It is important, however, to underline the limited amount of research in this field. Creative expression interventions were the most commonly used in refugee populations, but had the least steady results [54]. Cognitive behavioral therapeutic interventions showed more consistent and positive results than the music therapy and other creative programs [54].

10.9.2 Considerations

For schools with refugee students, it is important to provide culturally and linguistically appropriate services in response to the needs of these students and their families. Nevertheless, the limited body of research in this field leads to some concern because which and how services should be offered at schools for these young refugees is still a little ambiguous. On the basis of our description, we argue that interventions need some degree of tailoring to address the students' cultures or trauma experiences. Furthermore, it is necessary to provide training to teachers on the backgrounds, experiences, and potential mental health issues of refugee youth. Teacher involvement appears to be a very important factor for the academic engagement and achievements of young refugees [79]. Consequently, time-limited school-based interventions should not be regarded as a replacement for teacher involvement [80].

Refugee youth may consider school to be the place where they are "normal" children or adolescents again and as a safe place away from all the difficulties they face [15]. Consequently, by offering mental health services at school, in other words "by connecting these different worlds of the ecological territory", it is crucial to preserve school as a safe and fostering environment. There remain many challenges for schools to offer mental health services: confidentiality issues, funding, having adequately trained mental health school-based professionals, not overloading teachers and school staff with extra responsibilities and new tasks, and sustainability of the interventions. Finally, while the involvement of refugee parents or caregivers at school deserves extra attention, a more broader scope on preventive measures may be useful.

10.10 Concluding Remarks

Without disregarding the eminent resilience adolescent refugees demonstrate, it is important to note that they are considered at risk for developmental difficulties due to a series of circumstances in their home country, during flight, and/or in resettling in a host environment. As a result of disruptive experiences, including the separation from family members and familiar surroundings, they can show a variety of responses. In counteracting these normal responses to abnormal circumstances, they rely on supportive and facilitating interactions. As we have learned from the case of Rakim, the mere presence of a parent is not in itself a guarantee of adequate social support. Parents may offer a protective shield but also constitute a source of worry and stress. If they are present, caregivers do have the opportunity to provide their teenagers with adequate help. The vulnerability for development of psychosocial needs increases when social resources are missing. Particularly for adolescents, three domains of development are at stake: biological changes, autonomy and independence, and identity formation. Peers, family members, school, and church can all foster positive adjustment. At the same time, these social resources can also risk or jeopardize adaptation by inducing negative experiences.

In general, use of mental health services is low, and many barriers, such as stigma and sense of shame, are often associated. Recent insights on resilience and related factors supporting adjustment after turmoil, may help clinicians to better understand the multidimensionality of change and recovery in refugee adolescents. There may be harm or psychopathology in one domain of functioning while other domains have remained intact and can be utilized as a resource. Losses can turn into gains.

References

1. United Nations International Children's Emergency Fund. UNICEF data: monitoring the situation of children and women 2016. http://data.unicef.org/topic/child-migration-and-displacement/migration/. Accessed 10 April 2017.
2. van Os E, Kalverboer M, Zijlstra A, Post W, Knorth E. Knowledge of the unknown child: a systematic review of the elements of the best interests of the child assessment for recently arrived refugee children. Clin Child Fam Psychol Rev. 2016;19:185–203. https://doi.org/10.1007/s10567-016-0209-y.
3. Vitus K, Lidén H. The status of the asylum-seeking child in Norway and Denmark: comparing discourses, politics and practices. J Refug Stud. 2010;23:62–81. https://doi.org/10.1093/jrs/feq003.
4. Centraal Orgaan opvang asielzoekers. Personen in de opvang uitgesplitst naar leeftijd en land van herkomst. https://www.coa.nl/nl/over-coa/bezetting/personen-in-de-opvang-uitgesplitst-naar-leeftijd-en-land-van-herkomst2017. Accessed 11 April 2017.
5. United Nations. Convention on the rights of the child global trends: forced displacement in 2015. http://www.ohchr.org/EN/ProfessionalInterest/Pages/CRC.aspx. Accessed 20 February 2017.
6. United Nations High Commissioner for Refugees. UNHCR statistics–the world in numbers 2015. http://popstats.unhcr.org/en/overview. Accessed 15 April 2017.
7. United Nations High Commissioner for Refugees. Who we help. http://www.unhcr.org/who-we-help.html. Accessed 10 April 2017.
8. United Nations. Convention on the rights of the child. http://www.ohchr.org/EN/ProfessionalInterest/Pages/CRC.aspx. Accessed 11 April 2017.
9. Sameroff A. The transactional model. American Psychological Association: Washington; 2009.
10. Cicchetti D, Rogosch FA. A developmental psychopathology perspective on adolescence. J Consult Clin Psychol. 2002;70:6–20. https://doi.org/10.1037/0022-006X.70.1.6.
11. Kiser LJ, Black MM. Family processes in the midst of urban poverty: what does the trauma literature tell us? Aggress Violent Behav. 2005;10:715–50. https://doi.org/10.1016/j.avb.2005.02.003.
12. Figley CR, Kiser LJ. Helping traumatized families. New York: Routledge; 2013.
13. van Reisen M. The involvement of unaccompanied minors from Eritrea in human trafficking. 2016. http://194.0.234.211/wp-content/uploads/2016/08/the_involvement_of_unaccompanied_minors_in_ht.pdf. Accessed 22 Feb 2017.
14. Alegría M, Álvarez K, DiMarzio K. Immigration and mental health. Curr Epidemiol Rep. 2017:1–11. https://doi.org/10.1007/s40471-017-0111-2.
15. Sleijpen M, Mooren T, Kleber RJ, Boeije HR. Lives on hold: a qualitative study of young refugees' resilience strategies. Childhood. 2017. https://doi.org/10.1177/0907568217690031.
16. Nickerson A, Liddell BJ, Maccallum F, Steel Z, Silove D, Bryant RA. Posttraumatic stress disorder and prolonged grief in refugees exposed to trauma and loss. BMC Psychiatry. 2014;14:106. https://doi.org/10.1186/1471-244x-14-106.
17. Dyregrov A, Salloum A, Kristensen P, Dyregrov K. Grief and traumatic grief in children in the context of mass trauma. Curr Psychiatry Rep. 2015;17:1–8. https://doi.org/10.1007/s11920-015-0577-x.
18. Morgos D, Worden JW, Gupta L. Psychosocial effects of war experiences among displaced children in southern Darfur. OMEGA J Death Dying. 2008;56:229–53. https://doi.org/10.2190/OM.56.3.b.
19. van der Veer G. Counselling and therapy with refugees: psychological problems of victims of war, torture and repression. Oxford: John Wiley & Sons; 1992.
20. Crone E. Het puberende brein: over de ontwikkeling van de hersenen in de unieke periode van de adolescentie. Amsterdam: Prometheus; 2011.
21. Sleijpen M, Boeije HR, Kleber RJ, Mooren T. Between power and powerlessness: a meta-ethnography of sources of resilience in young refugees. Ethn Health. 2015;21:158–80.

22. Fazel M, Wheeler J, Danesh J. Prevalence of serious mental disorder in 7000 refugees resettled in western countries: a systematic review. Lancet. 2005;365:1309–14. https://doi.org/10.1016/S0140-6736%2805%2961027-6.
23. Fazel M, Reed RV, Panter-Brick C, Stein A. Mental health of displaced and refugee children resettled in high-income countries: risk and protective factors. Lancet. 2012;379:266–82. https://doi.org/10.1016/S0140-6736(11)60051-2.
24. Montgomery E. Trauma and resilience in young refugees: a 9-year follow-up study. Dev Psychopathol. 2010;22:477–89. https://doi.org/10.1017/S0954579410000180.
25. Reed RV, Fazel M, Jones L, Panter-Brick C, Stein A. Mental health of displaced and refugee children resettled in low-income and middle-income countries: risk and protective factors. Lancet. 2012;379:250–65. https://doi.org/10.1016/S0140-6736(11)60050-0.
26. Appleyard K, Osofsky JD. Parenting after trauma: supporting parents and caregivers in the treatment of children impacted by violence. Infant Ment Health J. 2003;24:111–25. https://doi.org/10.1002/imhj.10050.
27. Barnes M, Figley CR. Family therapy: working with traumatized families. In: Lebow JL, editor. Clinical family therapy. New Jersey: John Wiley & Sons, Inc.; 2005. p. 309–29.
28. Nickerson A, Bryant RA, Brooks R, Steel Z, Silove D, Chen J. The familial influence of loss and trauma on refugee mental health: a multilevel path analysis. J Trauma Stress. 2011;24:25–33. https://doi.org/10.1002/jts.20608.
29. Tull MT, Jakupcak M, Paulson A, Gratz KL. The role of emotional inexpressivity and experiential avoidance in the relationship between posttraumatic stress disorder symptom severity and aggressive behavior among men exposed to interpersonal violence. Anxiety Stress Coping. 2007;20:337–51. https://doi.org/10.1080/10615800701379249.
30. van Ee E, Kleber RJ, Mooren TT. War trauma lingers on: associations between maternal posttraumatic stress disorder, parent-child interaction, and child development. Infant Ment Health J. 2012;33:459–68. https://doi.org/10.1002/imhj.21324.
31. Weine S, Muzurovic N, Kulauzovic Y, Besic S, Lezic A, Mujagic A, et al. Family consequences of refugee trauma. Fam Process. 2004;43:147–60. https://doi.org/10.1111/j.1545-5300.2004.04302002.x.
32. Sleijpen M, Haagen J, Mooren T, Kleber RJ. Growing from experience: an exploratory study of posttraumatic growth in adolescent refugees. Eur J Psychotraumatol. 2016;7:28698. https://doi.org/10.3402/ejpt.v7.28698.
33. Montgomery E. Long-term effects of organized violence on young middle eastern refugees' mental health. Soc Sci Med. 2008;67:1596–603. https://doi.org/10.1016/j.socscimed.2008.07.020.
34. Smid GE, Lensvelt-Mulders GJ, Knipscheer JW, Gersons BP, Kleber RJ. Late-onset PTSD in unaccompanied refugee minors: exploring the predictive utility of depression and anxiety symptoms. J Clin Child Adolesc Psychol. 2011;40:742–55. https://doi.org/10.1080/15374416.2011.597083.
35. Figley CR. Treating stress in families. New York: Brunner/Mazel; 1989.
36. Bala J. Beyond the personal pain: integrating social and political concerns in therapy with refugees. In: Ingleby D, editor. Forced migration and mental health: rethinking the care of refugees and displaced persons. Boston: Springer; 2005. p. 169–82.
37. Walsh F. Strengthening family resilience. New York: Guilford; 2006.
38. Nadeau JW. Family construction of meaning. In: Neimeyer RA, editor. Meaning reconstruction and the experience of loss. Washington D.C.: American Psychology Association; 2003. p. 95–113.
39. Sutton V, Robbins I, Senior V, Gordon S. A qualitative study exploring refugee minors personal accounts of post-traumatic growth and positive change processes in adapting to life in the UK. Divers Equal Health Care. 2006;3(2):77–88.
40. Bala J, Kramer S. Intercultural dimensions in the treatment of traumatized refugee families. Traumatology. 2010;16:153–9. https://doi.org/10.1177/1534765610369262.
41. Ehntholt KA, Yule W. Practitioner review: assessment and treatment of refugee children and adolescents who have experienced war-related trauma. J Child Psychol Psychiatry. 2006;47:1197–210. https://doi.org/10.1111/j.1469-7610.2006.01638.x.

42. Reed R, Tyrer R, Fazel M. Treating forcibly displaced young people: global challenges in mental healthcare. In: Patel S, Reicherter D, editors. Psychotherapy for immigrant youth. Cham: Springer; 2016. p. 149–65.
43. Association. AP. Cultural formulation interview 2013. https://www.psychiatry.org/FileLibrary/Psychiatrists/Practice/DSM/APA_DSM5_Cultural-Formulation-Interview.pdf. Accessed 22 May 2017.
44. Isakson BL, Legerski J-P, Layne CM. Adapting and implementing evidence-based interventions for trauma-exposed refugee youth and families. J Contemp Psychother. 2015;45:245–53. https://doi.org/10.1007/s10879-015-9304-5.
45. Cicchetti D, Lynch M. Toward an ecological/transactional model of community violence and child maltreatment: consequences for children's development. Psychiatry. 1993;56:96–118. https://doi.org/10.1080/00332747.1993.11024624.
46. Betancourt TS, Meyers-Ohki SE, Charrow AP, Tol WA. Interventions for children affected by war: an ecological perspective on psychosocial support and mental health care. Harv Rev Psychiatry. 2013;21:70–91. https://doi.org/10.1097/HRP.0b013e318283bf8f.
47. Patel N, Kellezi B, Williams AC. Psychological, social and welfare interventions for psychological health and well-being of torture survivors. Cochrane Database Syst Rev. 2014;11:CD009317. https://doi.org/10.1002/14651858.CD009317.pub2.
48. Murray LK, Cohen JA, Ellis B, Mannarino A. Cognitive behavioral therapy for symptoms of trauma and traumatic grief in refugee youth. Child Adolesc Psychiatr Clin N Am. 2008;17:585–604. https://doi.org/10.1016/j.chc.2008.02.003.
49. Rousseau C, Measham T, Nadeau L. Addressing trauma in collaborative mental health care for refugee children. Clin Child Psychol Psychiatry. 2013;18:121–36. https://doi.org/10.1177/1359104512444117.
50. Shannon PJ, Wieling E, Simmelink-McCleary J, Becher E. Beyond stigma: barriers to discussing mental health in refugee populations. J Loss Trauma. 2015;20:281–96. https://doi.org/10.1080/15325024.2014.934629.
51. Bean T, Eurelings-Bontekoe E, Mooijaart A, Spinhoven P. Factors associated with mental health service need and utilization among unaccompanied refugee adolescents. Admin Pol Ment Health. 2006;33:342–55. https://doi.org/10.1007/s10488-006-0046-2.
52. Alegria M, Atkins M, Farmer E, Slaton E, Stelk W. One size does not fit all: taking diversity, culture and context seriously. Adm Policy Ment Health Ment Health Serv Res. 2010;37:48–60. https://doi.org/10.1007/s10488-010-0283-2.
53. Ellis BH, Lincoln AK, Charney ME, Ford-Paz R, Benson M, Strunin L. Mental health service utilization of Somali adolescents: religion, community, and school as gateways to healing. Transcult Psychiatry. 2010;47:789–811. https://doi.org/10.1177/1363461510379933.
54. Sullivan AL, Simonson GR. A systematic review of school-based social-emotional interventions for refugee and war-traumatized youth. Rev Educ Res. 2016;86:503–30. https://doi.org/10.3102/0034654315609419.
55. Ogden P, Minton K, Pain C. Trauma and the body: a sensorimotor approach to psychotherapy. New York: WW Norton & Company; 2006.
56. Klasen H, Crombag A-C. What works where? A systematic review of child and adolescent mental health interventions for low and middle income countries. Soc Psychiatry Psychiatr Epidemiol. 2013;48:595–611. https://doi.org/10.1007/s00127-012-0566-x.
57. Unterhitzenberger J, Rosner R. Case report: manualized trauma-focused cognitive behavioral therapy with an unaccompanied refugee minor girl. Eur J Psychotraumatol. 2016;7:29246. https://doi.org/10.3402/ejpt.v7.29246.
58. ter Heide F, Mooren TT, Knipscheer JW, Kleber RJ. EMDR with traumatized refugees: from experience-based to evidence-based practice. J EMDR Pract Res. 2014;8:147–56. https://doi.org/10.1891/1933-3196.8.3.147.
59. ter Heide FJJ, Mooren TM, van de Schoot R, de Jongh A, Kleber RJ. Eye movement desensitisation and reprocessing therapy v. stabilisation as usual for refugees: randomised controlled trial. Br J Psychiatry. 2016;209(4):311–8. https://doi.org/10.1192/bjp.bp.115.167775.
60. Cohen JA, Mannarino AP, Staron VR. A pilot study of modified cognitive-behavioral therapy for childhood traumatic grief (CBT-CTG). J Am Acad Child Adolesc Psychiatry. 2006;45:1465–73. https://doi.org/10.1097/01.chi.0000237705.43260.2c.

61. Deblinger E, McLEER SV, Henry D. Cognitive behavioral treatment for sexually abused children suffering post-traumatic stress: preliminary findings. J Am Acad Child Adolesc Psychiatry. 1990;29:747–52. https://doi.org/10.1097/00004583-199009000-00012.
62. Goenjian AK, Karayan I, Pynoos RS, Minassian D, Najarian LM, Steinberg AM, et al. Outcome of psychotherapy among early adolescents after trauma. Am J Psychiatr. 1997;154:536–42. https://doi.org/10.1176/ajp.154.4.536.
63. Unterhitzenberger J, Eberle-Sejari R, Rassenhofer M, Sukale T, Rosner R, Goldbeck L. Trauma-focused cognitive behavioral therapy with unaccompanied refugee minors: a case series. BMC Psychiatry. 2015;15:260. https://doi.org/10.1186/s12888-015-0645-0.
64. Neuner F, Catani C, Ruf M, Schauer E, Schauer M, Elbert T. Narrative exposure therapy for the treatment of traumatized children and adolescents (KidNET): from neurocognitive theory to field intervention. Child Adolesc Psychiatr Clin N Am. 2008;17:641–64. https://doi.org/10.1016/j.chc.2008.03.001.
65. Robjant K, Fazel M. The emerging evidence for narrative exposure therapy: a review. Clin Psychol Rev. 2010;30:1030–9. https://doi.org/10.1016/j.cpr.2010.07.004.
66. Onyut LP, Neuner F, Schauer E, Ertl V, Odenwald M, Schauer M, et al. Narrative exposure therapy as a treatment for child war survivors with posttraumatic stress disorder: two case reports and a pilot study in an African refugee settlement. BMC Psychiatry. 2005;5:7. https://doi.org/10.1186/1471-244X-5-7.
67. Schauer E, Neuner F, Elbert T, Ertl V, Onyut LP, Odenwald M, et al. Narrative exposure therapy in children: a case study. Intervention. 2004;2:18–32.
68. Oras R, de Ezpeleta SC, Ahmad A. Treatment of traumatized refugee children with eye movement desensitization and reprocessing in a psychodynamic context. Nord J Psychiatry. 2004;58:199–203. https://doi.org/10.1080/08039480410006232.
69. Measham T, Rousseau C, Nadeau L. The development and therapeutic modalities of a transcultural child psychiatry service. Can Child Adolesc Psychiatr Rev. 2005;14:68–72.
70. Montgomery E. Tortured families: a coordinated management of meaning analysis. Fam Process. 2004;43:349–71. https://doi.org/10.1111/j.1545-5300.2004.00027.x.
71. Dalgaard NT, Montgomery E. Disclosure and silencing: a systematic review of the literature on patterns of trauma communication in refugee families. Transcult Psychiatry. 2015;52:579–93. https://doi.org/10.1177/1363461514568442.
72. Price SJ, Price CA, McKenry PC. Families & change: coping with stressful events and transitions. Thousand Oaks: Sage; 2010.
73. Weine S, Kulauzovic Y, Klebic A, Besic S, Mujagic A, Muzurovic J, et al. Evaluating a multiple-family group access intervention for refugees with PTSD. J Marital Fam Ther. 2008;34:149–64. https://doi.org/10.1111/j.1752-0606.2008.00061.x.
74. Miller AB, Bixby CB, Ellis BH. School-based interventions. Psychotherapy for immigrant youth. Cham: Springer; 2016. p. 71–86.
75. DeSocio J, Hootman J. Children's mental health and school success. J Sch Nurs. 2004;20:189–96. https://doi.org/10.1177/10598405040200040201.
76. Wilkinson L. Factors influencing the academic success of refugee youth in Canada. J Youth Stud. 2002;5:173–93. https://doi.org/10.1080/13676260220134430.
77. Fazel M, Garcia J, Stein A. The right location? Experiences of refugee adolescents seen by school-based mental health services. Clin Child Psychol Psychiatry. 2016;21:368–80. https://doi.org/10.1177/1359104516631606.
78. Tyrer RA, Fazel M. School and community-based interventions for refugee and asylum seeking children: a systematic review. PLoS One. 2014;9(5):e97977. https://doi.org/10.1371/journal.pone.0097977.
79. Tucker CM, Zayco RA, Herman KC, Reinke WM, Trujillo M, Carraway K, et al. Teacher and child variables as predictors of academic engagement among low-income African American children. Psychol Sch. 2002;39:477–88. https://doi.org/10.1002/pits.10038.
80. Rousseau C, Beauregard C, Daignault K, Petrakos H, Thombs BD, Steele R, et al. A cluster randomized-controlled trial of a classroom-based drama workshop program to improve mental health outcomes among immigrant and refugee youth in special classes. PLoS One. 2014;9(8):e104704. https://doi.org/10.1371/journal.pone.0104704.

Psychotherapy and Psychosocial Support in Host Countries: State-of-the-Art and Emerging Paradigms

11

Boris Droždek and Derrick Silove

Abstract

Refugees may present with a constellation of mental health and psychosocial problems caused by a combination of exposure to violence and current and ongoing stress. In order to understand the complexity of their experiences, different models and frameworks have been developed. Most converge in attempting to provide an exhaustive and inclusive account of the diversity of mental health and existential impacts incurred as a consequence of exposure to often multiple human rights violations, experiences of forced migration and the stress of relocation. For those refugees in need of assistance for overt mental health problems, psychotherapeutic and psychosocial approaches have been developed, and these will be described together with suggestions and possible directions for future research.

11.1 Introduction

The refugee population in the contemporary world is at a record high and increasing. Over 244 million people are currently living outside of their country of origin [1], and the proportion of those migrating because of persecution, violence and human rights abuses is increasing [2]. In 2015 alone, over 1 million refugees fled to Europe by boat from Turkey and North Africa [3]. If, in theory, all refugees would relocate to one location, that "country" would be the fourth most populous in the

B. Droždek (✉)
PsyQ/Parnassia Group, Rosmalen/Eindhoven, The Netherlands
e-mail: drozdek@telfort.nl

D. Silove
Psychiatry, University of New South Wales, Sydney, NSW, Australia
e-mail: d.silove@unsw.edu.au

T. Wenzel, B. Droždek (eds.), *An Uncertain Safety*,
https://doi.org/10.1007/978-3-319-72914-5_11

world [4]. It is symbolic that for the first time, a refugee team participated in the 2016 Olympic Games, a powerful symbol of the determination of all asylum-seeking people to persist with maximizing their life potential: not only to survive but to make the best contributions they can in spite of their precarious circumstances. This endeavour is far from being readily accomplished given these persons' backgrounds of exposure to mass conflict and persecution and the ongoing uncertainties they confront in relation to their own and their families' futures.

This chapter will focus on several related issues: first, the psychosocial stressors that impact on the mental health of those seeking asylum outside of their country of origin, contemporary models for understanding the full complexity of the "refugee experience" and, finally, psychotherapies and psychosocial approaches applied to address mental health problems of these populations. Based on scientific evidence and clinical experience, we will attempt to provide a balanced overview and evaluation of the therapeutic approaches that work, for whom, in which settings and under what conditions. We will highlight the necessary ingredients of healing encounters with refugees while identifying ongoing dilemmas regarding elements of treatment that require to be further examined. Finally, we will offer suggestions and possible directions for research and development in the pursuit of investigating and refining psychotherapeutic and psychosocial approaches as the field makes progress into the future.

11.2 The "Refugee Experience" and Its Impacts on Mental Health

The migration trajectory can be divided into three phases: premigration experiences, the flight/forced migration period and the postmigration/resettlement phase. All components are associated with a set of specific psychosocial challenges and repeated exposure to violence, life-threatening events and more general stresses.

In the country of origin, refugees commonly are confronted with political violence, imprisonment and torture or are families of survivors, noting that the reported prevalence of exposure to these abuses amongst refugees in high-income host countries exceeds 30% [5]. More generally, refugee populations have been exposed to one or more of the broad experiences of war and related forms of mass conflict or persecution, loss of loved ones and belongings, social marginalization, discrimination and racism, fragmentation of communities and social capital, starvation, unemployment, disruption of social support and loss of roles and networks [6].

Migration from one country to another can be a risky and lengthy endeavour, often punctuated by repeated or chronic exposure to life-threatening situations and harsh living conditions. It is often the case that a refugee has to put his/her life and the lives of others, including family, at stake in order reach safety. A refugee may be apprehended by authorities while crossing state borders; imprisoned and tortured; be forced to travel through war-torn regions, thereby being exposed to additional violence; or be transported by dangerous forms of movement, across treacherous seas in unseaworthy or overcrowded boats or hidden in trucks for days without food and water. Flight is usually a financial burden for a refugee and/or the family, requiring compensation to be paid to unauthorized travel agents. Moreover, a refugee is often dependent on unscrupulous traffickers and their judgements and decisions. He/she runs the risk of extortion or enslavement, for example, being subject to human trafficking, prostitution or criminality in order to pay for the travel costs incurred.

Upon arrival to a host country, a refugee is confronted with a further set of new challenges and stressful life events, from the fraught pursuit of often lengthy procedure of seeking asylum which is found to worsen mental health [7–11] to adaptation problems once and if asylum is granted [12]. During the procedure of seeking asylum, asylum seekers live in constant fear of repatriation. They are commonly denied the right to work and attend lessons in the language of the host country, thereby preventing participation in meaningful activities in the country of residence. These conditions are deliberately imposed as a form of deterrence by the host government [13]. Further, complex legal provisions for establishing refugee status are often incomprehensible to asylum seekers, and the procedures themselves are opaque and stressful. Asylum seekers are often restricted in their access to social and medical services and compelled to live in group accommodation with basic resources and amongst strangers. At worst, asylum seekers may be held in detention centres under conditions of isolation, deprivation and potential for abuse [14]. Moreover, ongoing conflict in the region of origin means that family and kin remain at great risk, adding to the anxiety and fears experienced by the displaced person.

For those who are afforded formal refugee status, several challenges continue, including reaching competency in the host country language, achieving recognition of skills and qualifications and generally integrating into the new culture. However, the expectations from and demands by the host society concerning the ease and speed of integration of refugees may be unrealistic, many needing much more time to reorganize their lives due to the accumulation of a wide range of psychosocial stressors experienced throughout the prolonged premigration, migration and postmigration period. Postmigration stresses also include unemployment or underemployment; coping with multiple losses such as of social status, family ties, community and social support; limited opportunities for family reunification; the longer-term effects of uprooting; fear of culture extinction; discrimination and racism; and exposure to individual and society-wide hostility [15]. These stresses may be compounded by guilt arising from having migrated and unmitigated concerns about family left behind [16]. All these psychosocial factors have a potentially negative impact on the mental health of refugees [17]. Reinforcing of the "otherness" of refugees by a host society may be a further driver of mental health problems amongst refugees [18]. Moreover, research on a large sample of refugees [19] found that postmigration stressors also directly hinder their socioeconomic integration. It has been suggested that a loss of culture and home upon migration in combination with an unwelcoming environment in a host country may have a similar impact on mental health as torture or death of loved ones [20]. In that sense, there is a compounding of past torture and trauma by ongoing postmigration stresses after the initial relief of reaching a safe heaven, the consequence being substantial frustration and disillusionment that can increase risk of mental distress and disorder such as depression [21].

11.3 Mental Health Problems in Refugees

Although emphasizing herein the mental health impacts associated with the refugee experience, it is vital to acknowledge that the majority of refugees do not incur major mental health problems. Even for those who exhibit severe distress, time is a powerful healer. Refugees exhibit a natural resilience and capacity for spontaneous recovery, especially if given access to favourable postmigration environments. Nevertheless, even though only a minority develops overt mental health problems, the absolute numbers affected by these responses are substantial. Reviews of the existing body of research [17, 22–25] estimate that between 12 and 34% of refugees experience posttraumatic stress disorder (PTSD) and/or depression (often together with anxiety and somatic symptoms). Comorbidity is common and generally signifies great morbidity and a poorer outcome [26]. A minority of refugees develop a complex form of PTSD [27], especially those who have experienced a sequence of early childhood trauma such as sexual abuse and later exposure to political violence. Now included in the proposed classification in the International Classification of Diseases (ICD-11), complex PTSD is characterized by a distrustful and hostile attitude towards the world, estrangement, social withdrawal, feelings of emptiness and hopelessness, a chronic feeling of being threatened, disturbances in emotion regulation and a diminished and defeated sense of self [28]. Moreover, refugees may present with other anxiety disorders, complex forms of grief, somatoform disorders, explosive forms of anger, chronic pain, psychosis, personality changes and disorders, dissociative states and organic brain disorders (including head injury which may exacerbate conditions such as PTSD) [29, 30]. In general, these common mental disorders are twice as common in refugees as in comparable groups of economic migrants (approximately 40 vs. 21%) [31]. Moreover, refugees are ten times more likely to suffer from PTSD than age-matched native populations of host countries [22].

PTSD remains the most extensively studied mental health problem amongst asylum seekers and refugees. There is reasonable consistency in the literature [32] that PTSD is more strongly associated with exposure to man-made violence in the home country or during flight, whereas depression, anxiety and other adaptational problems are more closely related to post-migratory stressors, although this distinction is only relative. In general, cumulative stressors compound the effects of prior traumas and increase the risk of severity and chronicity of PTSD and other disorders [33].

It needs to be recognized that the validity of the PTSD concept has been challenged when applied as an indicator of mental disorder across cultures (and particularly amongst refugees), the claim being that there is a risk of medicalizing normative responses to socio-political challenges and threats and thereby obscuring the multitude of real-life challenges encountered in the ecological environment in which displaced persons find themselves [34, 35]. The worst potential outcome of this process is the risk of applying psychopathological labels to natural human responses to human rights violations, according to a narrow prism of the trauma paradigm [36]. The contrary position, now supported by extensive research, is that PTSD can be identified across a range of contexts and cultures and its acknowledgement can assist to explain and demystify mental health symptoms to survivors and their families.

In addition, in spite of its limitations, the PTSD concept can provide a common focus for communication, research and treatment [37]. A balanced position recognizes that at the normative level, post-traumatic stress symptoms such as intrusive memories, avoidance, numbing and hyperarousal represent normative survival responses to extreme threat, whereas at the other extreme, frank PTSD symptoms can become persistent and disabling [6]. Importantly, whereas trauma exposure initiates the PTSD reaction, ongoing human rights violations and psychosocial deprivations play a major role in shaping the prevalence and course of symptoms and associated functional impairment across conflict-affected populations [38]. Recognition of the impact of the ongoing eco-social and policy environment on symptoms underscores the importance of mental health professionals advocating strongly for just treatment and improvement in the living conditions and social context of refugees as a powerful tool to overcoming mental health symptoms, in addition to the benefits of offering therapy to the selective individuals in need of such interventions. In that regard, anthropological research [39] suggests that the priorities for survivors of human rights abuses are to achieve collective recognition and acknowledgement of the abuses they have experienced, restitution of lost property and, finally, restoration of a sense of existential safety. Other observers [34, 40, 41] have highlighted the urgency of focusing on ongoing postmigration rights and needs including denial of residency status, family separations, grief for the loved ones lost and inability to perform bereavement rituals, loss of social networks and cultural supports, poverty, intimate partner violence and barriers to work and self-sufficiency.

When refugees decide to seek assistance for their mental health problems, they experience a range of obstacles to obtaining recommended interventions, only minority being likely to be referred for appropriate treatment [42]. As suggested by Kirmayer et al. [16], these barriers include communication difficulties due to language and cultural differences, help-seeking behaviours that are not congruent with the customs of the host culture, presentations of symptoms and illness behaviour that are culture-specific and family factors (stigma, distrust of health systems, intergenerational differences in attitudes) that inhibit disclosure or the pursuit of effective action to address these issues. Stigma may be internalized concerning mental illness which in turn may shape a negative attitude towards help seeking and counselling [43]. Further, attitudes of the host society towards refugees, particularly the extent of acceptance versus treating members of minorities as alien, and perspectives shared by health professionals greatly influence the ease or otherwise of obtaining mental health care when there is a need.

11.4 Theoretical Frameworks for Understanding the Complexity of the Refugee Experience

In recent decennia, several authorities in the field have offered a range of models aimed at providing a comprehensive account of the diversity and contextual determinants of psychopathological outcomes following exposure to traumatic experiences amongst refugees. Contemporary models extend the focus beyond trauma exposure per se to a consideration of the complex interplay of multiple and reciprocal psychosocial, policy-related and ecological factors that simultaneously impact on the key domains of refugees' lives [44]. Theories draw on a pluralistic set of disciplines and schools of thought including the fields of systems theory, human rights, cultural psychiatry, migrant mental health and post-traumatic stress theory inter alia.

Khan's concept of cumulative trauma [45] depicts trauma as a product of a series of stressful experiences that accumulate over time in the interaction of an individual with the changing environment, a sequence of undermining events that may finally lead to the emergence of mental health problems. The author [45] introduced the dimensions of time and the interactive relationship between an individual and his/her surroundings into the discussion about trauma, thereby transforming the event (traumatic experience) into a process [46]. Later on, McEwen [47] introduced the notion of allostasis and allostatic load in understanding the psychobiology of stress. He described allostatic load as the physiological cost of making long-term adaptive shifts across a broad range of systems in order to match internal functioning to environmental demands. Thereby, allostasis became the most comprehensive account of regulatory accommodation to environmental demands and accumulated physiological cost over time. This concept enriched understanding of the interplay over time between context, current stressor exposure, internal regulation of bodily processes and health outcomes. This concept has also been used for understanding of the unfolding of PTSD phenomena [48].

In a similar vein, Keilson [49] introduced the concept of sequential traumatization. He suggested that there is no "post" in PTSD and that ongoing changes in the environmental/historical context of the individual survivor interact with traumatic experiences through time, recognizing that the quality and quantity of traumatic sequences can differ in various contexts and at different times across the lifespan [46]. These concepts are consistent with more recent recognition of the multiplicity of comorbid patterns associated with PTSD, each subtype being associated with a particular set of antecedents and ongoing stresses [50]. One possibility is that there is a continuum of reactions to trauma with the constellation of complex post-traumatic symptoms representing the extreme end of severity [51].

In order to explore and understand the interaction between the individual and environment, Bronfenbrenner [52] developed what is referred to as ecological systems theory. An individual is nested in "the ecological environment" described as a concentric arrangement of expanding levels/dimensions, each structure contained within the next. These structures are referred to as the micro- (intrapsychic), meso- (peer group, family, social life), exo- (society) and macrosystems ((sub)culture, belief systems, ideology). Individual development occurs within the context of a system of relationships that form the environment. Influences, within and between different dimensions/levels, are regarded as bidirectional, and changes or conflicts in any one dimension of the system ripple throughout other dimensions. According to this theory, although problems that individual refugee survivors present are defined as psychological or intrapsychic, these responses are simultaneously influenced by and interact with medical, social, political, cultural, existential or multidimensional influences. A mental health provider therefore should transcend the tendency to Cartesian thinking (mind-brain problems versus external world issues) and search for a broader conceptual frame which inculcates all these interacting components. This enables the clinician to examine the dynamic interplay of internal and external influences hindering or facilitating individual development and adaptation.

Hobfoll's [53, 54] conservation of resources (COR) theory views loss of resources as the key component in the process leading to mental health problems in refugees. The model presents an alternative to appraisal-based stress theories. This theory is based on the tenet that individuals strive to obtain, retain, protect and foster the things they value. The stress process occurs in the realm of social action, and it arises in situations where individuals face a threat of resource loss, where resources are actually lost or where an investment of resources fails to produce an expected return. COR theory provides tools to examine objective conditions out of which stressful demands are born. According to the COR theory, individuals accumulate resources in order to accommodate, withstand or overcome threats. These resources are personal, such as self-esteem; material, such as money; conditional, such as status; and social, such as support. Stressful or traumatic events consume these resources and augment one's sensitivity to subsequent stressors. COR theory analyses a flux of resources at times of stress, providing a framework for comparing the relative loss of resources with risk of adverse mental health outcomes.

Silove [6, 55] has proposed the adaption and development after persecution and trauma (ADAPT) model that identifies five core psychosocial pillars disrupted by conflict and displacement: safety, integrity of bonds and networks, systems of justice, roles and identities and systems of meaning and coherence. The traumas and stresses associated with the changing ecosystems experienced by refugees during the continuum of mass conflict, flight and resettlement involve a complex feedback loop of interaction between the individual psyche and the collective psychosocial environment; the natural response of the person and his or her group is to mount adaptive responses which, depending on internal or external factors or both, determine successful outcomes or the development of dysfunction and frank psychopathology [38]. Comorbid patterns can be understood in relation to the distinct pathways arising from disruptions of a combination of the five core psychosocial pillars, for example, severe and persisting insecurity tends to perpetuate PTSD symptoms and multiple traumatic losses; separations and material deprivations result in prolonged grief, separation anxiety and depression; and unmitigated injustices tend to generate persisting anger. Identifying the links that connect the disrupted psychosocial domains, the capacity of individuals and collectives to mount effective adaptive responses and the manifestations of psychopathology at the individual level is key to achieving a comprehensive understanding of the needs of refugees and to designing accurate preventive and clinical interventions that are synchronized with the specific history, culture and context of refugees populations.

Miller et al. [56] introduced the framework of social constructivism as an alternative to the widespread trauma-focused psychiatric epidemiology with war-affected populations and refugees. This framework represents a shift from searching for universal truths (the outsider, etic perspective) while trying to grasp the impacts of exposure to man-made violence to the perspective of understanding survivors' worldviews or lived experiences as they are rooted in their specific cultural contexts (the insider, emic perspective). The model emphasizes human agency in the creation of meaning and accentuates the role of the meaning-making process in mediating human responses to life adversities. These considerations point to the importance of: focusing on local idioms of distress, identification of local mental health concerns and priorities, understanding the effects of organized violence on multiple levels of the survivor groups cosmology or world views (in relation to the family, community, society), and understanding of local patterns of help-seeking behaviour. Furthermore, it is important to focus on identification of local resources that can promote healing and adaptation, and thereby to identify context relevant intervention strategies. While the trauma-focused approach presumes that helping individual survivor with PTSD complaints will positively influence functioning of survivor's family and community, the social constructivism framework suggests that improvement in functioning of a family and community will facilitate individual healing and adaptation.

Papadopoulos [57] introduced the trauma grid as a model which invites therapists to explore the entire range of refugees' reaction to adversities. He points out that exposure to traumatic experiences can cause a wide range of psychological wounds in survivors: from ordinary human suffering, via distressful psychological reactions involving stronger experiences of discomfort, to psychiatric disorders such as PTSD. The author introduces the notion of adversity-activated development (AAD) as a potentially positive effect of trauma. The notion of AAD means that a survivor becomes strengthened by exposure to adversity which may lead to individual transformation beyond previous understandings and expectations. The trauma grid assists therapists in distinguishing between a range of reactions to adversities, both positive and adverse. These reactions can occur simultaneously, and a survivor can experience damage in some and resilience or development in other functions.

Developmental psychopathology [58] offers a framework for a process-level understanding of mental health disorders. The model seeks to elucidate the interplay amongst the biological, psychological and social-contextual aspects of normal and abnormal development across the lifespan. This paradigm suggests the critical importance of adopting a developmental perspective on mental health, because psychopathology unfolds over time in a developing organism [59]. Its central focus is to investigate and describe the interactive processes that lead to the emergence and course of disturbed behaviour, since there are multiple pathways to similar manifest outcomes and different outcomes of the same pathway in development of mental health disorders. In relation to asylum seekers and refugees, this paradigm invites consideration of why someone develops psychopathology at a certain point in the lifespan and not earlier or later. In particular, it raises the important question why a trauma survivor may present with a late-onset PTSD, that is, the balance between resilience and post-traumatic vulnerability is disturbed in a manner that results in an adverse outcome only much later after exposure to traumatic experiences.

Building on the above-mentioned frameworks, Drožđek [60, 61] and Drožđek et al. [62, 63] have formulated the integrative contextual model for understanding and assessment of post-trauma mental health sequelae. This model merges the developmental and the ecological perspectives. It stresses that, in assessing and treating mental health problems, it is necessary for the clinician to simultaneously focus on the intrapsychic, biological, interpersonal and socio-political dimensions of human experience. This model underlines the importance of understanding the context of an individual as a dynamic system that can change over time, and it points out the bidirectional nature of the relationship between mental health disorders and context. Therefore, a mental disease diagnosis is viewed as a current reflection of a psychological imbalance, a mirror of one's lifelong dynamic struggle between sources of resilience and damage. A mental health professional is challenged to identify and evaluate the risk and the protective factors in both the developmental and the socio-environmental contexts of a patient, recognizing, thereby, the influence of culture on human psychology. The model suggests that assessing mental health disorders should resemble watching a movie about a patient's life trajectory in order to understand the onset of his/her mental health problems, a process that contrasts with taking a single snapshot at one point in time. In cases of refugees presenting with severe PTSD and an invalidating presence of current psychosocial stress, clinicians should aim at collecting information which will enhance understanding of the development of mental health problems across a patient's lifespan and in the ecological environment. They should be guided by a chain of causation principle in understanding the development of mental health problems which obliges them to question why a patient has developed psychopathology at a certain moment in his/her life, what has protected him/her from becoming sick earlier in life and which, previously present, sources of resilience may be strengthened in order to help the patient to get better. Although applying the integrative contextual model may be time-consuming, the authors argue that it may improve (1) assessment of patients' problems, (2) design and timing of interventions on different levels of ecological environment and (3) evaluation thereof. It is expected that the initial time investment will pay off later on in the course of treatment, as adequately tailored treatment strategies may produce better and more sustainable outcomes.

The approach of the person-centred psychiatry [64] aims at assessing both illness and health in patients' social and cultural context. Contrary to the "one-size-fits-all" approach in evidence-based psychiatry and psychology [65] which seeks general solutions that can be applied across patients, the person-centred approach aims to understand each patient as a unique individual exposed to a unique matrix of contextual determinants. Therefore, the person and not the disease should be the focus of clinical research and assistance.

More so than earlier editions, the recent, fifth edition of the *Diagnostic and Statistical Manual of Mental Disorders* (DSM) [66] acknowledges the importance of context and culture in psychiatric practice. The manual includes the Cultural Formulation Interview (CFI) based on the Cultural Formulation of Diagnosis (CFD) [67], which is an integrative approach to formulation that embraces a wide range of cultural and social issues relevant to understanding mental health problems across diverse cultures, a prerequisite to tailoring treatment options to each context. CFI can be used as a comprehensive assessment tool which inquires into the cultural definitions of problems that patients are presenting with: cultural perceptions of cause and the role of context; the support received from family, friends or community; the role of cultural identity; and cultural factors affecting self-coping, present and past help seeking, preferences for and barriers to care as well as clinician-patient relationship. This tool also provides information regarding explanatory models of sickness, illness prototypes, expectations of treatment, level of functioning, impact of social network on illness, psychosocial stressors, spirituality, religion and moral traditions and is designed for use with every patient in clinical practice.

Most recently, Kira and Tummala-Narra [68] have presented the development-based trauma framework (DBTF) as an emerging paradigm for psychotherapy with refugees. They point out the importance of focusing both on past and ongoing traumas in the treatment of refugees. Moreover, while trauma-focused therapies have focused primarily on trauma perpetrated by individuals, these authors stress the importance of paying attention to traumas perpetrated by institutions and social systems, as well as to transgenerational transmission of traumatic experiences involving a sense of collective identity. They suggest that the linear dose-dependent model for understanding post-traumatic impacts is insufficient in explaining the risk for developing psychopathology and stress the relevance of non-linear dynamics in a threshold model. Also, they include the notion of cumulative trauma disorder (CTD) as a framework for chronic and cumulative effects of refugee trauma and an alternative for the PTSD concept. The authors describe CTD as a trans-diagnostic cluster which may encompass a wide array of psychopathological phenomena comorbid with PTSD, such as psychosis, dissociation, depressive, anxiety and somatization disorders, and memory and executive function deficits. Consequently, trans-diagnostic interventions in psychotherapy should be developed, as the ones treating multiple disorders at the same time concerning their shared causes, commonalities, course and symptom maintenance [69].

To summarize, the above-mentioned models and frameworks are inspiring clinicians and theoreticians in the field of refugee mental health in their quest for a comprehensive understanding of the "refugee experience" and designing of adequate assistance approaches, but they still need to be submitted to further scientific evaluation. Although data supporting aspects of these models are already available, it seems virtually impossible to test all components of comprehensive models all at once. Future research will, therefore, be an incremental process in which aspects of these models will be assessed.

11.5 Psychotherapy with Refugees: The State-of-the-Art Overview of Approaches

Several systematic reviews and meta-analyses of psychological treatments for PTSD amongst asylum seekers and refugees [70–73] conclude that the effectiveness of these approaches is not yet firmly supported by scientific evidence. The most consistent evidence has been provided by studies on trauma-focused therapies, particularly narrative exposure therapy (NET) [74–77] and trauma-focused cognitive behavioural therapy (TFCBT) [78, 79]. In contrast, evidence for eye movement desensitization and reprocessing (EMDR) amongst refugees is limited [80]. However, most of the NET and TFCBT studies have been undertaken by a single or limited number of groups of researchers, making replication by independent research teams imperative [81]. As for refugee survivors of torture in particular, evidence for effectiveness of psychological therapies is of a very low quality and, if anything, suggests that these brief approaches provide no immediate improvement in PTSD, other forms of distress or quality of life in that specific group [82]. However, there is some evidence, yet to be fully confirmed, that NET and TFCBT confer moderate benefits in reducing PTSD and distress symptoms in torture survivors over the medium term of 6 months after treatment.

NET is based on the testimony therapy, an approach developed by Lira and Weinstein (published under the pseudonyms Cienfuegos and Monelli) [83] and applied in treatment of traumatized survivors of the Pinochet regime in Chile. It emphasizes the creation of a cohesive chronological narrative of a survivor's life trajectory, from birth to present. NET aims at integrating traumatic memory within the context of the individual life experience in order to bring coherence to fragmented memories, enhance cognitive reappraisal and processing of trauma through imaginal exposure and build adaptive internal schemas. Since it builds on an oral tradition of storytelling, it is suggested that NET is applicable across different cultural contexts [74]. While creating a narrative, NET uses past tense and usually includes many traumatic memories, while conventional exposure techniques make use of present tense and often involve just a single memory of the survivor's worst trauma. NET sessions typically last 90–120 minutes, offered once or twice weekly, with a total of five to ten sessions [83]. In a randomized controlled trial [84], NET has been found superior to stress inoculation training (SIT). A preliminary RCT study of NET in Iraqi refugees [85] suggests that as few as three sessions of NET reduced mental health symptoms and increased post-traumatic growth and well-being. Research [86] suggests that NET can be successfully delivered by lay counsellors and suitable for application in contexts where a shortage of psychotherapist is present. However, these optimistic research results should be approached with caution as data on sustainability of the treatment effects on longer terms are not available yet. Also, there are no data regarding risk for burnout in lay counsellors as they may operate outside of a health system or in circumstances of a non-existing health system.

Culturally sensitive TFCBT has been extensively studied in the past years [87–90], and the guidelines for its implementation with refugees have recently been published [91]. TFCBT aims at processing of traumatic memories and integrating them with normal autobiographical memories, thereby reducing distressing intrusions. Also, TFCBT addresses negative appraisals that are maintaining the sense of current threat in survivors' lives. In comparison with NET, this approach focuses more on direct and full emotional exposure and cognitive restructuring.

Although multimodal-phased treatment approaches are often used in clinical practice with refugees and have been recommended for this population [92], their effectiveness is not yet sufficiently supported by scientific research [72]. These approaches shift the emphasis away from PTSD towards a more holistic understanding of the "refugee experience", and they take into account both impacts of the resettlement environment and the capacity for resilience amongst refugee survivors [57, 93]. The first phase of the multimodal approach focuses on stabilization and strengthening of survivor's daily life skills. It includes interventions aiming at improving patients' safety and resources, developing capacities for emotional awareness and expression and increasing interpersonal and social competences. In the second phase, the review and reappraisal of trauma memories in an organized way take place. In this phase, the evidence-based trauma treatments such as cognitive behaviour therapy (CBT) [94], eye movement desensitization and reprocessing (EMDR) [95] or NET [96] can be applied. Phase 3 involves consolidation of treatment gains and focuses at enabling transition from the treatment to a life in the community. It is noted, however, that a study of a multimodal multidisciplinary treatment for refugee survivors of torture [97] suggested no clinically significant improvement related to the intervention in several indices of mental health. More recent research [98, 99] suggests that multimodal trauma-focused group treatments in a specialized refugee trauma treatment setting may reduce psychopathology in refugees both on the short and longer terms. A combination of carefully sequenced interventions may be useful in cases where a refugee is either unwilling or unable to confront traumatic memories immediately or is severely disturbed by PTSD and comorbid symptoms as well as by ongoing psychosocial stress. Also, more complex approaches to intervention are indicated where refugees hold culturally specific explanatory models for problems, a situation where common ground needs to be forged between the client's world view and that of the therapist who often adheres to models rooted in Western culture and science.

Although there is compelling clinical evidence that the refugee experience impacts profoundly on the cohesiveness and interconnectedness of families, suggesting that family interventions are highly relevant to comprehensive interventions, there remains a lack of evidence in support of the effectiveness of systemic family therapy, as a recent systematic review suggests [100].

There are several cogent reasons why a group approach to treatment is considered an important option for the treatment of PTSD amongst asylum seekers and refugees [98]. First, these populations commonly experience conditions of isolation, social withdrawal, and loss of connectedness with others. Both their psychological state and their living conditions make them vulnerable in relation to their capacity for interpersonal and social functioning. Second, loss of connectedness and isolation can be amplified by the context of forced migration, many contemporary host environments resulting in asylum seekers and refugees being socially marginalized and separated from familiar social networks and cultural frameworks and even being subject to ostracism and discrimination. Third, many asylum seekers and refugees originate from collectivist-oriented (sub)cultures [101] in which one's sense of self-worth and self-esteem is heavily dependent on interactions with and standing within the indigenous group. The quintessential collectivist notion of self in these contexts dictates that one realizes himself/herself as a person through others and through serving the community. The roles of the extended family and the wider network are, as a consequence, central to the person's sense of well-being and mental health. Being isolated and disconnected from a network of meaningful social contacts may lead to feelings of spiritual misery and disorientation with a loss of goals and a sense of meaning in life. Finally, a group approach has a pragmatic advantage in allowing service providers to meet the great demand for care presented by the ever-increasing number of refugees and asylum seekers requiring attention, especially in the perennial context of limited funding and resources that pertains in host countries worldwide.

A recent literaturereview [102] of group treatments made a distinction between various stages and models of group treatment, referred to as the supportive model, the stage one and the stage two groups, and group interventions that take place within a broader multidisciplinary treatment programme. Supportive approaches aim at building connections amongst group members, enhancing social support and breaking isolation. Stage one models focus both on present and past experiences, focusing on components of safety, support, rebuilding of social capital, trauma-focused education, anxiety and stress management techniques and skills in emotion regulation. Stage two groups also focus on past and present traumas and stresses, but they include more explicit sharing of the trauma narrative and processing of traumatic memories. In spite of these distinctions in models, there is little scientific evaluation to guide the therapist as to which of the range of components are effective and/or necessary to achieve positive outcomes. Kira et al. [103] suggest that informed principles of group therapy include homogeneity of group members in terms of gender and sometimes ethnicity, focus on past and present life challenges, flexible but structured sessions and community network building.

An early uncontrolled follow-up study of supportive group therapy with concentration camp survivors from Bosnia-Herzegovina [104] indicated some improvement in participants' mental health that was sustained up to 3 years after treatment. A randomized controlled study (RCT) of a school-based group psychotherapy programme for war-exposed adolescents in Bosnia-Herzegovina [105] further supported the effectiveness of the latter approach. Recently conducted controlled cohort studies [98, 99] have examined the short- and long-term effectiveness of a 1-year phase-based, trauma-focused, multimodal and multicomponent (group psychotherapy in combination with nonverbal therapies) group therapy with Iranian and Afghan asylum seekers and refugees within a day treatment setting. Throughout the treatment, advocacy activities were conducted by the therapists. These activities included writing of medical reports to support patients' claims for asylum, advising authorities working with asylum seekers and personnel in reception centres concerning approaches to reduce daily stressors on their clients and attempting to improve asylum seekers' life circumstances by strategic advocacy and interventions, for example, preventing unnecessary transfers from one reception centre to another, improvement of accommodation in terms of privacy, etc. The findings [98] suggest that this comprehensive approach to group therapy leads to a significant decrease in psychopathology compared with the waitlisted control group. Moreover, nonverbal therapies were found to have a distinct positive impact on the treatment outcomes. Different group modalities studied varied in a number of nonverbal therapy sessions applied in combination with group psychotherapy, and the outcomes were better in those modalities consisting of more nonverbal therapy sessions. In a further study [106] of the same treatment model, it was demonstrated that asylum seekers may benefit from group therapy regardless of whether they were subject to unstable living conditions, although, as predicted, obtaining refugee status during the course of the treatment led to improvements in treatment outcomes. Importantly, a unique 7-year follow-up study of this group treatment [99] showed a sustained improvement in psychopathology up to the 5-year mark. Over an even longer period of time, on average of 7.4 years, treatment gains were maintained, but the effect showed some attenuation starting from 5 years upon termination of the treatment.

A recent controlled trial of group cognitive processing therapy (CPT) [107] with Congolese female survivors of sexual violence was the first of its kind to compare group with individual treatment. Also, it examined the effects of this approach in a low-income, conflict-affected setting. The study suggested that group CPT, provided by community-based paraprofessionals, was more effective than individual supportive therapy in reducing PTSD, depression and anxiety symptoms and in improving overall functioning of the survivors. The effects of CPT were found to be substantial, and improvements were maintained 6 months following treatment.

Delivery of treatment for PTSD through the Internet is a new and seemingly promising approach. A recent meta-analysis of RCTs [108] with different populations of survivors shows that Internet-based CBT and expressive writing (EW) present promising results, although the number of studies is still low. Web-based CBT in written form was proven feasible and effective in a recent RCT study [109] with Arab patients in Iraq being submitted to ongoing war violence and human rights abuses. This intervention consisted of ten writing assignments over a 5-week period and was delivered by a team of Arabic-speaking therapists located in different countries in the world. Internet-based approaches may open new avenues for assisting survivors in contexts where conventional mental health-care provision is limited.

In addition to PTSD, depression has a high prevalence amongst refugees [25]. As a consequence, several studies have focused on the treatment of depression as well as of complicated grief in these populations. Recent meta-regression analyses [110, 111] support the effectiveness of psychotherapeutic interventions of various types for depression in general when applied across cultures and racial/ethnic groups. Effective interventions include CBT, interpersonal therapy (IPT), problem-solving therapy and behavioural activation therapy. In relation to complicated grief, there is a need for future research to examine whether cognitive behavioural approaches, in which cognitive restructuring and confrontation of the losses are core aspects, are as effective in refugee populations as has been demonstrated in other bereaved samples [112].

An important shift in focus is from treating established mental health problems to promoting mental health and resilience in refugees. Mazzetti [4], building on the knowledge within transactional analysis, distinguishes three sources of resilience in refugees: the ones shaped by individual premigratory psychosocial development and conditions (solidity of self, solidity and flexibility of cultural identity, effective attachment and coping styles, health condition), those linked with migration (preparation for migration and willingness to migrate, realistic expectations from migration, migration project achievement and effective re-elaboration postmigration) and the ones stemming from effective social support. In terms of interventions that may assist in resilience building amongst these populations and enhance social support, Kira and Tummala-Narra [68] recorded several factors including strengthening the collective by promoting contact with family, including extended family and networks, encouraging participation in religious rituals and activities, providing paths to express political ideologies and participation in the pursuit of just causes and seeking avenues to achieve a sense of justice and fairness. Interventions enhancing resilience in refugees have yet to be rigorously studied, methodological obstacles being formidable. Further consideration of the topic of resilience and the factors that can build that capacity in other survivors of trauma are described in greater detail elsewhere [113].

11.6 Important Ingredients of Psychotherapy with Refugees

The key aims of all psychotherapeutic interventions for refugees are to help them to regain control over their lives, restore self-efficacy and a sense of agency, reattach with humanity, make meaning out of traumatic experiences and suffering and regain hope for the future. Difficulties in these areas are strongly associated with symptoms of anxiety and depression, whereas addressing these issues results in reduction in psychopathology and post-traumatic growth [114]. The implications are that therapy aims to go beyond simply reducing symptoms of PTSD, depression and other comorbid conditions as treatment goals even though reduction in symptoms and associated suffering are important.

The role of the therapeutic relationship in psychotherapy with refugees and asylum seekers cannot be underestimated [115]. Applying a certain treatment technique would not immediately lead to success in healing unless survivors experience key ingredients in the therapeutic encounter, including a sense of trust, support, affirmation, respect, confidentiality and the confidence that they are being believed. Also, advocacy aimed at reducing the impact of current stressors in refugees' lives fosters faith in the therapist and adherence to therapy, as it proves that therapists are authentically interested in patients' existential uncertainties and daily life struggles. Deep professional compassion on behalf of the therapist has long been identified as the core healing factor in all therapeutic processes [116]. This compassion goes beyond the conventional notion of empathy in Western psychotherapy, in this context extending to the necessity of taking action in assisting and advocating for the person as an integral part of the intervention.

Also, as referred to earlier, caution is needed in adopting an excessively individual approach when working with sociocentric persons from collectivist-orientated cultures [21]. Cultural considerations together with human rights issues require that psychotherapists assisting refugees are obliged to reconsider and redefine their professional roles and boundaries. As Mazzetti [4] suggested, an excellent psychotherapist is one not restricted only to the office but a person who decides to be a social actor. A therapist should not only focus on the intrapsychic sequelae of exposure to violence and forced migration but recognize a multitude of problems refugees are facing on many levels in their ecological context. Therapists have a role in the creation and promotion of integrated multidisciplinary networks (including social workers, lawyers, city council, etc.) that provide services assisting refugees and asylum seekers. Also, as indicated, attention should be paid to the capacity of survivors to draw on their inner strengths and social networks to strengthen their resilience. All treatment approaches should be culture-sensitive and take into account differences in explanatory models of suffering across cultures. Cultural factors can affect the conception, manifestation, subjective explanation, coping strategies, help-seeking behaviour and prognosis of mental health problems in refugees [117]. Psychotherapists are expected to develop cultural competence [118], meaning that they should be aware of their own cultural values and beliefs, expand their knowledge of patient's cultural background and be able to intervene in appropriate and clinically meaningful ways. Cultural competence includes awareness of the impact of the clinician's own ethnocultural identity on patients, knowledge of the language and cultural background of groups seen in clinical practice and their interactions with mental health issues and treatment, the skills for working with particular groups, and the development of an organization or system that is capable of offering equity of access and outcome to diverse populations [119].

Therapists need to pay attention to both what refugee survivors share in sessions and that what remains untold. They should develop tolerance for "not knowing" and not always being in control over the treatment process and be ready to deal with ambiguities, uncertainties and cultural inhibitions to sharing emotionally burdened material [119].

11.7 Ongoing Dilemmas

One key issue that has remained in contention for decades is whether exposure to trauma memories during therapy, whether individual or group based, is essential to recovery from PTSD symptoms. While some advocate caution, others claim that all refugees with PTSD can be submitted to this form of treatment. Contrary to the conventional wisdom that exposure is necessary, a recent study by Markowitz et al. [120], although not with a refugee population, suggests that trauma-focused intervention is not necessary for recovery from PTSD. This study, the first of its kind, found that interpersonal therapy (IPT) is equal in effect to prolonged exposure for PTSD. This landmark finding raises further questions whether trauma-focused approaches should be so universally regarded as the gold standard for PTSD treatment in general. The importance of this issue to the refugee field is that there are individual survivors of trauma, particularly torture and related gross human rights abuses, who are unable or unwilling to confront the trauma memories or who require a substantial period of time building trust with the therapist in order to do so. A research by Kruse et al. [78] pointed out that war refugees being treated only with supportive and stabilizing interventions and without exposure to traumatic memories showed reduction of PTSD symptoms and somatoform disorders. However, in case that one chooses to apply a trauma-focused approach, the role of timing seems crucial [121]. Premature exposure to traumatic memories in counselling may reactivate traumatic reactions which survivors may be unable to handle because of high levels of ongoing and current stressors. It can also lead to a dropout from counselling as confronting traumatic memories for the sake of individual healing may not be perceived by survivors as a priority at a given time in their lives.

The other important ongoing discussion is whether the complexity of traumatic experiences in refugees causes complex PTSD. Courtois and Ford [27] suggested that complex traumatic experiences in refugees do not necessary cause complex PTSD with complex traumatic symptoms and that the complex form of PTSD is most often linked to refugees who have been submitted to early childhood trauma. This subgroup, requiring a phase-based treatment approach, seems to be relatively small [122]. Therefore, it is suggested that extensive stabilization, as in the phase-based PTSD treatments, should not be considered as a prerequisite for trauma-focused interventions in asylum seekers and refugees. This discussion has not yet come to an end. We suggest that the complexity of the "refugee experience" may be of another type than the complexity of mental health impacts in survivors of early childhood trauma and that stabilization is an important part of the treatment trajectory.

Further, it seems important to distinguish mental health problems caused by exposure to violence from those resulting from current and ongoing stress while assessing refugee patients and creating an adequate assistance approach addressing both sets of problems. Both sets of problems may resemble each other and refugees often present them in a package. However, these problems require different sets of interventions in order for refugee clients to be helped with. The "one-size-fits-all" approach should, therefore, be submitted to caution and critique [123].

Another important phenomenon in psychotherapy with refugees is anger management. Although anger and rage can be seen as a part of PTSD in the form of irritability, one should not always pathologize them. Refugees may be also angry because of chronic violation of their human rights both in country of origin and in host environment [124, 125]. As Murphy [126, 127] suggested, not feeling resentful upon violation of one's human rights conveys, emotionally, either that one does not think that he/she has rights or that one does not take these rights seriously. Whatever the origin of anger may be, survivors may lose control over it, act aggressively, then realize that they resemble their perpetrators and consequently feel ashamed, guilty and despaired [6].

Since refugees are often confronted with a spectrum of current life stressors, including ongoing violence in a country of origin, and they remain caring and worrying for those left behind, one may question the notion that this population presents with "post" in PTSD. It may be that clinicians assisting refugees are actually helping them to cope with an "ongoing" TSD, the reason why knowledge and experiences with other traumatized populations cannot be easily translated and applied in refugees.

The role of interpreters in the treatment of refugees is of vital importance and has attracted some research [128]. There are indications that the involvement of interpreters, often essential, can be associated with positive outcomes in treating PTSD patients with CBT. Also, Lambert and Alhassoon [71] conclude in their meta-analysis of trauma-focused treatments for refugees that across different studies no difference in outcome was found between sessions where an interpreter was used to facilitate communication and those without use of an interpreter. Unfortunately, in many treatment settings around the world, the use of qualified interpreters incurs additional costs and is therefore far from being a standard practice. The alternative, language matching of clients with therapists, has been found to be effective in retaining refugees in treatment but, perhaps surprisingly, does not impact clinical outcomes [129, 130].

11.8 Future Research Agenda

In our opinion, the major problem with current research is that inevitable biases may occur in the selection process and the types of survivors attending different services and participating in research endeavours. Moreover, the complex ecological factors that shape outcomes of treatment approaches are most often not taken into account in researching outcomes. The context and nature of the service greatly influence the subsection of the refugee population that attends for treatment. For example, a research sample of refugees presenting with some PTSD symptoms and looking for assistance in a conflict-affected country is a very different group of people than those assessed in a specialized service in a high-income country. The latter group may have received many interventions at primary care levels over several years and therefore is likely to be those with more severe, complex, comorbid disorders. The ecological, environmental factors presented at large in the section on the frameworks and models for understanding complexity of the "refugee experience" in both groups may be very different and yet not dealt with adequately within research designs. Therefore, comparing outcomes of treatment approaches to refugees across contexts and service models should be undertaken with utmost caution.

Future trials should evaluate interventions based on a local, emic understanding of trauma and psychological distress rooted in refugees' cultural backgrounds [70], although these approaches require extensive preparatory work and close collaboration between therapists and the source community. Empirical and clinical knowledge about which combinations of interventions may be effective and which may not should be studied, taking into account sampling and contextual factors that could influence outcomes. Moreover, symptom outcomes should be expanded beyond PTSD and depression to include a range of comorbid and/or multidimensional symptom patterns that are common amongst refugees. Outcomes should extend to nonsymptomatic effects of therapy including changes in quality of life, resilience, social integration, behaviour (such as aggression) and interpersonal relationships. As the American Psychological Association's (APA) Presidential Task Force on Evidence-Based Practice [131] suggests, "future research requires integration of RCTs with multiple streams of research evidence, including evidence of effectiveness in the context of translational research, that is, demonstrating that treatments that appear to be effective in controlled studies can be applied and sustained in real-life clinic and other settings where human and material resources are constrained".

11.9 Concluding Remarks

The treatment of asylum seekers and refugees is complex: these populations have experienced exposure to war and persecution, imprisonment and torture-related traumas in addition to extensive losses and disruptions associated with forced migration and secondary victimization in the postmigration environment. Culture, language, isolation, marginalization, lack of social support, poverty and other deprivations all can present major challenges in accessing and benefiting from therapy. Consideration of all these issues suggests [24, 93] that assisting asylum seekers and refugees requires a comprehensive approach that acknowledges the powerful impact of past experiences and the present context. In that sense, a broad rehabilitation framework makes sense, one that targets the full spectrum of psychological, societal, political, cultural, human rights-related and economic issues that affect the lives of refugees and asylum seekers in a dynamic and ever-changing pattern. Within such a treatment approach, evidence-based interventions should be combined with the nonmedical or so-called psychosocial interventions such as advocacy, assistance with language acquisition, skills in resettlement and support in pursuing legal, housing and other needs. Although nonevidence-based interventions are often used in services, there is an ethical obligation to subject them to appropriate testing, as models for integrating research into practice settings are now being clearly developed [131, 132]. An important issue to resolve in the asylum seeker and refugee field is the differential approach needed to treat relatively uncomplicated PTSD, which in other populations [123] is amenable to improvement following relatively short-term treatments (e.g. lasting 9 and 12 weeks) and the more complex forms of traumatic stress seen in many survivors attending clinics in high-income countries, who may need a longer and more comprehensive approach to treatment supplemented by practical support in overcoming life stressors, lack of social support and practical resettlement needs.

References

1. Unfpaorg. 1. Unfpaorg. Available from: http://www.unfpa.org/migration. Accessed 28 Jan 2017.
2. Priebe S, Giacco D, El-Nagib R. Public health aspects of mental health among migrants and refugees: a review of the evidence on mental health care for refugees, asylum seekers and irregular migrants in the WHO European region. Copenhagen: WHO Regional Office for Europe; 2016.
3. United Nations High Commissioner for Refugees (UNHCR). 1. UNHCR Refugees/Migrants Response–Mediterranean. Available from: http://data.unhcr.org/mediterranean/regional.php. Accessed 28 Jan 2017.

4. Mazzetti M. Trauma and migration: a transactional analytic approach toward refugees and torture victims. Transactional Analysis Journal. 2008;38(4):285–302.
5. Kalt A, Hossain M, Kiss L, Zimmermann C. Asylum seekers, violence and health: a systematic review of research in high-income countries. Am J Public Health. 2013;103(3):30–42.
6. Silove D. The psychosocial effects of torture, mass human rights violations, and refugee trauma: toward an integrated conceptual framework. J Nerv Ment Dis. 1999;187:200–7.
7. Hallas P, Hansen AR, Staehr MA, Munk-Andersen E, Jorgensen HL. Length of stay in asylum centres and mental health in asylum seekers: a retrospective study from Denmark. BMC Public Health. 2007;7:288–93.
8. Heeren M, Mueller J, Ehlert U, Schnyder U, Copiery N, Maier T. Mental health of asylum seekers: a cross-sectional study of psychiatric disorders. BMC Psychiatry. 2012;12:114–21.
9. Laban CJ, Gernaat HBPE, Komproe IH, Schreuders BA, Jong de JTVM. Impact of a long asylum procedure on the prevalence of psychiatric disorders in Iraqi asylum seekers in the Netherlands. J Nerv Ment Dis. 2004;192:843–51.
10. Mueller J, Schmidt M, Staeheli A, Maier T. Mental health of failed asylum seekers as compared with pending and temporarily accepted asylum seekers. Eur J Pub Health. 2010;21:184–9.
11. Ryan D, Benson C, Dooley B. Psychological distress and the asylum process: a longitudinal study of forced migrants in Ireland. J Nerv Ment Dis. 2008;196:37–45.
12. Silove DM, Steel ZP, Susljik I, et al. The impact of the refugee decision on the trajectory of PTSD, anxiety and depressive symptoms in asylum seekers: a longitudinal study. Am J Disaster Med. 2007;2(6):321–9.
13. Silove D, Steel Z, Watters C. Policies of deterrence and the mental health of asylum seekers in western countries. JAMA. 2000;284:604–11.
14. Steel Z, Momartin S, Silove D, Coello M, Aroche J, Tay KW. Two year psychosocial and mental health outcomes for refugees subjected to restrictive or supportive immigration policies. Soc Sci Med. 2011;72(7):1149–56.
15. Tummala-Narra P. Addressing political and racial terror in psychotherapy. Am J Orthopsychiatry. 2005;75:19–26.
16. Kirmayer LJ, Narasiah L, Munoz M, et al. Common mental health problems in immigrants and refugees: general approach in primary care. Can Med Assoc J. 2010;183(12):1–9. https://doi.org/10.1503/cmaj.090292.
17. Porter M, Haslam N. Predisplacement and postdisplacement factors associated with mental health of refugees and internally displaced persons. JAMA. 2005;294:602–12.
18. Ellis BH, Abdi SM, Lazarevic V, et al. Relation of psychosocial factors to diverse behaviors and attitudes among Somali refugees. Am J Orthopsychiatry. 2015;86(4):393–408. https://doi.org/10.1037//ort0000121.
19. Bakker L, Dagevos J, Engbersen G. The importance of resources and security in the socio-economic integration of refugees: a study on the impact of length of stay in asylum accommodation and residence status on socio-economic integration for the four largest refugee groups in the Netherlands. J Internat Migr Integr. 2014;15(3):431–48.
20. Silove D. The challenges facing mental health programs for post-conflict and refugee communities. Prehosp Disaster Med. 2004;19(1):90–6.
21. Bhugra D, Gupta S, Schouler-Ocak M, et al. EPA guidance mental health care of migrants. Eur Psychiatry. 2014;29:107–15.
22. Fazel M, Wheeler J, Danesh J. Prevalence of serious mental disorder in 7000 refugees resettled in western countries: a systematic review. Lancet. 2005;365:1309–14.
23. Hall BJ, Olff M. Global mental health: trauma and adversity among populations in transition. Eur J Psychotraumatol. 2016;7:31140. https://doi.org/10.3402/ejpt.v7.31140.
24. Schick M, Zumwald A, Knopfli B, et al. Challenging future, challenging past: the relationship of social integration and psychological impairment in traumatized refugees. Eur J Psychotraumatol. 2016;7:28057. https://doi.org/10.3402/ejpt.v7.28057.
25. Steel Z, Chey T, Silove D, Marnane C, Bryant RA, van Ommeren M. Association of torture and other potentially traumatic events with mental health outcomes among populations exposed to mass conflict and displacement. JAMA. 2009;302:537–49.

26. Momartin S, Silove D, Manicavasagar V, Steel Z. Comorbidity of PTSD and depression: associations with trauma exposure, symptom severity and functional impairment in Bosnian refugees resettled in Australia. J Affect Disord. 2004;80:231–8.
27. Courtois CA, Ford JD, editors. Treating complex traumatic stress disorder: an evidence-based guide. New York: Guilford Press; 2009.
28. Maercker A, Brewin CR, Bryant RA, et al. Proposals for mental disorders specifically associated with stress in the international classification of diseases-11. Lancet. 2013;381:1683–785.
29. Bhugra D. Migration and mental health. Acta Psychiatr Scand. 2004;109:243–58.
30. Buhmann CB. Traumatized refugees: morbidity, treatment and predictors of outcome. Dan Med J. 2014;61(8):84871.
31. Lindert J, Ehrenstein OS, Priebe S, Mielck A, Brahler E. Depression and anxiety in labour migrants and refugees. Soc Sci Med. 2009;69:246–57.
32. Lindencrona F, Ekblad S, Hauff E. Mental health of recently resettled refugees from the middle east in Sweden: the impact of pre-resettlement trauma, resettlement stress and capacity to handle stress. Soc Psychiatry Psychiatr Epidemiol. 2008;43:121–31.
33. Carswell K, Blackburn P, Barker C. The relationship between trauma, post-migration problems and the psychological well-being of refugees and asylum seekers. Int J Soc Psychiatry. 2011;57:107–19.
34. Bracken P, Giller J, Summerfield D. Psychological responses of war and atrocity: limitations and current concepts. Soc Sci Med. 1995;40(8):1073–82.
35. Patel N. Clinical psychology: reinforcing inequalities or facilitating empowerment? Int J Human Rights. 2003;7(1):16–29.
36. Patel N. The psychologisation of torture. In: Rapley M, Moncrieff J, Dillon J, editors. De-medicalising misery: psychiatry, psychology and the human condition. London: Palgrave Macmillan; 2011. p. 239–55.
37. Mezey G, Robbins I. Usefulness and validity of posttraumatic stress disorder as a psychiatric category. Br Med J. 2001;323:561–3.
38. Tay AK, Rees S, Chen J, Kareth M, Silove D. The structure of post-traumatic stress disorder and complex post-traumatic stress disorder amongst west Papuan refugees. BMC Psychiatry. 2015;15:111.
39. Lambourne W. Justice and reconciliation: postconflict peacebuilding in Cambodia and Rwanda. In: Abu-Nimer M, editor. Reconciliation, justice and coexistence: theory and practice. Lanham: Lexington Books; 2001. p. 311–38.
40. Miller KE, Worthington GJ, Muzurovic J, Tipping S, Goldman A. Bosnian refugees and the stressors of exile: a narrative study. Am J Orthopsychiatry. 2002;72:341–54.
41. Summerfield D. A critique of seven assumptions behind psychological trauma programs in war-affected areas. Soc Sci Med. 1999;48:1449–62.
42. Koenen KC, Goodwin R, Struening E, Hellman F, Guardino M. Posttraumatic stress disorder and treatment seeking in a national screening sample. J Trauma Stress. 2003;16:5–16.
43. Sohelian S, Inman A. Middle Eastern Americans: the effects of stigma on attitudes toward counseling. J Muslim Ment Health. 2009;4:139–58.
44. Porter M. Global evidence for a biopsychosocial understanding of refugee adaptation. Transcult Psychiatry. 2007;44:418–39.
45. Khan MMR. Das kumulative trauma. In: Khan MMR, editor. Selbsterfahrung in der Therapie: Theorie und praxis [The concept of cumulative trauma]. Munchen: Kindler; 1977. p. 50–70.
46. Becker D. Dealing with the consequences of organised violence in trauma work. In: Berghof handbook for conflict transformation. Berlin: Berghof Research Center for Constructive Conflict Management; 2004. p. 1–15.
47. McEwen BS. Protective and damaging effects of stress mediators. Semin Med Beth Isr Deaconess Med Cent. 1998;338(3):171–9.
48. Wilson JP, Friedman MJ, Lindy JD. Treatment goals for PTSD. In: Wilson JP, Friedman MJ, Lindy JD, editors. Treating psychological trauma and PTSD. New York: Guilford; 2001. p. 3–27.

49. Kielson H. Sequential traumatization in children. Jerusalem: Magnes Press Hebrew University; 1992.
50. Tay AK, Rees S, Chen J, Kareth M, Silove D. Corrigendum to "examining the broader psychosocial effects of mass conflict on PTSD symptoms and functional impairment amongst west Papuan refugees resettled in Papua New Guinea (PNG)". Soc Sci Med. 2015;138(13):70–8.
51. Resick PA, Bovin MJ, Calloway AL, et al. A critical evaluation of the complex PTSD literature: implications for DSM-5. J Trauma Stress. 2012;25:241–51.
52. Bronfenbrenner U. The ecology of human development: experiments by nature and design. 4th ed. Cambridge: Harvard University Press; 1981.
53. Hobfoll SE. Stress, culture and community: the psychology and philosophy of stress. New York: Plenum Press; 1998.
54. Hobfoll SE. The influence of culture, community, and the nested-self in the stress process: advancing conservation of resources theory. Appl Psychol Int Rev. 2001;50:337–421.
55. Silove D. The ADAPT model. Intervention. 2013;11(3):237–48.
56. Miller KE, Kulkarni M, Kushner H. Beyond trauma-focused psychiatric epidemiology: bridging research and practice with war-affected populations. Am J Orthopsychiatry. 2006;76(4):409–22.
57. Papadopoulos RK. Refugees, trauma and adversity-activated development. Eur J Psychotery Couns. 2007;9:301–12.
58. Cicchetti D, Toth SL. The past achievements and future promises of developmental psychopathology: the coming of age of a discipline. Child Psychol Psychiaty. 2009;50:16–25.
59. Sroufe LA. The place of development in developmental psychopathology. In: Masten AS, editor. Multilevel dynamics in developmental psychopathology, The Minnesota symposia on child psychology, vol. 34. Mahwah: Lawrence Erlbaum Associates; 2007. p. 285–99.
60. Droždek B. The rebirth of contextual thinking in psychotraumatology. In: Droždek B, Wilson JP, editors. Voices of trauma: treating survivors across cultures. New York: Springer; 2007. p. 1–25.
61. Droždek B. Challenges in treatment of posttraumatic stress disorder in refugees: towards integration of evidence-based treatments with contextual and culture-sensitive perspectives. Eur J Psychotraumatol. 2015;6:24750. https://doi.org/10.3402/ejpt.v6.24750.
62. Droždek B, Wilson JP, Turkovic S. Assessment of PTSD in non-western cultures: the need for new contextual and complex perspectives. In: Beck JG, Sloan DM, editors. The Oxford handbook of traumatic stress disorders. New York: Oxford University Press; 2012. p. 302–14.
63. Droždek B, Wilson JP, Turkovic S. Posttraumatic stress disorder (PTSD) and psychopathology in refugees: a reflective cross-cultural contextual view of mental health interventions. In: Elliott D, Segal UA, editors. Refugees worldwide. Westport: Praeger; 2012. p. 165–86.
64. Mezzich JE, Salloum IM, Cloninger CR, et al. Person-centered integrative diagnosis: conceptual basis and structural model. Can J Psychiatr. 2010;55:701–8.
65. Whitley R. Cultural competence, evidence-based medicine, and evidence-based practices. Psychiatr Serv. 2007;58:1588–90.
66. American Psychiatric Association (APA). Diagnostic and statistical manual of mental disorders. 5th ed. Washington, DC: APA; 2013.
67. Lewis-Fernandez R. Cultural formulation of psychiatric diagnosis. Cult Med Psychiaty. 1996;20:133–44.
68. Kira IA, Tummala-Narra P. Psychotherapy with refugees: emerging paradigm. J Loss Trauma. 2015;20:449–67.
69. Chu BC, Merson RA, Zandberg LJ, Areizaga M. Calibrating for comorbidity: clinical decision-making in youth depression and anxiety. Cogn Behav Med. 2012;19:5–16.
70. Crumlish N, O'Rourke K. A systematic review of treatments for post-traumatic stress disorder among refugees and asylum-seekers. J Nerv Ment Dis. 2010;198:237–51.
71. Lambert JE, Alhassoon OM. Trauma-focused therapy for refugees: meta-analytic findings. J Couns Psychol. 2015;62(1):28–37.
72. Nickerson A, Bryant RA, Silove D, Steel Z. A critical review of psychological treatments of posttraumatic stress disorder in refugees. Clin Psychol Rev. 2011;31:399–417.

73. Palic S, Elklit A. Psychosocial treatment of posttraumatic stress disorder in adult refugees: a systematic review of prospective treatment outcome studies and a critique. J Affect Disord. 2011;131:8–23.
74. Neuner F, Schauer E, Klaschik C, Karunakara U, Elbert T. A comparison of narrative exposure therapy, supportive counselling, and psychoeducation for treating posttraumatic stress disorder in an African refugee settlement. J Consult Clin Psychol. 2004;72(4):579–87.
75. Neuner F, Onyut PL, Ertl V, Odenwald M, Schauer E, Elbert T. Treatment of posttraumatic stress disorder by trained lay counselors in an African refugee setting: a randomized controlled trial. J Consult Clin Psychol. 2008;76(4):686–94.
76. Neuner F, Kurreck S, Ruf M, Odenwald M, Elbert T, Schauer M. Can asylum-seekers with posttraumatic stress disorder be successfully treated? A randomized controlled pilot study. Cogn Behav Therapy. 2010;39(2):81–91.
77. Robjant K, Fazel M. The emerging evidence for narrative exposure therapy: a review. Clin Psychol Rev. 2010;30:1030–9.
78. Kruse J, Joksimovic L, Cavka M, Woller W, Schmitz N. Effects of trauma-focused psychotherapy upon war refugees. J Trauma Stress. 2009;22(6):585–92.
79. Paunovic N, Ost LG. Cognitive-behavior therapy vs exposure therapy in the treatment of PTSD in refugees. Behav Res Ther. 2001;39(10):1183–97.
80. Ter Heide FJJ, Mooren TM, Knipscheer JW, Kleber RJ. EMDR with traumatized refugees: from experience-based to evidence-based practice. J EMDR Pract Res. 2014;8(3):147–56.
81. McFarlane CA, Kaplan I. Evidence-based psychological interventions for adult survivors of torture and trauma: a 30-year review. Transcult Psychiatry. 2012;49(3–4):539–67.
82. Patel N, Kellezi B, Williams ACDC. Psychological, social and welfare interventions for psychological health and well-being of torture survivors. Cochrane Database Syst Rev. 2014;11:CD009317. https://doi.org/10.1002/14651858.CD009317.pub2.
83. Schauer M, Neuner F, Elbert T. Narrative exposure therapy: a short-term treatment for traumatic stress disorders. 2nd ed. Cambridge: Hogrefe Publishing; 2011.
84. Hensel-Dittmann D, Schauer M, Ruf M, et al. Treatment of traumatized victims of war and torture: a randomized controlled comparison of narrative exposure therapy and stress inoculation training. Psychother Psychosom. 2011;80:345–52.
85. Hijazi AA, Lumley MA, Ziadni MS, Haddad L, Rapport LJ, Arnetz BB. Brief narrative exposure therapy for posttraumatic stress in Iraqi refugees: a preliminary randomized clinical trial. J Trauma Stress. 2014;27:314–22.
86. Gwozdziewycz N, Mehl-Madrona L. Meta-analysis of the use of narrative exposure therapy for the effects of trauma among refugee populations. Permanente J. 2013;17(1):70–6.
87. Hinton DE, Pham T, Tran M, Safren SA, Otto MW, Pollack MH. CBT for Vietnamese refugees with treatment-resistant PTSD and panic attacks: a pilot study. J Trauma Stress. 2004;17(5):429–33.
88. Hinton DE, Pham T, Tran M, Safren SA, Hofmann SG, Pollack MH. A randomized controlled trial of cognitive-behavior therapy for Cambodian refugees with treatment-resistant PTSD and panic attacks: a cross-over design. J Trauma Stress. 2005;18(6):617–29.
89. Hinton DE, Hofmann SG, Pollack MH, Otto MW. Mechanisms of efficacy of CBT for Cambodian refugees with PTSD: improvement in emotion regulation and orthostatic blood pressure response. CNS Neurosci Ther. 2009;15(3):255–63.
90. Otto MW, Hinton D, Korbly NB, et al. Treatment of pharmacotherapy-refractory posttraumatic stress disorder among Cambodian refugees: a pilot study of combination treatment with cognitive-behavior therapy vs sertraline alone. Behav Res Ther. 2003;41(11):1271–6.
91. Hinton DE, Jalal B. Guidelines for the implementation of culturally sensitive cognitive behavioural therapy among refugees and in global contexts. Intervention. 2014;12(1):78–93.
92. National Institute for Clinical Excellence (NICE). Post-traumatic stress disorder: the management of PTSD in adults and children in primary and secondary care. London: Gaskell; 2005.
93. Murray KE, Davidson GR, Schweitzer RD. Review of refugee mental health interventions following resettlement: best practices and recommendations. Am J Orthopsychiatr. 2010;80:576–85.

94. Hinton DE, Rivera EI, Hofmann S, Barlow D, Otto MW. Adapting CBT for traumatized refugees and ethnic minority patients: examples for culturally adapted CBT (CA-CBT). Transcult Psychiatry. 2012;49:340–65.
95. Shapiro F. Eye movement desensitization and reprocessing: basic principles, protocols, and procedures. 2nd ed. New York: Guilford Press; 2001.
96. Morina N, Maier T, Bryant R, et al. Combining biofeedback and narrative exposure therapy for PTSD and persistent pain in refugees: a pilot study. Eur J Psychotraumatol. 2012;3:17660. https://doi.org/10.3402/ejpt.v3i0.17660.
97. Carlsson JM, Reff Olsen D, Kastrup M, Lykke Mortensen E. Late mental health changes in tortured refugees in multidisciplinary treatment. J Nerv Ment Dis. 2010;198(11):824–8.
98. Drožđek B, Kamperman A, Bolwerk N, Tol WA, Kleber RJ. Group therapy with male asylum seekers and refugees with posttraumatic stress disorder: a controlled comparison cohort study of three day-treatment programs. J Nerv Ment Dis. 2012;200:758–65.
99. Drožđek B, Kamperman A, Tol WA, Knipscheer JW, Kleber RJ. Seven-year follow-up study of symptoms in asylum seekers and refugees with PTSD treated with trauma-focused groups. J Clin Psychol. 2014;70(4):376–87. https://doi.org/10.1002/jclp.22035.
100. Slobodin O, de Jong JTVM. Family interventions in traumatized immigrants and refugees: a systematic review. Transcult Psychiatry. 2015;0(0):1–20. https://doi.org/10.1177/1363461515588855.
101. Hofstede G. Cultures and organizations: software of the mind. London: McGraw-Hill; 1991.
102. Bunn M, Goesel C, Kinet M, Ray F. Group treatment for survivors of torture and severe violence: a literature review. Torture. 2016;26(1):45–67.
103. Kira I, Templin T, Lewandowski L, Ashby JS, Oladele A, Odenat L. Cumulative trauma disorder scale: two studies. Psychology. 2012;3:643–56.
104. Drožđek B. Follow-up study of concentration camp survivors from Bosnia-Herzegovina: three years later. J Nerv Ment Dis. 1997;185:690–4.
105. Layne CM, Saltzman WR, Poppleton L, et al. Effectiveness of a school-based group psychotherapy program for war-exposed adolescents: a randomized controlled trial. J Am Acad Child Adolesc Psychiatry. 2008;47:1048–62.
106. Drožđek B, Kamperman A, Tol WA, Knipscheer JW, Kleber RJ. Is legal status impacting outcomes of group therapy for posttraumatic stress disorder with male asylum seekers and refugees from Iran and Afghanistan? BMC Psychiatry. 2013;13:148.
107. Bass JK, Annan J, McIvor Murray S, et al. Controlled trial of psychotherapy for Congolese survivors of sexual violence. N Engl J Med. 2013;368:2182–91.
108. Kuester A, Niemeyer H, Knaevelsrud C. Internet-based interventions for posttraumatic stress: a meta-analysis of randomized controlled trials. Clin Psychol Rev. 2016;43:1–16.
109. Knaevelsrud C, Brand J, Lange A, Ruwaard J, Wagner B. Web-based psychotherapy for posttraumatic stress disorder in war-traumatized Arab patients: randomized controlled trial. J Med Internet Res. 2015;17(3):e71.
110. Van't Hof E, Cuijpers P, Waheed W, et al. Psychological treatments for depression and anxiety disorders in low- and middle-income countries: a meta-analysis. Afr J Psychiatry. 2011;14:200–7.
111. Unlu Ince B, Riper H, van't Hof E, Cuijpers P. The effects of psychotherapy on depression among racial-ethnic minority groups: a metaregression analysis. Psychiatr Serv. 2014;65(5):612–7.
112. Rosner R, Pfoh G, Kotoucova M. Treatment of complicated grief. Eur J Psychotraumatol. 2011;2:7995. https://doi.org/10.3402/ejpt.v2i0.7995.
113. Agaibi CE, Wilson JP. Trauma, PTSD, and resilience: a review of the literature. Trauma Violence Abuse. 2005;6:195–216.
114. Ford JD, Courtois C, van der Hart O, Nijenhuis E, Steele K. Treatment of complex posttraumatic self-dysregulation. J Trauma Stress. 2005;18:467–77.
115. Vincent F, Jenkins H, Larkin M, Clohessy S. Asylum-seekers' experiences of trauma-focused cognitive behaviour therapy for post-traumatic stress disorder: a qualitative study. Behav Cogn Psychother. 2013;41:579–93.

116. Mirdal GM, Ryding E, Essendorp Sondej M. Traumatized refugees, their therapists, and their interpreters; three perspectives on psychological treatment. Psychol Psychother Theory Res Pract. 2012;85:436–55.
117. Minas H, Silove D. Transcultural and refugee psychiatry. In: Bloch S, Singh BS, editors. Foundations of clinical psychiatry. 2nd ed. Melbourne: Melbourne University Press; 2001. p. 475–90.
118. Sue S, Zane N, Nagayama Hall GC, Berger LK. The case for cultural competency in psychotherapeutic interventions. Ann Rev Psychol. 2009;60:525–48.
119. Bala J, Mooren T, Kramer S. Cultural competence in the treatment of political refugees based on system approaches. Clin Neuropsychiatr. 2014;11(1):32–9.
120. Markowitz JC, Petkova E, Neria Y, et al. Is exposure necessary? A randomized clinical trial of interpersonal psychotherapy for PTSD. Am J Psychiatr. 2015;172(5):430–40. https://doi.org/10.1176/appi.ajp.2014.14070908.
121. Acaturk C, Konuk E, Cetinkaya M, et al. EMDR for Syrian refugees with posttraumatic stress disorder symptoms: results of a pilot randomized controlled trial. Eur J Psychotraumatol. 2015;6:27414. https://doi.org/10.3402/ejpt.v6.27414.
122. Ter Heide FJJ, Mooren TM, Kleber RJ. Complex PTSD and phased treatment in refugees: a debate piece. Eur J Psychotraumatol. 2016;7:28687. https://doi.org/10.3402/ejpt.v7.28687.
123. Cloitre M. The "one size fits all" approach to trauma treatment: should we be satisfied? Eur J Psychotraumatol. 2015;6:27344. https://doi.org/10.3402/ejpt.v6.27344.
124. Silove D. Torture and refugee trauma: implications for nosology and treatment of posttraumatic syndromes. In: Mak FL, Nadelson CC, editors. International review of psychiatry. Washington, DC: American Psychiatric Press; 1996. p. 211–32.
125. Silove D, Brooks R, Bateman Steel CR, et al. Explosive anger as a response to human rights violations in post-conflict Timor-Leste. Soc Sci Med. 2009;69(5):670–7.
126. Murphy JG. Moral epistemology, the retributive emotions, and the "Clumsy moral philosophy" of Jesus Christ. In: Bandes S, editor. The passions of law. New York: New York University Press; 1999. p. 149–90.
127. Murphy JG. Getting even: forgiveness and its limits. New York: Oxford University Press; 2003.
128. D'Ardenne P, Ruaro L, Cestari L, Fakhoury W, Priebe S. Does interpreter-mediated CBT with traumatized refugee people work? A comparison of patient outcomes in East London. Behav Cogn Psychother. 2007;35:293–301.
129. Birman D, Beehler S, Merrill Harris E, et al. International family, adult and child enhancement services (FACES): a community-based comprehensive services model for refugee children in resettlement. Am J Orthopsychiatry. 2008;78(1):121–32.
130. Cabral RR, Smith TB. Racial/ethnic matching of clients and therapists in mental health services: a meta-analytic review of preferences. Perceptions, and outcomes. J Couns Psychol. 2011;58(4):537–54.
131. Basoglu M. Rehabilitation of traumatised refugees and survivors of torture. Brit Med J. 2007;333:1230–1.
132. Carlsson J, Sonne C, Silove D. From pioneers to scientists. J Nerv Ment Dis. 2014;202(9):630–7.

Special Situations: Places of Immigration Detention

12

Joost Jan den Otter, Thomas Wenzel, Bernadette McGrath, Andres Leal Osorio, and Boris Drožđek

Abstract

The detention of migrants and asylum seekers has become a common practice in both developing and high-economy regions. The fact of detention but also the conditions of detention are the subject of much criticism. They have been shown to frequently violate international human rights standards and to have an adverse impact on the psychological health and, later, the integration of migrants. In this chapter the authors outline standards and risks, based on research data and a case example, but also alternatives to detention as outlined by UNHCR.

12.1 Introduction

This chapter focusses—by intention—on a broader group of people: those who meet the International Federation of Red Cross and Red Crescent Societies' (IFRC) definition of a migrant and who are deprived of their liberty solely because of their undocumented or irregular status. The IFRC definition reads:

J. J. den Otter (✉)
WPA Section on Psychological Consequences of Torture and Persecution, Geneva, Switzerland

T. Wenzel
World Psychiatric Association Scientific Section,
Psychological Aspects of Persecution and Torture, Geneva, Switzerland
e-mail: drthomaswenzel@web.de

B. McGrath · A. L. Osorio
Overseas Services to Survivors of Torture and Trauma, Adelaide, SA, Australia
e-mail: bmcgrath@osstt.org.au

B. Drožđek
PsyQ/Parnassia Group, Rosmalen/Eindhoven, The Netherlands
e-mail: drozdek@telfort.nl

T. Wenzel, B. Drožđek (eds.), *An Uncertain Safety*,
https://doi.org/10.1007/978-3-319-72914-5_12

> Migrants are persons who leave or flee their habitual residence to go to new places—usually abroad—to seek opportunities or safer and better prospects. Migration can be voluntary or involuntary, but most of the time a combination of choices and constraints are involved. Their policy includes, among others, labour migrants, stateless migrants, and migrants deemed irregular by public authorities. It also concerns refugees and asylum seekers, notwithstanding the fact that they constitute a special category under international law.[1]

Figures published in 2016 indicate that the total number of international migrants reached 244 million[2] with the total number of refugees worldwide estimated at 19.5 million,[3] the highest number since World War II. Developing regions hosted 86% of the world's refugees with the top three refugee-hosting countries being Turkey with 1.6 million refugees, followed by Pakistan (1.5 million) and Lebanon (1.2 million). While the Global Detention Project[4] has published detention profiles on dozens of countries, to date there has been no comprehensive study that documents immigration detention practices (both pre-admission detention and pre-removal detention) globally.

Flynn argues that before the 1980s, immigration detention appeared to have been used largely as an ad hoc tool, employed mainly by wealthy states. Guantánamo Bay (long before its more notorious role as the detention site for alleged "unlawful combatants" in the "War on Terror") was one of the world's first offshore immigration detention facilities used to deter asylum seekers and prevent "alien smuggling". The Australian "Pacific Solution" which aimed to prevent asylum seekers and unauthorised migrants from reaching Australian territory and claiming asylum by intercepting vessels and detaining asylum seekers and unauthorised migrants in offshore facilities was inspired by the Guantanamo example. Nowadays, immigration detention has become an established modus operandi all over the globe. There are several reasons behind the detention of migrants: because of their irregular or unauthorised mode of arrival, to prevent movement during asylum claims determination procedures, before return after due process, or in response to perceived threats to public order [1].

With respect to the conditions in immigration detention facilities, several international NGOs such as Amnesty International, Human Rights Watch and the Global Detention Project together with a number of (inter)national monitoring bodies including the ombudsman, National Preventive Mechanism and European Committee for the Prevention of Torture have raised concerns regarding the arbitrariness of the detention, the lack of access to appropriate health care, the lack of identification and protection of vulnerable cases (such as victims of torture) and the general conditions within detention (which will be discussed later in this chapter). Special attention is paid to the conclusion of the Special Rapporteur on Torture

[1] IFRC Policy on Migration 2009 available at https://media.ifrc.org/ifrc/document/migration-policy/ last accessed 10 June 2017.

[2] United Nations, Department of Economic and Social Affairs, Population Division (2016). International Migration Report 2015: Highlights (ST/ESA/SER.A/375).

[3] United Nations High Commissioner for Refugees 2015.

[4] http://www.globaldetentionproject.org/.

regarding the detention of children. This report states: *Immigration detention practices across the globe, whether de jure or* de facto, *put children at risk of cruel, inhuman or degrading treatment or punishment. Furthermore, the detention of children who migrate to escape exploitation and abuse contravenes the duty of the State to promote the physical and psychological recovery of child victims in an appropriate environment.*[5] The Special Rapporteur recommends: *Therefore, States should, expeditiously and completely, cease the detention of children, with or without their parents, on the basis of their immigration status. States should make clear in their legislation, policies and practices that the principle of the best interests of the child takes priority over migration policy and other administrative considerations.*[6]

Twelve countries recently joined a global initiative aimed at (a) ending the practice of children being held in places of immigration detention, (b) ensuring that alternatives to detention are available in law and implemented in practice and (c) ensuring that the conditions of detention, where detention is necessary and unavoidable, meet international standards.[7] When it comes to meeting international standards, the World Medical Association in its recent Buenos Aires Resolution urges governments and local authorities to ensure access to adequate health care as well as safe and adequate living conditions for all, irrespective of their legal status. Moreover, it calls on National Medical Associations and physicians to actively support and promote the right of all people to receive medical care on the basis of clinical need alone and to speak out against legislation and practices that are in opposition to this fundamental right.[8] In the United Nations Standard Minimum Rules for the Treatment of Prisoners (the Mandela Rules),[9] health care in prison and the roles and responsibilities of health professionals working in places of detention are further clarified (rules 24–35). Apart from their role in providing individual medical care, health-care professionals are, in conjunction with others, responsible for identifying vulnerable individuals (including victims of torture or ill-treatment (rule 30b and 34)) and reporting to the prison authorities whenever a prisoner's physical or mental health has been or will be injuriously affected by continued imprisonment or by any

[5] Monitoring Places of Detention: Seventh annual report of the United Kingdom's National Preventive Mechanism 2015–16 available at http://www.justiceinspectorates.gov.uk/hmiprisons/wp-content/uploads/sites/4/2014/07/6.2808_NPM_AR2015-16_v4_web.pdf; Greece: A blue print for despair. Human rights impact of the EU-Turkey deal available at https://www.amnesty.org/en/documents/eur25/5664/2017/en/; Systemic Indifference available at https://www.hrw.org/sites/default/files/report_pdf/usimmigration0517_web_0.pdf.

[6] United Nations Report of the Special Rapporteur on torture and other cruel, inhuman or degrading treatment or punishment, Juan E. Méndez A/HRC/28/68 available at http://www.ohchr.org/EN/HRBodies/HRC/RegularSessions/Session28/Documents/A_HRC_28_68_E.doc.

[7] [UNHCR Global Strategy–Beyond Detention 2014–2019, Progress Report, August 2016, available at: www.unhcr.org/detention].

[8] WMA Council Resolution on Refugees and Migrants Adopted by the 203rd WMA Council Session, Buenos Aires, April 2016 available at https://www.wma.net/policies-post/wma-council-resolution-on-refugees-and-migrants/.

[9] https://www.unodc.org/pdf/criminal_justice/UN_Standard_Minimum_Rules_for_the_Treatment_of_Prisoners.pdf.

condition of imprisonment (rule 33). Last but not least, health professionals working in places of detention (or a public health entity) have a responsibility to regularly inspect and provide advice to the prison authorities in relation to the provision of food, hygiene and sanitation and general conditions. As elaborated further in this chapter, it is evident that these different roles and responsibilities are not always met by the health professionals and/or respected by the authorities.

An example described in detail by Newman [2, 3] is the case of CR, a permanent Australian citizen speaking her native language (German). CR ended up in an immigration detention centre and was placed in a "behaviour management unit" (de facto solitary confinement) where the signs and symptoms of her psychosis and disorganisation were not properly recognised by the centre staff and hence not diagnosed as a mental illness. Only after being recognised by her relatives as a result of media coverage was she transferred to a mental health facility and provided with appropriate treatment. A later inquiry by Palmer concluded that "the inadequacy of psychiatric services did not inspire confidence in the integrity of the system" and demonstrated that there was a "clear lack of management and quality control oversight of the service delivery process".[10] The enquiry led to substantial changes in the management of detention facilities in Australia including the monitoring of facilities by independent health experts which were subsequently eroded in the context of changing political and community attitudes.

Immigration detention is a form of *administrative* detention, which means that the deprivation is ordered by the executive branch of the government—rather than the judiciary—and implemented without judicial oversight or review. Immigration detention should be of a non-punitive nature and should only be used as a last resort after considering alternatives (see, e.g. From Deprivation to Liberty, Alternatives to Detention in Belgium, Germany and the United Kingdom[11]). However, as Grange's analysis shows [4], states worldwide frequently do not respect the different UN treaties they have ratified in relation to immigration detention with a number of concerns being raised in relation to the practice of detention itself, particularly the detention of vulnerable groups, and in relation to the conditions within detention facilities including the limited access to health-care providers or services. In an increasing number of states, immigration detention facilities for asylum seekers and unauthorised migrants are now more restrictive than criminal correction facilities and yet lacking the necessary judicial safeguards.[12]

[10] M.J. Palmer: Inquiry into the circumstances of the Immigration Detention of Cornelia Rau; Report, Canberra Commonwealth of Australia, 2005.

[11] Jesuit Refugee Service Europe, (December 2011). Available at http://idcoalition.org/jrs-europe-report.

[12] Working Group on Arbitrary Detention, Report of the Working Group on Arbitrary Detention, 59, U.N. Doc. A/HRC/13/30 (Jan 18, 2010).

12.2 Mental Health Impacts of Detention

The detrimental effects of prolonged detention on mental health have been studied by several authors. Recently Filges et al. published a review following up on a series of studies published over the last few decades which indicates the deterioration of mental health due to detention [5]. The mental health issues associated with detention have been known for a considerable time having first been raised more than 30 years ago in a critical paper by Goodwin [6] and later on by Summerfield [7]. The severe psychological consequences of detention have been documented in refugees generally and especially amongst those with previous exposure to trauma for whom the risk of re-traumatisation is high. Australia in particular has been criticised for its adoption of potentially re-traumatising immigration detention strategies, first in 1991 [8] and then again in 2001, in a call taken up by several key medical journals [9–11], though similar problems are increasingly observed also in European countries [12]. Many authors have drawn attention to the special needs of vulnerable groups including pregnant and nursing women [13, 14], survivors of torture [15] and children [12, 16–23].

A number of further publications in the health-care and medical fields (see [5] for a meta-analysis) include case publications [24, 25] and several clinical studies. In one longitudinal study, Keller et al. examined 70 detained asylum seekers in the USA. Results indicated high rates of anxiety in 77%, depression in 86% and depression and posttraumatic stress disorder (PTSD) in 50% of the sample at baseline. These findings suggest that the sample population may be vulnerable and unfit for detention due to health reasons, especially in the case of PTSD symptoms. The authors further demonstrated that these symptoms were significantly correlated with the length of time spent in detention. At follow-up, released participants showed marked reductions in all psychological symptoms, while those still in detention were more distressed than at the baseline [26, 27]. Steel et al. used a structured psychiatric interview with ten families detained for more than 2 years and reported that all adults and children met diagnostic criteria for at least one current psychiatric disorder. Further, a threefold increase in psychiatric disorders in adults and a tenfold increase in children was established subsequent to detention, with trauma-specific symptoms related to exposure to trauma within detention. The authors also observed "the majority of parents felt they were no longer able to care for, support, or control their children" [19]. Ishikawa [28]. examined a group of 55 Afghan asylum seekers in Japan, 18 (33%) of whom had previously been detained, using the Hopkins Symptom Checklist 25 and the Harvard Trauma Questionnaire. The level of trauma exposure and other characteristics of those who had been detained was not significantly different from those who had not been detained; however the symptom scores of anxiety, depression and PTSD were higher amongst the group who had been previously detained, a trend that was confirmed by a multiple regression analysis of factors. In a study of 49 Persian-speaking refugees with temporary protection visas living in Sydney, Australia, Momartin [28] produced findings that indicated that past experiences of stress in detention contributed to adverse psychiatric outcomes [29]. Steel assessed post-traumatic stress disorder (PTSD), major depressive episodes and indices of stress related to past trauma, detention and temporary protection status in 241 Arabic-speaking Mandaean refugees in Sydney, a substantial percentage (60%) of this local ethnic population group. Past immigration detention and ongoing temporary protection each contributed independently to the risk of ongoing PTSD, depression and mental health-related disability, with longer periods in detention being associated with more severe mental health disturbances. The impact appeared to be severe as it had persisted for an average of 3 years following release [30].

In a pilot study in the UK, Lorek used the Strengths and Difficulties Questionnaire with 11 out of a group of 24 detained children (aged between 3 months and 17 years) [31]. A high level of symptom was identified in all children (and their nine parents) with eight of these children meeting the criteria for treatment by a mental health professional. Robjant et al. [31] conducted a major study comparing 67 detained asylum seekers, 30 who had previously been imprisoned within the UK for criminal offences and 49 who were living in the community. The authors used standard instruments, the Hospital Anxiety and Depression Scale (HADS) and the Impact of Event Scale-Revised (IES-R), and found the highest symptom rates in detained asylum seekers. They also found a complex effect on depression scores indicating interaction between the lengths of time spent in detention and prior exposure to interpersonal trauma [32]. The results of one of the first systematic literature reviews undertaken on the issue published by Robjant [33] revealed high rates of clinical symptoms correlating with time in detention and moderate improvement but also persistence of symptoms after release. In a follow-up study with 104 refugees from Iran and Afghanistan in Australia, Steel compared refugees released from immigration detention on Temporary Protection Visas ($n = 47$) with those resettled in Australia under the Humanitarian Program having been granted Permanent Protection Visas prior to arrival ($n = 57$). Based on standard instruments like HTQ and HSCL, the results confirmed a high number of symptoms and persistent problems with integration and everyday life amongst those on Temporary Protection Visas who had been detained [34]. Using the same instruments, Cleveland et al. documented significant psychiatric deterioration even after a short period of detention in a sample of 122 detained and 66 non-detained adult asylum seekers in Montreal and Toronto, Canada [35]. Graf used the Brief Jail Mental Health Screening in a validation study with the WHO standard CIDI interview with 80 inmates at a Swiss detention centre and found high rates (76%) of at least one mental health disorder according to the CIDI, with higher rates for phobic and post-traumatic stress disorders (23%) as compared to general prison groups [36]. Young re-analysed the Australian Human Rights Commission mental health screening data and reported that longer periods in detention were associated with higher self-reported depression scores, particularly in women. Moreover, about 50% of those who completed the Harvard Trauma Questionnaire had post-traumatic stress disorder symptoms [37]. And finally, in an important study commissioned by the Australian Department of Immigration and Border Protection, an analysis of health records held by the Department revealed an initial improvement in physical and mental health amongst asylum seekers held in immigration detention followed by a significant deterioration, firstly in physical health and, after 12 months, in mental health [38].

The research results lead to the following main conclusions:

- The impact of detention on mental health in itself is substantial and tends to persist even after release.
- Vulnerable sub-groups present with higher symptom rates.
- Vulnerable sub-groups are apparently not sufficiently identified, supported or protected (see also Wenzel et al. in this book).
- Stress and trauma-related disorders are characteristic for but not limited to asylum seekers.
- The overall high rates of trauma spectrum symptoms in particular form an argument against detention in itself and plead for alternative options with full access to health-care services.

Further, it might be argued that:

- Governments using detention have to implement a careful initial medical screening and follow-up monitoring in order to assess health needs and to avoid detention of groups with high vulnerability, including most refugees, and use immigration detention only as a last resort suggested in the UNHCR strategy[13] and documents mentioned below.
- Governments should be held accountable for health and other problems resulting from detention.

12.3 The Role of Health Professionals

Detention and other restrictions on the freedom of migrants, including asylum seekers before, during or after a legal claims determination process, have become critical issues frequently involving serious violations of appropriate standards of treatment and human rights. Health professionals could play a crucial role in addressing issues that might affect the (mental) health of migrant detainees, if they, with the support of their National Medical Associations, were able to fully implement the Mandela Rules (or similar rules, e.g. the European Prison Rules). They would then be able to identify individuals with vulnerabilities (e.g. those who have been victims of torture or ill-treatment, or a contagious disease) and bring them to the attention of the authorities as well as ensure continuity of medical care by a specialist in or outside the place of detention. For this to occur governments would

[13] Beyond Detention, A Global Strategy to support governments to end the detention of asylum seekers and refugees, UNHCR. Available at http://www.unhcr.org/53aa929f6.

need to (a) recognise the right of patients to receive the care deemed necessary by a physician, (b) respect and uphold the obligation of physicians to administer treatment on the basis of clinical need alone and (c) ensure physicians have adequate time and sufficient resources to assess the detainees' physical and psychological conditions.[14]

Within any detention system, there will be conflicts between the security paradigm of the detaining authorities and the health paradigm of the health professionals. Hence there should be ample consideration of the conflict (express or implied) between the physician's professional obligations to a patient and their contractual obligations to the prison administration or the state authority, commonly known as dual loyalty.[15] Gatherer et al. recommend that government health authorities should provide and be accountable for health-care services in prisons and should advocate for healthy prison conditions and that specific training for health professionals working in prisons should be offered on a standard basis. Moreover, all health staff should have complete professional independence and should preferably be employed by a health authority independent of the prison administration. The right of physicians and other health professionals to practice their profession in accordance with their professional codes of conduct and ethics should be clearly understood and accepted. Finally, prison health services should not be isolated but should be integrated into regional and national health systems [39].

Recently, a broad lack of concern by some governments with regard to the role and ethical obligations of physicians drawing attention to the situation of detained persons [40, 41] has been identified and has been taken up in the Royal Australasian College of Physicians Position Statement on refugee and asylum seeker health [42] . This document provides good guidance on the health needs of asylum seekers. The special chapter on detention in the Statement summarises the position as follows:

> "Held detention is harmful to the physical and mental health of people of all ages in the short and long term. People face profound uncertainty, hopelessness and fear for their future, which, in combination with the detention environment and lack of meaningful activity, contribute to high rates of mental health problems, self-harm and attempted suicide. Held detention represents a significant breach of human rights, including the right to liberty, to not be detained, and the right to health (page 16)".

Other tools and documents which can be used in order to protect vulnerable groups and improve conditions for detainees include the European Asylum Support Office (EASO) "tool for identification of persons with special needs",[16] the UNHCR

[14] WMA Council Resolution on Refugees and Migrants Adopted by the 203rd WMA Council Session, Buenos Aires, April 2016. Available at https://www.wma.net/policies-post/wma-council-resolution-on-refugees-and-migrants/.

[15] Dual Loyalty & Human rights in health professional practice. Physicians for Human Rights (2003).Availableathttp://physiciansforhumanrights.org/library/reports/dual-loyalty-and-human-rights-2003.html.

[16] https://ipsn.easo.europa.eu/easo-tool-identification-persons-special-needs. Accessed 19 Jun 17.

Heightened Risk Identification Tool and User Guide,[17] the UNHCR/APT/IDC guide "Monitoring Immigration Detention: Practical Manual"[18] and the IDC handbook *There are Alternatives: A Handbook for Preventing Unnecessary Immigration Detention*[19]. Finally, in considering alternatives for detention, it is important to recognise the value of family life and family cohesion, not only as a fundamental human right but also as an important protective influence on psychological health and recovery from traumatic stress resulting from earlier life experiences.

In a position paper, the UNHCR has further summarised recommendations based on international humanitarian law ("Back to Basics: The Right to Liberty and Security of Person[20]"). These recommendations were taken up in the conclusions of the "Second Global Roundtable on Reception and Alternatives to Detention—Summary of Deliberations[21]". The assessment tools provided by the UNHCR (see Wenzel et al. in this volume) can assist in important steps including priority placement in alternative housing and prohibition of the use of detention in the most vulnerable groups, like minors and survivors of torture. The relevant UNHCR manual[22] lists a number of concrete alternatives that might have to be modified based on the situation in a specific country and include:

- Private accommodation and rental housing.
- Living with immediate family, friends or relatives.
- Living with members of the host community.
- Government-funded housing.
- Private housing funded by charities.
- Open reception centres for asylum seekers.
- Open centres for recognised refugees.
- Shelters run as part of humanitarian aid.
- Shelters for groups experiencing a common vulnerability factor, such as unaccompanied or separated children, survivors of family violence, and trafficked persons. Shelters for the homeless may be an option in emergency circumstances.
- Foster families or homes.
- Centres for migrants and asylum seekers preparing to depart the country.

An example of the successful implementation of one such alternative is the Community Detention Program implemented in Australia over the last few years. Under this programme, the majority of people in immigration detention for whom there are no security concerns are able to live in the community. While still subject

[17] http://www.refworld.org/docid/46f7c0cd2.html. Accessed 19 Jun 17.

[18] http://www.apt.ch/en/resources/monitoring-immigration-detention-practical-manual/. Accessed 19 Jun 17.

[19] http://idcoalition.org/publication/there-are-alternatives-revised-edition/. Accessed 19 Jun 17.

[20] http://www.refworld.org/docid/4dc935fd2.html. Accessed 19 Jun 17.

[21] http://www.refworld.org/docid/55e8079f4.html. Accessed 19 Jun 17

[22] http://www.refworld.org/pdfid/57f21f6b4.pdf. Accessed 1 Jun 17.

to a number of restrictions, they are able to access services and participate in community life and activities, thus mitigating some of the more harmful effects of closed detention.[23]

The UNHCR manual screening questions give a good indication of the factors that should be considered:

Separation from parents, family and guardians:

- Is the child separated from her/his parents or customary primary carers?
- Where are the child's parents or customary primary carers? If in the country of arrival, are there any impediments to their being reunited?
- Who is the child travelling with and does the child feel safe with them?
- What guardianship/legal representation and care arrangements need to be established?
- What assistance is required to restore family links, and how can this assistance be accessed?
- Ask the unaccompanied or separated child: "Tell me about your parents and other family members. What are the best/most difficult aspects of your life at present? What supports do you have/need?".

12.4 Hunger Strike as Example of Special Problems in Detention

Hunger strikes [9, 16, 43] and self-injurious behaviour [21, 44] have frequently been mentioned as special problems in detention and should not be misunderstood as signs of psychiatric disorders like eating or borderline disorder. Often it is a form of protest by people who lack any other ways of making themselves heard. In refusing nutrition for a significant period, they hope to obtain certain goals by inflicting negative publicity on the authorities. These phenomena have also been observed in detained asylum seekers and refugees [43, 45–47]. The support of persons on hunger strike in accordance with ethical and medical standards is a complex challenge [48–52] and includes giving information and support, offering consensual measures of treatment to reduce health risks [53, 54], monitoring and careful refeeding and rehabilitation after the end of a hunger strike by experienced experts [55]. Non-consensual forced feeding of mentally competent detainees on hunger strike has been advocated or used [56], even in case of children [16]. However, the involvement of physicians is clearly prohibited by the WMA Declaration of Malta [43] and can be seen as an ethical challenge in "dual loyalty" situations when under pressure from authorities, as well as participation in torture.

Physicians should be aware of their responsibility to differentiate between the possibility that the hunger strike or other self-injurious behaviour is a form of protest against human rights abuses including torture or inhuman and degrading

[23] http://www.refugeecouncil.org.au/getfacts/seekingsafety/asylum/detention/key-facts/. Accessed 17 Jul 17.

treatment or that it may indicate undiagnosed or untreated health-care needs. Physicians are obliged by international ethical standards to take necessary action against abuses and torture in particular and report on such problems. The UN/WMA Istanbul Protocol (see again Wenzel et al. in this book) should be used in documentation of these cases.

12.5 A Case Example: Australia

The majority of published articles regarding the detention of asylum seekers and unauthorised migrants (more than 20 according to the MEDLINE standard database only), which we partly have reviewed in this chapter, deal with human rights violations in the context of detention in Australia or in Australian offshore processing facilities. The following case example illustrates many of the issues described in these articles.

12.5.1 The Waiting Game: Detention in Australian Offshore Immigration Detention Facilities

12.5.1.1 History and Overview

The Australian Government first introduced mandatory detention for non-citizens who arrived in Australia without a visa in 1992. The numbers of unauthorised asylum seekers arriving by boat remained generally low before rising sharply in 1999 and continuing to climb. In 2001, the Government brought in a suite of policies intended to stop unauthorised boat arrivals. Known as the "Pacific Solution", policies included the excision of some island territories from the Australian migration zone and the offshore processing of asylum claims. Asylum seekers arriving by boat to any of these excised territories were sent to Australian-funded detention centres on Nauru and on Manus Island in Papua New Guinea, rather than being allowed to claim asylum in Australia. Following the introduction of these policies, the number of boat arrivals dropped considerably. Then in 2007, a new government dismantled the "Pacific Solution" and closed the detention facilities on Manus Island and Nauru. Over the next few years, the number of boat arrivals increased significantly until August 2012; the Australian Government once again introduced legislation allowing offshore processing and reopening the detention centres on Nauru and Manus Island. A new government introduced further measures including the ruling that after July 19, 2013, any asylum seeker reaching Australia by boat would *never* be resettled in Australia. All boat arrivals would be sent to either Manus Island or Nauru for processing and, if and when their claim for refugee status was recognised, they would be offered permanent resettlement in Papua New Guinea or, for those transferred to Nauru, temporary resettlement in Nauru (for up to 20 years) or resettlement in Cambodia. Papua New Guinea, Nauru and Cambodia are all are developing countries with poor to non-existent health and mental health services little in the way of social or economic infrastructure able to support refugee resettlement. These policies have had the effect of "stopping the boats" but have also resulted in approximately 2000 men, women and children, being held indefinitely on Nauru and Manus Island.

The accommodation for asylum seekers on both islands is overcrowded, unsuited to the prevailing hot and humid climate and provides almost no privacy for couples and families, or for individuals seeking some time alone. On Nauru detainees live in canvas army tents or vinyl marquees with bunk beds separated by tarpaulin walls into "rooms" for couples and family groups. The marquees for families with children have some air-conditioning, but for the most part, the only cooling available is from large portable fans. These tents hold as many as 40 people and can reach temperatures of up to 45 °C during the day. On Manus Island the men live in marquees or converted containers or modular style accommodation. Only some of the accommodation is air-conditioned. Basic medical and mental health services (including torture and trauma counselling) as well as legal support, language classes and welfare services are provided at both locations. Supports and services notwithstanding, the UNHCR reports that conditions at the facilities fall short of international protection standards by failing to provide (a) a fair and efficient system for assessing refugee claims, (b) safe and humane conditions of treatment in detention and (c) adequate and timely solutions for recognised refugees.[24]

12.5.1.2 Impact of Detention

It has been well documented that arbitrary, protracted and indefinite detention is profoundly destructive of resilience and mental health. For survivors of torture and trauma in particular, immigration detention may replicate past experiences of imprisonment, torture and other forms of violence. During April 2016 a group of expert medical consultants convened by the UNHCR surveyed self-selected groups of asylum seekers and refugees on Nauru and Manus Island.[25] On Manus Island, 88% of respondents and, on Nauru, 83% of respondents were found to be suffering from a depressive or anxiety disorder and/or post-traumatic stress disorder. This compares with the rate of moderate to high psychological distress amongst asylum seekers living in the Australian community (61% for major depressive disorder (MDD) and 52% for post-traumatic stress disorder (PTSD) according to the study by Hocking et al. [57]) and rates of between 35% and 46% amongst newly settled refugees.[26]

[24] http://www.unhcr.org/news/latest/2013/11/52947ac86/unhcr-reports-harsh-conditions-legal-shortcomings-pacific-island-asylum.html. Accessed 17 Jul 2017.

[25] Submission by the Office of the United Nations High Commissioner for Refugees to the Australian Senate Legal and Constitutional Affairs Committee in relation to the Inquiry into the Serious Allegations of Abuse, Self-Harm and Neglect of Asylum Seekers in Relation to the Nauru Regional Processing Centre and any Like Allegations in Relation to the Manus Regional Processing Centre; 12 November 2016.

[26] David Marshall, National Centre for Longitudinal Data, Building a New Life in Australia: The Longitudinal Study of Humanitarian Migrants; Data Highlight No. 2/2015 https://www.dss.gov.au/sites/default/files/documents/09_2015/data-highlight-n0-2-2015-bnla_pdf.pdf; cited in UNHCR Submission (see above).

12.5.2 Challenges and Problems

There is a complex and dynamic interaction between initial trauma and the subsequent impact of situational stressors and secondary trauma. Over time it becomes impossible to distinguish between symptoms that are the result of a history of torture and trauma and symptoms that are the result of prolonged detention, separation from family and ongoing uncertainty and anxiety about the future. Exposure to traumatic and even violent events such as major riots (one on Nauru which resulted in the complete destruction of the detention facility and the other on Manus Island which resulted in the murder of an asylum seeker by a local centre employee), hunger strikes, the deaths of two asylum seekers caused by delays in accessing the level of medical care required and numerous incidents of self-harm and suicide (including the public self-immolation and subsequent death of a refugee on Nauru) have a profound impact on the entire asylum seeker/refugee community. The increase in symptoms associated with post-traumatic stress is apparent even amongst those not directly involved in the events. Suicide attempts increase as asylum seekers use their lives and bodies to express their distress and attempt to influence the system, no matter what the consequences. Self-harm becomes another way of regaining some control, "I cut myself to relieve some of the pressure of this place, it feels good because I can control the pain, it is one of the few things they can't take away from me".

Detainees commonly express apprehension about their personal safety. There are frequent reports of verbal abuse, harassment, intimidation, bullying, theft, physical assaults and, occasionally, sexual assaults. Many report that they are afraid to make formal complaints or report crimes. Some are concerned that they will be accused of making "false" complaints or attempting to "make trouble" which they fear may in turn jeopardise their protection claims. Others have lost confidence that anything can or will be done about their complaints, while others avoid making complaints due to family or cultural reasons. Victims feel exposed and unsafe because they fear they cannot be protected from retaliation in the isolated closed community of the detention centre. This is of particular concern in relation to women and children or LBGTI (lesbian, gay, bisexual, transgender) people reporting sexual harassment or assault. People who are already experiencing symptoms of traumatic stress are likely to find recovery extremely challenging in these circumstances.

Children in detention are always particularly vulnerable with presentations including bed-wetting, nightmares, anxiety and emotional dysregulation, depression and the imitation of adult self-harming behaviours. In these situations children are frequent witnesses to the distress of adults around them and are often obliged to take on responsibilities beyond their level of maturity. The availability of schooling and other activities is limited. Parents, unable to shield their children from the physical and emotional stressors inherent in this environment, consistently express concerns for their development and wellbeing. Many, overwhelmed by the living conditions and ongoing uncertainty regarding their future, find their capacity to look after their children diminished as a result of their own deteriorating mental health.

Over the past few years, Australian Government policy in relation to asylum seekers has changed frequently in response to shifting political agendas and legal challenges. This has resulted in confusion, anger and a loss of trust that adds to and compounds previous trauma. The term "detention fatigue" is used to describe the symptomology of individuals who have been within detention or a detention-like environment for a prolonged period of time. Commonly reported symptoms include sleep deprivation; cognitive impairment; deterioration in the ability to regulate emotions; persistent negative beliefs about oneself and the world; loss of identity and meaning; profound helplessness and hopelessness; distorted self-blame; persistent feelings of fear, anger, guilt, and shame; detachment from others; psychosomatic complaints; suicidal ideation; and chronic intense anxiety and depression, all of which indicate high levels of distress. Comments, such as "I left a certain death in my country to die slowly here", are common.

Freedom goes beyond the ability to move freely, and in the case of people in detention, normal freedoms are stripped away. Inflexible and arbitrary rules, constant surveillance, high security fencing and uniformed guards contribute to an oppressive prison-like atmosphere. Asylum seekers go from being resourceful, self-sufficient individuals to people who have almost no control over their day-to-day lives, let alone any control over issues profoundly affecting their future life or the lives of their children. People become demoralised to the point where they cede control of their lives to the institution. This results in very low levels of energy and motivation, the loss of ability to plan or think hopefully about the future, rigid thinking and a reduced tolerance for change, a reduced interest or ability to participate in daily activities and a reduced sense of self-efficacy. Expressions of a profound sense of "moral injury" are also common; anger at being arbitrarily denied access to asylum in Australia; anger at the injustice of being "locked up and treated like criminals" when no crime has been committed; frustration at the delays and inconsistent information in relation to the processing of claims; anxiety about if, where and when they will be offered permanent resettlement; and anguish at separation from their families all contribute to a profound sense of hopelessness and powerlessness. One counsellor reported, "It is a terrible thing to witness–seeing people lose their hope to the point where it is like having an empty shell in front of you, where clients are only fixated on their pain with no hope, goals or dreams for the future, a total absence of future, barely living, simply cocooned in and by their pain".

12.5.3 Supports and Services

Prolonged detention and uncertainty about their future means that asylum seekers cannot move on from their past and therefore continue to relive it. The level of physical discomfort, the lack of privacy and the ongoing uncertainty and lengthy delays in gaining access to durable settlement solutions are significant factors in the widespread deterioration of physical and mental health. Providing counselling and other mental health supports to asylum seekers in long-term detention or detention-like conditions requires an approach that recognises that exposure to trauma is current and ongoing and in this context may serve only to ameliorate rather than remedy.

The impact of protracted detention and institutionalisation has significant implications for post-detention adjustments with the psychological consequences posing significant impediments to transitioning and managing the challenges of resettlement. Recovery from trauma is rarely if ever possible in situations where people continue to experience the environment as unsafe and unsupportive; for asylum seekers in detention, the journey to safety is not yet over.

Conclusion

A number of binding international standards supported by specific documents including but not limited to those by the UN either prohibit detention of vulnerable groups like children and torture survivors or at least limit the use of detention. The severe and potentially long-term effects on physical and mental health and on integration underline the need for priority to be given to less restrictive alternatives. If detention is used, special care must be given to respect standards including access to health care, protection from abuse, protection of family life and other fundamental human rights. In June 2017 an AU$70 million conditional settlement deal was reportedly reached in a class action brought on behalf of 1905 detainees who were held at the Manus Island detention centre, one of the Australian offshore processing centres. The defendants to the proceedings were Australian Government and the detention centre's contracted infrastructure and security providers.[27] This can be seen as an important step in holding governments responsible for the treatment of asylum seekers and refugees as the conditions in transit or reception countries should not be a continuation of persecution or abuse experienced in war regions or under oppressive regimes.

[27] https://www.slatergordon.com.au/media-centre/media-releases/70-million-settlement-reached-manus-island-class-action published 14 Jun 17. Accessed 17 Jul 17.

References

1. Flynn M. There and back again: on the diffusion of immigration detention. Journal on Migration and Human Security. 2014;2(3):32.
2. Newman LK, Dudley M, Steel Z. Asylum, detention, and mental health in Australia. Refug Surv Q. 2008;27(1):17.
3. Newman L. Seeking asylum—trauma, mental health, and human rights: an Australian perspective. J Trauma Dissociation. 2013;14(2):213–23.
4. Grange M. MI. When is immigration detention lawful? The monitoring practices of UN human rights mechanisms. 2017.
5. Filges TME, Kastrup M, Jørgensen A-MK. The impact of detention on the health of asylum seekers: a systematic review. Campbell Systematic Reviews. 2015;13:104.
6. Goodwin-gill GS. International law and the detention of refugees and asylum seekers. Int Migr Rev. 1986;20(2):193–219.
7. Summerfield D, Gorst-Unsworth C, Bracken P, Tonge V, Forrest D, Hinshelwood G. Detention in the UK of tortured refugees. Lancet. 1991;338(8758):58.
8. Silove D, McIntosh P, Becker R. Risk of retraumatisation of asylum-seekers in Australia. Aust N Z J Psychiatry. 1993;27(4):606–12.
9. Silove D, Steel Z, Watters C. Policies of deterrence and the mental health of asylum seekers. JAMA. 2000;284(5):604–11.

10. Silove D, Steel Z, Mollica R. Detention of asylum seekers: assault on health, human rights, and social development. Lancet. 2001;357(9266):1436–7.
11. Steel Z, Silove DM. The mental health implications of detaining asylum seekers. Med J Aust. 2001;175(11–12):596–9.
12. Williams B, Cassar C, Siggers G, Taylor S. Medical and social issues of child refugees in Europe. Arch Dis Child. 2016;101(9):839–42.
13. Mannion M. Behind the wire: nursing in a detention centre. Aust Nurses J. 1992;21(10):22–4.
14. Pregnant asylum seekers in detention. Pract Midwife. 2002;5(11):7.
15. Woodhead M. Australian doctor challenges government over child detention "torture". BMJ. 2016;352:i550.
16. Mok A, Nelson EA, Murphy J, Hampson A, Hendriks JH. Children on hunger strike: child abuse or legitimate protest? BMJ. 1996;312(7029):501–4.
17. Zwi KJ, Herzberg B, Dossetor D, Field J. A child in detention: dilemmas faced by health professionals. Med J Aust. 2003;179(6):319–22.
18. Shields L, Stathis S, Mohay H, van Haeringen A, Williams H, Wood D, et al. The health of children in immigration detention: how does Australia compare? Aust N Z J Public Health. 2004;28(6):513–9.
19. Steel Z, Momartin S, Bateman C, Hafshejani A, Silove DM, Everson N, et al. Psychiatric status of asylum seeker families held for a protracted period in a remote detention centre in Australia. Aust N Z J Public Health. 2004;28(6):527–36.
20. Newman LK, Steel Z. The child asylum seeker: psychological and developmental impact of immigration detention. Child Adolesc Psychiatr Clin N Am. 2008;17(3):665–83.
21. Hodes M. The mental health of detained asylum seeking children. Eur Child Adolesc Psychiatry. 2010;19(7):621–3.
22. Dudley M, Steel Z, Mares S, Newman L. Children and young people in immigration detention. Curr Opin Psychiatry. 2012;25(4):285–92.
23. Isaacs D. Nauru and detention of children. J Paediatr Child Health. 2015;51(4):353–4.
24. McGorry P. Asylum seeking and mandatory detention. The psychological consequences. Aust Fam Physician. 2002;31(3):275–8.
25. Koopowitz LF, Abhary S. Psychiatric aspects of detention: illustrative case studies. Aust N Z J Psychiatry. 2004;38(7):495–500.
26. Keller AS, Ford D, Sachs E, Rosenfeld B, Trinh-Shevrin C, Meserve C, et al. The impact of detention on the health of asylum seekers. J Ambul Care Manage. 2003;26(4):383–5.
27. Keller AS, Rosenfeld B, Trinh-Shevrin C, Meserve C, Sachs E, Leviss JA, et al. Mental health of detained asylum seekers. Lancet. 2003;362(9397):1721–3.
28. Ishikawa E. Nihon no nanmin ukeire: sono keii to tenbou [Acceptance of refugees in Japan: history and prospects]. In: Komai H, editor. Koza guroubaruka suru nihon to imin mondai dai 1 kan: kokusaika no nakano imin seisaku no kadai [Lectures on globalizing Japan and problems of immigrants, vol. 1, problems of immigrant policy in globalization]. Tokyo: Akashi Shoten; 2002. p. 207–51.
29. Momartin S, Steel Z, Coello M, Aroche J, Silove DM, Brooks R. A comparison of the mental health of refugees with temporary versus permanent protection visas. Med J Aust. 2006;185(7):357–61.
30. Steel Z, Silove D, Brooks R, Momartin S, Alzuhairi B, Susljik I. Impact of immigration detention and temporary protection on the mental health of refugees. Br J Psychiatry. 2006;188:58–64.
31. Lorek A, Ehntholt K, Nesbitt A, Wey E, Githinji C, Rossor E, et al. The mental and physical health difficulties of children held within a British immigration detention center: a pilot study. Child Abuse Negl. 2009;33(9):573–85.
32. Robjant K, Robbins I, Senior V. Psychological distress amongst immigration detainees: a cross-sectional questionnaire study. Br J Clin Psychol. 2009;48(Pt 3):275–86.
33. Robjant K, Hassan R, Katona C. Mental health implications of detaining asylum seekers: systematic review. Br J Psychiatry. 2009;194(4):306–12.

34. Steel Z, Momartin S, Silove D, Coello M, Aroche J, Tay KW. Two year psychosocial and mental health outcomes for refugees subjected to restrictive or supportive immigration policies. Soc Sci Med. 2011;72(7):1149–56.
35. Cleveland J, Rousseau C. Psychiatric symptoms associated with brief detention of adult asylum seekers in Canada. Can J Psychiatr. 2013;58(7):409–16.
36. Graf M, Wermuth P, Hafeli D, Weisert A, Reagu S, Pfluger M, et al. Prevalence of mental disorders among detained asylum seekers in deportation arrest in Switzerland and validation of the Brief Jail Mental Health Screen BJMHS. Int J Law Psychiatry. 2013;36(3-4):201–6.
37. Young P, Gordon MS. Mental health screening in immigration detention: a fresh look at Australian government data. Australas Psychiatry. 2016;24(1):19–22.
38. Green JP, Eagar K. The health of people in Australian immigration detention centres. Med J Aust. 2010;192(2):65–70.
39. Gatherer A, Enggist S, Møller L. The essentials about prisons and health. In: Enggist S, editor. Prisons and health. Copenhagen: WHO; 2014. p. 1–5.
40. Berger D. Australia's law to gag doctors with concerns about asylum seekers is a failure of democracy. BMJ. 2015;350:h3256.
41. Smith P. Australia backs down over jail terms for doctors who speak out about abuse of asylum seekers. BMJ. 2016;355:i5681.
42. Paxton GA, Cherian S, Zwi KJ. The royal Australasian college of physicians position statement on refugee and asylum seeker health. Med J Aust. 2015;203(4):176–7.
43. Kenny MA, Silove DM, Steel Z. Legal and ethical implications of medically enforced feeding of detained asylum seekers on hunger strike. Med J Aust. 2004;180(5):237–40.
44. Cohen J. Safe in our hands? A study of suicide and self-harm in asylum seekers. J Forensic Legal Med. 2008;15(4):235–44.
45. Silove D, Curtis J, Mason C, Becker R. Ethical considerations in the management of asylum seekers on hunger strike. JAMA. 1996;276(5):410–5.
46. Roggla G. Medically enforced feeding of detained asylum seekers on hunger strike. Wien Klin Wochenschr. 2005;117(11-12):436.
47. Dahlberg J, Dahl V. Asylum seekers on hunger strike–how far does the patient's right to refuse treatment go? Tidsskr Nor Laegeforen. 2015;135(1):45–7.
48. Lazarus JA. Physicians' ethical obligations to hunger strikers. BMJ. 2013;346:f3705.
49. Irmak N. Professional ethics in extreme circumstances: responsibilities of attending physicians and healthcare providers in hunger strikes. Theor Med Bioeth. 2015;36(4):249–63.
50. Karni T. Hunger striking inmates and detainees, and medical ethics. Isr Med Assoc J. 2015;17(3):179–81.
51. Caenazzo L, Tozzo P, Rodriguez D. Hospitalized hunger-striking prisoners: the role of ethics consultations. Med Health Care Philos. 2016;19(4):623–8.
52. Druml C, Ballmer PE, Druml W, Oehmichen F, Shenkin A, Singer P, et al. ESPEN guideline on ethical aspects of artificial nutrition and hydration. Clin Nutr. 2016;35(3):545–56.
53. Getaz L, Rieder JP, Nyffenegger L, Eytan A, Gaspoz JM, Wolff H. Hunger strike among detainees: guidance for good medical practice. Swiss Med Wkly. 2012;142:w13675.
54. Chalela JA, Lopez JI. Medical management of hunger strikers. Nutr Clin Pract. 2013;28(1):128–35.
55. Eichelberger M, Joray ML, Perrig M, Bodmer M, Stanga Z. Management of patients during hunger strike and refeeding phase. Nutrition. 2014;30(11–12):1372–8.
56. Kalk WJ. Guantanamo force feeding trial: the US is wrong to medicalize hunger striking. BMJ. 2015;350:h669.
57. Hocking DC, Kennedy GA, Sundram S. Mental disorders in asylum seekers: the role of the refugee determination process and employment. J Nerv Ment Dis. 2015;203(1):28–32.

13 Promoting Health of Refugees in and through Sport and Physical Activity: A Psychosocial, Trauma-Sensitive Approach

Clemens Ley and María Rato Barrio

Abstract

While psychosocial interventions are underlined by most international models of refugee health care, few guidelines exist so far as to the implementation of specific programmes. In this chapter, a resource-oriented, trauma–sensitive approach to sport and physical activity is presented, aiming to promote health and psychosocial support among refugees. We first provide an overview of research on sport and physical activity with linguistically and culturally diverse migrants and with refugees from conflict regions in 'new societies' as well as in refugee camps. Furthermore, we outline some initiatives from the sport for development and peace field and different body- and movement-based approaches with people living with posttraumatic stress disorder. We then present some key issues relating to the implementation of sport and physical activity for promoting health and psychosocial support. Finally, we draw some conclusions regarding research needs and practical implications.

13.1 Introduction

While psychosocial interventions in prevention and rehabilitation of psychological and medical problems in refugees are underlined by most international models of refugee support and health care, such as the WHO's Mental Health and Psychosocial Support (MHPSS) (see [1]), few guidelines exist so far as to the implementation of specific programmes. Sport and physical activity programmes have been proposed

C. Ley (✉)
Institute of Sport Science, University of Vienna, Vienna, Austria

M. R. Barrio
NGO Asociación para la cooperación, la convivencia y la investigación, Madrid, Spain
e-mail: mariaratobarrio@yahoo.es

T. Wenzel, B. Droždek (eds.), *An Uncertain Safety*,
https://doi.org/10.1007/978-3-319-72914-5_13

as low-barrier approaches that can be easily offered in most settings; however, often it remains unclear how psychosocial processes and health benefits are facilitated in these programmes.

In order to discuss how sport and physical activity can contribute to psychosocial support and health in refugees, we first present an overview of related fields of research, from the relevant aspects of the relatively well-researched fields of sport with culturally and linguistically diverse (CALD) migrants and intercultural sport programmes to the specific aspects of sport with refugees. While some research emerged about sport with refugees from conflict regions, seeking asylum in 'new societies' (i.e. in culturally and linguistically diverse countries), few data are available on internally displaced people (IDP) or people living in refugees camps and hostels in neighbouring (often conflict-affected) countries.

Second, we discuss critical issues for implementing sport and physical activity with refugees coming from or living in (post-)conflict regions. Thereby, we distinguish basic orientations and goals as well as potential psychosocial processes and health effects of sport and physical activity from a resource-oriented and trauma-sensitive perspective. Finally, we draw some conclusions and recommendations for psychosocial support and promotion of health in and through sport and physical activity.

While acknowledging the many benefits of sport and physical activity on health, we also advert to the ambivalent nature of sport and physical activity, that is, that they are not healthy per se and that negative effects may occur as well. It is paramount to analyse risks and to avoid negative effects of sport and physical activity, e.g. an injury may be a big burden and an additional stress for refugees from or in (post-)conflict regions. Nevertheless, we consider that the positive effects outweigh the negative ones. Participation in (health-oriented) sport and physical activity is crucial in the face of the many negative effects of sedentary behaviour and non-participation (e.g. isolation, social exclusion, physical illnesses). There is a need to discuss critically how we can maximise the positive effects and minimise the negative ones. This chapter aims to contribute to this discussion.

In this chapter, we do not discuss the effects of sport and physical activity on physical health and on the prevention and rehabilitation of physical disorders which may be relevant for refugees (see [2]). Our focus in this contribution remains on psychosocial support and mental health. While many refugees participate in sport and physical activity that are available in the host country for everybody, some refugees may not participate in these activities, as the setting, activities or interaction do not fit to their needs. In order to contribute to stimulating participation and inclusion in and through sport and physical activity, we propose in this chapter a *trauma-sensitive* approach to sport and physical activity. Having said this, we do not aim to direct the main focus on trauma but to take trauma-related aspects into consideration for a resource-oriented approach to sport and physical activity with refugees from and in (post-)conflict regions.

13.2 Overview of the Field and Research

In the following, we provide an overview of related fields of research, pointing out some relevant aspects from studies with CALD migrants and with refugees in CALD host countries as well as in refugee camps. Furthermore we present some research from the sport for development and peace (SDP) field in post-conflict regions and about diverse body- and movement-based interventions with people living with posttraumatic stress disorder (PTSD). Due to the low participation in sport and physical activity, we finalise this section with an overview of correlates for participation in sport and physical activity and the concept of (movement-related) health literacy. We conclude from the overview some questions, before we discuss in the next section key issues for the practical implementation of sport and physical activity with refugees from or in (post-)conflict regions.

13.3 Sport with CALD Migrants

Sport programmes with culturally and linguistically diverse (CALD) population groups and migrants often aim at assimilation or inclusion (e.g. from a multi- or intercultural perspective) [3, 4]. These programmes are frequently based on the assumptions that sport is a universal language, a bridge between cultures and a provider of social support. While some evidence was provided for the social and inclusive effects of sport (mostly applied in a modified manner and/or connected to other interventions) [5–8], other authors questioned the role of sport for inclusion [9] and pointed out its ambivalent nature; sport can be exclusive and inappropriate in some contexts, e.g. if different sociocultural notions, norms or behaviours are ignored; violence and aggression are reported in sport settings as well [10–13]. Thus, sport seems not to be automatically beneficial but to have a great potential of providing benefits, if adequately used. Sport clubs may provide a place for accumulating social capital, both in culturally 'mixed' (i.e. multi-ethnic) and 'separated' (i.e. mono-ethnic) sport clubs [14], e.g. by providing bridging and bonding processes [10] or by gaining contacts, knowledge and skills [14]. It seems crucial for sport clubs to reflect on barriers for participation and on assimilative and exclusionary discourses and practices and to allow multiple forms of belonging to be granted in community sport [11]. Furthermore, it seems beneficial for sport programmes which aim to promote intercultural living together to direct the focus on the similarities among the culturally diverse participants in order to stimulate identifying processes before dealing with feelings of *otherness* or *strangeness,* providing processes for mutual understanding and enrichment from the differences [8]. Despite the potential benefits, participation in sport and physical activity is in general low in CALD migrant populations [10, 15, 16].

13.4 Sport and Physical Activity with Refugees

Refugees' background and current situation may differ from other CALD migrants owing to their experiences of forced migration, e.g. due to persecution, war, torture and violence. Refugees from conflict regions have often suffered from extreme and traumatic experiences, which caused, e.g. loss, grief, separation from the family and friends, as well as a high prevalence of mental health disorders, i.e. PTSD, depression and anxiety disorders ([17, 18]; see [19]). Besides migratory and post-migratory stressors (e.g. continued insecurity and vulnerability, violence, detention or deportation), acculturation challenges are added, at least in those refugees that seek protection in a 'new society' [17, 20].

13.4.1 Sport with Refugees from Conflict Regions (Living in CALD Host Countries)

Although many sport initiatives were recently created in cultural and linguistically diverse (CALD), economically developed host countries such as EU countries or Australia in the recent years and decades, using sport to 'welcome' and to integrate refugees, only few scientific studies and evaluations were published. Spaaij [11] discussed participation of Somali refugees in community football clubs in Australia, their sense of belonging and boundaries of inclusion/exclusion through ethnographic fieldwork. He concluded, on the one hand, that in mono-ethnic sport clubs, the Somali refugees 'have more power to "grant" belonging, and it is within this context that they may experience their sport involvement as a temporary escape from tense social relations in other societal domains' ([11], cf. [21]). On the other hand, he concluded that multi-ethnic football clubs may promote both social integration, by providing greater opportunities for building social relationship between refugees and other population groups and producing new forms of belonging, and societal exclusion, through exclusionary and discriminatory discourses and practices against minority ethnic groups in football clubs [11].

Whitley et al. [17] analysed a sport-based youth development programme for refugees in the United States, based on the Teaching Personal and Social Responsibility Model (cf. [22]), within a framework for acculturation [20]. The authors presented qualitative data from interviews that showed refugees' positive experiences in the programme that may aid in the resettlement and acculturation process [17].

Harris [23] engaged South Sudanese refugee youths, who were resettled to the United States, in a Dance Movement Therapy programme. Traditional movements and dances were combined with rituals and coping mechanisms of the South Sudanese Dinka culture, achieving an improvement in solidarity, group cohesion and preventive and recovering capacities, particularly in reference to the body-mind split and their refugee situation, i.e. being away from their home country and beyond the armed conflict atmosphere they suffered.

The research project *Movi Kune—moving together* investigated therapeutic processes and health effects of sport and exercise with refugees, survivors of war and torture, in Austria [24–27], discussing diverse processes and effects, as well as strengths and limitations, of sport and exercise as adjunctive therapy in refugees with posttraumatic stress symptoms. These four examples showcase the wide range of different approaches, goals and interventions using sport and physical activity, as well as diverse research conducted in refugee populations.

13.4.2 Sport in (Post-)Conflict Regions and Refugee Camps

In the so-called *sport for development and peace* (SDP) field, some knowledge about psychosocial and health effects of SDP projects was provided in recent years, including studies in the aftermath of disasters (e.g. [28–30]), in post-conflict contexts (e.g. [8, 12, 31–34]) and in refugee camps (e.g. [35, 36]). For post-conflict and post-disaster contexts, the model of salutogenesis (e.g. [37]) and the concept of resilience (e.g. [23, 38]) were used so far as two frameworks for conceptualising psychosocial support and health-oriented sport and physical activity. For example, Henley [38] reviewed theories and practices of international community-based resilience programmes using sport and play to help children to manage adversities in their life. The authors concluded that 'sport and physical activity can have a stabilizing impact on most children through supporting and encouraging their resilience processes, with resilience being described as the process of, and capacity for, successful adaptation despite challenging or threatening circumstances' [38].

However, the SDP field faces major challenges in post-conflict regions to establish evidence for health effects, which often are perceived to be achieved automatically and universally, i.e. independent from how sport is implemented and contextualised [39]. One of the few rigorous studies in this field was conducted by Richards et al. ([39], cf. [40]) in Northern Uganda, a civil war-torn region. The authors critically discuss several challenges to research in this post-conflict context and validity in spite of their efforts to adapt to local circumstances [39, 40]. They concluded from their single-blinded randomised controlled trial (RCT) that 'there is no evidence that voluntary competitive sport-for-development interventions improve physical fitness or mental health outcomes in post-conflict settings' [39]. They even reported some adverse impact of the football-based intervention on the mental health of the participating boys (aged 11–14 years). One of their explanations of this adverse impact related to the coaches' and participants' focus on football performance and competition in a post-conflict context where the 'only previous reference point for physical contest was armed conflict' [39]. These results confirm the ambivalent nature of sport and that the health effects are not gained automatically; thus a critical reflection on the tools and specific strategies for providing psychosocial support is needed (cf. [12]).

The crucial role of the sport leaders and coaches and the creation of a supportive environment within a culture-sensitive approach were concluded in various studies, for example, with women who suffered violence in post-conflict Guatemala [41] or with traumatised children and youth in the aftermath of the earthquake in Bam, Iran [28]. In the handbook 'Moving Together—Promoting Psychosocial Well-Being Through Sport and Physical Activity', these aspects are also thematised, e.g. how to ensure safe and healthy interventions and sociocultural appropriateness and how to be a good facilitator; unfortunately, the handbook does not provide a description of the scientific sources underlying their proposal, probably due to its focus on practitioners [42]. The description of scientific or experience-based sources would however be useful to determine the origin and foundation of the proposed strategies, processes and effects, e.g. in which context the knowledge was acquired, with whom the strategies were successfully applied.

Although many sport-related initiatives target refugee camps (e.g. [43, 44]), ranging from providing sport materials or organising once-off tournaments, to a more prolonged engagement in the fields through capacity building, life-skills training, HIV-prevention or organisation of regular sport and sport development activities, few of them seem to target specifically health or psychosocial support through sport and physical activity (cf. [12]). Moreover, little is known about the processes and effects of sport and physical activity on people living in refugee camps. Refugee camps are often located in active conflict areas, affected by prevailing conflicts and instability, and in the social-political and military circumstances of the region. People living in refugee camps were and/or are often exposed to extreme events and sources for trauma, due to the high level of violence, sexual abuse, armed robbery and conflicts in the camp, as well as to the limited resources available to cope with this situation [45]. Minimal access to shelter, food, water, education, recreation, health care and psychosocial support are frequently reported in refugee camps [45].

In the framework of a broader study [46], interviews and observation were conducted by the authors in the Kakuma refugee camp in Northern Kenya. The results exemplified the ambivalent nature of sport in this camp, being an arena for educational opportunities and meaningful recreation, as well as an arena for violence and conflicts [46]. Prevailing psychosocial problems and conflicts among refugees in camps and hostels seem to get visible in sport. The problems may get worse, if sport is not adequately used and adapted to the post-conflict context and risks. However, sport may also provide an opportunity to address these problems (cf. [12]), providing psychosocial support in and through sport and physical activity.

13.4.3 Sport, Physical Activity and Health of Refugees

Independently from the location, i.e. whether people seek refuge in their own countries (as internal displaced people) and in refugee camps or escape to other potential host countries ('new societies'), sport programmes need to consider their state of health. Health is affected by pre-, peri- and post-migratory experiences and stressors (e.g. violence, torture, persecution, discrimination, separation from family), as well as by a lack of resources (e.g. loss of social network, limited access to health care, educational and occupational opportunities, language barriers, unfamiliar environment). This disbalance between stressors and available resources often results in major health problems, i.e. a high prevalence of posttraumatic stress (PTSD), depression and anxiety disorders, and problems in sleeping, concentration, presence and motivation (see [1, 19]) as well as physical health problems (see [2]). Health status impacts on their inclusion, e.g. isolation or avoidance behaviour as a result of PTSD may reduce social interaction with others. In turn, this lack of inclusion may negatively impact on their health state, e.g. feeling lonely and excluded from social interaction [47]. Thus, a certain level of well-being, health and stability can be considered a prerequisite for inclusion and participation in sport and physical activity.

Yet, the health status is often not considered and addressed in sport projects with refugees. As a result, it is likely that sport projects may reach out only to healthy refugees, thus to be *exclusive*, as an involuntary selection of participants may take place (cf. [32]). Thus, addressing health issues determines to an important degree the effectiveness, appropriateness and inclusiveness of the sport initiatives with refugees from conflict areas. Despite the lack of studies in refugee populations and in post-conflict context, participation in physical activity has been shown to be beneficial in promoting physical and mental health in other population groups and in supporting psychosocial support and recovery processes in people with mental illness [48–50] and also in people suffering from PTSD.

13.5 Sport and Exercise with People Suffering from PTSD

More research has been done on the effects of exercise with a broader range of people diagnosed with PTSD, including combat veterans and people suffering from other *traumatic* events (e.g. sudden death of a nearby person, severe accident or diagnosis of illness). Health status and recovery processes may differ according to the nature of the *trauma* and the pre- and post-*trauma* situation, e.g. availability of and access to resources or stability and supportiveness of the environment [51]. Refugees from conflict regions often have suffered from prolonged exposition to multiple traumatic events and additional stressors during and after forced migration, which may result in a severe PTSD with comorbidities (i.e. a *complex PTSD*) [51].

In the following, we present three systematic reviews including different types of physical activity used with different population groups with PTSD, aiming to point out the potential benefits of physical activity for refugees' health as well to the different and complementary approaches to physical activity. A quantitative meta-analysis, including four RCTs, reported a small to moderate effect size of exercise on reducing PTSD symptoms and depression symptoms in people with PTSD [52]. According to the available data, the authors proposed the inclusion of aerobic and resistance training as well as yoga-based exercises as adjunctive treatments [52]. In fact, yoga has in recent years received an increased attention in the treatment of PTSD [53] and a trauma-sensitive yoga approach has emerged [54–56]. Van der Kolk et al. [53] concluded from a 10-week RCT with 64 women suffering from chronic, treatment-resistant PTSD that 'yoga significantly reduced PTSD symptomatology, with effect sizes comparable to well-researched psychotherapeutic and psychopharmacologic approaches'.

Levine and Land [57] presented a systematic meta-synthesis of qualitative findings, including nine studies on Dance Movement Therapy for individuals with *trauma*, concluding four crucial themes for effective movement-based interventions: '(a) creating awareness of the mind-body connection; (b) increasing the range of movement (for the purpose of efficacy, empowerment, and reclaiming the body); (c) creating a new and healthy relationship with the self, therapist, or group through the movement process; and (d) creating a new and healthy relationship with movement' [57].

Caddick and Smith [58] conducted a systematic review, including 11 quantitative and qualitative studies, about the impact of physical activity on the well-being of combat veterans in the aftermath of physical and/or psychological combat *trauma*. The authors synthesised the benefits of a wide range of different types of sport and physical activity (e.g. adventure sports, Paralympic sports, sport and exercise camps) on subjective and psychological well-being. They concluded various processes and effects: active coping and doing things again (after inactivity), focus on abilities, positive affective experience (enjoyment, relaxation, energising effects, restorative power), improved quality of life, increased determination and inner strength, sense of achievement and accomplishment, social well-being (positive social interactions, shared experiences, supportive relationships) and source of motivation for living [58]. Combat veterans have a high prevalence of PTSD due to their experiences of war. Therefore, the reviewed studies may be interesting for refugees from conflict regions as well, and similar processes may be expected. However, conversely to refugees, combat veterans generally return to their previous sociocultural and political environment and often have access to psychosocial support systems and resources which may help in living with the heavily burden of war experiences and PTSD.

Though not exclusively linked to the situation of refugee, war experiences or post-conflict context, several initiatives were undertaken to consider *trauma* in sport-based interventions. Adapting trauma-informed psychotherapy approaches to play structures, Bergholz et al. [59] and D'Andrea et al. [60] described practical principles for *trauma*-informed sport programmes with youth, including the provision of a safe space, integration of local cultural practices, long-term engagement, meaningful relationships and skilled youth worker. The authors also provided examples of coaching techniques aiming to promote healing, e.g. *trauma*-sensitive communication and skills development, and day-to-day programme practices, emphasising the crucial role of the coach. Similar principles are presented in a manual on *trauma*-informed sport and play with women [61]. The authors present key principles as well as concrete strategies and activities, aiming to provide guidance for practitioners [61].

13.6 Other Body- and Movement-Based Approaches in Trauma Therapy

The literature on body- and movement-based work on health issues of refugees or people living with PTSD comes from a wide range of therapeutic orientations, partly unclear differentiated and delimitated, showing a very heterogeneous field of approaches. Besides the already mentioned sport- and exercise-orientated approaches, e.g. using exercise [62–67], sports and games [24, 28, 37, 59, 60] and psychomotor and play therapy [68, 69], other body- and movement-based work includes body awareness and mindfulness-based approaches, e.g. using yoga [53, 54, 70], qigong and t'ai chi [71], and psychotherapeutic approaches, e.g. creative and art therapies [72–77], Dance Movement Therapy [23, 57, 78–83], movement psychotherapy [84, 85], integrative movement therapy [86–89], concentrative movement psychotherapy [90–92] and other body psychotherapies [93–99]. Many of these approaches are based on similar principles. For example, most of them consider cultural aspects and rituals, provide lived experiences and encounters with one's own body and self, address the reciprocal relationship between psychological and corporal aspects, combine non-verbal and verbal techniques and work in the *here and now*. Mindfulness, body awareness and practice of presence are recurrent mentioned, as well as the importance of the therapeutic relationship.

> A holistic view on the human organism and the interconnections between body, psyche and soul justify, within the integral approaches of trauma related work, the use of a diversity of methods and techniques from the area of body-psychotherapy, body and movement centred work, Gestalt-therapy, creative therapy, the work with inner/internal images, as well as psychodrama. [100]

13.7 Participation of Refugees in Sport and Physical Activity

Refugees and CALD migrants, as well as people suffering from PTSD, tend to have low levels of physical activity and low rates of participation in sport and exercise [15, 101, 102]. Refugees often disengage in sport and physical activity as a consequence of migration, resettlement and acculturation challenges and/or of traumatic experiences (cf. [15]). Also through the onset of PTSD the person may become inactive, even though he/she has participated previously in sport and exercise [102]. Disengagement and inactivity may be caused by various health-related factors, e.g. a general low level of motivation or listlessness, feelings of isolation, fatigue and high levels of stress as well as by PTSD symptoms, depression and anxiety [15, 103–105]. For example, sleep disturbance is frequent among refugees from conflict regions; low sleep quality is associated with lower physical activity in people with PTSD [106].

Physical inactivity can be seen as the consequence of avoidance behaviour as well [57]. Sport and physical activity can produce bodily sensations, such as increased heart rate, muscle tension or pain, sweating or shortness of breath, which may remind the participants to stressful or traumatic experiences and make him/her stop or avoid the activity (see Sect. 13.13.1). De Assis et al. [102] argue that 'subjects diagnosed with PTSD stop participating in society and no longer take part in activities they used to enjoy; this inaction may lead to depression and social isolation'. They found out that people with PTSD preferred to choose individual sports over group activities like soccer, handball and dancing after the onset of PTSD, even though they had been involved in team sports before. Such choices are affected by the consequences of PTSD, fear, anxiety, attachment disorder or social isolation and may point to avoidance behaviour as well [102]. Hence, social interaction could have important positive benefits for people living with PTSD, if adequately implemented, including acting as a motivational force for participation.

We can distinguish social-ecological and psychological correlates of physical activity. Important social-ecological barriers for participation include lack of social support, lack of information or knowledge, unfamiliarity with the environment, diverse cultural and religious beliefs, socioeconomic problems and structural barriers. Important psychological correlates for participation include self-efficacy beliefs and attitudes towards physical activity, which however may be marked by sociocultural norms and practices [15, 16]. Acknowledging the potential benefits of sport and physical activity, a fundamental goal should be to increase habitual levels of physical activity and participation in sport [52].

To address low participation and dropouts, the health literacy approach has recently gained more recognition, also in the field of sport and physical activity [107, 108]. Refugees tend to have a low health literacy, i.e. having more difficulties to access, understand, appraise or apply health information [109, 110]. Health literacy seems strongly influenced by linguistic, religious and cultural factors, e.g. culture-specific knowledge or attitudes towards seeking professional support, as well as by structural barriers, e.g. to access health care, preventive services and support networks. An increase in health literacy may augment the efficient use of health care, sustainability of the health outcomes and adherence to health behaviour as well as foster autonomy, empowerment and social inclusion [111]. The concept of health literacy seems crucial to provide the step from receiving health care to self-regulating health behaviour. Therefore, the acquisition of critical *knowledge* (e.g. about the effects of sport and exercise), relevant *competences* (e.g. fitness, movement skills and body awareness) and *motivation* (e.g. positive attitudes towards physical activity and self-efficacy beliefs) to comply with health recommendations seems crucial for promoting self-regulated participation in sport and physical activity.

13.8 Conclusive Remarks from the Overview of Research

Concluding, we propose three challenges for the practical implementation of sport and physical activity with refugees from or in (post-)conflict regions:

1. While we acknowledge the potential *health benefits* of sport and physical activity for refugees, we have to question how we can best facilitate sport and physical activity with refugees in order to achieve these benefits. Which basic orientation and types of sport and physical activity are appropriate in which settings to provide psychosocial support? Which goals, motives and needs of the participants are crucial to address? Which processes and strategies are to be implemented to achieve the desired benefits?
2. While we acknowledge the importance of *participation in sport and physical activity*, we have to question how participation can be initiated and maintained. How to increase participation in sport and physical activity? How to make sport inclusive? How to consider sociocultural aspects and to facilitate a positive intercultural encounter? How to increase autonomous motivation and reduce social-ecological barriers?

3. While we acknowledge the *ambivalent nature of sport*, we have to question how to maximise the positive effects and minimise negative effects or risks. Which organisational aspects and cautions have to be considered? How to make sport and physical activity safe? How to adapt sport and physical activity to refugees' current health state, migratory background and experiences, as well as to possible stress-inducing aspects or *trauma* triggers?

13.9 Key Issues for the Promotion of Health in and through Sport and Physical Activity with Refugees: A Resource-Oriented, Trauma-Sensitive, Psychosocial Approach

In the following, we highlight some key issues for planning and implementing health-orientated sport and physical activity with refugees escaping from or living in (post-)conflict regions. We propose a resource-oriented and trauma-sensitive approach, aiming to improve health and psychosocial support as well as the conditions for inclusion in and through sport and physical activity. Therefore, we first present diverse basic notions of sport and physical activity, possible settings, goals and contents. Second, we describe the basic principles of a psychosocial perspective, including resource orientation and culture-sensitiveness. Third, we discuss the need for a trauma-sensitive approach and highlight organisational aspects concerning the provision of safe space, potential triggers of stress and the trauma-sensitive coach. Finally, we highlight some potential processes and health effects of sport and physical activity from a psychosocial perspective.

We do not distinguish who is implementing the activities, e.g. if refugees are leading the initiative, other CALD migrants or members of the host country, or all together. We argue that certain knowledge, experiences, sensitivity and competences are required for planning, implementing and facilitating psychosocial processes and health effects in and through sport and physical activity and for adopting an inclusive, resource-oriented and trauma-sensitive approach. Therefore, a joint initiative from people with different background, knowledge and experiences would probably be the best.

While we attempt to base the discussion on existing literature, we also give some examples from our experiences and field work made in various post-conflict contexts, e.g. from a psychosocial intervention through movement, games and sport (*APM programme*) with women and children who suffered violence in post-conflict Guatemala [8, 37, 41, 112]; from field visits in various African countries, including in the *Kakuma refugee camp* and Southern Sudan [46]; and from the sport and exercise therapy programme *Movi Kune—Moving Together* with war and torture survivors in Austria [24–27].

13.10 Basic Notions of Sport and Physical Activity

In the following section, we argue that various approaches to sport and physical activity are possible, influenced by the basic orientations of sport and physical activity (more therapeutic or recreational, physical or psychosocial), the setting and resources available (e.g. refugee camp, health centres), the goals and needs of the target population, as well as the competences of the facilitators or coaches (see Sect. 13.12). While referring to the polyvalent use of the activities, we present possible contents, combining bodily and verbal techniques.

13.10.1 Diverse Orientations, Goals and Settings

In the previous overview of the field, we presented various body- and movement-based approaches, including (a) sport- and exercise-orientated approaches, e.g. using exercise, sports and games and psychomotor and play therapy; (b) body awareness and mindfulness-based approaches, e.g. using yoga, qigong and t'ai chi; and (c) psychotherapeutic approaches, e.g. creative and art therapies, Dance Movement Therapy, integrative movement therapy and body psychotherapy. Thus, various approaches and types of physical activity are used in the field. They may be distinguished by their basic orientations and goals (see Fig. 13.1) (cf. [113, 114]); however they also present many similarities. Furthermore, in practice, the actual implemented orientation and goals strongly depend on the needs of the participant in that particular moment, e.g. the need for distraction versus the disposition for exposure to somatic sensations (see Sect. 13.13).

More than which type of physical activity is utilised, we have to consider how the tool, i.e. sports and physical activities, is employed, e.g. which strategies are applied to achieve the desired goal. For example, playing football can be recreational (e.g. to keep people busy), but it also can be used in recovery (e.g. to achieve therapeutic goals or to promote health) (cf. [115]). Furthermore, the different approaches are complementary and may enrich each other by learning from each other and providing interdisciplinary offers according to the needs and goals of the affected person.

Goals of health-oriented sport and physical activity with refugees from conflict regions could include (cf. [24]):

- To increase physical, behavioural, cognitive and emotional activation as well as relaxation (to improve psychophysiological regulation, motivation and active coping with arousals and stressors)
- To strengthen physical fitness, e.g. cardiorespiratory endurance, resistance to fatigue and muscle strength (to feel more energised and strong, and to improve physical functioning)

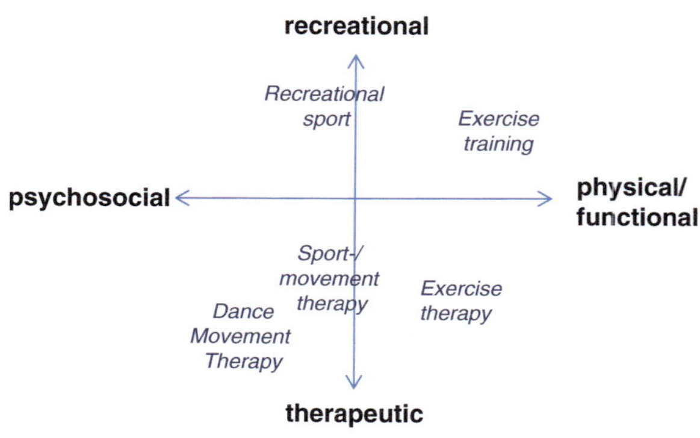

Fig. 13.1 Mapping of different basic notions and goals

- To increase sport and exercise skills, e.g. basketball skills (to facilitate positive experiences, distraction or catharsis, as well as to support inclusion in sport)
- To augment flexibility, mobility and coordination (e.g. to reduce muscle tensions, stiffness).
- To improve body awareness and mindfulness (to foster a healthy relationship with own body and self)
- To foster positive affective experiencing (e.g. joy) and affect regulation (e.g. coping with anxiety, fears, pain sensations, frustration or depressive moods)
- To provide subjective meaningful experiences of mastery and control, as well as internal attribution of success (to improve self-efficacy as a health outcome and a motivational force)
- To facilitate momentary experiencing and attentional focus on the present 'here and now' (to provide a respite, e.g. from PTSD symptoms like intrusive memories from the past)
- To improve cognitive performance (e.g. concentration, perception, appraisal, thinking, memory)
- To improve motivation and volition to initiate and maintain physical activity as well as self-regulation and self-control competences (to increase participation and adherence to physical activity)
- To facilitate social interaction and mutual support, e.g. among participants (to reduce isolation and to activate or augment social competences and social capital; to construct relationships and relatedness; and to stimulate social inclusion).

According to the goals and needs of the participant, the *setting* for sport and physical activity can be quite different, e.g. group or individual offers, clinical or non-clinical (community) setting and closed or open setting. The setting depends on the local sociocultural context, resources and opportunities as well. For example:

- A community-based setting could include health-oriented sport and physical activity programmes at a youth centre, school, sport organisation or NGO, providing health as well as recreational and inclusive benefits.
- An outpatient (day clinic/health centre) or inpatient (hospital, clinic, rehabilitation centre) centre may include offering sport and physical activity as an adjunctive therapy for people living with PTSD and for people at risk of developing a mental health problem, individually or in group, in own infrastructures or in nearby sport and exercise facilities.

The leaders of the activities can be from the refugee, CALD migrants or host country populations or include several of the mentioned population groups, working, participating and playing jointly together. Thus, the setting can be a culturally 'mixed' (multi-cultural) or 'separated' (mono-cultural) [11, 14]. The choice of the setting, types of physical activity and goals will depend on the target group, e.g. if the participants are:

- Children, youth or adults
- All people (integrative, health promotion approach), people at risk (preventive approach) or exclusive groups of people with trauma (therapeutic approach)

In this chapter, we focus on adults and youth. For the discussion on the use of sport and physical activity with refugee children, we have to refer to further literature (e.g. see [50, 60, 65, 68, 69, 112, 116]).

13.10.2 Types of Physical Activity

All kind of different types of physical activity can be used, ranging from endurance, resistance, strength, coordination and mobilisation exercises to sports or modified sports, games, dance and movement improvisations, traditional games as well as respiration and relaxation techniques, yoga exercises and body awareness, grounding and mindfulness exercises.

The choice of the activities depends on various aspects, including:

- The formation and experiences of the coach(es), facilitator(s) or leader(s)
- The abilities, skills and constraints of the participants
- The group dynamics
- The motives and interests of the participants
- The characteristics of the activity (incentives, complexity, risks and safety)
- The resources available (facilities, space, materials, financial aspects)
- The suitability in regards to culture-sensitiveness and trauma-sensitiveness

However, it is crucial to adapt and modify the activities according to sociocultural backgrounds, individual and collective needs and specific goals. Adapting sport and physical activity includes, for example, the modification of the task, challenge and rules; the required speed, amplitude and forms of movement; the material, space and time; as well as the number of participants and roles and the degree and manner of interaction.

The activity should provide an optimal challenge for each participant. Therefore, good observation skills are paramount for the coaches/facilitators/leaders in order to continuously adapt the activities to the current situation and needs of the individuals and group dynamics.

Furthermore, as it was observed during creative and sport activities in psychosocial interventions of *War Child Holland* in Kosovo, the war-affected and displaced children 'tend to communicate and express themselves by playing, rather than talking' [117]. Sport and physical activity offer an outstanding opportunity for other forms of expression, through body language, movement and behaviour, and thus an opportunity for observation and getting to know the *other* [46, 118]. Therefore these means may be particularly useful for children or adults who do not want to speak about experiences or who have difficulties to express themselves verbally (cf. [1]).

A typical session could include:

- A warm-up, e.g. using a small game or continuous fast walking or running
- Exercises for physical fitness, e.g. resistance and endurance training, coordination and mobility exercises or sport-specific training

- Modified sports, dance or movement improvisations
- A cool-down, e.g. stretching, breathing and relaxation exercises

Bergholz et al. [59] strongly recommended a consistent practice plan. This practice plan should contain, for example, thoughtful transitions, a body- and brain-based warm-up and cool-down and intervals of both high activity and recovery, allowing an adequate psychophysiological arousal regulation throughout the session (cf. [24]).

13.10.3 Combining Verbal and Non-verbal Techniques

Many authors recommended combining non-verbal with verbal techniques [74, 82, 85–87, 91, 119–121]. Besides generally combining physical activity and verbal communication (e.g. using person-centred communication), other forms of using both non-verbal and verbal techniques may include directing verbally the attentional focus on certain processes, facilitating experiences of the body in motion and reflecting about these lived experiences (verbalising bodily experiences), comparing observation of corporal as well as verbal expression, using creative or arts techniques (e.g. painting momentary emotions while moving around) or prompting to verbally describe momentary bodily sensations (e.g. muscle tensions while stretching or breathing).

Case 1: Active Participation in the APM Programme [34, 37]
In Guatemala, the history of racism and discrimination, suffered particularly by the Mayan population, as, for example, the 36 years of civil war including systematic ethnic massacres, persists still today in a more subtle form. As in many other conflicts, in Guatemala, misuse of power, oppression, violence, discrimination and social-political influences target to control the people, to maintain or obtain more power (over people, natural resources, economy, etc.) and to destroy educational and sociocultural structures, families and lives. In this complex situation, one of the most affected groups of population in Guatemala is the women, especially Mayan women in rural areas.

The *psychosocial intervention through movement, games and sport for women* (APM) focused, among other health-related aspects [37], on mutual support in group setting, active learning processes and coping skills of women survivors of violence [34]. In the analysis of the processes of the APM intervention, the active and participative character of the programme became manifest, making it being perceived different from other interventions: 'Sometimes they invite us to a workshop and this is somehow boring and we nearly fall asleep. But this workshop is well, quite active. We have a lot of fun and forget our problems'. Having an experience in a game or modified sport was combined with verbal reflection about that experience and possible learning. For example, a participant explained: 'For me, the course seemed to be very dynamic, very enjoyable, where women—even without knowing how to read, without knowing how to write—talked, participated and commented'; 'This was like a school for me, because it was through games [...]; because each game had its reason to be and after finishing a game, the dynamic, there was always a reflection'.

The participating women had the opportunity to express feelings and to face problems directly or indirectly, personalised or anonymously, in a protected and supportive environment. For example, in one session, we started with storytelling, where the women related together an imaginary story about a woman who was at home when the husband came home drunk. Afterwards they played the story and in the process they complemented and extended the story, as they analysed more in detail the situation and searched for solutions while acting. One participant described it in the following way: 'We did a dramatization (...) and then the women felt themselves supported, those who were victims, and then among them, they themselves gave conclusions. Among themselves, they found out how to denounce this mistreatment and not to keep quiet (...). In this way the woman saw herself in her process'. Similar results were obtained by other participatory group activities, such as role playing, games and modified sport activities. The results of these techniques showed how realistic situations were imitated, inducing 'real' feelings and experiences in the 'here and now'. The search for alternatives and solutions in these situations was lived in an active way and in a participative process. This process was not limited to a theoretical reflection about the problem and its possible solutions, but, rather, the women experienced it themselves by directly participating in these activities [37].

13.11 A Psychosocial Approach

13.11.1 Psychosocial Perspective

A psychosocial perspective in sport and physical activity emphasises psychological and social factors rather than biological factors. A psychosocial perspective recognises that the causes and consequences of illness as well as the recovery processes are influenced by psychosocial aspects. For example, important risk factors for myocardial infarct are psychosocial in nature (e.g. stress, depression); at the same time, in the aftermath of a myocardial infarct, depression and anxiety are frequently diagnosed. Thus, a psychosocial perspective is based upon a holistic concept of health.

In psychosocial interventions, the participants are holistically looked at with their life history, their sociocultural background, their social environment (family, friends, community) and the mutual influence on all factors that have played a role in the traumatisation process [122]. For example, survivors of war and torture often had to experience an extreme lack of power and a strong dependence on the perpetrators; in addition, very close persons, e.g. their own parents, were helpless in these situations as well [122].

Therefore, a psychosocial intervention aims to support the individual, family and communities in their endeavours, empowering them to cope with the stressors and to care for one and each other. In doing so, individual and community resources augment, which encourages recovery and strengthen their abilities to deal with future challenges as well. Thus, psychosocial support aims to strengthen resilience within individuals, families, groups and communities. Thereby, psychosocial support can be both preventive (i.e. increasing mental health as protector for illness) and curative (i.e. supporting individuals or groups to deal with existing psychosocial problems and mental disorders).

Case 2: Observations in Southern Sudan [46]
In August 2004, in Southern Sudan, where most people had experienced violence or/and were forced to use it during the long conflict, we observed the following on several occasions in sports being played: Militant authoritarian conducts were shown by players, as well as dictation of individually self-made rules and harsh games. Very little interaction took place between team players: In volleyball they were playing directly over the net like tennis; in football and in basketball, single players were trying to beat all others on his/her own; all were running behind the ball; there was little cooperation between players; everybody was on his/her own. We had the impression that there was also little sense of confidence and trust between them; everybody was looking 'only' after himself/herself. Without doubt, in sport and recreation you could observe personal and social behaviours; these behaviours might have been learnt during the conflict as strategies to survive and to protect oneself or as a reaction to violence they have suffered. Unfortunately, there were a very limited number of well-prepared coaches, educators and leaders available, making it difficult to use sport and recreation for personal and social development. However, the sport field would be a crucial place to provide psychosocial support.

13.11.2 Resource Orientation and Connecting Efforts

A psychosocial perspective is based upon a resource orientation and empowerment. Resource orientation refers in trauma therapy particularly to stabilisation, which is fundamental throughout the trauma therapy, e.g. for coping with trauma exposure. Promoting and activating resources support the participants in their potential for self-healing and dealing with (trauma-related) stressors [122]. Resource orientation implies being sensitive about trauma and symptoms, though not to primarily focus on them. Resource orientation aims to shift the focus on strengths instead of weakness and to empower and strengthen capacities and skills. Therefore, from such a perspective, sport and physical activity departs from what participants can do and focuses primarily on the prevailing skills and competences and aims to improve them.

A psychosocial perspective is based upon a holistic concept of health. There exist different understandings and sociocultural notions of what health means in practical terms for each person; however, it is widely accepted (at least in theory) that health includes the dimensions of physical, mental and social health. Sport and physical activity may increase resources in all three dimensions. A holistic concept of sport and physical activity encompasses *physical exercising* (physical dimension), *experiencing* (psychosocial dimension) and *learning* (educational dimension) processes, which may work at the same time. For example, while playing basketball, one is exercising the body, learns or improves skills and experiences emotions (e.g. fun, frustration) or social interaction (e.g. support from the team). Thus, we should make a polyvalent use of one and the same activity (cf. [113]), stimulating psychosocial processes and health effects and applying concrete strategies to achieve the desired health effects (see examples in Sect. 13.13).

Despite the potential benefits and complementary use of different approaches, sport and physical activity offers are limited in attending the current needs of the participants and thus should be combined or connected with other support activities. One option would be connecting the participant to other offers, i.e. providing information about and referral to support offers (e.g. individual counselling, therapy offers, etc.) from other stakeholders (e.g. health centres), and thus working in an interconnected support network and not be standing isolated from other support initiatives. Another option would be to combine activities, e.g. providing counselling, examinations or health education on the spot (e.g. in the sport facility) and working alongside or side by side or integrated in the same activities. Combining offers aims to work together more intensively achieving a more holistic and integrated support and benefitting from the strengths of each support. For example, sport and physical activity can sometimes reach where speaking cannot reach, e.g. due to language barriers; difficulties in interpersonal communication, motivational or sociocultural barriers; or because the person does not want to speak or is not used to speaking about certain sensations or experiences. Sport and physical activity may reach and engage people who do not go to doctors or do not participate in psychotherapy programmes. They can be good mediators and a catalyst for other interventions. The sport field can be a platform for other support activities, including health education and health care.

13.11.3 Cultural-Sensitivity and Intercultural Encounter

Sociocultural norms and practices influence on the practice of sport and physical activity and differ among CALD population groups. Besides the many similarities, values, norms and practices differ among cultures, within the individual cultures and from generation to generation [123]. For example, it is common in some cultures not to talk about something happening within the family and to conceal certain emotions and experiences. This may happen to protect themselves and the family from exclusion and loss of honour. Furthermore, also symptoms and related behaviour patterns can vary from culture to culture [123]; the same holds true for the motives, barriers and lived experiences in sport and physical activity. For example, the influence of religious beliefs and faith on participation in sport and physical activity were perceived differently, either supportive or prohibitive or non-influential [15]. Some requirements in sports (e.g. uniform) are considered inappropriate in regard to different sociocultural norms and practices [15]. In general, men do more physical activity in leisure time than women. Women seem to face more barriers for participation in sport, including contradictions between the perceived value of sport practice and sociocultural norms and practices [15]. Sport is often dominated by young men and thus can be exclusive. Often, initiatives for promoting gender equality aim to provide access for women to the often men-dominated sports or to provide exclusive sport and physical activity offers for girls and women, aiming empowerment [124]. However, we should not only aim to empower and include girls and women but also to address the relational element of gender, e.g. changing the gender relationships and gendered experiences within the sporting context [124].

Thus, gender relationships and different sociocultural norms and practices have to be considered in designing sport and physical activity for psychosocial support. For example, taking care of children and family members can inhibit physical activity for women [15] and requires timing the activities according to their possibilities (e.g. when children are in school) or offering child care at the same time. In some settings, gender-separated spaces may be required [24, 42] and may be valued more adequate by the participants (see also Sect. 13.12.1). Thus, a culture-sensitive approach involves also an adaptation of the setting to diverse cultural and religious norms and practices.

Working with refugees requires openness for other sociocultural reference systems. Aspects such as perceiving, feeling, appraising, thinking, expressing, etc. are culture-marked. Sociocultural differences in perceptions and interpretations can lead to misunderstandings. An awareness and critical reflection of one's own culture (i.e. decentring processes) and of one's own perceptions about *other* cultures is an important prerequisite for a productive intercultural encounter and should be stimulated in the group as well [8, 123]. In addition to mutual appreciation and respect, identification with the *other(s)* should be promoted through focusing on commonalities, shared values, norms and practices. For example, traditional games could be presented by the participants and similarities among the games and inherent values discussed [8]. On the basis of a certain degree of identification with the *other(s)*, enrichment through the differences and sociocultural diversity should be facilitated. Therefore, a certain degree of openness and curiosity is needed, e.g. by showing sincere interest in the culture of the person concerned. Finally, knowledge about the *othe(r)s* is important as well and learning from each other should be stimulated [8, 125].

Feelings of strangeness commonly occur in culturally diverse groups and should be acknowledged and dealt with [125], e.g. by speaking about them individually or in a positive group environment, in order to prevent conflicts. This may include also clarifying misunderstandings, encouraging to ask questions and to dialogue. Paying attention to non-verbal communication, bodily contact, interpersonal distance and sensitive body zones, which may differ among culture and personal background, is particularly important for sport and physical activity programmes (cf. [42]).

Particularly if sport and physical activity is provided by economically developed CALD countries (such as EU countries, United States, or Australia) in refugee camps in developing countries, it is important that the planning and implementation of sport and physical activity are based on participants' local circumstances, culture and thinking, led by the needs, interests and goals of the target population, including shared decision-making, and enriched by mutual learning and respectful interaction of all stakeholders and participants. An understanding of the practices and sociocultural values of sport, games and physical activity in the local context is needed before planning interventions. The influence of modern sports as well as the setting of the promotion of traditional games and sports (e.g. their promotion outside of their sociocultural setting) should be critically reflected in each context. Harris [23], who implemented dance and movement therapy with Sudanese refugees in United States of America and with youth in Sierra Leone, highlighted the importance of cultural relevance: 'Dance Movement Therapy (DMT) interventions, if designed to promote cultural relevance and community ownership, may enhance healing among African adolescent survivors of war and organised violence'. Schaeffer [119] reached the same conclusion as Harris with regard to the importance of adapting dance and movement therapy to sociocultural context of the refugees, in this case, at a psychosocial centre in Düsseldorf (Germany).

Case 3: Cultural Activities in Southern Sudan [46]
In a conflict-torn, rural village of Southern Sudan, with many internal displaced people, Ley and Barrio [46] conducted interviews and observation at the premises of the Salesians of Don Bosco, concluding that traditional and cultural activities, especially dance, games and music, were used, preserving and promoting cultural identities of the different ethnic groups living in the village. Knowledge was exchanged and friendships were promoted among the diverse cultural groups. Using their cultural activities helped the Salesians' coaches to come close to the youth and to start working together from what they like.

13.12 A Trauma-Sensitive Approach

13.12.1 Sense of Safety and Safe Space

Providing a sense of safety and a protected safe space is paramount for psychosocial support through sport and physical activity. The sense of safety was not only shattered in the conflict area before migration but also during forced migration and asylum seeking in a host country or while staying in a refugee camp. Refugees often have to expect a deportation for a long time and live in constant uncertainty and anxiety [122]. Providing a sense of safety and a protected space allows the participants to experience one's own and others' perceptions and behaviour, to reassess sensations and to experiment alternative experiences and effects of behaviour. Therefore, the space for sport and physical activity should be safe with regard to physical and psychosocial hazards.

The construction and adaptation of the space should consider diverse cultural and religious norms and practices. Taking into mind sociocultural norms and practices as well as trauma-related and gender-discriminatory experiences (e.g. gender-based violence, maltreatment, oppression, sexual abuse), gender-separated spaces may provide in some settings a better option and may be valued more safe and trustworthy by the participants, allowing a higher degree of participation, possibility to move more liberally (i.e. with less restrictions/restraints from social norms and practices) and to express oneself more openly. Accordingly, it has also to be questioned if the space should be closed and protected from observers or not necessarily. The *Moving Together* handbook gives some useful recommendations for providing a safe space for children [42].

The facilities should be appropriate, for example, closed rooms without a way out should be avoided. There should always be an exit option and the possibility for (temporal) withdrawal from the activity. Environmental risks and dangers should be minimised and injuries should be prevented. Over- and underload, which can lead to injury, fear, frustration, demotivation or dropout, should be avoided. Accordingly, the physical and psychological resilience must always be taken into account in the planning and implementation; activities have to be adapted accordingly.

Providing a clear framework and a stable structure seems beneficial for perceiving safety and control. Using recurrently rituals and a uniform progression of the sessions provides a known structure. Transparency about what is proposed and why helps to avoid surprises and mistrust. For example, at the beginning of the session, one can provide a preview of the planned activities and explain what participants can expect from the session. At the end of the session, a retrospective of the lived experiences and happenings can be stimulated and feedback and time for reflection be provided. Providing accurate information from the beginning (with support by interpreters if required) and clearly agreed rules seem crucial for a sense of safety and control as well.

A sense of control and self-determination is to be emphasised against the experiences of external determination and being exposed, e.g. to feelings of helplessness and impotence. Self-determination is promoted by augmenting a sense of autonomy, competence and relatedness [126]. Furthermore, sport and physical activity can be used to facilitate experiences of control. Experiencing control as well as perceiving own competences and skills, e.g. in/through mastery experiences, may provide an improvement in self-efficacy (see Sect. 13.13.5) and improves the sense of safety.

Independently if the coaches or leaders are members of the host country or refugees, they should be competent in the sports and physical activities, in observing needs and dynamics and adapting accordingly the activities. They also have to be competent in issues related to the background and current situation of the participating refugees and to be culture sensitive and knowledgeable in trauma-related issues, detecting possible triggers for distress and in acute crises interventions. According to a person-centred communication, competences related to acceptance, basic appreciation, empathy and congruence are required in order to provide a supportive and trusting relationship and positive climate for interaction. Traumatic experiences often lead to loss of confidence in themselves and in other people [122]. Therefore, the task of psychosocial support should be to restore this confidence successively through an adequate setting and relationship, which builds on verbal and non-verbal messages. The probability of a successful outcome in effective psychosocial intervention is increased by a trusting relationship. However, we should note transparently that the relationship (with a therapist or coach/facilitator/leader) is often limited in duration and (from therapist and coach) independent relationships need to be promoted (e.g. through strengthen social capital).

13.12.2 Potential Stress and Trauma Triggers in Sport and Physical Activity

Stress-inducing aspects should be appraised for each person and avoided as far as possible. Stress-inducing aspects could be, for example, references to military and drills, cellar rooms, materials or locations that may remind to a traumatic event (e.g. ropes, water, forest, certain music), noise, suddenly disturbing unauthorised persons (entering and endangering the safe space), stress-inducing competition in sport, feelings of too little control over the situation (e.g. the need to close the eyes during a relaxation exercise) and lack of information (e.g. what happens, what is expected, is there an alternative option or a way to opt-out?). Giving clear information and the highest possible level of subjective control seems paramount to prevent and mitigate stress-triggering factors. Uncertainty generates stress and helplessness; perceived control over the situation, possibilities for action and own choices as well as individual available knowledge (information) counteract this, by generating a sense of safety. Individual conversations with the participants may help, in addition to a close observation, to avoid the activation of potential triggers. Adequate communication, control of group dynamics and professional planning and implementation of the activities minimise the likelihood that such events will occur. The sport and physical activity should be adapted and modified according to potential trauma triggers, for example, to provide the option to perform relaxation procedures with the eyes open, to keep the outgoing paths from the specific location open, to make body contact and distance between bodies cautious and to allow temporal or complete withdrawal at any time.

Despite professionally planned and implemented sport and physical activity sessions, unexpected and unpredictable triggers of traumatic experiences can also occur. Also the interoceptive exposure to bodily sensations may trigger negative or fear-induced reactions (see Sect. 13.13.1). The presence of a trauma expert could ensure the mitigation and coping of stress and possible crises intervention; further referral to additional, free support is to be provided. Early detection and interception of crises as well as the prevention and transformation of stressors and conflicts have priority. Corresponding prevention and emergency plans should be established upfront.

13.12.3 The Trauma-Sensitive Coach, Leader or Facilitator

There is crucial agreement among researchers and practitioners that the coaches, leaders or facilitators and their relationship with the participants determine to a high degree the success of the intervention (e.g. [28, 38, 46, 59–61]). For example, Ley et al. [24] described practical strategies and skills of coaches, facilitators and leaders for facilitating sport and exercise with refugees, war and torture survivors. Similarly, Bergholz et al. [59] provided thoughtful insights on trauma-informed coaching in sport-based interventions, giving concrete examples of coaching techniques and day-to-day programme practices. The authors also gave some important recommendations for coaches in performance-focused programmes and competition, e.g. to primarily focus on progress, to coach the players on the bench and rather not the current players in the game (rather let them play), to take care in moments of substitutions of players and reframe players' possible negative assumptions about substitution, to design an individual competition schedule and to seize on situations that merit reframing or an informal encounter [59]. The authors emphasised that the sport-based programme must be will-designed by the coach, as 'the competitive sport experience could actually create a kind of stress and pressure that might trigger players and potentially exacerbate the existing trauma' [59].

The coaches need to be competent in sport and physical activity as well as in psychosocial and trauma-related aspects and preferably work in pairs in order to be able to observe and react to the momentary experiences of each participant. The coach should be aware of own limitations and work in the frame of his/her own capacities. If a (psycho)therapeutic approach is taken and exposure to trauma is aimed, a well-experienced *trauma* expert should (co-)facilitate or take part in the sport and physical activity programme and offer additional counselling and support.

Besides basic competences—including sport- and physical activity-related knowledge and experiences (e.g. training principles), planning and implementing skills, competences in observing and adapting the contents to the needs and dynamics, communication skills and competences in facilitating meaningful experiences, group processes and knowledge transfer—a *trauma-sensitive* coach should have additional specific competences, including the knowledge, skills and experiences [24, 59]:

- To provide a safe space, to stimulate a sense of safety and to continuously monitor possible risks (e.g. providing a stable structure, clear and shared rules and behaviour codes; see Sect. 13.12.1) as well as to identify possible stressors or trauma triggers (e.g. managing possible exposure to negative bodily experiences; see previous section).

- To observe and identify behaviour that may be related to trauma, e.g. stress reactions, difficulties in affect regulation, sudden disengagement, difficulties in attention, avoidance behaviour, difficulties in the interaction with the other participants, etc., and to react accordingly, e.g. to adapt the activities or change the setting; to provide calmness; to reconstruct a sense of safety; to prevent or transform a potential conflict; to direct attentional focus, e.g. on resources; and to provide individual counselling and/or referral to other support offers.
- To identify, promote and activate resources, skills and strengths of each participant, including to facilitate (self-)awareness processes, e.g. perception of self and collective efficacy (i.e. belief in own competences or group abilities).
- To facilitate experiences which are subjectively meaningful for the participant and accord with the psychosocial needs, health, motives and goals of each participants and the group, including positive affective experiences and mastery experiences.
- To observe and optimise the challenges of the activities, avoiding underload (e.g. causing boredom, cognitive distraction from the task) as well as overload (e.g. causing anxiety, frustration), and to adequately regulate psychophysiological arousal levels throughout a session (phases of high activation as well as of recovery and relaxation).
- To motivate and actively engage the participants, without forcing, e.g. through coach-player power relations; this includes providing the opportunity to withdraw (temporally or completely) without negative consequences and the choice to opt-out and to opt-in at any time.
- To direct purposefully participants' attentional focus in one or another direction (e.g. on body awareness or task performance), to provide moments for introspection (e.g. to pause and get aware of bodily sensations) and to stimulate individual and collective reflection on perceptions, experiences, behaviours or happenings (e.g. verbal reflection in pairs after an exercise, a break for group discussion to reflect on a certain happening, naming or drawing momentary emotions or using bodily expression of emotions).
- To regulate the degree of social and bodily interaction according to the individual needs and sociocultural norms and practices and to foster the inclusion of each participant according to the individual skills and momentary health.
- To construct trustworthy and meaningful relationships that are transparent about reliability and stability over time.
- To adequately communicate with the participants, based on empathy, acceptance and congruency. Bergholz et al. recommended a CLEAR communication: 'Calming voice and tone; Listen deeply; Explain HOW and WHY you are doing what you're doing; Ask engaging questions; Reduce outside "noise"' [59].

13.13 Processes and Effects

In the following, we discuss potential processes and effects of a polyvalent use of sport and physical activity. We first present possible effects of directing attentional focus on bodily sensations (exposure) or away from bodily sensations (distraction).

Second, we discuss processes relating to experiencing positive affective states, mastery experiences and flow experiences as well as group processes. Finally, we highlight the importance of an active participation and motivation for adherence to sport and physical activity practices.

13.13.1 Exposure to Bodily Sensations and Body Awareness

The bodies of refugees from conflict regions may be affected in multiple ways. On the one hand, the bodies may have been direct objects of physical violence. On the other hand, psychological stress or trauma may have *somatised* in the body, resulting, for example, in recurring somatic complaints that remain without a physical explanation (e.g. trauma-related pain sensations). Chronic muscle contraction, back and neck hardening, chronic pain and unnatural body postures are frequent symptoms as well. Thus, the body remembers physical and psychological wounds. Traumatic experiences exert an influence on the neurobiological level and are linked with permanent neuronal and hormonal changes. As a consequence, hyperarousal and hyper-reactivity are prevalent. Healthy embodiment and body awareness, the possibility of experiencing security and pleasure in the body and the capacity to feel grounded and centred may be impaired [88, 89, 127, 128].

Thus, working with and through the body is important [128]. The body is used in psychotherapy as access point for trauma exposure; however, the body can also be used for stabilisation and resource activation. For example, yoga provides processes of body awareness and mindfulness, which has shown to be beneficial for dealing with somatic arousals and for increasing attention, emotional awareness and affect tolerance [53]. Yoga may be supportive in restoring the inner balance and the interplay of muscles, nerves and organs, e.g. through the practice of body postures, introspection and the control of breathing [54, 129]. However, body awareness and mindfulness can also be facilitated through many other physical activities.

Case 4: Body Awareness and Mindfulness in the *Movi Kune* Programme [27]
In the sport and exercise programme *Movi Kune—moving together* with war and torture survivors, various participants achieved to observe momentary inner experiences and to describe them; at the same time, an increased acting with awareness was observable in many participants [27]. These findings point towards processes of increased body awareness and mindfulness. However, several factors were noted that constrained body awareness and mindfulness processes, e.g. attentional focus was not maintained, or certain preconditions were not met, e.g. a sense of safety and confidence and readiness for exposure to bodily sensations. Some participants seemed to avoid any exposure to somatic sensation, particularly in the men group, performing the exercises without taking care about their body or without describing bodily sensations when asked. This avoidance behaviour may aim to protect the *traumatised* body; however, sociocultural norms and practices (i.e. speaking about sensations) may have influenced as well in the disposition to body awareness [27].

In sport and physical activity, an interoceptive exposure to bodily sensations seems implicit [130]. It seems hardly avoidable to be exposed to bodily sensations in sport and physical activity. Thus, we have to be aware of these processes, as exposure to possible negative sensations (e.g. pain sensations) may occur and may lead to stress reactions, fear and feelings of insecurity or provoke avoidance behaviour and dropout [27]. Negative sensations may also restrain task performance and mastery experiences [25]. However, directing attentional focus on somatic sensations in a safe space may provide positive bodily experiences as well, counteracting the negative ones, and may provide the opportunity to reassess (habituated) negative associations, e.g. to experience that fast heartbeat is not necessarily related to distress or a traumatic event (as a psychophysiological stress reaction) [27]. Thus, somatic experiences during sport and physical activity may demonstrate the non-threatening nature of bodily sensations. In that way, exercise has shown to reduce anxiety sensitivity [131].

The attentional focus can be verbally directed on somatic sensations, by asking the participant to listen to the body during physical activity, e.g. perceiving the heartbeat, breathing or muscle efforts, or compare perceptions in different moments, e.g. before and after running. However, attentional focus is also influenced interoceptively, e.g. by pain sensations. Exercises for body awareness should be provided with sufficient time for introspection and—if possible—with verbalisation processes.

Besides processes relating to exposure to somatic sensations, body awareness and mindfulness, we should not forget to stimulate positive bodily experiences, which means feeling (again) pleasure in the body and experiencing the body as a resource. This may help to strengthen a healthy relationship with the body and improve the body-mind unity [27, 57].

Case 5: Exposure to Somatic Experiences in the Sport and Exercise Programme *Movi Kune—Moving Together* with War and Torture Survivors [27]

In the physical exercises, the participants were exposed to perceive somatic sensations, both positive and negative ones. Various participants described negative sensations, e.g. pain sensations, tensions or perception of own physical limitations. These negative sensations constrained in many cases their task performance; frequently the observers noted reactions like suddenly stopping the exercise, negative emotional expressions or stress reactions. Data analysis suggested that in some cases the bodily sensations, e.g. fast heartbeats or pain sensation, reminded the participants of past (traumatic) experiences and triggered distress. However, the exposure to existing negative sensations also provided a therapeutic opportunity as the exposure took place in a safe space and the participating *trauma* experts took care about them. This provided the participants the opportunity to get more aware about (negative) sensations and then to reassess the sensations while experiencing positive bodily sensations and learning alternative ways to deal with them. Many participants improved body and self- awareness and expressed to have learnt more about bodily processes and effects as well as about how to use exercise for coping with pain and stress or for emotional regulation. Various participants reported a change from the beginning to the end of the programme: of their negative perceptions of their body and self, e.g. through perceiving their own competences and coping skills, or of their initial negative association between exercising and pain, which have contributed to deal better with pain sensations.

13.13.2 Distraction from Problems or Trauma-Related Thoughts: A Respite

Instead of directing the attentional focus on bodily sensations, stimulating exposure, as discussed in the previous section, we can also direct the attentional focus away from bodily sensations, stimulating a distraction effect [25]. Sport and physical activity may provide distraction from problems, recurrent negative thoughts, intrusive memories from the past or (*trauma*-related) pain sensations [25, 26]. This distraction effects may lead to a reduction in the personal burden and acute stress level [113, 132, 133]. For example, Caddick et al. [134] concluded from their qualitative study with combat veterans that surfing can induce a respite from trauma symptoms. Refugees may benefit from a distraction effect of sport and physical activity regarding post-migratory stressors, e.g. feelings of insecurity, worries about the situation in the home country and people they had to leave behind or fears of deportation or intrusive memories from the past. The distraction from these thoughts also may allow them to be more in the present ‘here and now’.

Distraction from negative or stressful thoughts or sensations may be achieved best through activities they enjoy and that require certain degree of attention and activation. In our studies [25, 26], the attentional focus away from bodily sensations was achieved through attractive, active activities, particularly, dancing, sports and games, which required full attention for task performance. Similar to flow experiences (see below), distraction may rely on an adequate challenge, i.e. being the demands of sport and physical activity in balance with the perceived skills, avoiding over- and underload [25, 26].

13.13.3 Experiencing Joy and Positive Affective States

Experiencing joy and pleasure may have an energising and restorative effect and influences positively motivation and adherence to sport and physical activity [25, 58]. Joy can be considered the antithesis of PTSD and depression. It is more probable to experience positive affective states when the task challenge is optimal, i.e. when the demands of the tasks are adequate to the skills of the persons, and mastery experiences are achieved [25, 26].

Among the therapies and psychosocial interventions, sport and physical activity may seem particularly suited to provide experiences of joy. This seems to be particularly true, if the sport and physical activity are oriented on the needs and motives of the participants, i.e. when the subjective incentives of the sport and physical activity fit the motives of the person (cf. [135]). Thus, from this perspective, it is more convenient to do activities the person wants and enjoys to do, i.e. the activities subjectively fit to the person's needs and interest (perceived benefit). Furthermore, overload (frustration, fear, worries) and underload (boredom) should be avoided as well as negative bodily sensations as they may trigger negative affective states (see also Sects. 13.12 and 13.13.1).

13.13.4 Group Experiences

Sport and physical activity in groups may help to improve a sense of belonging, tackling feelings of loneliness and isolation. Group environment also can contribute to the construction of confidence, particularly if positive feedback or support comes from other participants (cf. [102, 134]). Being physically active in a group may also provide joy:

> By bringing the [combat] veterans together and immersing them in a common activity, surfing helped to overcome social isolation and temporarily relieved the problems associated with PTSD. Indeed, (…) positive social interactions (e.g., encouragement, laughter, support) occurring between veterans while in the water helped to create a feeling of respite. Furthermore, the participants spoke of a sense of security they felt around other veterans. They were able to let their guard down around people who understood and accepted them, which enabled them to relax and enjoy the activity of surfing. [134]

Social interaction, trust in others and the building of relationships, however, may be affected by the often extreme pre-, peri- and post-migratory experiences, e.g. the sudden separation from or loss of important attachment persons (e.g. close friends or family members) and social networks, the lack of stable and reliable relationships as well as the experiences of human rights violations, torture and violence [136]. Furthermore:

> many trauma survivors struggle with challenges to sense of meaning and justice in the face of shattered assumptions about prevailing justice in the world due to the way in which they were either exposed to traumatic events (e.g., being sent to a war they perceive as senseless, being an innocent victim) or treated during the post-traumatic aftermath (e.g., via discriminatory distribution of resources). [136]

These experiences may influence upon the social and bodily interaction in sport and physical activity, dependently how far a sense of safety and control may be provided. Thus, care should be taken that the practice of sport and physical activity is taking place in a positive, safe and trustworthy group environment, providing the opportunity to get (slowly) out of isolation and to socialise with others in the degree each one wants to do or can do. In that regard, Levine and Land expressed:

> With many victims of trauma, building a healthy physical relationship, both with oneself and with others, is difficult. The use of movement in a group setting creates opportunities for connections with others, which is an inherent part of the therapeutic process. (…) Togetherness in a healthy and safe shared space is often the impetus for relationship building. [57]

Case 6: The Role of Group Experiences in a Single Case Study [25]
Rashid is a refugee from a South Asian country, whose parents were murdered in front of him and who then escaped and finally got to Austria. At this moment, he was still under-aged. He was diagnosed with a complex PTSD and recurrent depression.

According to his therapist, Rashid could not establish any solid relationship or tangible friendship in the sport and exercise group *Movi Kune*, and also the colleagues with whom he was later going to the fitness club 'were not directly friends; it was more like *being in the same boat*'. Yet, Rashid seemed to enjoy the regular contact with the other participants. He even emphasised the sharing of positive emotions as something he most liked about the programme: 'Laughing, laughing together with others cheerfully'. His therapist highlighted 'his joy when the people came to meet each other; this was something really astonishing'.

Rashid was for a long time introverted and would not look at anybody. The interaction within the group was determined by doing exercise and sport together, but no further communication took place. In addition, communication with some participants was hindered by them speaking different languages. Yet, the simple fact that the practice of exercise and sport was taking place in a group environment and not individually was much valued by Rashid; being asked what was special about the programme, we answered: 'The group, being together, that was good (…). Here you are accepted, you are together. If you are strong or weak, that doesn't matter'. Furthermore, he also got positive feedback from others on several occasions, which helped his sense of belonging, thereby tackling feelings of loneliness and isolation and establishing confidence. This may seem a small step, but its meaningfulness is becoming more visible, when we consider that Rashid had missed out on stable relationships since his childhood and had an attachment disorder, PTSD and recurrent depression.

A good planning and adaptation of the activities to the social needs of the participants and the group dynamics are paramount in order to stimulate participation of all participants and prevent exclusion of a participant. Each participant should be able to participate with his/her skills and capacities and to find a role in the group. A selection of activities that stresses cooperation above competition may be beneficial if competition is taking too serious and provides conflicts (cf. [59]). Cooperative games and modified sports may allow social interaction without forcing to speak about oneself.

Furthermore, the interventions should be long-lasting or connected to long-lasting opportunities for sport and exercise, e.g. in sport clubs, fitness centres, etc. that may provide sustainable opportunities for further social interaction and inclusion, and thus the construction of stable relationships.

13.13.5 Mastery Experiences and Self-Efficacy Beliefs

The experiences of mastery and accomplishments may impact on the perception of self-efficacy, as one becomes more aware of own competences and skills. Experiences of mastery and accomplishments are crucial sources of self-efficacy beliefs, which may be endorsed by feedback, encouragement and positive affective experiences as well [137]. Thereby, it is important that the mastery experiences and accomplishments are valued as subjective meaningful and attributed to the competences of oneself and not to external factors, such as luck. Thus, the mastery experience and accomplishments should be perceived as the consequence of own actions, behaviour or competences. Feedback and encouragement from coaches, facilitators or leaders as well as from other participants may endorse the development of self-efficacy beliefs [137]. An adequate balance between the demands of the physical activity tasks and the perceived skills, i.e. an individual optimal challenge, is momentous for facilitating subjective meaningful mastery experiences and successful task performance.

A strong self-efficacy belief is an important health outcome (e.g. improved self-concept and well-being) as well as a motivating force (e.g. perceiving that one can do it, one can achieve the goals) increasing the possibility to maintain physical activity practices on long term [65, 137]. Mastery attempts also may serve to increase enjoyment in the activity as well as activation, which may result in perseverance in performing exercise, in volition to resist fatigue and thus finally in better performance [137, 138].

13.13.6 Flow Experiences

The concept of flow was shaped predominately by Csikszentmihalyi, who described flow as a 'state in which people are so involved in an activity that nothing else seems to matter; the experience itself is so enjoyable that people will do it even at great cost, for the sheer sake of doing it' [139]. Flow is an autotelic experience, an intrinsically rewarding experience and, thus, a powerful motivating force. A flow experience is often described with the following elements: balance between demands and skills (challenge), clear goals and direct feedback, sense of control, enhanced concentration, merging of action and awareness, a distorted sense of time and a loss of self-consciousness [139]. Flow experiences are also associated to positive affective states during or after—as a result of—successful task performance [139].

Flow experiences may provide health benefits through directing the person's attentional focus away from problems and worries about illness, reducing negative affective states and thoughts, contributing to positive sensations and experiences, improving self-concept and subjective control and thus enhancing well-being and quality of life [26, 140, 141]. These benefits may be achieved at least for the duration of the activity, providing a respite and recovery processes [26]. Further benefits of flow experiences are the experiencing of momentary task performance, being more present in the 'here and now' (versus intrusive memories and flashbacks from the past) and the perceived mastering of the challenge [26]. Another benefit is the autotelic character of flow, which may increase motivation for adopting and maintaining physical activity [141].

These potential benefits of flow advocate the provision of adequate tasks and settings that facilitate the occurrence of flow while minimising possible hindering factors. However, entering in a flow state seems not to be as easy. An optimal challenge with an adequate work load and somatic arousal level is required. Furthermore, the sense of safety plays a central role, as it is a precondition for full immersion in the activity, for positive affective states and fluent performance of the movement and thus for a flow experience [26, 142]. The momentary subjective well-being and affective experiencing of the task, events and setting may influence the occurrence of flow [26, 142].

Hindering factors include task- and setting-related triggers of discomfort, fear or worries, stress and flashbacks from the past. Another factor that may hinder the occurrence of flow is a low level of activation and concentration during the task. Depressive moods, anxiety, sleeping problems, fatigue or side effects of medication may inhibit activation and full concentration; hyperarousal may inhibit an optimal arousal level for flow experiences as well [26, 143].

Thus, to facilitate flow experiences in sport and physical activity with refugees, it seems important to foster a feeling of safety and confidence and to be aware of task- and setting-related aspects that could trigger stress or negative affective experiences. Clear information and explanations of the tasks must be provided so that attention is not required at higher cognitive levels—as this would hinder full concentration on the task—and that a sense of safety, control and optimal challenge prevails.

Case 7: Flow Experiences in the *Movi Kune* Programme [26]

In the *Movi Kune* programme, Flow was observed mainly during sports, games, movement improvisations or dancing. These activities seemed very motivating for the participants; activation and pleasure were observed more frequently. In these tasks, the attentional focus was probably more on the overall performance and not on bodily sensations or isolated movement performance. It seemed as in this programme the physical exercise tasks (strength, flexibility or coordination training) could not capture the full attention and concentration of the war and torture survivors, giving them time and space to get distracted from the task and thinking about other things, like pain sensations; thus, these exercises (or the way how these exercises were performed) did not facilitate flow experiences in this group.

Remarkably, the same activity facilitated flow in one and stress reactions in another moment. The current personal situation, perceived environment and present events influenced upon the occurrence of flow during a certain task.

13.13.7 Active Participation and Active Coping

In sport and physical activity people are active, not passive. The participants are not *only* listening or talking about an aspect; they are also experiencing, perceiving and expressing themselves with their own body in motion. They engage actively with and in physical activity; nobody moves and trains their body for them; they bring themselves in motion: physically, emotionally and socially. Thus, the participants can get into action, experience new things, observe changes, search for their own solutions and experiment alternative behaviours.

Being active seems very important for refugees, as they are put in a rather passive role, e.g. during the asylum seeking process. They often express the wish to be active. Being active may stimulate active coping with challenges in daily living; motivation to perform daily activities, e.g. learning the local language; and self-healing processes, e.g. coming out of trauma-related stiffness and isolation [58]. Therefore, it seems beneficial that refugees are engaging actively—and not *only* as participants—in shaping the sessions or the organisation of sport and physical activity. As many refugees have been physically active before migration or before a certain event, they may be experienced as coaches, facilitators or leaders as well. Refugees should be encouraged and empowered to take an active role, to be coaches, facilitators and leaders in sport and physical activity, if they wish to do so.

Case 8: Active Participation: Experiences from the *Kakuma Refugee Camp* [46]
Free time is in abundance in the refugee camp due to a general lack of jobs and recreational possibilities. Therefore, sport and recreational offers aim to facilitate and to share cheerful experiences and to make a meaningful use of the free time. Thus, sport and recreational activities were used together with educational activities and leadership training to bring people together and to teach them to prevent or transform conflicts and to promote peace. However, sport and recreational activities also boosted the motivation in the educational activities and reduced even the dropout rate in the professional training, pointing towards a more generalised activation and motivation. Furthermore, it was hoped that the experiences and capacities gained during these activities would also help the refugees to engage in an active reconstruction of their home countries once they are able to return [46].

13.13.8 Motivation and Participation in Sport and Physical Activity

A truly active and empowered participation of the refugees may also strengthen the senses of autonomy and competence. The senses of autonomy and competence are central elements of the self-determination theory and are crucial for autonomous motivation and self-determined participation in sport and physical activity [58, 126, 138].

This may lead to a certain independency from currently offered programmes as well. Independency is aimed, particularly if the offered programme is limited in duration. The participant should be empowered through gaining knowledge, skills and participation in decision-making and thus be able to maintain autonomously the sport and physical activity practices. An active participation could include planning, shaping and implementing sessions or leading the programme and may also favour identification processes and perceived ownership.

The aspects of empowerment and knowledge transfer are also targeted within the concept of health literacy (see Sect. 13.7). Three main competences should be acquired in order to strengthen one's movement-related health literacy and, as a consequence, increase the chance of self-maintained participation in health-oriented sport and physical activity [108]:

1. Persons with high *control competence* can plan and modify the implementation of physical activity to optimise personal health benefits [108]. Learning processes that stimulate functional and comprehensive knowledge, particularly on health effects, on principles of training and adequate performance and on local physical activity opportunities (e.g. spaces, offers, support), can contribute to the acquisition of control competences.
2. 'Persons with high *movement competence* can adequately meet the direct movement-related requirements of everyday physical activities as well as health sports activities' [108]. Movement competences, including, e.g., psychomotor, exercise and sport skills, physical fitness and body-movement awareness, are fundamental for the practice of health-orientated physical activity as well as for participation in sport groups and thus for inclusion. These competences can be acquired through regular physical training.
3. 'Persons with high physical activity-specific *self-regulation competence* can ensure regularity of physical activity for lasting effects on health and wellbeing' [108]. This competence refers to an autonomous regulation of own motivation and volition to initiate and maintain physical activity. Crucial motivational and volitional correlates are self-efficacy beliefs, attitudes towards physical activity and outcome expectancies, self-determined intentions, action and coping, planning and self-monitoring [144, 145]. Furthermore, the person should also be able to find a (optimal) fit according to one's motive structure and the subjective incentives of the corresponding sport and physical activity, i.e. to find a sport and physical activity that fits to himself/herself [108].

Important motivational and volitional correlates are mapped in process or stage models, such as the Transtheoretical Model, the Health Action Process Approach (HAPA) or the MoVo Process Model, which provide a structured foundation for behaviour change interventions [144, 145]. Behaviour change techniques to promote participation in physical activity are well researched and theory-based as well [16, 146–148]. The behaviour change wheel may be a useful tool to design corresponding physical activity interventions [149].

Self-efficacy belief is one of the strongest correlates of physical activity participation [144]. Sources of self-efficacy beliefs are experiences of mastery and accomplishments, feedback, encouragement and positive affective experiences [137] (see Sect. 13.13.5). Furthermore, autonomous motivation, i.e. intrinsic regulated motivation, is considered crucial for adopting and maintaining sport and physical activity practices [138, 150]. For example, flow experiences are intrinsically rewarding (see above) and thus foster autonomous motivation. Therefore, coaches should consider the individual motives and goals of refugees to practise sport and physical activity and try to foment intrinsic regulated motivation accordingly [138]. Experiencing positive effects of the physical activity influences on the outcome expectancy and thus may stimulate the continued motivation to practise sport and physical activity again and again. Action and coping planning and self-monitoring are important correlates for the volitional phase, i.e. to put into practice the intention and to maintain practising sport and physical activity [144, 145]. Coaches should support the participants in planning actions (e.g. when to exercise where and with whom) and coping with their individual barriers. The latter includes also planning to deal with barriers, both individual, e.g. depressive moods, pain sensations or discomfort, and social-ecological ones, e.g. different sociocultural practices or stress-inducing situations. In that regard, the aspects discussed under the Sect. 13.12, e.g. to provide a safe space, to consider potential triggers of stress and exposure to feared bodily sensations as well as to adopt a culture-sensitive approach, play a crucial role also for maintaining physical activity practices. For example, it seems beneficial that motivation for initiating participation comes through individuals from the same culture as well [16]. Finally, a sense of belonging, social capital and social inclusion may foster a maintained participation in sport and physical activity as well [10, 11, 14, 151].

13.14 What Comes Next: Future research?

As described in the overview of research, we still lack of evidence of the multifaceted health benefits of sport and physical activity, as well as of the responsible factors for change, i.e. the underlying processes and effects. The few studies that have been conducted in the field suggest that we face a quite complex mix of diverse factors and challenges influencing the various psychosocial processes and health effects of sport and physical activity, calling for more research in this area. For example, a more in-depth understanding and comparison among the diverse physical activity intervention approaches may serve to give an insight about which approaches and strategies are most beneficial in which moments and settings and how to interconnect them.

Further studies should also try to target the whole range of refugee with different backgrounds. For example, many of the examples we used in the discussion of key issues originated from our studies with war and torture survivors, i.e. refugees suffering from PTSD; results from these studies may not be generalised to the whole refugee population. There is a particular paucity of knowledge about sport and physical activity with refugees in post-conflict regions and in refugee camps.

Furthermore, we should critically analyse the optimal environment and conditions for sport and physical activity with refugees to maximise the health benefits and minimise risk or negative experiences. It is paramount to analyse (and avoid) negative effects of sport and physical activity, e.g. an injury may be a big burden and an additional stress for refugees from or in (post-)conflict regions.

Future research may focus on the relationship between promoting health and social inclusion in and through sport and physical activity, as well. In this regard, movement-related health literacy may be a motor for connecting health care, empowerment, participation and social inclusion.

Finally, we need to investigate more comprehensively the motives of refugees to practise sport and physical activity and how to stimulate motivation and volition to sport and physical activity in the light of the background and current situation of refugees. This is decisive in order to stimulate and maintain participation and inclusion in sport and finally to achieve the health benefits of regular participation in sport and recommended physical activity levels.

13.15 Summary and Practical Recommendations

In this chapter, we highlighted some key issues for planning and implementing health-oriented sport and physical activity with refugees from or living in (post-) conflict regions. We proposed a psychosocial approach to sport and physical activity, including a resource orientation and a culture-sensitive perspective. We also included a trauma-sensitive approach, responding to the extreme and often traumatic experiences of many refugees from conflict regions. With a trauma-sensitive approach, we do not aim to direct the main focus on trauma but to take trauma-related aspects into consideration in a resource-oriented, psychosocial approach to sport and physical activity with refugees. We discussed critical issues such as the provision of safe space and a sense of safety, potential trigger of stress and the need for well-qualified, trauma-sensitive coaches.

Finally, we highlighted some potential processes and health effects of sport and physical activity from a psychosocial perspective. We can direct the attentional focus in sport and physical activity on different aspects, stimulating different processes. On the one hand, the attentional focus can be directed away from somatic sensations, providing a distraction effect or—under certain conditions—even flow experiences. This distraction from negative thoughts and body sensations may provide positive affective states, mastery experiences and (behavioural) activation. These experiences also may impact positively on the motivation for participation and self-determined maintenance of sport and physical activity. In addition these experiences may also be relating to positive group experiences, a sense of belonging and social inclusion.

On the other hand, the attentional focus may also be directed towards bodily sensations; moreover, an implicit interoceptive exposure to bodily experiences is probable in sport and physical activity. Thus, the participants will be exposed in sport and physical activity to bodily sensations, which include positive and negative ones. Dealing with negative sensations is paramount, particularly if they refer to trauma triggers or feared somatic sensations. Consequences include stress reactions, anxiety or avoidance behaviour and dropout. Therefore a trauma-sensitive approach is crucial. However, in a safe space, exposure to bodily experiences can also be an opportunity to reassess negative associations, experience positive bodily sensations and improve body awareness and mindfulness. This in turn may help to strengthen a healthy relationship with the body and the perception of the body and physical activity as resources. Besides a trauma-sensitive approach, we consider a resource orientation paramount for psychosocial support through sport and physical activity.

Another crucial factor is the active participation of refugees, including various degrees from participation in shaping the activities to leading the initiative. Refugees should be empowered to take an active role, to be coaches, facilitators and leaders in sport and physical activity, e.g. through facilitating participation in training courses to obtain official licences or providing specific training courses, which however should result in job opportunities as well, recognising their important active role they can play.

References

1. Wenzel T, Völkl-Kernstock S, Wittek TU, Baron D. Identifying needs, vulnerabilities, and resources in refugee persons and groups. In: Wenzel T, Drožđek B, editors. An uncertain safety. Cham: Springer International; 2018.
2. Kühnel M, Drožđek B, Wenzel T. Medical aspects of health care: reflections from the field experience in European countries and an overview of the basic health needs. In: Wenzel T, Drožđek B, editors. An uncertain safety. Cham: Springer International; 2018.
3. Henry I, Amara M, Aquilina D. Multiculturalism, interculturalism, assimilation and sports policy in Europe. In: Henry I, Institut of Sport and Leisure Policy, editors. Transnational and comparative research in sport: globalisation, governance and sport policy. Abingdon: Taylor & Francis; 2007.
4. Barrio MR, Ley C. La promoción intercultural a través del deporte en contextos postbélicos. Anduli Rev Cienc Soc. 2012;11:101–16.
5. Amara M, Aquilina D, Argent E, Betzer-Tayar M, Coalter F, Henry I, et al. The roles of sport and education in the social inclusion of asylum seekers and refugees: an evaluation of policy and practice in the UK, European year of education through sport, report to DG Education and Culture, European Commission. Institute of Sport and Leisure Policy Loughborough University, University of Stirling; 2005.
6. Barrio MR, Giess-Stüber P. Review of project evaluations aiming the promotion of interculturalism through sport. Freiburg im Breisgau, Germany: Albert-Ludwigs-Universität Freiburg; 2012. p. 241.
7. Barrio MR, Ley C. Interculturalism through physical activity and sports in cooperation for development. Int J Sport Soc. 2010;1(1):271–83.
8. Barrio MR, Ley C. Potentialities and challenges of an intervention model to promote intercultural processes in post-conflict contexts. In: Gilbert K, Bennett W, editors. Sport, peace and development. Champaign, IL: Common Ground; 2012. p. 163–76.
9. Spracklen K, Long J, Hylton K. Leisure opportunities and new migrant communities: challenging the contribution of sport. Leis Stud. 2015;34(1):114–29.
10. Walseth K. Bridging and bonding social capital in sport—experiences of young women with an immigrant background. Sport Educ Soc. 2008;13(1):1–17.

11. Spaaij R. Refugee youth, belonging and community sport. Leis Stud. 2015;34(3):303–18.
12. Ley C, Barrio MR. Movement, games and sport in psychosocial intervention: a critical discussion of its potential and limitations within cooperation for development. Intervention. 2010;8(2):106–20.
13. Darnell SC. Conflict, education and sport. Responses, cautions and questions. Confl Educ. 2011;1(1):1–7.
14. Janssens J, Verweel P. The significance of sports clubs within multicultural society. On the accumulation of social capital by migrants in culturally "mixed" and "separate" sports clubs. Eur J Sport Soc. 2014;11(1):35–58.
15. O'Driscoll T, Banting LK, Borkoles E, Eime R, Polman R. A systematic literature review of sport and physical activity participation in culturally and linguistically diverse (CALD) migrant populations. J Immigr Minor Health. 2013;16(3):515–30.
16. Caperchione CM, Kolt GS, Mummery WK. Physical activity in culturally and linguistically diverse migrant groups to Western Society. Sports Med. 2009;39(3):167–77.
17. Whitley MA, Coble C, Jewell GS. Evaluation of a sport-based youth development programme for refugees. Leisure/Loisir. 2016;40(2):175–99.
18. Hebebrand J, Anagnostopoulos D, Eliez S, Linse H, Pejovic-Milovancevic M, Klasen H. A first assessment of the needs of young refugees arriving in Europe: what mental health professionals need to know. Eur Child Adolesc Psychiatry. 2016;25(1):1–6.
19. Drožđek B, Silove D. Psychotherapy and psychosocial support in host countries: state-of-the-art and emerging paradigms. In: Wenzel T, Drožđek B, editors. An uncertain safety. Cham: Springer International; 2018.
20. Ha J-P, Lyras A. Sport for refugee youth in a new society: the role of acculturation in sport for development and peace programming. S Afr J Res Sport Phys Educ Recreat. 2013;35(2):121–40.
21. Spaaij R. Beyond the playing field: experiences of sport, social capital, and integration among Somalis in Australia. Ethn Racial Stud. 2012;35(9):1519–38.
22. Whitley MA, Gould D. Psychosocial development in refugee children and youth through the personal–social responsibility model. J Sport Psychol Action. 2011;1(3):118–38.
23. Harris DA. Dance/movement therapy approaches to fostering resilience and recovery among African adolescent torture survivors. Torture. 2007;17(2):134–55.
24. Ley C, Lintl E, Movi Kune Team. 'Movi Kune – gemeinsam bewegen': Bewegungstherapie mit Kriegs- und Folterüberlebenden ('Movi Kune – moving together': movement and exercise therapy with war and torture survivors). Spectrum. 2014;26(2):71–97.
25. Ley C, Barrio MR, Koch A. "In the sport I am here": a qualitative study on therapeutic processes and health effects of sport and exercise. Qual Health Res. 2018;28(3):491–507.
26. Ley C, Krammer J, Lippert D, Barrio MR. Exploring flow in sport and exercise therapy with war and torture survivors. Ment Health and Phys Act. 2017;12:83–93.
27. Ley C, Barrio MR. Centrando la atención en las sensaciones corporales en un programa físico-deportivo terapéutico (directing attentional focus towards somatic sensations in sport and exercise therapy). Rev Psicol Deporte. 2017;26(4):17–21.
28. Kunz V. Sport as a post-disaster psychosocial intervention in Bam, Iran. Sport Soc. 2009;12(9):1147–57.
29. ICSSPE. Sport and physical activity in post-disaster intervention. Berlín: ICSSPE - International Council of Sport Science and Physical Education; 2008.
30. Gschwend A, Selvaraju U. Psycho-social sport programmes to overcome trauma in post-disaster interventions. An overview. Biel/Bienne: Swiss Academy for Development; 2007. 31p.
31. Richards P. Soccer and violence in war-torn Africa: soccer and social rehabilitation in Sierra Leone. In: Armstrong G, Giulianotti R, editors. Entering the field: new perspectives on world football. Oxford: Berg; 1997.
32. Richards J, Foster C. Sport-for-development interventions: whom do they reach and what is their potential for impact on physical and mental health in low-income countries? J Phys Act Health. 2013;10(7):929–31.

33. Barrio MR, Ley C. Methodologies for evaluating the use of sport for development in post-conflict contexts. In: Henry I, Ko L-M, editors. Routledge handbook of sports policy. London: Routledge; 2013. p. 289–302.
34. Ley C, Barrio MR. Active learning and self-supporting processes through sport, games and participatory activities with women who suffered violence. In: Gilbert K, Bennett W, editors. Sport, peace and development. Champaign, IL: Common Ground; 2012. p. 355–66.
35. Munro B. Sport for peace and reconciliation. Young peacemakers in the Kakuma refugee camp and Mathare slums in Kenya; 2012. p. 71–86.
36. Prytherch H, Kraft K. The psychosocial impact of capoeira for refugee children and youth. The University of East London; 2015.
37. Ley C, Barrio MR. Movement and sport therapy with women in Guatemalan context of violence and conflict. Body Mov Dance Psychother. 2011;6(1):145–60.
38. Henley R. Resilience enhancing psychosocial programmes for youth in different cultural contexts: evaluation and research. Prog Dev Stud. 2010;10(4):295–307.
39. Richards J, Foster C, Townsend N, Bauman A. Physical fitness and mental health impact of a sport-for-development intervention in a post-conflict setting: randomised controlled trial nested within an observational study of adolescents in Gulu, Uganda. BMC Public Health. 2014;14:619.
40. Richards JA, Foster C. Evaluating the impact of a sport-for-development intervention on the physical and mental health of young adolescents in Gulu, Uganda - a post-conflict setting within a low-income country; 2012.
41. Ley C, Barrio MR. Evaluation of a psychosocial health programme in the context of violence and conflict. J Health Psychol. 2013;18(10):1371–81.
42. Wiedemann N, Ammann P, Bird M, Engelhardt J, Koenen K, Meier M, et al. Moving together – promoting psychosocial well-being through sport and physical activity. Copenhagen: International Federation of Red Cross and Red Crescent Societies Reference Centre for Psychosocial Support; 2014.
43. Maharmeh Y. Street football at the Jordan refugee camp. J Sci Med Sport. 2013;16:e83.
44. Korsik A, Ivarsson V, Nakitanda OA, Pérez Rosas LR. Implementing sports in refugee camps. Lausanne: AISTS & UNHCR; 2013. 68p.
45. Vossoughi N, Jackson Y, Gusler S, Stone K. Mental health outcomes for youth living in refugee camps: a review. Trauma Violence Abuse. 2016:1524838016673602. https://doi.org/10.1177/1524838016673602.
46. Ley C, Barrio MR. Sport and recreation as educational and diagnostic tools: Don Bosco's vision and the Salesians' mission in Eastern and Southern Africa. In: Gilbert K, Bennett W, editors. Sport, peace and development. Champaign IL: Common Ground; 2012. p. 141–50.
47. Lincoln AK, Lazarevic V, White MT, Ellis BH. The impact of acculturation style and acculturative hassles on the mental health of Somali adolescent refugees. J Immigr Minor Health. 2015;18(4):771–8.
48. Carless D, Douglas K. Sport and physical activity for mental health. Chichester: Wiley; 2010. 181p.
49. Rosenbaum S, Tiedemann A, Sherrington C, Curtis J, Ward PB. Physical activity interventions for people with mental illness: a systematic review and meta-analysis. J Clin Psychiatry. 2014;75(9):964–74.
50. Henley R, Schweitzer I, de Gara F, Vetter S. How psychosocial sport & play programs help youth manage adversity: a review of what we know & what we should research. Int J Psychosoc Rehabil. 2007;12(1):51–8.
51. Drožđek B. Challenges in treatment of posttraumatic stress disorder in refugees: towards integration of evidence-based treatments with contextual and culture-sensitive perspectives. Eur J Psychotraumatol. 2015;6(1):24750.
52. Rosenbaum S, Vancampfort D, Steel Z, Newby J, Ward PB, Stubbs B. Physical activity in the treatment of post-traumatic stress disorder: a systematic review and meta-analysis. Psychiatry Res. 2015;230(2):130–6.
53. Van der Kolk BA, Stone L, West J, Rhodes A, Emerson D, Suvak M, et al. Yoga as an adjunctive treatment for posttraumatic stress disorder: a randomized controlled trial. J Clin Psychiatry. 2014;75(6):e559–65.

54. Emerson D. Trauma-sensitive yoga in therapy: bringing the body into treatment. 1st ed. New York: W. W. Norton; 2015. 196p.
55. Clark CJ, Lewis-Dmello A, Anders D, Parsons A, Nguyen-Feng V, Henn L, et al. Trauma-sensitive yoga as an adjunct mental health treatment in group therapy for survivors of domestic violence: a feasibility study. Complement Ther Clin Pract. 2014;20(3):152–8.
56. Nolan CR. Bending without breaking: a narrative review of trauma-sensitive yoga for women with PTSD. Complement Ther Clin Pract. 2016;24:32–40.
57. Levine B, Land HM. A meta-synthesis of qualitative findings about dance/movement therapy for individuals with trauma. Qual Health Res. 2016;26(3):330–44.
58. Caddick N, Smith B. The impact of sport and physical activity on the well-being of combat veterans: a systematic review. Psychol Sport Exerc. 2014;15(1):9–18.
59. Bergholz L, Stafford E, D'Andrea W. Creating trauma-informed sports programming for traumatized youth: core principles for an adjunctive therapeutic approach. J Infant Child Adolesc Psychother. 2016;15(3):244–53.
60. D'Andrea W, Bergholz L, Fortunato A, Spinazzola J. Play to the whistle: a pilot investigation of a sports-based intervention for traumatized girls in residential treatment. J Fam Violence. 2013;28(7):739–49.
61. Ammann P, Matuska N. Women on the move. Trauma-informed interventions based on sport and play. A toolkit for practitioners. Biel/Bienne: Swiss Academy for Development (SAD); 2014.
62. Diaz A, Motta RW. The effects of an aerobic exercise program on posttraumatic stress disorder symptom severity in adolescents. Int J Emerg Ment Health. 2007;10(1):49–59.
63. Goldshtrom Y, Korman D, Goldshtrom I, Bendavid J. The effect of rhythmic exercises on cognition and behaviour of maltreated children: a pilot study. J Bodyw Mov Ther. 2011;15(3):326–34.
64. Manger TA, Motta RW. The impact of an exercise program on posttraumatic stress disorder, anxiety, and depression. Int J Emerg Ment Health. 2005;7(1):49–57.
65. Motta RW, McWilliams ME, Schwartz JT, Cavera RS. The role of exercise in reducing childhood and adolescent PTSD, anxiety, and depression. J Appl Sch Psychol. 2012;28(3):224–38.
66. Newman CL, Motta RW. The effects of aerobic exercise on childhood PTSD, anxiety, and depression. Int J Emerg Ment Health. 2007;9(2):133–58.
67. Rosenbaum S, Nguyen D, Lenehan T, Tiedemann A, van der Ploeg HP, Sherrington C. Exercise augmentation compared to usual care for post traumatic stress disorder: a randomised controlled trial (The REAP study: Randomised Exercise Augmentation for PTSD). BMC Psychiatry. 2011;11(1):115.
68. Webb NB. Play therapy with children in crisis: individual, group, and family treatment. 3rd ed. New York: Guilford Press; 2007. 513 p.
69. Volmer J. Psychomotorik und Psychotrauma - Körper und Bewegung als therapeutisches Agens in der Arbeit mit körperlich misshandelten und sexuell missbrauchten Kindern. In: Beudels W, Hammer R, Hamsen R, Kuhlenkamp S, Volmer J, editors. Bewegung in der lebensspanne. Lemgo: Verl. Aktionskreis Literatur und Medien; 2008. p. 234–50. (Psychomotorik; vol. 6).
70. Telles S, Singh N, Balkrishna A. Managing mental health disorders resulting from trauma through yoga: a review. Depress Res Treat. 2012:401513. https://doi.org/10.1155/2012/401513.
71. Grodin MA, Piwowarczyk L, Fulker D, Bazazi AR, Saper RB. Treating survivors of torture and refugee trauma: a preliminary case series using Qigong and T'ai Chi. J Altern Complement Med. 2008;14(7):801–6.
72. Carey L. Expressive and creative arts methods for trauma survivors. London: Jessica Kingsley; 2006. 224p.
73. Chapman L, Morabito D, Ladakakos C, Schreier H, Knudson MM. The effectiveness of art therapy interventions in reducing post traumatic stress disorder (PTSD) symptoms in pediatric trauma patients. Art Ther. 2001;18(2):100–4.
74. Gray AEL. Expressive arts therapies: working with survivors of torture. Torture. 2011;21(1): 39–47.
75. Harris DA. The paradox of expressing speechless terror: ritual liminality in the creative arts therapies' treatment of posttraumatic distress. Arts Psychother. 2009;36(2):94–104.

76. Lyshak-Stelzer F, Singer P, Patricia SJ, Chemtob CM. Art therapy for adolescents with posttraumatic stress disorder symptoms: a pilot study. Art Ther. 2007;24(4):163–9.
77. Meekums B. Creative group therapy for women survivors of child sexual abuse: speaking the unspeakable. London: Jessica Kingsley; 2000. 221p.
78. Devereaux C. Untying the knots: dance/movement therapy with a family exposed to domestic violence. Am J Dance Ther. 2008;30(2):58–70.
79. Gray AEL. The body remembers: dance/movement therapy with an adult survivor of torture. Am J Dance Ther. 2001;23(1):29–43.
80. Gray AEL. Dancing in our blood. Dance/movement therapy with street children and victims of organized violence in Haiti. In: Jackson N, Shapiro-Lim T, editors. Dance, human rights and social justice: dignity in motion. Lanham, MD: Scarecrow Press; 2008. p. 222–36.
81. Harris DA. Pathways to embodied empathy and reconciliation after atrocity: former boy soldiers in a dance/movement therapy group in Sierra Leone. Intervention. 2007;5(3):203–31.
82. Koch SC, Weidinger-von der Recke B. Traumatised refugees: an integrated dance and verbal therapy approach. Arts Psychother. 2009;36(5):289–96.
83. Singer A. Interactions between movement and dance, visual images, etno and physical environments: psychosocial work with war-affected refugees and internally displaced children and adults. In: Jackson NM, Phim TS, editors. Dance, human rights, and social justice: dignity in motion. Lanham, Maryland: Scarecrow Press; 2008. p. 237–52.
84. Callaghan K. Movement psychotherapy with adult survivors of political torture and organized violence. Arts Psychother. 1993;20(5):411–21.
85. Callaghan K. In limbo: movement psychotherapy with refugees and asylum seekers. In: Dokter D, editor. Arts therapists, refugees and migrants reaching across borders. London: Jessica Kingsley; 1998.
86. Endel G. Therapeutische arbeit unter kriegsbedingungen. Integr Bewegungstherapie. 1996;1:30–2.
87. Koop II. Narben auf der Seele. Integrative Traumatherapie mit Folterüberlebenden. Z Polit Psychol. 2000;8(4):561–85.
88. Koop II. Das Leibparadigma in der Traumatherapie. Erfahrungen aus der Arbeit mit traumatisierten Flüchtlingen und Gefolterten. Integr Bewegungstherapie. 2002;1:4–9.
89. Petzold HG. Body narratives - Traumatische und Posttraumatische Erfahrungen aus Sicht der Integrativen Therapie. Integr Bewegungstherapie. 1999;1:24–30.
90. Karcher S. Körpererleben und Beziehungserleben - Konzentrative Bewegungstherapie mit Überlebenden von Folter. Psychother Im Dialog. 2000;1:28–37.
91. Karcher S. Body psychotherapy with survivors of torture. In: Drozðek B, Wilson JP, editors. Broken spirits: the treatment of traumatized asylum seekers, refugees, war and torture victims. New York: Taylor & Francis; 2004. p. 403–18.
92. Schmitz U, Sachsse U. Konzentrative Bewegungstherapie (KBT) zur Traumabewältigung: ein handlungsorientierter Ansatz. Göttingen: Vandenhoeck & Ruprecht; 2004.
93. Forester C. Your own body of wisdom: recognizing and working with somatic countertransference with dissociative and traumatized patients. Body Mov Dance Psychother. 2007;2(2):123–33.
94. Price C. Dissociation reduction in body therapy during sexual abuse recovery. Complement Ther Clin Pract. 2007;13(2):116–28.
95. Levine PA. Waking the tiger: healing trauma: the innate capacity to transform overwhelming experiences. Berkeley, CA: North Atlantic Books; 1997.
96. Levine PA. In an unspoken voice: how the body releases trauma and restores goodness. Berkeley, CA: North Atlantic Books; 2010. 388p.
97. Langmuir JI, Kirsh SG, Classen CC. A pilot study of body-oriented group psychotherapy: adapting sensorimotor psychotherapy for the group treatment of trauma. Psychol Trauma Theory Res Pract Policy. 2012;4(2):214–20.
98. Payne P, Levine PA, Crane-Godreau MA. Somatic experiencing: using interoception and proprioception as core elements of trauma therapy. Front Psychol. 2015;6:93.

99. Eckberg M. Victims of cruelty: somatic psychotherapy in the treatment of posttraumatic stress disorder. Berkeley, CA: North Atlantic Books; 2000. 274p.
100. Joachim I. Psychosoziale und psychotherapeutische Arbeit mit Überlebenden sexualisierter Gewalt im Kontext von Krieg und Krisen. In: medica mondiale e.V., Griese K, editors. Sexualisierte Kriegsgewalt und ihre Folgen Handbuch zur Unterstützung traumatsierter Frauen in verschiedenen Arbeitsfeldern. Frankfurt am Main: Mabuse; 2006. p. 375–412.
101. Wieland ML, Tiedje K, Meiers SJ, Mohamed AA, Formea CM, Ridgeway JL, et al. Perspectives on physical activity among immigrants and refugees to a small urban community in Minnesota. J Immigr Minor Health. 2015;17(1):263–75.
102. de Assis MA, de Mello MF, Scorza FA, Cadrobbi MP, Schooedl AF, da Silva SG, et al. Evaluation of physical activity habits in patients with posttraumatic stress disorder. Clinics. 2008;63(4):473–8.
103. Busch AM, Ciccolo JT, Puspitasari AJ, Nosrat S, Whitworth JW, Stults-Kolehmainen MA. Preferences for exercise as a treatment for depression. Ment Health Phys Act. 2016;10:68–72.
104. Hemmis L, de Vries H, Vandelanotte C, Short CE, Duncan MJ, Burton NW, et al. Depressive symptoms associated with psychological correlates of physical activity and perceived helpfulness of intervention features. Ment Health Phys Act. 2015;9:16–23.
105. Stubbs B, Vancampfort D, Rosenbaum S, Ward PB, Richards J, Soundy A, et al. Dropout from exercise randomized controlled trials among people with depression: a meta-analysis and meta regression. J Affect Disord. 2016;190:457–66.
106. Talbot LS, Neylan TC, Metzler TJ, Cohen BE. The mediating effect of sleep quality on the relationship between PTSD and physical activity. J Clin Sleep Med. 2014;10(7):795–801.
107. Dominick GM, Dunsiger SI, Pekmezi DW, Marcus BH. Health literacy predicts change in physical activity self-efficacy among sedentary Latinas. J Immigr Minor Health. 2012;15(3):533–9.
108. Sudeck G, Pfeifer K. Physical activity-related health competence as an integrative objective in exercise therapy and health sports – conception and validation of a short questionnaire. Sportwissenschaft. 2016;46(2):74–87.
109. Wångdahl J, Lytsy P, Mårtensson L, Westerling R. Health literacy among refugees in Sweden – a cross-sectional study. BMC Public Health. 2014;14:1030.
110. Lee HY, Lytle K, Yang PN, Lum T. Mental health literacy in Hmong and Cambodian elderly refugees: a barrier to understanding, recognizing, and responding to depression. Int J Aging Hum Dev. 2010;71(4):323–44.
111. Sørensen K, Van den Broucke S, Fullam J, Doyle G, Pelikan J, Slonska Z, et al. Health literacy and public health: a systematic review and integration of definitions and models. BMC Public Health. 2012;12(1):80.
112. Espejo MJC, Ley C. Música y movimiento en contextos de violencia: Procesos educativos y terapéuticos. Rev Música Educ. 2013;26(95):24.
113. Hölter G. Bewegungstherapie bei psychischen Erkrankungen: Grundlagen und Anwendung. 1st ed. Deutscher Ärzte-Verlag: Köln; 2011. 626p.
114. Ley C. Die Situation von Bewegung und Sport als Rehabilitationsmaßnahmen in Spanien. Bewegungstherapie Gesundheitssport. 2007;23(4):146–52.
115. Magee J, Spaaij R, Jeanes R. "It's recovery united for me": promises and pitfalls of football as part of mental health recovery. Sociol Sport J. 2015;32(4):357–76.
116. Meier M. Zum ersten Mal im Leben umarmt. In: Dieckhoff P, editor. Kinderflüchtlinge. Wiesbaden: VS Verlag für Sozialwissenschaften; 2010. p. 169–81.
117. Wertheim-Cahen T, Euwema M, Nabarro M. Trees coloured pink. The use of creativity as a means of psychosocial support for children in Kosovo: an ongoing learning process. Intervention. 2005;3(2):112–21.
118. Kalksma-Van Lith B, et al. Psychosocial interventions for children in war-affected areas: the state of the art. Intervention. 2007;5(1):3–17.
119. Schaeffer E. Tanz- und Bewegungstherapie mit traumatisierten Flüchtlingen. Z Psychotraumatologie. Psychol Med. 2004;2:43–59.

120. Abdallah-Steinkopff B. Psychotherapeutische Behandlung traumatisierter Flüchtlingskinder bei Refugio München. In: Interkulturelle Verständigung Dokumentation der Fachtagung Mir geht's doch gut – Jugend, Kultur und Salutogenese. München: Sozialreferat Landeshauptstadt München; 2001.
121. Suchanek G. Körpertherapie und Psychotrauma. na; 2003.
122. Joachim I. Grundlagen(wissen) für die Arbeit mit Überlebenden sexualisierter Kriegsgewalt. In: medica mondiale e.V., Griese K, editors. Sexualisierte Kriegsgewalt und ihre Folgen Handbuch zur Unterstützung traumatsierter Frauen in verschiedenen Arbeitsfeldern. Frankfurt am Main: Mabuse; 2006. p. 175–83.
123. Maercker A. Posttraumatische Belastungsstörungen. Berlin: Springer; 2013.
124. Megan Chawansky. New social movements, old gender games?: locating girls in the sport for development and peace movement. In: Anna Christine Snyder, Stephanie Phetsamay Stobbe, Critical aspects of gender in conflict resolution, peacebuilding, and social movements Emerald; Bingley, 2011. p. 121–134.
125. Gieβ-Stüber P, Barrio MR, Ley C. Physical education and sports as tools to promote intercultural living together. Some bases for a trans-national research project. In: Lidor R, Schneider K-H, Koenen K, editors. Proceedings sport as a mediator between cultures. Berlin: International Council of Sport Science and Physical Education - ICSSPE/CIEPSS; 2012. p. 81–96.
126. Deci EL, Ryan RM. Self-determination theory: a macrotheory of human motivation, development, and health. Can Psychol. 2008;49(3):182–5.
127. Rothschild B. The body remembers: the psychophysiology of trauma and trauma treatment, vol. xvi. W. W. Norton: New York; 2000. 190p.
128. Van der Kolk BA. The body keeps the score: brain, mind, and body in the healing of trauma. New York: Viking; 2014. 443p.
129. Härle D. Körperorientierte Traumatherapie: sanfte Heilung mit traumasensitivem Yoga (TSY), vol. 2015. Paderborn: Junfermann; 2015. 290p.
130. Fetzner MG, Asmundson GJG. Aerobic exercise reduces symptoms of posttraumatic stress disorder: a randomized controlled trial. Cogn Behav Ther. 2015;44(4):301–13.
131. Asmundson GJG, Fetzner MG, DeBoer LB, Powers MB, Otto MW, Smits JAJ. Let's get physical: a contemporary review of the anxiolytic effects of exercise for anxiety and its disorders. Depress Anxiety. 2013;30(4):362–73.
132. Faulkner G, Sparkes A. Exercise as therapy for schizophrenia: an ethnographic study. J Sport Exerc Psychol. 1999;21:52–69.
133. Stoll O, Ziemainz H. Laufen psychotherapeutisch nutzen Grundlagen, Praxis, Grenzen. Berlin: Springer; 2012.
134. Caddick N, Smith B, Phoenix C. The effects of surfing and the natural environment on the well-being of combat veterans. Qual Health Res. 2015;25(1):76–86.
135. Ley C, Krenn B. Erhebung sportartspezifischer Motivausprägungen bei sportlich aktiven Personen mit dem Berner Motiv- und Zielinventar (BMZI). Diagnostica. 2017;63:1–12.
136. Hobfoll SE, Watson P, Bell CC, Bryant RA, Brymer MJ, Friedman MJ, et al. Five essential elements of immediate and mid-term mass trauma intervention: empirical evidence. Focus. 2009;7(2):221–42.
137. Samson A, Solmon M. Examining the sources of self-efficacy for physical activity within the sport and exercise domains. Int Rev Sport Exerc Psychol. 2011;4(1):70–89.
138. Teixeira P, Carraça E, Markland D, Silva M, Ryan R. Exercise, physical activity, and self-determination theory: a systematic review. Int J Behav Nutr Phys Act. 2012;9(1):78.
139. Csikszentmihalyi M. Flow: the psychology of optimal experience. New York: Harper & Row; 1990.
140. Chilton G. Art therapy and flow: a review of the literature and applications. Art Ther. 2013;30(2):64–70.
141. Reinhardt C, Wiener S, Heimbeck A, Stoll O, Lau A, Schliermann R. Flow in der Sporttherapie der Depression – ein beanspruchungsorientierter Ansatz. Bewegungstherapie Gesundheitssport. 2008;24(4):147–51.

142. Jackson SA, Ford SK, Kimiecik JC, Marsh HW. Psychological correlates of flow in sport. J Sport Exerc Psychol. 1998;20(4):358–78.
143. Weinberg RS, Gould D. Foundations of sport and exercise psychology. 6th ed. Champaign, IL: Human Kinetics; 2014.
144. Schwarzer R. Modeling health behavior change: how to predict and modify the adoption and maintenance of health behaviors. Appl Psychol. 2008;57(1):1–29.
145. Fuchs R, Seelig H, Göhner W, Burton NW, Brown WJ. Cognitive mediation of intervention effects on physical exercise: causal models for the adoption and maintenance stage. Psychol Health. 2012;27(12):1480–99.
146. Mabweazara SZ, Ley C, Leach LL. Physical activity interventions for the management of chronic disease in low-income populations: a systematic review. Afr J Phys Act Health Sci. 2016;22(2.1):348–64.
147. Johnston M, Francis J, Hardeman W, Eccles M. From theory to intervention: mapping theoretically derived behavioural determinants to behaviour change techniques. Appl Psychol. 2008;57(4):660–80.
148. Michie S, Johnston M. Theories and techniques of behaviour change: developing a cumulative science of behaviour change. Health Psychol Rev. 2012;6(1):1–6.
149. Michie S, van Stralen MM, West R. The behaviour change wheel: a new method for characterising and designing behaviour change interventions. Implement Sci. 2011;6(1):42.
150. Vancampfort D, Stubbs B, Venigalla SK, Probst M. Adopting and maintaining physical activity behaviours in people with severe mental illness: the importance of autonomous motivation. Prev Med. 2015;81:216–20.
151. Spaaij R. Building social and cultural capital among young people in disadvantaged communities: lessons from a Brazilian sport-based intervention program. Sport Educ Soc. 2012;17(1):77–95.

Language Barriers and the Role of Interpreters: A Challenge in the Work with Migrants and Refugees

14

Maria Kletečka-Pulker, Sabine Parrag, Boris Drožđek, and Thomas Wenzel

Abstract

The quality of services for migrants and refugees depends to a substantial part on the quality of communication. Particularly in refugees, who usually have no realistic opportunity to acquire the language of the host country before their flight and might be distressed or traumatised, experienced interpreters are required. However, these are frequently not available or not integrated so far in healthcare or legal services. Untrained translators or family members are frequently used instead. The chapter explores legal and medical risks attached to different strategies regarding the use of interpreters and the differences between trained and untrained translators. It further gives an overview of standards and alternatives to address this important challenge in refugee care.

14.1 Introduction

Communication is a key element in human coexistence. When persons involved are refugees, communication is particularly vital due to their vulnerability. It is essential that no language barriers exist, particularly in situations where

M. Kletečka-Pulker (✉) · S. Parrag
Institute for Ethics and Law in Medicine, Medical University of Vienna, Vienna, Austria
e-mail: maria.kletecka-pulker@univie.ac.at; sabine.parrag@univie.ac.at

B. Drožđek
PsyQ/Parnassia Group, Rosmalen/Eindhoven, The Netherlands
e-mail: drozdek@telfort.nl

T. Wenzel
World Psychiatric Association Scientific Section,
Psychological Aspects of Persecution and Torture, Geneva, Switzerland
e-mail: drthomaswenzel@web.de

T. Wenzel, B. Drožđek (eds.), *An Uncertain Safety*,
https://doi.org/10.1007/978-3-319-72914-5_14

individuals face obligations or consequences in legal and medical procedures as a result of their statements. Consequently, for a long time experts have demanded that professional interpreter services should be established for the healthcare and other sectors [1–6].

14.2 Interpreters in Legal Proceedings (Judicial and Executive Branches)

Communication and language are particularly important in legal proceedings. Incomplete or incorrect communication can have significant negative consequences. In asylum proceedings in particular, oral statements provided by the parties involved often constitute the key evidence and are decisive to the outcome of proceedings.

In the following discussion, we will use the European legal framework as an example to demonstrate necessary safeguards. In the EU law, recital 13 of the Council Directive (CD 2005/85/EC) specifies the right to the services of an interpreter [7]. In order to meet the specifications of a "fair trial", as laid out in article 6, paragraph 3 of the ECHR, EU directive 2010/64/EU lays out the right of every accused to interpretation and translation services during legal proceedings. This directive sets the minimum standards, valid throughout the EU, for the right to interpreting services and translations in criminal proceedings and proceedings relating the execution of the European arrest warrants. This was the first step in a series of measures to set EU-wide minimum standards on procedural rights. The action was followed in 2012 by the directive on the right to information in criminal proceedings. Consequently, professional interpretation and translation are considered to be essential. Due to possible risks associated with actions such as denial of protection and refoulement (e.g. to a state where a person was tortured), the same standards should apply in asylum cases and other legal procedures.

In addition to legal provisions, training standards are necessary to ensure a reliable quality of interpretation and translation services. They must reflect the specific subject areas encountered by an interpreter. The UNHCR has responded by providing a training programme called project QUADA ("Qualitätsvolles Dolmetschen im Asylverfahren", lit. "Quality Interpretation in the Asylum Process")[1] for translators in asylum and other similar cases. Project QUADA is organised into 12 learning modules. They include basic information on the legal aspects of protection and the asylum process, ethics, techniques, special challenges, such as working with vulnerable groups, and strategies to protect oneself from psychological impacts while working with traumatised clients. The handbook and training programme are user-friendly, they utilise graphic media, and have been tested in different settings. This project can serve as an important model for capacity building in other areas.

[1] www.unhcr.org/dach/at/trainingshandbuch (*Authors*: Annika Bergunde, Sonja Pöllabauer)

14.3 Interpreters in Migrant and Refugee Healthcare

Many important areas require the aid of translation and interpretation services. One such area is the healthcare sector for which there are few, if any, national regulations regarding this issue. Translation and interpretation services are crucial during mass emergencies and displacements and in larger displaced persons' (DP) camps or similar settings. Often the legal and professional frameworks providing for guidelines and quality assurance are unclear, or no applicable legal requirements exist for healthcare settings. Vital medical treatments needed in emergencies are usually given priority, and no sanctions might be expected when no professional interpretation or translation is offered, even when legal safeguards might apply. This cannot be considered as an acceptable situation. In host countries, there is often uncertainty and a lack of clarity with regard to who is responsible for bearing the costs of interpretation services. Consequently, mostly unqualified, ad hoc interpreters, including relatives of patients or multilingual employees, are frequently used in daily practice. Thereby, new media are also employed to provide for professional interpreting via telephone or video conferencing [8]. Both options will be explored later on in this chapter.

Communication problems are not only awkward, time-consuming, and unpleasant for all parties involved, they may also result in inferior support [9] and medical care [10, 11]. Language barriers and barriers to understanding can lead to incorrect care provision, particularly in medical emergency situations. Factors such as class affiliation, lack of health literacy, culturally specific concepts of health and illness, and culturally specific variations in attitudes to prevention and understanding of the role of a healthcare system play here a decisive role [12–15] (see also [16, 17]). Consequently, important information about relevant healthcare services and their benefits/importance in maintaining health is often not adequately transmitted leading to a reduced use of such services. D'Avanzo [18] interviewed a random sample of 75 refugees in a US city and observed an expressed willingness to seek healthcare more frequently if interpreters were available in healthcare facilities and to change healthcare sites in order to gain access to an interpreter. In addition, a lack of mutual understanding may lead to a lower patient adherence or compliance with treatment [19, 20]. Patients may also run an increased risk of being treated differently, e.g. by being more frequently exposed to invasive procedures as compared to non-invasive procedures [21]. Last but not least, lack of sufficient communication gives rise to legal problems in providing comprehensive clarification to patients and in gaining their consent for treatment [22].

14.4 Differences Between Professional and Ad Hoc Interpreters

There are, in general, no guidelines applicable for the settings in which it is not possible to plan the use of interpreters in advance. Therefore, born out of necessity, other solutions are frequently applied in order to establish communication.

A special challenge can be observed in, the already mentioned, use of untrained or otherwise ad hoc interpreters [23–26], such as family members or unqualified members of the refugee community. This option may be sometimes hard to avoid due to a lack of access to or unavailability of trained personnel. However, it can be sufficient or even a preferred solution in less sensitive settings, as it involves community members and persons with cultural competence in a shared process. Yet, it is not acceptable in situations where exact and competent communication and confidentiality issues are of paramount interest.

14.5 Professional Interpreters

The assumption that general language competence, which many ad hoc interpreters display, is sufficient for interpreting is one of the primary misunderstandings. Professional interpreters should also possess translational competence [27, 28]. Studies in translation science largely agree that persons lacking a professional background in the subject and without a formal training are not suitable for use as interpreters [29].

It is important to point out that there is a fundamental difference between translation and interpretation. These two terms must be clearly defined first, as they are often incorrectly assumed to be synonymous. The key difference is that "translation [is] the written conversion of a text, whereas interpreting is the oral conversion of the spoken word" [30]. Consequently, interpreting is also used to denote the professional activity, whereas the designation used for lay persons involved in this process is, increasingly, that of a *language mediator* [26].

Professional interpreters are qualified in a series of skills, usually acquired during a tertiary level education. Pöchhacker [27] specifies the three key competences which professional interpreters should acquire: *language competence*, *cultural competence*, and, most importantly, *translational competence*. In addition to mastery of at least two languages (language competence), a professional interpreter must have a thorough understanding of the respective culture, its specific cultural behaviour patterns, and their significance in communicative interactions (cultural competence) (Fig. 14.1).

In many cases, the competence to work as a (professional) interpreter is regarded as sufficient where the first two competences are present. However, the true qualification required in order to practise the profession is represented by the last of the acquired competences, the translational competence, which "[...] is based on language and cultural competence and includes, above all, the cognitive and linguistic interaction with the particular field of knowledge, specialist area or subject of the communication in question" [27]. Thus, translational competence consists of both interpretation competence, the "ability to convert communication content" (ibid), and interpreter competence, the "ability to behave in a professional manner in an interpreting situation both before and afterwards (pre-/post interaction)" [27].

Translational competence allows interpreters to reproduce precisely and completely all statements, with a summary provided only in agreement with partners in

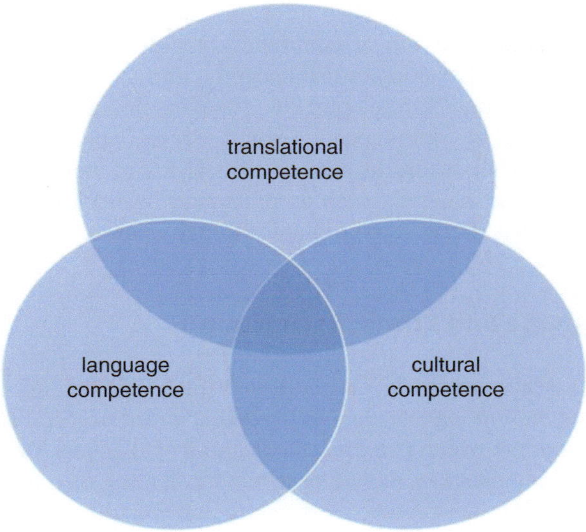

Fig. 14.1 Model of professional interpreter competences

a dialogue. This allows dialogues to be reproduced in the first-person form, literally in the "voice of the other", while an ad hoc interpreter usually uses the third-person form with a frequent use of reporting verbs ("she says") [5]. This competence allows statements of any length to be consecutively interpreted, as professional interpreters are able to draw on the technique of note-taking. However, it is still the case that shorter statements are always more conducive to direct interaction between parties in a dialogue.

Another key trait of professional interpreters, especially in healthcare ("medical interpreters", MI) [31–33], is their avoidance of expression of personal opinion, commentaries and assessments, and their adherence to the principle of impartiality with respect to the content of a dialogue or a communication partner. In addition, a professionally trained interpreter with a master's degree in the subject is also able to expand his/her specialist vocabulary permanently in order to support interpreting activities [27].

Interpreter impartiality and neutrality are the fundamental principles of the interpreting profession. As any party in a dialogue may regard the interpreter as more partial to its own side, or perceive the interpreter as an advocate on its behalf, the risk of tension within a medical dialogue or legal setting may heighten. As such, it is important to be aware of the potential challenges posed by a triadic and, particularly, by an interpreted dialogue.[2]

The non-verbal aspects of the setting provide a key framework for interaction with clients from different cultures. They may be grouped into:

[2] See also the Swiss Office of Public Health [34] on the characteristics of trialogues and the shifting balance of conversation in interpreted dialogues [34].

(a) General aspects of a setting, such as seating arrangements, persons involved, cultural habits, and the aim of communication (like personal history taking, treatment, family counselling or legal negotiation).
(b) Non-verbal behaviour [35] as a parallel (complementing) information source.
(c) Alternative modes of communication where, for example, printed text must be substituted by other media in case of illiteracy. The latter challenge can be addressed through materials such as illustrated healthcare tables in order to communicate basic healthcare problems through images.

14.6 Language and Ethnic Background

Transnational displacement aside, even locally displaced populations within a country or region can present with regional differences, different social stratification, or multilanguage settings which can cause substantial challenges. These may lead to difficulties in communication, including misunderstanding of crucial information, incomplete translation/interpretation, irritation, and mistrust. In conflict environments in particular, having a different accent can reduce confidence in interpreters, can be experienced as hostile and arrogant, or may lead to perceiving of disclosure as dangerous. All this impedes conducting an efficient interview or establishing a productive working relationship [36, 37] (see also [16]).

14.7 Specific Aspects of the Work with Refugee People

14.7.1 Culture and Trauma

Limiting the focus to culture as the only decisive factor in a particular form of health behaviour can be reductive and may pose a series of risks. When patients' personal situation is ignored, there exists a danger of stereotypical generalisation overlooking many important factors [38]. Working with refugees, therefore, requires not only a detailed knowledge of their cultural or medical backgrounds but also experience and specific strategies to deal with for example traumatic stress-related issues [39]. This is important as high trauma loads have been demonstrated to result in a higher need for support in communication in medical settings and make access to efficient translation necessary [40]. Further, knowledge of cultural idioms of distress [41, 42] is required to recognise culture-specific stress or trauma-related symptoms. They should be correctly translated and explained by the interpreter.

Former refugees who become interpreters may be confronted with their own personal history of trauma while doing their work. However, a qualitative study by Johnson with a group of such interpreters in the UK [43] drew attention to the potentially positive aspects of their work for posttraumatic growth. The authors concluded that "A sense of shared victimisation provided a protective backdrop from which the participants could make sense of the personal traumas they had experienced. The role of interpreting was important as it helped maintain cultural identity". A study by Splevins et al. yielded similar results [44]. The role of interpreters as cultural mediators has also been underlined by many authors (see, e.g., LaMancuso et al.) [45]. On the other side, retraumatisation of such interpreters is a risk factor not to be neglected and should be addressed by proper observation, supervision, and training [46].

Results of a recent meta-analytic review [47] demonstrated no differences in trauma-related psychotherapy outcome between sessions with and without the use of an interpreter. This finding is not easy to interpret and can be perceived either as an argument in favour or as the one against the use of interpreters in this specific setting. Further, Jensen et al. [48] have reported a case study of successful exposure therapy with a torture survivor with the help of an interpreter. More research should be done as the needed quantity of trained psychotherapists being fluent in the languages spoken by their clients, outnumbers by far capacities in both countries of origin and in host countries, even when only level IV interventions from the WHO model (see [49]) are considered.

Confidentiality is yet another key issue that speaks in favour of trained interpreters. Legal or cultural frameworks guaranteeing confidentiality in privileged situations at the levels expected in the EU or the USA, are almost non-existing in most other countries and it cannot therefore be expected from ad hoc interpreters from third countries to follow them. Clients' experiences of persecution may also lead to an—often healthy—mistrust in interpreters from other ethnic or religious groups. Background screening and monitoring of interpreters, particularly those involved in asylum cases, must ensure that they are not only aware of but also respect confidentiality issues and do not report on to home governments because of their political conviction or employment as informants. This problem must be addressed and resolved in order to ensure adequate communication in sensitive situations.

The interpreter's own unresolved personal issues, such as a history of unresolved trauma or interethnic adversities, can lead to distorted or incomplete interpretations, stress or inadequate behaviour (acting out) causing missing appointments, incomplete translation, and aggressive or arrogant behaviour.

Measures to be taken in order to prevent the above mentioned problems should include:

- Training (in a system like UNHCR's QUADA described earlier in this chapter, adapted for healthcare settings)
- Screening of prospective interpreters for prior major problems and vulnerabilities, ethnic or political bias
- A strategy for preventing problems that includes either intervision or supervision
- Staff management measures such as rotational or controlled shifts
- Mutual support and monitoring, possibly including a "buddy" system
- Low barriers to accessing peer counselling and treatment and avoidance of stigma

14.8 Ad Hoc Interpreters

When an interpreter has no professional training, the term "ad hoc interpreter" is used [26]. Ad hoc interpreters may be divided into several groups. In each case, it must be considered that the translation process involving ad hoc interpreters might lead to incorrect translations, particularly when legal or healthcare vocabulary is unknown to them. Also in the case of sensitive matters, such as reports on violence, torture, or sexuality, information cannot always be shared or could lead to distress or even indirect trauma or burnout in an ad hoc interpreter. Flores et al. [50] compared interpreter errors and their potential consequences in encounters with professional, ad hoc, and in "no interpreter" settings, and demonstrated that the use of professional interpreters resulted in a significantly lower likelihood of errors.

14.8.1 Children and Adolescents as Language Mediators

The above-mentioned difficulties are particularly present when children have the role of language mediators, as they are highly vulnerable to indirect trauma or in confrontation with age-inadequate subjects. Children might also suffer from being exploited in domestic conflicts. In the presence of children, parents may be hesitant to share information on traumatic events experienced, but also on a culture-dependent range of issues, such as sensitive medical subjects, gender issues, domestic violence, mortality, family problems, or other experiences that might conflict with their role as parents [25, 51–54]. Despite broad consensus on the wide range of problems, the use of children and adolescents as language mediators is often perceived as essential or unavoidable in order to quickly and directly overcome language barriers in everyday life [55–57]. Furthermore, refusing their assistance would result in huge delays, additional expenditure, and a potential conflict with parents who may perceive inclusion of family members as translators as a good practice even in sensitive settings [57].

Findings from the "video interpretation in healthcare" pilot project published in 2015 indicated that 81% of healthcare professionals (n = 144) in the sample used children as language mediators [56]. Another study concluded that children and adolescents are most frequently used as language mediators in healthcare and social services in Vienna, Austria [58]. Ebden et al. [59] looked into the interpreting services provided by children and other family members. They concluded that at least 16% of the questions rated as simple were incorrectly interpreted or not interpreted at all. This figure was rising up to 82% for more complex questions. Anatomical terms and symptoms were most often inaccurately or incorrectly interpreted. Furthermore, there were major difficulties in translating specialist terminology, e.g. confusing breathlessness with asthma. Moreover, healthcare personnel had no means of checking whether the information interpreted by language mediators was correct or complete. Most of them had the impression that dialogues had been interpreted by ad hoc interpreters without problems with the content been completely and correctly transmitted. All this leads to a false sense of security in health professionals [25, 60].

Although many studies have demonstrated a degree of risk associated with the use of children and adolescents as interpreters, as well as unreliability of the outcomes, there has been almost no change in the daily practice. In addition, services of foreign language employees and relatives or friends of patients as language mediators have been preferred to those of professional interpreters, as booking a professional interpreter was perceived as time-consuming [61].

It should be noted that multilingual children and adolescents can use their, so-called, "innate" ability to interpret effectively only when the context of a dialogue lies within their linguistic horizons and range of experience [62]. But when interpreting in a medical context or for public authorities, it is particularly easy for a child's limited horizons to be exceeded. This is usually because they are unable to assign meaning to medical terms in a source language and are then unable to provide a corresponding translation [57, 63, 64]. Parents of bilingual children often tend to hold unrealistic expectations of children's language competence, unconsciously exposing these children to a high degree of psychological pressure. In contrast, in the, so-called, "protected" contexts, such as conversations at home with friends or acquaintances, or out shopping, this activity can certainly have a positive impact on the child's personal development [52, 57].

Additionally, using children and adolescents as language mediators can strongly change interfamilial roles and lead to shifts in power relationships. The risk for children and adolescents to suffer from linguistic and psychological overload while being used as language mediators, particularly in unprotected contexts, should not be underestimated. Moreover, the proven increased rate of mistranslations represents a liability risk for the particular institution involved [25, 51, 52, 62].

As the use of children and adolescents may constitute a form of "invisible language work", it is worth investigating whether this should be regarded as child labour. Ahamer [52] explored this question in detail and compellingly argued that time is a valuable resource: "Although this is an activity undertaken by lay persons – not in terms of professionalism, but in relation to the required expenditure of resources – it represents potential financial savings for institutions and parents and therefore corresponds to an activity which equates to work". Orellana [65] has also stressed the major contribution made by children and adolescents in their role as interpreters, an activity from which parents or relatives, as well as institutions and society itself, profit. The decisive question is not "whether the children work, but how visible their work is". Taking on this role as interpreter is usually not considered out of the ordinary, and children receive little or no acknowledgement for it. It would be worthwhile taking a differentiated approach to the role children play here rather than viewing them exclusively as beneficiaries of educational and social systems [52]. Accordingly, one could conclude that, working as interpreters, translators, cultural and language mediators, bilingual children and adolescents of parents with a migration background have been making a substantial contribution to the informal health economy for decades, thereby "contributing" significantly to the society even at this young age [57].

From a legal perspective, using children as ad hoc interpreters raises the question of potentially unlawful employment of children, as well as the question of potential threats to child welfare [66]. At this point, it should be stated that children should not be used as interpreters in sensitive settings and that institutions or organisations involved in refugee care should carry the responsibility to provide alternatives, like trained interpreters or video remote interpreting.

14.8.2 Adult Relatives or Third Persons as Language Mediators

The use of adult relatives and multilingual employees without specific training is often problematic as there can be no reliance on the quality and completeness of their translation. Moreover, this type of work is not a part of the multilingual employees' job description. In case that an employee makes an error, this could have ramifications in terms of employment and insurance regulations. These errors might be seen as a lesser risk in emergency situations but deserve serious consideration in more permanent settings. However, many institutions and NGOs still rely on internal resources in order to overcome language barriers. Implementing this alternative requires a clear regulation of framework conditions (clarification of use, remuneration, courses and advanced training, supervision, legal aspects). It is particularly important to raise awareness that language competence alone is no longer a sufficient qualification for quality interpretation and that interpretation is a highly responsible task involving training, additional time, and emotional distress.

14.8.3 Reverting to a Shared Third Language (e.g. English)

Often attempts are made to use a third, shared language, increasingly English, in communication with patients. A key problem, hereby, is that helpers often hugely overestimate their own foreign language abilities. Switching to a third language is equally problematic for patients for whom this is not a native language either. Consequently, a basic communication problem is simply shifted, and the risk of communication problems increases rather than decreases.

14.8.4 Translated Information Materials

Oral transmission of information can, and should, be supported and complemented with printed material translated into foreign languages. However, supporting materials only serve to complement oral clarification required by law. Attention should be paid to the quality of translated materials as this may vary markedly. Although a very wide range of often high-quality translations are available in many fields, they do not cover all topics yet. Excellent educational material available in different languages can be downloaded free of charge from websites of the Swiss association *Interpret*,[3] as well as of the Austrian Federal Ministry of Health and Women's Affairs (https://www.bmgf.gv.at/home/Service/Broschueren/), though the range of subjects is limited.

14.8.5 Translation Programmes

Free electronic on- or offline translation programmes are a relatively new tool designed to overcome language barriers. They are easily available, for example, on

[3] www.inter-pret.ch/de/home-1.html

smartphones used by migrants today as communication hubs. Translation tools may provide assistance, particularly for scarcer languages, and can be quickly and easily used to clarify organisational queries in a daily medical setting. However, caution should again be exercised, as reliability of these tools is currently limited. It is certainly not advisable to conduct a consent dialogue using a translation programme alone, as there is a clear risk of error due to the nature and limitations of such programmes.

14.9 Professional Solutions: On-Site Interpreters vs. Alternatives

14.9.1 On-Site Interpreters

Finding professional strategies for overcoming language barriers should be given a high priority. The conventional solution is to use a local, professional interpreter, who is qualified based on the principles described earlier. Quite clearly, the advantages gained are directly visible—a barrier-free interpreting. One possible disadvantage may be that the interpreter becomes overburdened by emotional distress or is biased in some cases.

In addition to on-site interpreting, language barriers can be further overcome by using tools such as telephone or video interpreting. The key advantages of these remote solutions are increased temporal and spatial flexibility they facilitate.

14.9.2 Telephone Interpreting

A well-established strategy applied, for instance, in Switzerland and Australia is telephone interpreting. It facilitates access to interpretation services using pre-existing equipment, thereby minimising technical efforts involved. A recent qualitative study on telephone interpreting from the US draws attention to special considerations in using this tool with refugees [8]. The most important issues reported by the interpreters were (1) the importance of developing trust between the interpreter and the client and that (2) working with refugees requires more attention from the interpreter. Further, in his recent survey Wang [67] took a deeper look at telephone interpreting and the interpreter's perceptions of suitability, remuneration, and quality in healthcare.

14.9.3 Video Interpreting

Compared to other remote methods, video interpreting is the method which simulates the face-to-face situation most precisely by enabling non-verbal communication [68, 69] and by ensuring that cultural aspects expressed in the form of gestures and mimics are not being ignored [69]. Additionally, interpreting visual indicators may explain inconsistencies at the verbal and non-verbal message levels and help preventing misunderstandings. Appropriate non-verbal reactions of the interpreter may have a positive effect on the person whose narrative is being interpreted [68]. This is an important factor in building trust between the interpreter and the client. It also supports an uninterrupted flow of conversation despite being a remote solution. In situations where a declaration of consent must be obtained, consideration of mimics and gestures is particularly important [68].

Video interpreting, as an innovative means of overcoming language barriers in the healthcare sector, has for a long time been a fixed component of care provision for foreign language patients in several countries including the US. However, it is only recently that steps have been taken to establish a professional video interpreting service in the German-speaking world [56].

As part of the project already mentioned, an Austrian study [56] evaluated the use of professional interpreters integrated into the physician-patient dialogue via video conferencing in a technically uncomplicated manner. The majority of the research sample evaluated the tool as very helpful. Increased efficiency and reliance on the precision of translation were perceived as particularly positive aspects. In addition, it was an ideal means of ensuring neutrality and objectivity of interpretation in terms of spatial and emotional closeness and distance between the interpreter and the patient.

Confidence gained by being able to access correct and complete interpretation played a significant role in increasing employees' satisfaction and in ensuring patient safety. Using a video interpreter allowed employees to complete their tasks to their usual quality standard and, above all, independently of physical presence and availability of a third-party language mediator. Video interpreting received also the highest rating for quick and flexible availability and is perceived as a very good method for overcoming communication barriers in a way that assures quality of translation.

This method may not, however, be the most suitable one for every setting. For scheduled treatments, the use of on-site professional interpreters is the ideal solution as they can be booked in advance. Even where employees, team members, and accompanying persons serving as language mediators are able to cover the interpretation demand, organisational and institutional framework conditions should guarantee a constant level of quality and safety in the care of patients who do not speak the host countries' language [56].

Last but not least, promising research results, increasing awareness of the problem, and a growing openness to new solutions have provided the opportunity to develop and improve the professional and innovative video interpreting system. Today this system is used by numerous institutions in the healthcare, social, and justice sector in Austria, Germany, and Switzerland and covers approximately 72 different languages. Six hundred qualified interpreters are involved in this network across the EU, offering availability in the core languages for up to 24 h at only 120 s' notice. Since November 2015, video interpreting has been available in the city of Hamburg which chooses a comprehensive container solution to provide refugees with medical care. Germany's first vaccination van for refugees started in Berlin in November 2016 and provides video interpreting, too. In Austria, video interpreting is used to provide medical care in police detention centres, which predominantly house detainees pending deportation and detainees with criminal convictions [70].

14.10 Translation of Standardised Materials

In translation of standardised materials and diagnostic tools, such as medical and psychological questionnaires, culture-specific adaptation and (re)validation is required (also discussed by Wenzel et al. [16]). Particularly for critical issues, a complete revalidation process has been recommended, including professional translation and validation in a comparable population [71]. A practical alternative has been developed, using common translation—retranslation procedures [72, 73]. These might consist of a simple A-B-A model, which is based on translation by a bilingual, ideally professional, translator. If differences are observed in language A after retranslation, the text should be adapted until the results are sufficiently identical when again retranslated from language B. Care should be taken in choosing bilingual translators. They should belong to the same ethnic group as the person being questioned and should be aware of differences in language used by different social groups. Ideally, they will have a professional understanding of translation sciences and the field/topic in question. Qualitative methods, such as focus groups, can be a relatively simple but efficient tool for improving results and can be conducted at the onset or later on to address translation problems.

14.10.1 A Case Example

In a study conducted in former Yugoslavia, we (TW) observed an unusual problem occurring when the Harvard Trauma Questionnaire (HTQ) [71] was applied. While many participants reported that they had been subjected to torture, their specific life circumstances made this finding improbable. A focus group yielded the information that the subjects felt helpless in face of continuous exposure to the hostile and degrading enemy propaganda in public media and have experienced this as torture. While the generally accepted legal definition of torture was obviously not been fulfilled, the results yielded a better understanding of the impact and needs of the patient group in question and avoided misinterpretation of the results.

14.11 Conclusions: Barrier-Free Communication—A Leadership Task

Language and communication are not only essential and fundamental components of every legal process but are also of great importance in almost every area of life, including healthcare. Language barriers are a particular source of error in work with migrants and refugee people, as well as a liability risk, a factor about which the affected professions must particularly be made aware of. Alternatives, like ad hoc interpreters that are used in emergencies, should not become a standard and should be avoided as much as possible due to medical, psychological, and legal risks involved. New approaches like video-based models and training programmes like the UNHCR's QUADA should be further developed and integrated into legal and healthcare systems. Finally, introduction of quality assured measures for overcoming language barriers increases safety of both parties in a dialogue and reduces costs. As a result, all directly or indirectly involved, both interpreters and patients, as well as NGOs, institutions, and authorities responsible for them, can benefit from systematically organised, professional interpreting services. However, in order to achieve this, "[...] there must be increasing awareness on all sides that using qualified interpreters is not a luxury, but rather a mark of an open society" [74], as demanded by Rasky in an article summarising challenges in the present healthcare systems.

References

1. Pöchhacker F. Krankheit, Kultur, Kinder, Kommunikation: Die Nichte als Dolmetscherin. Curare Z Medizinethnol. 2008;31(2–3):133–42.
2. Kalra J. Medical errors and patient safety. Strategies to reduce and disclose medical errors and improve patient safety. In: Sonntag O, Plebani M, editors. Patient Safety. Berlin: Walter de Gruyter; 2011. p. 113.
3. Johnstone M, Kanitsaki O. Culture, language, and patient safety: making the link. Int J Qual Health Care. 2006;18(5):383–8.
4. van Rosse F, de Bruijne M, Suurmond J, Essink-Bot ML, Wagner C. Language barriers and patient safety risks in hospital care. A mixed methods study. Int J Nurs Stud. 2016;54:45–53.
5. Menz F. Ärztliche Gespräche mit PatientInnen mit geringen Deutschkenntnissen. In: Peintinger M, editor. Interkulturell kompetent. Ein Handbuch für Ärztinnen und Ärzte. Wien: Facultas Verlag; 2011. p. 225–35.
6. Flores GL, Laws MB, Mayo S, Zuckerman B, Abreu M, Medina L, Hardt EJ. Errors in medical interpretation and their potential clinical consequences in pediatric encounters. Pediatrics. 2003;111(1):6–14.
7. Matti E, Rienzner M. Dolmetschen und Übersetzen im Asylverfahren. Migralex. 2013;11(1): 2–13.
8. Dubus N. Interpreters' subjective experiences of interpreting for refugees in person and via telephone in health and behavioural health settings in the United States. Health Soc Care Commun. 2016;24(5):649–56.
9. Dressler D, Pils P. A qualitative study on cross-cultural communication in post-accident inpatient rehabilitation of migrant and ethnic minority patients in Austria. Disabil Rehabil. 2009;31(14):1181–90.
10. Colucci E, Minas H, Szwarc J, Guerra C, Paxton G. In or out? Barriers and facilitators to refugee-background young people accessing mental health services. Transcult Psychiatry. 2015;52(6):766–90.
11. Bird S. Lost without translation. Aust Fam Physician. 2008;37(12):1023–4.
12. Richter M, Hurrelmann K. Gesundheitliche Ungleichheit. Grundlagen, Probleme, Perspektiven. Wiesbaden: VS Verlag für Sozialwissenschaften; 2009.
13. Razum O. Gesundheit von Migranten: Hintergründe. In: Deutscher Ethikrat, editor. Migration und Gesundheit Kulturelle Vielfalt als Herausfoderung für die medizinisch Versorgung, Tagungsdokumentation. Berlin; 2010. pp. 21–7.
14. Löschke-Yaldiz K, Özsoy S, San E, Ünsal S, Keegan N. "Gesund in allen Sprachen". Health Literacy bei MigrantInnen. In: Wolf H, Endler M, Wimmer-Puchinger B, editors. Frauen Gesundheit Soziale Lage. Wien: Facultas Verlag; 2010. p. 143–54.
15. Kutalek R. Kulturelle Aspekte von Gesundheit und Krankheit: Medizinanthropologische Ansätze. In: Peintinger M, editor. Interkulturell kompetent Ein Handbuch für Ärztinnen und Ärzte. Wien: Facultas Verlag; 2011. p. 23–38.
16. Wenzel T, Völkl-Kernstock S, Wittek TU, Baron D. Identifying needs, vulnerabilities, and resources in refugee persons and groups. In: Wenzel T, Drožđek B, editors. An uncertain safety. Cham: Springer International; 2018.

17. Kühnel M, Droždek B, Wenzel T. Medical aspects of health care: reflections from the field experience in European countries and an overview of the basic health needs. In: Wenzel T, Droždek B, editors. An uncertain safety. Cham: Springer International; 2018.
18. D'Avanzo CE. Barriers to health care for Vietnamese refugees. J Prof Nurs. 1992;8(4): 245–53.
19. StatistikAustria. Sozio-demographische und sozio-ökonomische Determinanten von Gesundheit. Auswertungen der Daten aus der Österreichischen Gesundheitsbefragung 2006/2007. Wien; 2008.
20. StatistikAustria. Migration & Integration. Zahlen. Daten. Indikatoren 2014. Wien; 2014.
21. Tate RC, Kelley MC. Triage in the Tower of Babel: interpreter services for children in the prehospital setting. Pediatr Emerg Care. 2013;29(12):1280–2.
22. Kletecka-Pulker M. Therapieverzicht in der Chirurgie aus der Sicht einer Juristin. Chirurgie. 2017;1:24–5.
23. Rosenberg E, Leanza Y, Seller R. Doctor-patient communication in primary care with an interpreter: physician perceptions of professional and family interpreters. Patient Educ Couns. 2007;67:286–92.
24. Meyer B. How untrained interpreters handle medical terms. In: Mason I, editor. Triadic exchanges studies in dialogue interpreting. Manchester: St. Jerome; 2001. p. 87–106.
25. Meyer B, Pawlack B, Kliche O. Family interpreters in hospitals: good reason for bad practice? MediAzioni. 2010;10:297–324.
26. Marics A. "Miš fa:him walla e:?" Ein diskursanalytischer Beitrag zum Laiendolmetschen. In: Grbić N, Pöllabauer S, editors. Kommunaldolmetschen/Community Interpreting Probleme – Perspektiven – Potenziale Forschungsbeiträge aus Österreich. TRANSÜD. Arbeiten zur Theorie und Praxis des Übersetzens und Dolmetschens. 21st ed. Berlin: Frank & Timme GmbH Verlag für wissenschaftliche Literatur; 2008.
27. Pöchhacker F. Dolmetschen. Konzeptuelle Grundlagen und deskriptive Untersuchungen. Tübingen: Stauffenburg Verlag; 2000.
28. Pöllabauer S. "I don't understand your English, Miss". Dolmetschen bei Asylanhörungen. In: Kaindl K, Pöchhacker F, editors. Translationswissenschaft. Band 2. Tübingen: Gunter Narr Verlag; 2005.
29. Pöchhacker F. KrankenhausdolmetscherInnen: Bedarf, Probleme, Perspektiven. In: Rasky E, editor. Gesundheit hat Bleiberecht: Migration und Gesundheit; Festschrift zum Anlass des 10-jährigen Bestehens des Ambulatoriums Caritas Marienambulanz in Graz. Wien: Facultas. WUV; 2009. p. 117–23.
30. Europäische Kommission. Übersetzen und Dolmetschen: Mit Sprachen arbeiten. Broschüre; 2009. http://www.universitas.org/uploads/media/MitSprachenArbeiten.pdf.
31. White K, Laws MB. Role exchange in medical interpretation. J Immigr Minor Health. 2009;11(6):482–93.
32. VanderWielen LM, Enurah AS, Rho HY, Nagarkatti-Gude DR, Michelsen-King P, Crossman SH, et al. Medical interpreters: improvements to address access, equity, and quality of care for limited-English-proficient patients. Acad Med. 2014;89(10):1324–7.
33. Partridge R, Proano L. Communicating with immigrants: medical interpreters in health care. Med Health Rhode Island. 2010;93(3):77–8.
34. BAG BfGS. Sprachliche Brücken zur Genesung. Interkulturelles Übersetzen im Gesundheitswesen der Schweiz. Bern: Bundesamt für Gesundheit; 2011.
35. Bramberg EB, Sandman L. Communication through in-person interpreters: a qualitative study of home care providers' and social workers' views. J Clin Nurs. 2013;22(1–2):159–67.
36. Kutalek R. Diversity competence in medicine: equity, culture and practice. Wien Klin Wochenschr. 2012;124:3–9.
37. Ferguson W, Candib L. Culture, language, and the doctor-patient relationship. Fam Med Community Health. 2002;34(5):353–61.
38. Zielke-Nadkarni A. Gesundheits- und Krankheitskonzepte. In: Domenig D, editor. Transkulturelle Kompetenz. Lehrbuch für Pflege-, Gesundheits- und Sozialberufe. Bern: Verlag Hans Huber; 2007. p. 191–204.

39. Crosby SS. Primary care management of non-English-speaking refugees who have experienced trauma: a clinical review. JAMA. 2013;310(5):519–28.
40. Wagner J, Burke G, Kuoch T, Scully M, Armeli S, Rajan TV. Trauma, healthcare access, and health outcomes among Southeast Asian refugees in Connecticut. J Immigr Minor Health. 2013;15(6):1065–72.
41. Nichter M. Idioms of distress revisited. Cult Med Psychiatry. 2010;34(2):401–16.
42. Kohrt BA, Rasmussen A, Kaiser BN, Haroz EE, Maharjan SM, Mutamba BB, et al. Cultural concepts of distress and psychiatric disorders: literature review and research recommendations for global mental health epidemiology. Int J Epidemiol. 2014;43(2):365–406.
43. Reich PJ, Boyle MG, Hogan PG, Johnson AJ, Wallace MA, Elward AM, et al. Emergence of community-associated methicillin-resistant Staphylococcus aureus strains in the neonatal intensive care unit: an infection prevention and patient safety challenge. Clin Microbiol Infect. 2016;22:645–e1.
44. Splevins KA, Cohen K, Joseph S, Murray C, Bowley J. Vicarious posttraumatic growth among interpreters. Qual Health Res. 2010;20(12):1705–16.
45. LaMancuso K, Goldman RE, Nothnagle M. "Can I ask that?": perspectives on perinatal care after resettlement among Karen refugee women, medical providers, and community-based doulas. J Immigr Minor Health. 2016;18(2):428–35.
46. Fischman Y. Secondary trauma in the legal professions, a clinical perspective. Torture. 2008;18(2):107–15.
47. Lambert JE, Alhassoon OM. Trauma-focused therapy for refugees: meta-analytic findings. J Couns Psychol. 2015;62(1):28–37. https://doi.org/10.1037/cou0000048.
48. Jensen BS. Treatment of a multitraumatized tortured refugee needing an interpreter with exposure therapy. Case Rep Psychiatry. 2013;2013:197323.
49. Weissbecker I, Hanna F, El Shazly M, Gao J, Ventevogel P. Integrative mental health and psychosocial support interventions for refugees in humanitarian crisis settings. In: Wenzel T, Drožđek B, editors. An uncertain safety. Cham: Springer International; 2018.
50. Flores G, Abreu M, Barone CP, Bachur R, Lin H. Errors of medical interpretation and their potential clinical consequences: a comparison of professional versus ad hoc versus no interpreters. Ann Emerg Med. 2012;60(5):9.
51. Weisskirch R. Child language brokers in immigrant families: an overview of family dynamics. MediAzioni. 2010;10:68–87.
52. Ahamer V. Unsichtbare Spracharbeit. Jugendliche Migranten als Laiendolmetscher. Integration durch "Community Interpreting". Bielefeld: Transcript Verlag; 2012.
53. Guske I. Familial and institutional dependence on bilingual and bicultural go-betweens – effects on minority children. MediAzioni. 2010;10:325–45.
54. MacFarlane A, Dzebisoca Z, Karapish D, Kovacevic B, Ogbebor F, Okonkwo E. Arranging and negotiating the use of informal interpreters in general practice consultations: experiences of refugees and asylum seekers in the west of Ireland. Soc Sci Med. 2009;69:210–4.
55. Cohen S, Moran-Ellis J, Smaje C. Children as informal interpreters in GP consultations: pragmatics and ideology. Sociol Health Illn. 1999;21(2):163–86.
56. Kletecka-Pulker M, Parrag S. Endbericht "Qualitätssicherung in der Versorgung nichtdeutschsprachiger PatientInnen – Videodolmetschen im Gesundheitswesen". Ein Pilotprojekt der Österreichischen Plattform Patientensicherheit und des Instituts für Ethik und Recht in der Medizin an der Universität Wien; 2015.
57. Schmidt-Glenewinkel A. Kinder als Dolmetscher in der Arzt-Patienten-Interaktion. Berlin: Frank & Timme Verlag für wissenschaftliche Literatur; 2013.
58. Pöchhacker F. Kommunikation mit Nichtdeutschsprachigen in Wiener Gesundheits- und Sozialeinrichtungen: MA 15, Dezernat für Gesundheitsplanung; 1997.
59. Ebden P, Bhatt A, Carey OJ, Harrison B. The bilingual consultation. Lancet. 1988; 331(8581):347.
60. Pöchhacker F. Dolmetschen – ein Kinderspiel? Eine klinische Fallstudie. Textcontext. 2000;14(2):153–79.

61. Langer T, Schaper K, Gupta S, Porst R, Ostermann T. Sprachbarrieren in der Betreuung von Patienten mit Migrationshintergrund – Ergebnisse einer Pilotstudie zu den Erfahrungen von Kinder- und Jugendärzten. Klin Padiatr. 2013;225:96–113.
62. Rajič K. "Die Familienaußenminister". Kinder als Sprach- und KulturmittlerInnen – eine empirische Erhebung. In: Grbić N, Pöllabauer S, editors. "Ich habe mich ganz peinlich gefühlt" Forschungen zum Kommunaldolmetschen in Österreich: Problemstellungen, Perspektiven und Potentiale. Graz: Selbstverlag, Institut für Theoretische und Angewandte Translationswissenschaft; 2006. p. 139–78.
63. Saleh M. Kinder als DolmetscherInnen im medizinischen Bereich. Graz: Karl-Franzens-Universität Graz; 2013.
64. Kuljuh E. Kinder als Dolmetscher/innen. In: Pöllabauer S, Prunč E, editors. Brücken bauen statt Barrieren Sprach- und Kulturmittlung im sozialen, medizinischen und therapeutischen Bereich. Graz: Selbstverlag, Institut für Theoretische und Angewandte Translationswissenschaft; 2003. p. 143–8.
65. Orellana MF. The work kids do: Mexican and Central American immigrant children's contributions to households and schools in California. Harv Educ Rev. 2001;71(3):366–89.
66. Fischer-Czermak C. in Kletečka/Schauer, ABGB-ON1.02 § 170 (Stand 1.7.2013, rdb.at).
67. Wang J. 'Telephone interpreting should be used only as a last resort.' Interpreter's perceptions of the suitability, remuneration and quality of telephone interpreting. Perspectives. 2017:17.
68. Felgner L. Zur Bedeutung der nonverbalen Kommunikation im gedolmetschten medizinischen Gespräch. In: Andres D, Pöllabauer S, editors. "Spürst du, wie der Bauch rauf-runter?" Fachdolmetschen im Gesundheitsbereich. München: Meidenbauer; 2009. p. 45–70.
69. Saint-Louis L, Friedman E, Chiasson E, Quessa A, Novaes F. Testing new technologies in medical interpreting. Somerville: Cambridge Health Alliance; 2003.
70. SAVD Videodolmetschen GmbH. Available from: http://www.videodolmetschen.com.
71. Mollica RF, Caspi-Yavin Y, Bollini P, Truong T, Tor S, Lavelle J, The Harvard Trauma Questionnaire. Validating a cross-cultural instrument for measuring torture, trauma, and posttraumatic stress disorder in Indochinese refugees. J Nerv Ment Dis. 1992;180(2):111–6.
72. Combaluzier S, Gouvernet B, Menant F, Rezrazi A. [Validation of a French translation of Krueger's personality inventory for DSM-5 in its brief form (PID-5 BF)]. Encephale. 2016. https://doi.org/10.1016/j.encep.2016.07.006.
73. Gautam S, Nijhawan M, Kamal P. Standardisation of hindi version of goldbergs general health questionnaire. Indian J Psychiatry. 1987;29(1):63–6.
74. Rásky E. Blockierte Verständigungswege. Das österreichische Gesundheitswesen ÖKZ. 2010;51(01–02):26–8.

15 Mental Health and Well-Being of the Staff Supporting Refugees: How to Deal with Risks?

Rosa Izquierdo, Nino Makhashvili, Boris Drožđek, and Thomas Wenzel

Abstract

The aim of this chapter is to address impacts of the work with refugees on mental health of helpers, in particular humanitarian aid workers. These assist vulnerable populations on a daily basis and often in challenging environments. Organizations providing assistance to refugees are responsible for mental health and well-being of their staff, since the staff is exposed to situations it would have not been exposed to otherwise. A set of measures and internationally accepted standards for prevention and protection of mental health in humanitarian aid workers and in emergency settings are presented and discussed. Moreover, a Georgian research study of the helpers' mental health and related issues is illustrating situation in the field in connection with the provided background information.

R. Izquierdo (✉)
GLOCARIS-Glocal Minds Rosa Izquierdo S.L., Bilbao, Spain
e-mail: rizquierdo@cop.es

N. Makhashvili
Mental Health Resource Center, Ilia State University, Tbilisi, Georgia
e-mail: nino.makhashvili.1@iliauni.edu.ge

B. Drožđek
PsyQ/Parnassia Group, Rosmalen/Eindhoven, The Netherlands
e-mail: drozdek@telfort.nl

T. Wenzel
World Psychiatric Association Scientific Section,
Psychological Aspects of Persecution and Torture, Geneva, Switzerland
e-mail: drthomaswenzel@web.de

T. Wenzel, B. Drožđek (eds.), *An Uncertain Safety*,
https://doi.org/10.1007/978-3-319-72914-5_15

15.1 Introduction

> "Consider what goes on in your mind when you bear witness as your client talks about a traumatic experience. Owing to your brain's gift for vivid imagery, you are likely to picture what your client went through. Like your client, you may later be haunted by these images, at daytime or during your sleep. Owing to your empathy and penchant for emotional contagion, you may experience some degree of distress, potentially sharing in the full range of emotions: fear, anger, despair, and the rest. Like your client, you may feel guilty about your emotional and physiological responses (i.e. feeling guilty for your vengeful fantasies or sexual arousal). Like your client, your cognitive assumptions may be shattered. Like your client, you may become sensitised, and more reactive rather than less reactive to subsequent stressors. Just as it is for your client, the therapeutic work you are doing may constitute a reminder of your past trauma" ([1], pp. 376–77).

Humanitarian aid workers and human service providers in conflict and post-conflict settings are exposed to a number of stressors and traumatic events that may result in stress-related illness. Over the last 10–15 years, the environment in which humanitarian assistance has been implemented has changed resulting in workers increasingly being targeted by violence. During the last decade [2], intentional violence has become the leading cause of death (67.4%) among aid workers in complex emergencies, followed by death due to motor vehicle accidents (17%). Two other causes were disease and natural causes responsible for 8% of deaths. The murders of aid workers that took place over the last 5 years in East Timor, Central Africa, Chechnya, Afghanistan, and Iraq illustrate the dangers of violent physical assault in conflict and post-conflict nations.

Workers may also suffer more mundane stressors related to difficult situations in post-conflict societies. Living conditions are often poor, with a lack of privacy and of separation between work and living space and with intermittent or nonexistent running water and electricity. The job may require traveling on hazardous roads with unreliable means of transportation. International workers may also be exposed to a culture shock. Access to medical care is often limited, and evacuation in case of personal illness or injury may be difficult. In addition to these difficult working conditions, international aid workers are separated from their social support network. Separation from family and friends for extended periods of time may be a stressor in itself. Furthermore, communication with the outside world may be limited due to a lack of access to phone lines, e-mail, and international newspapers or television.

At the same time, national staff involved in humanitarian aid may have to deal with an additional set of specific stressors, like loss of family members due to an armed conflict [2]. These workers are often selected from the same population that the humanitarian agency serves and may have been exposed to traumatic events directly related to the events which have precipitated the humanitarian intervention. In contrast to international staff, national staff generally cannot go home to a safe place and stable environment when their assignment is over.

The stressors for national staff can be compounded with previous traumatic experiences. For example, in June 2000, a study [2] conducted by the Centers for Disease Control and Prevention (CDC) in Kosovo among 410 international and 429 Kosovar Albanian aid workers from 22 humanitarian organizations found that national staff had higher rates of post-traumatic stress disorder (PTSD) than their international counterparts. This is understandable because these workers had been exposed for 10 years to an environment of oppression, persecution, ethnic killings, and hatred. Shortly after the end of the war in 1999, the remaining national mental health care workers started a center for rehabilitation of trauma and torture victims, and mental health staff were providing care to the victims of the conflict. At the same time, most of the national staff themselves had suffered from the consequences of the conflict.

All staff and volunteers providing assistance to refugees and migrants on the move will be repeatedly exposed to narratives of terror and personal tragedy. Confrontations with horror, danger, and human misery are emotionally demanding and have a potential to affect mental health and well-being of the workers. Helpers may experience moral anguish regarding choices they have to make in their daily work. They may also live and work under physically demanding and unpleasant working conditions, characterized by heavy workloads, long hours, and within difficult security constraints. These stressors may have adverse consequences such as anxiety and depressive feelings; psychosomatic complaints; over-involvement with beneficiaries; callousness; apathy; self-destructive behavior, such as alcohol or other substance abuse; and interpersonal conflicts. However, for many workers, the greatest stress comes from insufficient managerial and organizational support [3].

Humanitarian workers should be alert to signs of stress in themselves and colleagues. Team managers should monitor their staff, through informal observation and periodic routine inquiry or by organizing informal or formal group stress evaluation sessions. A supportive, inclusive, and transparent organizational climate protects staff and volunteers. Humanitarian organizations should aim to improve their performance in staff support and to reduce differential support practices for national and international staff [3]. Thereby, individual differences such as gender, age, culture, and experience should be taken into consideration.

The United Nations High Commissioner for Refugees (UNHCR) has recently published a survey [4] regarding well-being and mental health of their staff. The survey explored the impact of three psychosocial hazards that are characteristic of the UNHCR workplace:

1. Exposure to traumatic experiences, as the populations of concern to humanitarian organizations reside in environments deeply affected by insecurity and risks. The ensuing psychological trauma and its prevention have been the centerpiece of many psychosocial support strategies which have included preparation for traumatic situations, resilience building, critical incident interventions, and end-of-assignment debriefings. In the UNHCR alone, a number of recommendations of the MHPSS (Mental Health and Psychosocial Support) report (2013) focused on dealing with the prevention of PTSD and on supporting critical incident stress.
2. Exposure to secondary trauma through working directly with people of concern. Years of observations by the Staff Welfare Officers (SWO) in the UNHCR found that continuous exposure to the traumatic experiences of people of concern through interviews, assessments, and translation can have a profound impact, both positive and negative, on employees.
3. Effort-reward imbalance (ERI) linked to organizational factors.

Although the effort-reward imbalance theory does not capture all organizational stressors (such as interpersonal relationships or type of work), it was considered to be relevant enough for the UNHCR's environment. Global prevalence of 72% of respondents being at risk for the ERI confirmed that assumption.

When a traumatic incident occurs, there is an increased risk for post-traumatic stress disorder (PTSD), a fact also confirmed by this UNHCR study [4]. However, when, in addition to that, there is an imbalance between efforts and rewards, the risk for PTSD seems to further increase. Therefore, it is not just trauma that leads to PTSD outcomes, the ERI seems to play a mediating role in this relationship. The survey suggested that the UNHCR needs to consider organizational stressors and support systems to help build resilience, along with the trauma prevention and response mechanisms in their staff members. The response should include recognition of an incident and its impact by the managers, being accompanied by administrative procedures, and ensure a subsequent posting that takes into account earlier staff's experiences, to mention just a few options. All these are important elements in meeting the "reward" criteria. Life-threatening situations highlight the limits that a person is not necessarily willing to cross but is nevertheless exposed to. Not being supported following critical incidents in the manner described above tends to create a sense of resentment and frustration in the staff, complicating recovery from trauma. Unfortunately, some of administrative processes that are not in the UNHCR's control, such as the service incurred compensation plans, have been notorious for adding to the injury.

Further, the importance of work-related stressors in mental health can be corroborated by data from the Staff Welfare Section [4]. In 2014, the Staff Welfare Officers (SWO) registered 4506 actions with staff and affiliate workforce. The most common reason for staff to contract individual support of the SWOs was linked to the working conditions category (workload, lack of clarity of roles, etc.) accounting for 31% of all actions taken. This is way above the 16% of actions linked to cases of personal problems and/or family-related concerns. Finally, 14% of all actions were related to cases involving security incidents and trauma. This confirms the assumption that organizational stressors must be considered seriously.

15.2 Coping with Stress

Coping is a behavior that is designed to prevent, delay, avoid, or manage tension and stress [5]. It is intertwined with one's social and emotional resources and one's emotional and psychological tools. Most individuals learn individualized ways of dealing with stress, but they usually follow a pattern of:

- Avoidance
- Alteration
- Management
- Prevention
- Control of undue emotional expression

Coping mechanisms may take three different forms:

1. The individual may attempt to change the source of strain or stress. This action presumes knowledge and perception of its causes. Attention is focused on changing a situation before strain or stress occurs.
2. The individual may attempt to redefine a situation in order to control a degree of stress and lessen or buffer its impact. Redefinition is a means of managing significance and gravity of the problem situation. Cognition and perception are important in this process.
3. The individual may attempt to manage stress so he/she can continue to function as normally as possible. This includes denial, withdrawal, passive acceptance, undue optimism, avoidance, or even magical thinking.

According to the literature ([4], pp. 141–45), a distinction can be made between the positive and the negative coping skills. The positive ones are:

- Ability to orient oneself rapidly
- Planning of decisive action
- Mobilization of emergency problem-solving mechanisms
- Appropriate use of assistance resources
- Ability to deal simultaneously with affective dimensions of the experience and the tasks that must be carried out
- Appropriate expression of painful emotions
- Acknowledgment of pain, without obsession with troubled feelings
- Development of strategies to convert uncertainty into manageable risk
- Acknowledgment of increased dependency needs and seeking, receiving, and using assistance
- Tolerance of uncertainty without resorting to impulsive action
- Reaction to environmental challenges and recognition of their positive value for growth
- Use of nondestructive defenses and modes of tension relief to cope with anxiety

On the other hand, the negative coping skills are:

- Excessive denial, withdrawal, retreat, and avoidance
- Frequent use of fantasy and poor reality testing
- Impulsive behavior
- Venting rage on weaker individuals and creating scapegoats
- Being overdependent, clinging, and counter-dependent behavior
- Inability to evoke caring feelings from others
- Emotional suppression, leading to "hopeless-helpless-giving up" syndrome
- Use of hyper-ritualistic behavior with no purpose
- Fatigue and poor regulation of the rest-work cycle
- Addiction
- Inability to use support systems

When normal coping no longer works, different forms of mental health disbalance may occur. For the purpose of this chapter, we will limit ourselves to stress reactions, including burnout, acute stress reactions, and PTSD. These reactions are characterized by physical (sleep disturbance, nightmares, aches and pains, appetite and digestive changes, lowered resistance to colds and infection, persistent fatigue), emotional (mood swings, feeling unstable, anxiety, fear of recurrence, depression, grief, irritability, hostility, self-blame, shame, fragility, feeling vulnerable, numbness, detachment, fear of "contaminating" loved ones when sharing difficult experience, irritability, and lack of resistance to frustration), cognitive (intrusive memories, reactivation of previous traumatic events, preoccupation with the event, increased rigidity, resistance to new ideas, difficulty making decisions), behavioral (avoidance of reminders of the event, social relationship disturbances, difficulty connecting with "outsiders" and/or colleagues, lowered activity level, increased use of alcohol and drugs as a self-medication for depression and anxiety, loss of enthusiasm, avoidance of work, frequently late, lower productivity), and spiritual complaints ("Why me?" struggle, increased cynicism, loss of self-confidence, loss of purpose, renewed faith in higher being, profound existential questioning, loss of belief in cooperative spirit of mankind, disillusionment, loss of meaning, loss of life's objectives, feelings of alienation, changes in one's value system). All these reactions may have an obviously negative impact on one's professional functioning.

15.3 Impact of Stress on the Staff

The stress and support balance depicted in Fig. 15.1 ([2], p. 162) shows the equilibrium between factors that place stress on an individual and those that lessen it, also known as mitigating factors. Job-related and other stressors may result in burnout among aid workers and human service providers if no adequate and effective mitigating factors are in place, e.g. organizational support, supervision, self-care resources, and adequate training and education, to counterbalance these stressors. On the one hand, every effort should be made aiming at minimizing stressors, and on the other hand, mitigating factors should be instituted to decrease the risk for burnout.

Although humanitarian aid workers are generally able to adapt to acute and chronic stressors in their work, a disbalance between stress and mitigating factors impacts their mental health. Compassion fatigue, burnout, and hazardous alcohol drinking seem to be the most frequently observed consequences of a mental health disbalance.

Compassion fatigue is an understandable consequence of providing care to those who have experienced extreme or traumatic stressors. As compassion is one of the most important ingredients in encounters with survivors, its gradual lessening over time together with hopelessness, a decrease in experiences of pleasure, constant stress and anxiety, sleeplessness or nightmares, and a pervasive negative attitude can occur in helpers. Also, helpers may exhibit feelings of being overwhelmed by the work, which should be distinguished from feelings of fear associated with the work.

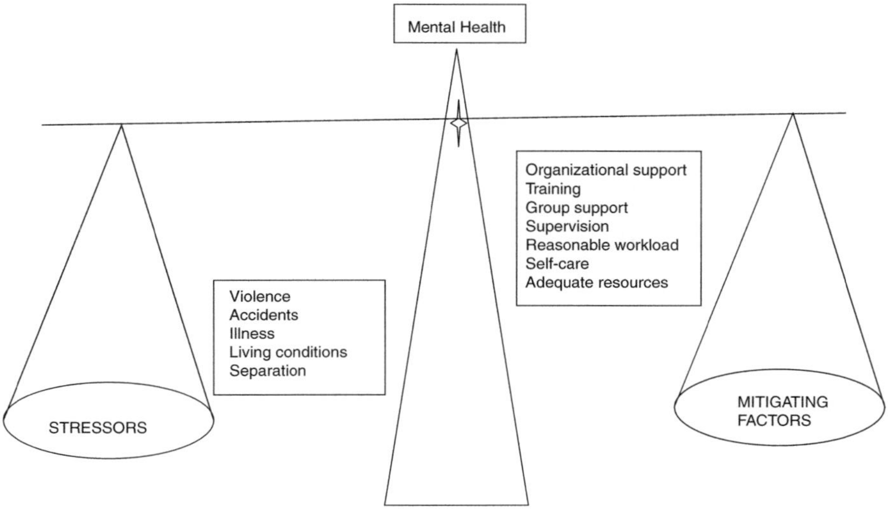

Fig. 15.1 Balance of stressors and mitigating factors in humanitarian aid workers and human service providers

There is no universally accepted definition of burnout. However, some researchers describe it as a psychological syndrome involving chronic emotional and interpersonal stressors that individuals experience in the workplace [6, 7]. Burnout refers to a complex of psychological responses to the stressors related to constant interaction with people in need. For instance, it can occur when nurses struggle to maintain high levels of empathy and caring in work situations where unrealized and unrealistic expectations are likely [8].

Two major contributors can explain the experience of burnout at work. These are the persistent imbalance of demands over resources and the conflict between personal values of employees and organization's values [9, 10]. Burnout is still predominantly considered as a social problem, but it has also been increasingly used as a diagnostic criterion in the medical world. The burnout diagnosis requires following symptoms to appear over a period of 2 weeks and in relation to work: (1) persistent and increased fatigue or weakness after a minimal effort, (2) a minimum of two distress symptoms (i.e., irritability, inability to relax), and (3) absence of other disorders such as mood or anxiety disorders (ICD-10) [2]. Those who experience burnout may suffer from sleep disturbances, work/family conflicts, physical illness, and substance abuse [11].

Last but not least, the recent UNHCR survey [4] of well-being and mental health of the staff reported that 25% of the respondents were classified as being at risk for hazardous alcohol drinking. Alcohol use is common in many societies as a means to enjoy oneself, relax, or unwind. It can play a big role within families, social groups, and traditions. Therefore, it is sometimes difficult to know how much alcohol consumption is too much. When people use alcohol as a coping mechanism to numb themselves from experiencing strong negative emotions or painful life circumstances, problems may arise. Controlled and moderate usage can quickly become abuse when it compromises one's own health and safety or that of those around. Hazardous alcohol use can lead to dangerous decisions, harmed relationships, and work and legal problems. Moreover, it can quickly lead to alcohol dependence, a condition in which a person feels that he/she needs alcohol just to survive.

15.4 Recent Research

The most comprehensive analysis of well-being of the staff working with refugees has consequently been recently undertaken by the UNHCR [4]. 2431 respondents participated in the study, accounting for 21% of the UNHCR's staff and its affiliate workforce. It was the first-ever comprehensive survey of risk for mental health outcomes, and it has focused on measuring the risk for anxiety, depression, PTSD, secondary stress, and burnout dimensions (emotional exhaustion (EE), personal accomplishment (PA), and depersonalization). In addition, the survey measured two behavioral outcomes: hazardous alcohol use and use of mental health services.

The objectives of the survey were to obtain baseline data on the prevalence of risk for mental health and behavioral outcomes among the UNHCR's workforce; to understand how these risks are related to the psychological hazards, such as exposure to traumatic events, exposure to working with people of concern, and exposure to workplace stress; and to help prioritize the focus of the Staff Welfare Section to where the needs are.

The results showed that the effort-reward imbalance (ERI), as a measure of workplace stress, had the strongest predictive value of risk for all mental health outcomes (anxiety, depression, PTSD, secondary stress, and burnout dimensions), but not for behavioral outcomes (hazardous alcohol drinking). The individuals at risk for ERI had a higher risk for mental health problems than those who reported experiencing traumatic situations. Exposure to traumatic events had a strong predictive value of risk for PTSD and secondary trauma and could also marginally predict the risk of depersonalization as a burnout dimension. Finally, this study found that as many as 38% of the respondents who worked directly with people of concern were at risk for secondary traumatic stress. As for other mental health and behavioral outcomes, the study found a significant and relatively strong relationship with burnout (respondents working with people of concern were less likely to be classified as being at risk for diminished personal accomplishment), hazardous alcohol use (respondents not working with people of concern were more at risk for hazardous alcohol use), and a weak relationship with the risk for anxiety (respondents working with people of concern were only marginally more likely to be classified at risk for developing anxiety). Working with people of concern could potentially be a positive factor in mental health, yet the level of risk for secondary traumatic stress and burnout might undermine this potential.

Most participants were somewhat to very satisfied with their jobs (43.8% somewhat satisfied and 35.7% very much satisfied). Job satisfaction was found to be moderately and negatively correlated to anxiety, depression, PTSD, secondary stress, and emotional exhaustion. This means that as job satisfaction increases, the chance of being at risk for these mental health outcomes decreases.

Given a high proportion of the staff being classified as at risk, percentage of the respondents who indicated that they needed to consult health services was understandably high (48.8%), yet only 26.4% of them actually consulted a mental health service. Of those at risk for each of the mental health and behavioral outcomes, as many as one third did not believe that they needed to contact a mental health service. Among those at risk who did feel a need for support, only a half sought help, mostly from mental health services within the United Nations (including UNHCR). The reason for this lack of uptake on an expressed need to consult mental health services warrants further investigation.

The main recommendations of the survey are in line with the goal of the UNHCR's People Strategy 2016–2021, issued recently [2], in which care and support for staff is one of the four key strategic goals. The survey emphasizes the importance of sustaining and further strengthening of the measures in place for support to colleagues following traumatic events, focusing on staff working in high-risk environments and particularly on national staff. In addition, the UNHCR should prioritize developing two corporate strategies to further enhance the staff's well-being in the organization: reduction of ERI and supporting staff working directly with people of concern. In that context, further qualitative research to obtain a more detailed understanding of ERI and of the use of mental health services should be foreseen.

15.5 How to Provide a Healthy Workplace?

A healthy workplace is not an added value, but a must. The World Health Organization (WHO) has in 2003 [3] published a widely used document describing a healthy workplace model for humanitarian aid workers that provides clear guidance on the basic standards and on the more elaborated elements. It is a comprehensive model of thinking and acting that addresses several important issues.

Organizations should consider their organizational systems and identify pitfalls and ways to aid helpers in accomplishing their goals. Thereby, they should always bear in mind that the helpers' needs are their own needs and that the constraints encountered in staff when performing their jobs are directly connected to the type of activities they are engaged in, exposing themselves to circumstances they would not be exposed to without the already mentioned working relationship. Besides making work interesting, often rewarding, and highly vocational, organizations should not minimize or indefinitely postpone staff rights.

Personnel working voluntarily with refugees put themselves in volatile, hazardous, or even intensely hostile locations, in order to support determination of their organization and of their own to operate and offer help in contexts where issues such as stability, security, the rule of law, humanitarian action, conflict resolution, human rights defense, and minimum living standards guarantee are a 24/7 challenge.

Employers and organizations are, therefore, morally and legally bound to ensure that their duty of care obligations are fulfilled. Duty of care is a complex term that the Voluntary Guidelines on the Duty of Care to Seconded Civilian Personnel structure around five standards that organizations need to consider and fulfill [12]. These are:

1. *Legal and regulatory compliance*: What are the relevant national and international legal and regulatory requirements to health, safety, and security of secondees?
2. *Safety and security risk management*: What kind of information does a seconding organization need to have, regarding safety and security risk management of a peace operation, in order to second staff with good conscience?
3. *Informed consent*: What kind of information does seconding and staff-receiving organizations need to provide to seconded personnel in order to allow secondees to make an informed decision about being deployed?
4. *Competent workforce*: What kind of experience, skills, and competencies does seconded personnel need to bring along in order to contribute to a success of a mission?
5. *Quality management*: How can seconding and staff-receiving organizations continually work on improving processes and measures for the benefit of their personnel, including work-related physical and psychosocial risks, promotion and support of healthy behaviors, and broader social and environmental determinants?

Therefore, a healthy workplace is the "one in which workers and managers collaborate to use a continual improvement process to protect and promote health, safety and wellbeing of all workers and sustainability of the workplace by considering the following, based on identified needs:

- health and safety concerns in the physical work environment;
- health, safety and wellbeing concerns in the psychosocial work environment including organization of work and workplace culture;
- personal health resources in the workplace (support and encouragement of healthy lifestyles by the employer);
- ways of participating in the community to improve the health of workers, their families and members of the community;
- minimizing stressors and risks that can be avoided" ([13], p. 11).

15.6 International Standards: Actions to Be Undertaken

An important step in protecting and enhancing mental health and well-being of humanitarian aid workers was the formulation of the Inter-Agency Standing Committee (2007) (IASC) Guidelines on Mental Health and Psychosocial Support in Emergency Settings [14]. This document presents a set of measures which are considered to be the golden standard in the field of humanitarian emergency work and are therefore also discussed in further chapters of this book. For the purpose of this chapter, we will shortly present the most relevant sections of the guidelines.

1. *Prepare staff for their jobs and for the emergency context*:
   (a) Ensure that national and international staff receive information on (a) their jobs (see key action 4 below) and (b) the prevailing environmental and security conditions and possible future changes in these conditions. Provide to international staff (and, when appropriate, to national staff) information on the local sociocultural and historical context, including:
   - Basic knowledge of the crisis and the world view(s) of the affected population
   - Basic information on local cultural attitudes and practices and systems of social organization
   - Basic information on staff behaviors that may cause offense in the local sociocultural context

   (b) Ensure that all staff receive adequate training on safety and security.
   (c) Ensure that all staff are briefed on a spectrum of stress identification (including but not restricted to traumatic stress) and stress management techniques and on any existing organizational policy for psychosocial support to staff.
   (d) Ensure that experienced field management staff are available.
2. *Facilitate a healthy working environment*:
   (a) Implement the organization's staff support policy, including a rest and recuperation (R&R) provision. When the environment provides no opportunities for non-work-related activities, then consider organizing a higher frequency of R&R opportunities.
   (b) Ensure appropriate food and hygiene for staff, taking into account their religion and culture.
   (c) Address excessive, unhealthy living practices, such as heavy alcohol use by workers.
   (d) Facilitate some privacy in accommodation (e.g. if possible, provide separate work and living places).
   (e) Define working hours and monitor overtime. Aim to divide the workload among staff. If a 24-hour, 7-days-a-week work pattern is essential in the first weeks of an emergency, then consider rotating staff in shifts. Eight-hour shifts are preferable, but if that is not possible, shifts should be no longer than 12 h. Twelve hours on and 12 h off is tolerable for a week or two during emergency situations, but it would be helpful to have an extra half-day added to rest schedules about every 5 days. The hotter or colder an environment, or the more intense the stress, the more breaks are required.
   (f) Facilitate communication between staff and their families and other preexisting support mechanisms.

3. *Address potential work-related stressors*:

   - Ensure clear and updated job descriptions.
   - Define objectives and activities.
   - Confirm with staff that their roles and tasks are clear.
   - Ensure clear lines of management and communication.

- Evaluate daily the security context and other potential sources of stress arising from the situation.
- Ensure sufficient supplies for staff security (bulletproof vests, communication equipment, etc.).
- Ensure equality between staff (national, international, lower and higher management) in the personal decision to accept security risks. Do not force national staff to take risks that international staff are not allowed or not willing to take.
- Organize regular staff or team meetings and briefings.
- Ensure adequate and culturally sensitive technical supervision (e.g. clinical supervision) for mental health and psychosocial support staff.
- Build teams, facilitate integration between national and international staff, and address intra-team conflict and other negative team dynamics.
- Ensure appropriate logistical backup and supply lines of materials.
- Ensure that members of senior management visit field projects regularly.

4. *Integrated support systems*

Activities and programming should be integrated as far as possible. Proliferation of stand-alone services, such as those dealing only with rape survivors or only with people with a specific diagnosis, such as PTSD, can create a highly fragmented care system. Activities that are integrated into wider systems (e.g. existing community support mechanisms, formal/nonformal school systems, general health services, general mental health services, social services, etc.) tend to reach more people, are often more sustainable, and tend to carry less stigma.

Apply a human rights framework through mental health and psychosocial support activities.

Example: Occupied Palestinian Territory, 2000

Adolescents agreed to use an adolescents' forum to advocate for their rights with Palestinian decision-makers; to use media to explain their situation, rights, and views on what should be done; to work as trained volunteers in health facilities; to conduct recreational activities for younger children; and to establish a peer-to-peer help.

5. *Conduct a multi-sectoral participatory assessment of protection threats and capacities*:
   (a) Conduct a situation analysis of protection concerns.
   (b) Conduct assessments in an ethical and appropriately participatory manner.
   (c) Include in the team members of the affected group who are trained and supported, provided they are viewed as impartial and it is safe for all involved.
   (d) Determine whether it is acceptable to discuss sensitive protection issues either with people individually or in group settings.
   (e) Identify in a range of settings (e.g. camps, routes followed by people collecting water or firewood, nonformal education sites, markets) protection threats

such as gender-based violence (GBV), attacks on civilians, forced displacement, abduction, recruitment of minors, trafficking, exploitation, hazardous labor, landmines, exposure to HIV/AIDS, and neglect of people in institutions.

However, avoid using a checklist approach, which may "blind" assessors to other or emerging protection threats.

(f) Avoid causing harm, ask questions such as:
- What factors cause the violence and who are the perpetrators?
- Are the perpetrators still present and are they intimidating local people or those who would offer protection?
- Has family separation occurred? Is it still happening?
- Where are separated or unaccompanied children?
- What has happened to elderly/disabled people?
- What has happened to those living in institutions and hospitals?
- What are the current safety/security concerns?
- Analyze local capacities for protection, asking questions such as:
- In the past, how did groups in the community handle protection threats such as these present now, and what are people doing at present?
- How has the crisis affected protection systems and coping mechanisms that were previously active?
- Where are those who would normally provide protection?
- Are some of the presumed protective resources—such as police, soldiers, peacekeepers or schools—creating protection threats?

6. *Facilitate the process of community identification of priority actions through participatory rural appraisal and other participatory methods*:

All communities contain effective, naturally occurring, psychosocial supports and sources of coping and resilience. Nearly all groups of people affected by an emergency include helpers to whom people turn for psychosocial support in times of need. In families and communities, steps should be taken at the earliest opportunity to activate and strengthen local supports and to encourage a spirit of community self-help. A self-help approach is vital, because having a measure of control over some aspects of their lives promotes people's mental health and psychosocial well-being following overwhelming experiences. Affected groups of people typically have formal and informal structures through which they organize themselves to meet collective needs. Even if these structures have been disrupted, they can be reactivated and supported as a part of the process of enabling an effective emergency response. Strengthening and building on existing local support systems and structures will enable locally owned, sustainable, and culturally appropriate community responses. In such an approach, the role of outside agencies is less to provide direct services, but to facilitate psychosocial supports and build capacities of locally available resources.

Discuss with key actors or community groups:

- Organizations that were once established in order to confront crisis and that may be reactivated
- Mechanisms (rituals, festivals, women's discussion groups, etc.) that have helped community members in the past to cope with tragedy, violence, or loss
- How the current situation has disrupted social networks and coping mechanisms
- How people have been affected by the crisis
- What priorities people should address in moving toward their vision of the future
- What actions would help people to achieve their priority goals
- What successful experiences of other organizations have been noticed in their and neighboring communities

7. *Provide short, participatory training sessions where appropriate, coupled with follow-up support*:

Where local support systems are incomplete or are too weak to achieve particular goals, it may be useful to train community workers, including volunteers, to perform tasks such as:

- Identifying and responding to the special needs of community members who are not functioning well
- Developing and providing supports in a culturally appropriate way
- Providing basic support, i.e. psychological first aid, to those acutely distressed after exposure to extreme stressors
- Creating mother-child groups for discussion and to provide stimulation for smaller children
- Assisting families, where appropriate, with problem-solving strategies and knowledge about child-rearing
- Identifying, protecting, and ensuring care for separated children
- Including people with disabilities in various activities
- Supporting survivors of gender-based violence
- Facilitating release and integration of boys and girls associated with fighting forces and armed groups
- Setting up self-help groups
- Engaging youth, e.g. in positive leadership, organizing youth clubs, sports activities, conflict resolution dialogue, education on reproductive health, and other life skills training
- Involving adults and adolescents in practical, purposeful, common interest activities, e.g. constructing/organizing shelters, organizing family tracing, distributing food, cooking, sanitation, organizing vaccinations, and teaching children
- Referring affected people to relevant legal, health, livelihood, nutrition, and social services, if appropriate and available

8. *Make psychological support for survivors of extreme stressors available*:
   (a) Most individuals experiencing acute mental distress following exposure to extremely stressful events are best supported without medication. All aid workers, and especially health workers, should be able to provide very basic psychological first aid (PFA). PFA is often mistakenly seen as a clinical or emergency psychiatric intervention. Rather, it is a description of a humane, supportive response to a fellow human being who is suffering and who may need support. PFA is very different from psychological debriefing in that it does not necessarily involve a discussion of the event that caused the distress. PFA encompasses:
      - Protecting from further harm (in rare situations, very distressed persons may take decisions that put them at further risk of harm). Where appropriate, inform distressed survivors of their right to refuse to discuss the events with (other) aid workers or with journalists.
      - Providing the opportunity for survivors to talk about the events, but without pressure. Respect the wish not to talk and avoid pushing for more information than the person may be ready to give.
      - Listening patiently in an accepting and nonjudgmental manner.
      - Conveying genuine compassion.
      - Identifying basic practical needs and ensuring that these are met.
      - Asking for people's concerns and trying to address these.
      - Discouraging negative ways of coping (specifically discouraging coping through use of alcohol and other substances, explaining that people in severe distress are at much higher risk of developing substance use problems).
      - Encouraging participation in normal daily routines (if possible) and use of positive means of coping (e.g. culturally appropriate relaxation methods, accessing helpful cultural and spiritual supports).
      - Encouraging, but not forcing, company from one or more family member or friends.
      - As appropriate, offering possibility to return for further support.
      - As appropriate, referring to locally available support mechanisms or to trained clinicians.
   (b) In a minority of cases, when severe acute distress limits basic functioning, clinical treatment will probably be needed (for guidance, see *Where There Is No Psychiatrist* under Key Resources ([14], pp. 119–20)). If possible, refer a patient to a clinician trained and supervised in helping people with mental disorders. Clinical treatment should be provided in combination with (other) formal or informal supports.
   (c) With regard to clinical treatment of acute distress, benzodiazepines are greatly overprescribed in most emergencies. However, this medication may be appropriately prescribed for a very short time for certain specific clinical problems (e.g. severe insomnia). Nevertheless, caution is required as use of

benzodiazepines may sometimes quickly lead to dependence, especially among very distressed persons. Also, various experts have argued that benzodiazepines may slow down a recovery process after exposure to extreme stressors.

(d) In most cases, acute distress will decrease naturally, without outside intervention, over time. However, in a minority of cases, a chronic mood or anxiety disorder (including severe PTSD) will develop. If the disorder is severe, it should be treated by a trained clinician as a part of the minimum emergency response. If the disorder is not severe (e.g. one is able to function and tolerate suffering), then the person should receive appropriate care as a part of a more comprehensive aid response. Where appropriate, support for these cases may be given by trained and clinically supervised community health workers (e.g. social workers, counselors) linked to health services.

The most common approach [15] to lowering stress in humanitarian aid workers upon exposure to traumatic incidents or distressful situations is to set up peer support groups in which staff members can share and ventilate their feelings and seek solutions. The group approach has the advantage of building a team spirit in those facing difficult conditions and providing collective support for those who may be more vulnerable at any given moment. It is recognized that when support groups function well:

- The stressors are accepted as real and legitimate.
- The problem is viewed as a problem for the entire group and not as a problem that is limited to the individual.
- The general approach to the problem is to seek solutions, not to assign blame.
- There is a high level of tolerance for individual disturbance.
- Support is expressed clearly, directly, and abundantly in the form of praise, commitment, and affection.
- Communication is open and effective; there are few sanctions against what can be said. The quality of communication is good, and messages are clear and direct.
- There is a high degree of cohesion.
- There is a considerable flexibility of roles, and individuals are not rigidly restricted from assuming different roles. Resources—material, social, and institutional—are utilized efficiently.
- There is no subculture of violence (emotional outbursts are not a form of violence).
- There is no substance abuse.

Broadly used techniques following critical incidents can be used in distressful situations encountered by helpers working with refugees, in order to enhance resilience and psychological recovery. They can be executed on a group level and outside of the incident scene, in a place considered safe by the participants.

Two different and complementary techniques include [16]:

The emotional deactivation (defusing)

The defusing consists of a group encounter, brief and semi-structured, which usually takes place after a critical incident. It is a process that allows those who have been involved in a critical incident to describe what has happened and to talk about their immediate reactions. In the aftermath of such an incident, the emotions of sadness, anxiety, fear, frustration, etc. are so intense that people prefer to deny them. The defusing facilitates immediate expression of emotions in order to start emotional recovery of the professional and to prevent intensity of emotions from interfering with his/her rest. The defusing must take place within hours of the event and should be short and direct. It is a psychological intervention in which a person, not necessarily a psychologist, facilitates a responder in a traumatogenic event to express everything he/she needs: sensations, emotions, thoughts, etc. Likewise, during this process, information and resources are provided to handle the situation adequately.

Organization of the memory (debriefing)

Memory of an event that had a strong emotional impact is sharp and intense but incomplete and unclear as to what actually happened in the space-time sequence of the event. This prevents participants from integrating what has happened and seeing it in terms of a past event. Looking back at what has happened and sharing memories, is a means to regain aspects of the story of which one is unaware and to facilitate creation of a more complete and coherent memory. This technique can be applied individually and/or in a group setting and should take place at least 48–72 h after the event occurred. The technique is not a psychotherapy, but it is based on the principles of crisis intervention and on the idea that an individual has sufficient resources to manage his/her own crisis. It is very important that the debriefing is conducted by staff with training and experience in the technique in order to prevent re-traumatization of the helper.

9. *Learn about cultural, religious, and spiritual supports and coping mechanisms.* Once rapport has been established, ask questions such as:

- What do you believe are the spiritual causes and effects of the emergency?
- How have people been affected culturally or spiritually?
- What should happen when people have died?
- Are there rituals or cultural practices that could be conducted, and what would be the appropriate timing for them?
- Who can best provide guidance on how to conduct these rituals and handle a burial of bodies?
- Who in a community would greatly benefit from specific cleansing or healing rituals and why?
- Are you willing to advise international workers present in this area on how to support people spiritually and how to avoid spiritual harm?

If feasible, make repeated visits to build trust and learn more about religious and cultural practices. Also, if possible, confirm information collected by discussing it with local anthropologists or other cultural guides with an extensive knowledge of local culture and practices.

10. Adapt the information to address specific needs of subgroups of the population as appropriate.

Different subgroups within a population may have particular ways of coping that are different from those of the population in general. Develop separate information on positive coping mechanisms for subgroups as appropriate (e.g. men, women, and (other) specific groups at risk: see Chap. 1). Consider including a special focus on "children's coping" and "teenagers' coping," noting in the latter that short-term coping methods such as drinking or taking drugs are likely to cause long-term harm.

Last but not least, it is of utmost importance that social interventions continue after the acute emergency, including promotion of functional, culture-sensitive coping mechanisms. Moreover, efforts should be directed toward establishing a more comprehensive range of community-based mental health interventions in a post-conflict setting. The type of proposed intervention should take into account emotional needs of the helpers.

15.7 A Case Study: Mental Health of Helpers in Georgia

The first-ever study of secondary traumatic stress and professional burnout in helpers assisting internally displaced persons and refugees in Georgia was carried out in 2015 [17]. Its aims were to explore relationships between secondary traumatization (ST) and professional burnout (PB), empathy and quality of life, exposure to trauma narratives, coping strategies, and mechanisms for preventing PB, including organizational measures.

Participants were mental health professionals from various services in the country. They were all involved in assisting refugees and internally displaced persons subjected to abuse and ill-treatment, survivors of torture and cruel treatment, ex-prisoners, childhood trauma survivors, ambiguous loss trauma survivors (family members who lost their dear ones without any trace), and children survivors of abuse, neglect, and violence experiences. The services operate through multidisciplinary teams, both at treatment centers and via field work. The number of clients per service differs from 200 to 600 per year.

The instruments used in the study were as follows: Professional Quality of Life Scale (ProQOL) [18, 19], Empathy Questionnaire [20], Coping Styles Questionnaire [21], and a questionnaire designed for the purpose of the study in order to collect information on the type of services that a professional is offering to clients, whether a professional is directly exposed to trauma narrative, and which measures they undertake to deal with professional stress.

The sample of the study consisted of psychiatrists (16.7%), psychologists and psychotherapists (43%), social workers (16.7%), and medical doctors, nurses, and lawyers (23.3%). Response rate was 84%. A total of 30 helpers participated in the study (27% female and 3% male). The average working experience in a trauma center was 7 years, while on average total working experience was 13 years.

The average score on the ProQOL was 40.13, which is considered to be an average level of professional satisfaction. PB score was 29.87, suggesting a moderate level of burnout. As for ST, the average score was 24.33, indicating a moderate and acceptable degree of ST.

Dominant coping styles were rational (28.13) and detached (20.00) coping, while avoidant (14.07) and emotional (13.3) coping strategies were less evident. Thus, the sample was using more adaptive than maladaptive coping.

3.3% of the respondents were directly and very often exposed to traumatic narratives in their daily work, and 13.3% were exposed frequently. 53.3% of the sample reported that they were not listening to clients' stories often, while 30% was rarely exposed to trauma narratives.

3.3% of the respondents were frequently attending intervision sessions, 13.3% were engaged often in such sessions, 20.0% attended them occasionally, and 63.3% rarely took part in them.

As for supervision sessions, 50% of the sample reported that they rarely attended, 33.3% attended occasionally, 33.3% were engaged often, and 6.7% attended supervision very often.

Majority of the respondents (53.3%) cared about their health (physical and mental) rarely, 27.7% occasionally, 16.7% often, and only 3.3% cared about their health on a regular basis. The list of measures taken to care about one's health included socialization (73.3%), physical activities/exercise (56.7%), relaxation (56.7%), having fun (46.7%), professional help seeking (13.3%), reading (13.3%), and other (46.7%).

The respondents have also evaluated measures for staff care taken by their respective organizations. They indicated that only 13.3% of the organizations take care and implement relevant measures of prevention on a regular basis, while 6.7% indicated that such measures were never implemented. Interventions implemented by the organizations were supervision (36.7%), intervision (26.7%), informal socialization (36.7%), education and trainings (6.7%), and others (23.3%).

The medium indexes of ST and PB in those who were directly exposed to clients' narratives/trauma histories were, respectively, 29.6 and 34.4, while in those who have seldom listened to such stories, the indexes were, respectively, 24.0 and 29.31.

The survey illustrated that the average PB level in helpers who were seldom engaged in intervision was 28.63 and for ST 23.05, while, interestingly, these levels in helpers who were often engaged in such interventions reached 33.2 and 29.8, respectively.

The average index of ST among those who were engaged in supervision sessions also showed interesting dynamics: the ST score among those who often took part in SV was 29.2, in those who seldom attended 22.4, and in those who occasionally attended, it was 24.0.

In helpers who rarely took care about their health (physical and mental), the professional satisfaction level was 41.4, and the ST score was 19.60, while these levels were 42.44 and 26.78 among those who often and regularly payed attention to their health needs.

The statistical analysis illustrated further that TS was in high correlation with PB (Pearson coefficient 0.602 ($P < 0.05$) (see Fig. 15.2)) and that the correlation between empathy and PB was also positive/medium (Pearson coefficient 0.47 ($P < 0.05$)), as well as between empathy and ST (Pearson coefficient 0.423 ($P < 0.05$) (see Figs. 15.3 and 15.4)).

The study illustrated that the Georgian professionals who assist refugees and other traumatized populations exhibit medium levels of ST and PB, as well as average levels of professional satisfaction. The data suggested that they, despite average scores, are still at risk for ST and PB. This group is inclined to adaptive coping and

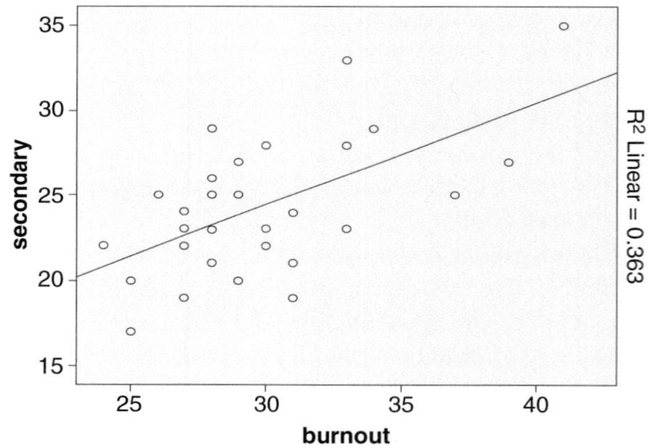

Fig. 15.2 Secondary traumatization and professional burntout

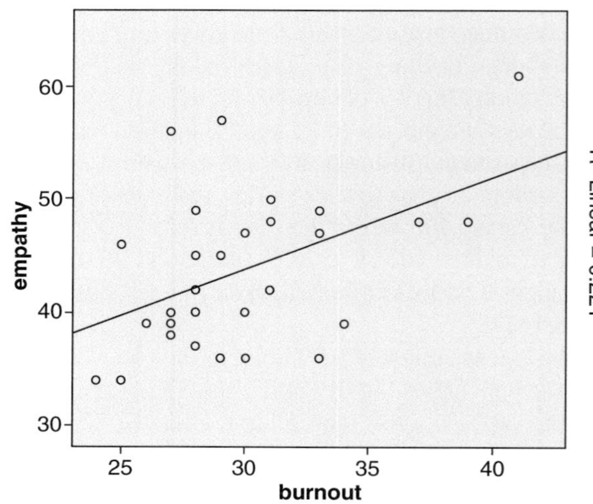

Fig. 15.3 Empathy and professional burnout

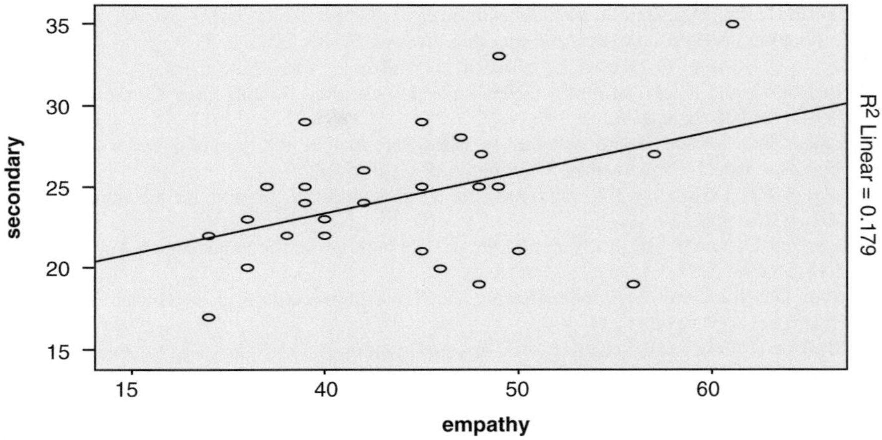

Fig. 15.4 Correlation of empathy and secondary traumatization

also pays attention to their physical and mental health needs. The positive associations were revealed among empathy and ST and PB, as well as direct exposure to trauma histories: those who directly worked with clients are at higher risks of ST and PB then other helpers involved in case management only.

The surprising finding of higher scores of ST and PB among helpers who were engaged in intervision and supervision sessions probably indicates a need and drive among those feeling more affected by the work to seek collegial consultancy and support, though this finding needs further exploration.

Conclusion

An organizational culture founded on a supportive attitude and environment toward employees has a very important role in approaching mental health of humanitarian workers. It is not sufficient to focus on coping mechanisms of the individual helpers. The manner in which an organization engages with its staff in order to communicate reassurance, commitment, and respect is vital. Without that, any psychosocial support to employees will fail to improve their mental health. Identification and facilitation of other protection mechanisms are also needed when helpers are exposed to abnormal situations, which may overwhelm their coping capacities.

References

1. Allen JG. Traumatic relationships and serious mental disorders. New York: Wiley; 2001.
2. Mollica RF, Guerra R, Bhasin R, Lavelle J, editors. International Congress of Ministers of Health for Mental Health and Post-Conflict Recovery. Book of the best practices. Trauma and role of mental health in post-conflict recovery; 2004. pp. 87–265.

3. World Health Organization. Mental health in emergencies: mental and social aspects of health in populations exposed to extreme stressors. Geneva: WHO; 2003. p. 37.
4. Suzic D, Roslyn T, Jachens L, Mihalca L, Wairoa Z, Brossard-Salazar C, editors. Staff well-being and mental health in UNHCR. Geneva: United Nations High Commissioner for Refugees; 2016. p. 110–1.
5. Cohen RE. Mental health services in disasters: manual for humanitarian workers. Pan American Health Organization: Washington, D.C; 2000. 92 p.
6. Cordes CL, Dougherty TW. A review and an integration of research on job burnout. Acad Manag Rev. 1993;18:621–56.
7. Maslach C, Leiter MP. Early predictors of job burnout and engagement. J Appl Psychol. 2008;93:498–512.
8. Blair DT, Ramones VA. Understanding vicarious traumatization. J Psychosoc Nurs Ment Health Serv. 1996;34(11):24–30.
9. Maslach C, Leiter MP, Schaufeli WB. Measuring burnout. In: Cooper CL, Cartwright S, editors. The Oxford handbook of organizational well-being. Oxford: Oxford University Press; 2009. p. 86–108.
10. Schaufeli WB, Leiter MP, Maslach C. Burnout: 35 years of research and practice. Career Dev Int. 2009;14(3):204–20.
11. Swider B, Zimmerman R. Born to burnout: a meta-analytic path model of personality, job burnout, and work outcomes. J Vocat Behav. 2010;76(3):487–506.
12. Merkelbach M, Kelly V, Berghe V, editors. Voluntary Guidelines on the Duty of Care to Seconded Civilian Personnel. Swiss Federal Department of Foreign Affairs (FDFA), Stabilisation Unit (SU) and Center for International Peace Operations (ZIF); 2017.
13. World Health Organization. Healthy workplaces: a model for action: for employers, workers, policymakers and practitioners. Geneva: World Health Organization WHO; 2010. p. 11.
14. IASC. Guidelines on mental health and psychosocial support in emergency settings. Geneva: Inter-Agency Standing Committee; 2007. p. 119–20.
15. Árpád B, Da Victoria Lobo A, Hoxha-Beganovic RD, Jaffé P, Motus N, Szilárd I, Tudorache D, Venelinova R, Weekers J. The mental health of trafficking in human beings – a set of minimum standards. Budapest: International Organization for Migration IOM; 2004. p. 141–5.
16. Urruzuno JM, Espinosa I, Izquierdo R, De la Puerta C. Manual Psicosocial para intervinientes en Emergencias. Academia vasca de policía y Emergencia; 2012. pp. 75–6.
17. Latibashvili T. Secondary traumatization and professional burn-out [master's thesis]; 2015 [unpublished].
18. Stamm BH. Professional quality of life: compassion satisfaction and fatigue [Internet]. Version 5; 2009 [Cited April 12, 2017]. Available from www.isu.edu/~bhstamm or www.proqol.org.
19. Stamm BH. The concise ProQOL manual [Internet]. 2nd ed. Pocatello; 2010. Available from http://ProQOL.org.
20. Baron-Cohen S, Wheelwright S. The empathy quotient: an investigation of adults with asperger syndrome or high functioning autism, and normal sex differences. J Autism Dev Disord. 2004;34(2):163–75.
21. Rogers D, Jarvis G, Najarian B. Detachment and coping: the construction and validation of a new scale for measuring coping strategies. Personal Individ Differ. 1993;15(6):619–26.

Part III

Physical Health: From Refugee Camps to the Health Care System in Host Countries

Medical Aspects of Health Care: Reflections from the Field Experience in European Countries and an Overview of the Basic Health Needs

16

Michael Kuehnel, Boris Drožđek, and Thomas Wenzel

Abstract

This chapter aims at presenting a basic introduction to primary health-care needs of refugees during transit and in camps. These include challenges like emergency and first-line treatments, water preparation, hygiene and vaccinations but also recognition of long-term health-care-related needs. The chapter is based on the international standards and on practical (field) experience with the refugees recently arrived in Europe. However, it does not intend to replace handbooks on refugee and migrant medicine.

16.1 Introduction

When refugees reach a host country, their struggle for health and well-being continues, and their lives remain precarious. Besides general risks to physical and psychological health conditions, health of refugees can be complicated by pre-existing conditions contracted in their home countries, illnesses picked up during flight and those related to specific living conditions in a host country. On top of this, refugees bring with their sociocultural backgrounds and medical habits which can be as diverse as countries and regions they originate from are. Understanding these backgrounds and habits is essential in providing effective aid.

M. Kuehnel (✉)
Water, Sanitation and Hygiene (WASH), Public Health and Tropical Medicine, Vienna, Austria

B. Drožđek
PsyQ/Parnassia Group, Rosmalen/Eindhoven, The Netherlands
e-mail: drozdek@telfort.nl

T. Wenzel
World Psychiatric Association Scientific Section,
Psychological Aspects of Persecution and Torture, Geneva, Switzerland

T. Wenzel, B. Drožđek (eds.), *An Uncertain Safety*,
https://doi.org/10.1007/978-3-319-72914-5_16

To keep refugees healthy, the camps within a host country must meet basic needs, like water, showers, toilets and waste management, basic medical services, as well as maintenance of the minimum quality standards of these services. Any crisis situation responses described in the following chapter should not only respect medical and psychosocial needs of refugees, but also the respective human rights standards, as outlined in several other chapters in this book (see, e.g. [1–3]).

16.2 Flight

Observing the 2016 flight routes which refugees have used in order to reach Europe, three main routes can be defined:

- The first one is the, so-called, Balkan Route that goes via Turkey and Greece, up to the north of Europe, with refugees travelling on foot, by cars, trucks or trains [4, 5].
- After the Balkan Route was closed, the second route arose and quickly gained in popularity—the one by boat from Turkey to the Greek islands. After the contract signed between the European Union (EU) and Turkey, this route was also made almost unavailable.
- The third route many refugees have chosen is to cross the Mediterranean Sea by boat, from Libya to the Italian island of Lampedusa. This is the nearest EU territory, approximately 300 km away from the North African coast.
- Other routes are continuously developing and are expected to carry further specific risks and conditions with.

On the routes across land, refugees were, where possible, assisted by different NGOs (mainly the local Red Cross, Caritas, Medécins sans Frontières (MSF) and others [5]) which were taking care of their basic needs in transit, though frequently without support of local governments, and having to deal with a shortage of food, medical support and sometimes clothes for refugees in need.

The route across the Mediterranean Sea was the most dangerous one. In 2016 alone, more than 5000 people officially died trying to reach the EU.[1] They have used boats which were unsuitable for the trip and overloaded with people, being the main reasons why many of them sunk. Numerous NGOs also began to use ships in order to take care of the refugees on boats and to guide them safely to Italy or Malta. The first author was part of a team on such a ship in November 2016. Based on observations in rescuing more than 1100 people in 14 days, the most common diseases observed in the rescued refugees were:

- Hypothermia, because of duration of the journey and weather conditions (more than 200 out of 1100)
- Burns from fuel and added chemicals (more than 20 out of 1100)

[1] International Organization for Migration, recent data at https://www.iom.int, accessed 1.7.2017

- Scabies (more than 30 out of 1100)
- Breathing problems because of aspiration of fuel and/or sea water (5 out of 1100)
- Minor injuries which people sustained because of their flight (such as blisters, feeling exhausted, hypoglycaemia)

Pasta [6] reported that in the 378 refugees rescued and taken to hospitals in Lampedusa (Italy) between January 2011 and June 2014, women were hospitalised almost exclusively for obstetric-gynaecological problems and men were hospitalised mainly for "bone fractures, burns, dehydration, infectious diseases, suicide attempts, and, … for CO poisoning of people locked in the holds of boats", with 20 cases of tuberculosis. Another study [7], using data collected from 2656 refugees between May and September 2015 from a German Naval Force frigate, observed that 16.9% of them were classified as "medical treatment required" at first assessment. The authors found dermatological diseases in 55.4, followed by internal diseases in 27.7 and trauma in 12.1% of the sample. The authors also observed that the first preliminary assessment to identify those in need of treatment was usually correct, as status of those being healthy did not change at a later evaluation.

When taking refugees on board, NGOs should be aware of the minimum standards of medical treatment they can provide and of the minimum requirements necessary to keep refugees healthy, for example, serving hot tea to prevent hypothermia and providing clothes, blankets and other objects. The standards developed by the Sphere Project can, hereby, be used as a guideline.[2]

WHO has summarised the characteristic challenges in such mass emergencies (Fig. 16.1).

16.3 Transitional and Permanent Refugee Camps

After reaching a safe heaven, refugees are most often settled in refugee camps. These can be of a transitional or of a permanent character. A comparison of transitional and permanent camps in Central Europe, Africa, Asia or other places can reveal a variety of different needs and standards. The minimum requirements which should be kept worldwide are again described in the Sphere Handbook, which suggests standards for the different environments [8].

16.3.1 Transitional Camps

Transitional camps are defined by their ability to produce a safe place for refugees, "a shelter which provides a habitable covered living space and a secure, healthy living environment, with privacy and dignity, to those within it, during the period between a conflict or natural disaster and the achievement of a durable shelter solution" [9, 10].

[2] www.sphereproject.org/handbook/, accessed 1.7.2017

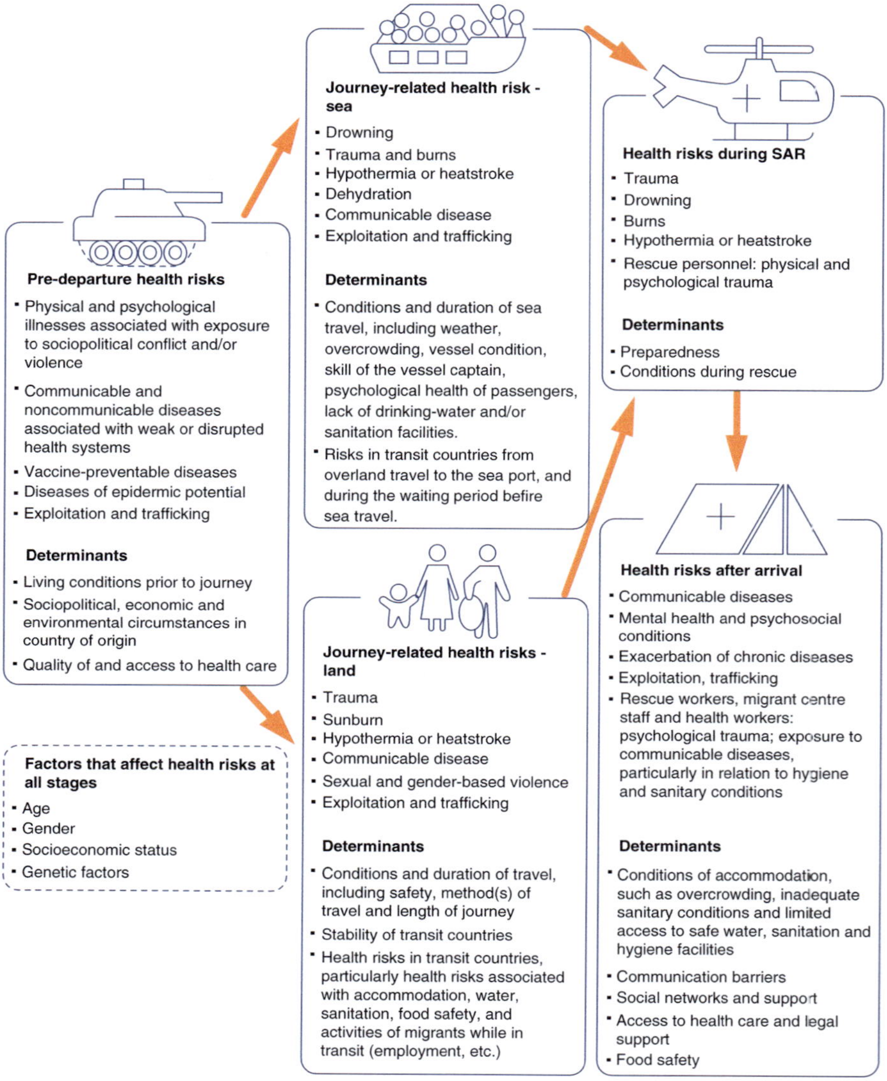

Fig. 16.1 An overview of health risks in refugees. From: Toolkit for assessing health system capacity to manage large influxes of refugees, asylum seekers and migrants, ISBN 978 92 890 5203 0, ©World Health Organization 2016, also online at www.who.org

To (Fig. 16.2) understand the basic hygiene needs in transitional camps, we have to divide them into two types:

(a) Transitional camps in which people stay for one or two nights. People on the move usually arrive, have a shower, a meal and a sleep, and then move on.

(b) Transitional camps in which people stay for an undetermined longer period of time. This period can last from several days up to several months, but still the camp is not considered to be a permanent settlement (Fig. 16.3).

16.3.2 Permanent Camps

Permanent camps have structures and sociocultural aspects different from the transitional ones. The residents usually try to build up and modify camps in order to

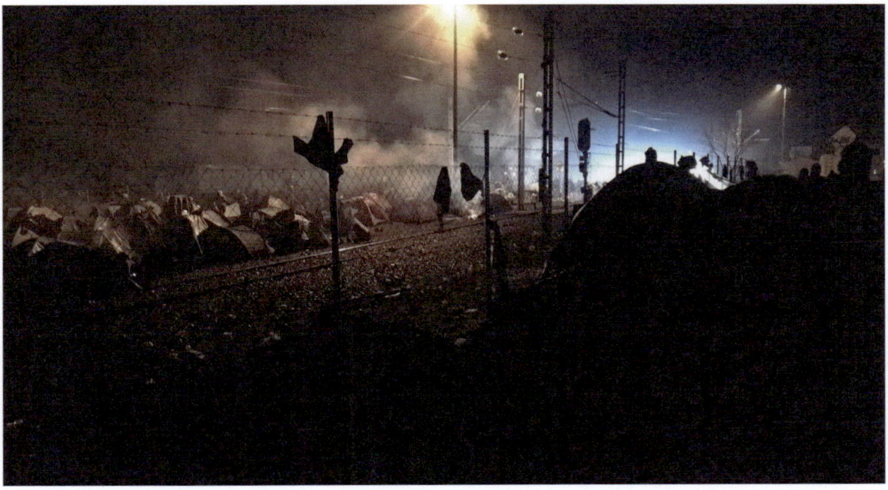

Fig. 16.2 Idomeni, Greece, February, 2016

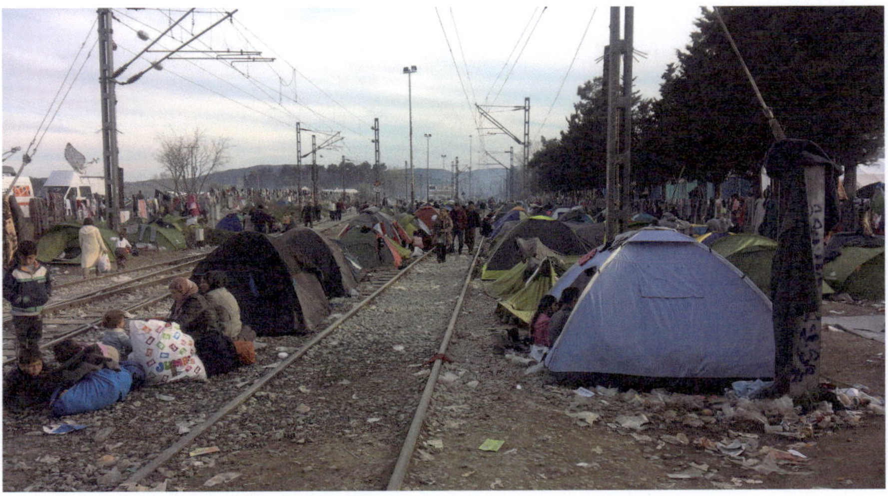

Fig. 16.3 Idomeni, Greece, February, 2016

create an environment in which they feel comfortable. Often these camps resemble a small village with its own communal life and structures but also with specific problems as, for example, in Jordan [11, 12].

16.3.3 Community-Based Approaches

A community-based approach [12] is a synonym for involving people living in the area in which camps are to be built in planning and activities, as outlined in several other chapters in this book. Local population might fear the newcomers arriving from a different country and/or having a different religion or a skin colour. Perhaps even more of an issue is a belief that the newcomers may bring with "new" diseases, like tuberculosis, malaria or even Ebola.

Therefore, local population living next to the camp should be informed about risks of contracting illnesses. Most of their fears may be unrealistic. Illnesses like dengue, malaria, yellow fever or others transmitted via vectors, like the *Anopheles* mosquito, need a vector for transmission. While in Turkey or Greece, infection may be possible because the vector can grow locally, absence of the vector in, for example, middle Europe means that there is no risk whatsoever for spreading of these diseases.

Some illnesses, like tuberculosis, are more prevalent within a refugee community than in the general population [13]. Refugees living in close quarters, as they do in camps, can be more easily exposed to germs which are transmitted via air or droplet. This leads to high rates of infection within the camps, but not necessarily outside. In this case, vectors are not needed for transmission, and close exposure to an infected individual is crucial for transmitting a disease [14].

16.4 Culture and Medical Background

16.4.1 Medical Systems

Health-care system in refugees' countries of origin and their medical "culture" in terms of the use of health care should be taken into account. They are a part of refugees' background, and they shape their expectations from and participation in the health-care system of a host country.

Using Austria as an example for European host countries, the key health indicators in countries where the most refugees in Austria originated from in 2015 are listed below:

Maternal mortality rate	
Syria	68/1000
Iraq	50/1000
Afghanistan	396/1000
Austria	4/1000

Infant mortality rate	
Syria	112/1000
Iraq	27/1000
Afghanistan	66/1000
Austria	31/1000
Under the age of 5 mortality rate	
Syria	13/1000 (2015)
Iraq	32/1000 (2015)
Afghanistan	91/1000 (2015)
Austria	4/1000 (2015)[3]

These key indicators suggest that Syria had a more developed health-care system compared to Iraq and Afghanistan. Comparing medical systems that refugees have been accustomed to in their home countries can help understanding their expectations from health-care systems and help seeking in host countries. In 2016, Syrian refugees explained the health-care system in their country before the war to the first author: "Visiting a hospital was the cheapest way of getting a treatment. This service was free of charge for people. Visiting a general practitioner had to be paid by a patient. This is one of the reasons why Syrian refugees prefer visiting hospitals".

The health-care system in Afghanistan was different, as reported in the World Health Organization's (WHOs) recent "Health System Profile Afghanistan".[4] This document summarised its key features: "After the collapse of the Taliban regime the health system passed the emergency and conflict period and now is in the post-conflict and developmental phase. For the first three years of the transitional Islamic state of Afghanistan, the health system was more prevention focused and more emphasis was placed on the delivery of the "Basic Package of Health Services"". Iraq has other severe problems that can illustrate specific difficulties in the region, as outlined in the WHO Health System Profile for this country: "There is no reported history of [the] existence of a social health insurance system.… Financing in general and since the fall of the last regime in 2003 is through the Ministry of Finance except for some limited number of beds in nursing homes mainly in Baghdad and some few governorates, where patients are being charged for admissions and medical interventions".[5]

16.4.2 Cultural Differences: Body and Psyche

Some refugees in a camp may consequently want to visit hospitals or outpatient departments for treatment of minor problems. Others may demand antibiotics, special services or examinations for no apparent medical reason, just because they have

[3] Worldbank: http://data.worldbank.org/, accessed 1.07.2017

[4] apps.who.int/medicinedocs/documents/s17666en/s17666en.pdf, accessed 1.07.2017

[5] apps.who.int/medicinedocs/documents/s17295e/s17295e.pdf, accessed 1.07.2017

been used to this approach in their home countries. They can also be anxious or non-compliant with treatment schedules based on their cultural health belief models (a factor explored in more detail by Kienzler et al. [15]). For example, it is quite common in the Middle East to receive an intramuscular injection of particular antibiotics, like penicillin. On the other hand, health professionals in the most parts of Europe prefer to administer this antibiotic orally. Therefore, refugees who are not accustomed to taking this medication orally may show a very low compliance with their antibiotic treatment.

Migrants and refugees may also frequently seek help of traditional healers or use traditional drugs instead of treatment by "Western" medicine ("alternative" use of traditional medicines) [16, 17]. Von Andel [18] documented, for example, the reported use of more than 140 different plants in a study based on interviews with 210 first- and second-generation Surinamese migrants in the Netherlands. A parallel, complimentary treatment can lead to complications, especially when the herbs used conflict with biomedical treatment procedures. Therefore, unclear composition and possible toxicity of herbal medicines being a part of traditional healing practices and health belief systems [19] should be taken into consideration when delivering treatment (see also [15]), as observed by Ramzan and colleagues among migrants from Pakistan in Denmark [20]. In most countries there is also an illegal market for drugs, and refugees may buy and use not clearly labelled, habit forming or else inadequate medications. Differences in the cytochrome system [21–24] involved in the metabolisation of drugs [25] and some traditional herbal medicines are a further common but frequently neglected problem in refugees, as documented, for example, in the Hmong refugees [21]. Such ethnic differences in drug metabolism must be considered in most areas of medical treatment, including haemostaseology [26]. Unexpected side effects, complications or either increase or decrease of plasma levels of medical drugs can be observed as a result of this problem [21, 25].

16.4.3 Somatic Symptoms?

A patient's selective presentation with "somatic" symptoms due to a stigma of suffering from mental health problems, like in a depressed person [27–29], might lead to establishing of a psychiatric diagnosis of "somatoform" or "conversion" disorder according to the DSM or ICD systems (defined as a divergence between physical findings and a degree of suffering reported by a patient). However, this presentation might also be seen as a cultural idiom of distress or a culture-based representation style (cultural formulation) of a common mental health problem, as described again by Kienzler et al. [15]. Still, not all apparently "psychosomatic" syndromes should be seen as an exclusion diagnosis for somatic disorders. In some ethnic groups, somatic disorders common in a geographical region can also be experienced and presented as "psychological" culture-bound syndromes or idioms of distress [30], as demonstrated by Volpato [31] for the "Eghindi" syndrome caused by osmotic imbalance and salt intake in the Western Saharan refugees.

16.4.4 Health Literacy

The important concept of health literacy [32, 33] should be applied with care and might include a necessary learning process in both a patient and a health-care professional in a transcultural, culture-sensitive setting. This was earlier proposed by Na et al. [34], who argued for a "culturally responsive framework for mental health literacy". Traditional medicines, their related practices and health belief systems are usually developed as a part of a comprehensive cultural system [35] reflecting adaptation processes of a group in a certain physical, psychological, and social environment. Cultural health belief systems are dynamic and change over time, as demonstrated by Carruth in Somalia, who perceives them as "changing and pluralistic health cultures" instead of static concepts [17]. They should be understood, respected and discussed together with a patient, although international standards might require challenging such concepts held in a refugee community.

Awareness of such background factors helps in understanding refugees' needs and fears, and assists with creating adequate strategies for integration of refugees into a health-care system of a host country.

16.5 Medical Help

When large numbers of refugees arrive in host countries having no adequate governmental plan or response, as is the case in the most EU countries at the moment, a challenge arises as of how to deal with a substantial demand for medical help in a refugee population. The UNHCR guidelines, as discussed by Weissbecker et al. [1], are not always followed upon nor immediately implemented by local partners or governments. In many host countries, NGOs are helping refugees with their health needs in the beginning. However, the longer a crisis situation lasts, the less volunteers can be mobilised. In the early phase of a crisis, people mostly feel compassionate with fate of refugees. But after some time, compassion may decrease, and a local government of a host country has to take over all major tasks in a coordinated way. Depending on a number of refugees, local country policies and a capacity of a health-care system, some host countries can provide refugees with access to regular, basic or emergency health-care services (e.g. in Germany). In other host countries, it is possible to provide refugees with a full access to a local public health-care system (e.g. in Austria). If the last option is not possible, special plans need to be created and put in place in order to ensure refugees' well-being.

16.5.1 Non-governmental Organisations (NGOs)

NGOs like the Red Cross, Caritas, Medécins sans Frontières or Medécins du Monde are quite fast in responding to emergencies due to their experience, resources and efficient action plans. They usually help without prejudice. NGOs have financial resources, equipment and medical staff, which is paid or works on a voluntary basis.

In the beginning of a crisis situation, a basic health-care unit (BHCU) is usually set up, followed by a more specific aid programme.

There are two options regarding recruitment of NGO staff:

1. Staff can be recruited from a local population.
2. Staff is recruited from abroad and shipped in for an average stay between 4 weeks and several months.

The strategy of recruitment depends on strengths and capacities of a health-care system in a host country as the main aim of an intervention is twofold:

1. To build an adequate health-care system for refugees
2. To avoid weakening of a national health system

In 2016, the first author worked in Greece for the Red Cross BHCU, which was responsible for three refugee camps next to Kilkis. The staff consisted mostly of foreign medical professionals, because the Greek health-care system was fragile at the time. Employing Greek doctors would have weakened their national health system, as the Red Cross paid doctors higher wages than were those of the Greek colleagues in hospitals. It may have caused a lack of medical professionals within the Greek health-care system and led to longer waiting lists for the local population seeking medical assistance. Further, tensions fanned by rumours, social or other media networks can be created in cases where a local population perceives refugees as being privileged with regard to medical care access. Therefore, Red Cross wanted to avoid this problem by hiring foreign staff only.

16.5.2 Voluntary Staff

This staff includes medical doctors, nurses, aid nurses, midwives and paramedics of all kinds. In the beginning of an emergency situation, there is usually a strong response of professionals who are willing to work for free. The longer an emergency lasts, the less interest it generates. Therefore, it is important to establish as soon as possible a "second line" of paid medical staff which can take over the tasks from volunteers. However, replacing voluntary work system with an employment-based system may create challenges. It is important to avoid that volunteers get an impression that they have being replaced and are "not needed anymore". A reward system for volunteers should be established. This system should not necessarily be a financial one, but include other forms of acknowledgement. In long-term camps and in refugee camps in host countries, health-care professionals from the refugee community might be identified and included in medical teams (see [2]).

16.6 Setting Up a Refugee Camp: Basic Needs

16.6.1 Basic Hygiene Needs

In a recent review on this issue, the Sphere Handbook concludes [36]: "People require spaces where they can bathe in privacy and with dignity. If this is not possible at the household level, separate central facilities for men and women will be needed… Washing clothes, particularly children's clothes, is an essential hygiene activity; cooking and eating utensils also need washing. The number, location, design, safety, appropriateness and convenience of facilities should be decided in consultation with the users, particularly women, adolescent girls and persons with disabilities" (Fig. 16.4).

16.6.2 Water

16.6.2.1 Water Quantity

People need water for daily use. According to their habits, cultural origin and background, the amount of water needed may differ [37] (Table 16.1):

Table 16.1 Basic survival water needs (Sphere)

Survival needs: water intake (drinking and food)	2.5–3 L/day	Depends on the climate and individual physiology
Basic hygiene practices	2–6 L/day	Depends on social and cultural norms
Basic cooking needs	3–6 L/day	Depends on food type and social and cultural norms
Total basic water needs	7.5–15 L/day	

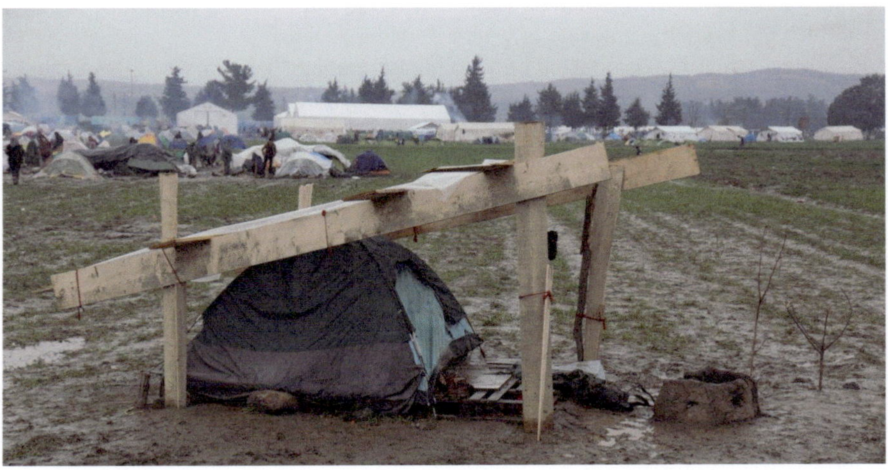

Fig. 16.4 Idomeni, Greece, February, 2016

16.6.2.2 Water Quality

The quality of drinking water should match that of household water, meaning that there should be no coliform bacteria in 100 mL of drinking water. Faecal coliform bacteria are a sign of contamination of water with human faeces. If water does not reach this standard, an alternative way of water disinfection [38], like chlorination [39] with a residual of chlorine (minimum 0.3–0.5 mg/L), should be effectuated. Drinking water should have just a small turbidity and at best no smell at all. While these guidelines are for drinking and for cooking water, water used for showering and washing clothes does not have to reach the same, high standards. If there are different types of water in a camp, they must be clearly separated from each other and labelled accordingly.

16.6.2.3 Water Availability

Water should be available within 500 m of the living quarters in a camp. A maximum queuing time of 30 min should not be exceeded, and therefore there should be enough water taps.

Refugees must be sensitised regarding reliability of water sources [40, 41]. Here as well, their background is very important. While in many European countries and in many parts of the US tapped water fulfils the minimum standards of drinking water, this might not be the case in other parts of the world where refugees come from. In these cases, refugees should be instructed that drinking tap water incurs no health risks.

If tapped water is unavailable or undrinkable, an alternative solution should be provided.

Water can be treated in different ways:

- Chlorination: (as described above): This can be done either on a household level with chlorine tablets or powder or at a water source. When treated at a water source, water must have a higher concentration of active chlorine because water pipes have to be disinfected as well. Storage in hot climates and transportation reduce the available chlorine in water.
- Boiling: When water is boiled on wood, an average of 1 kg of wood is needed to boil 1 L of water. In huge camps, the use of this method can quickly deplete resources.
- Ceramic filter [42, 43]: Using ceramic filters is a very effective but expensive solution for water disinfection. The advantage of this solution is that the filter needs to be bought just once and can be used for an unlimited number of times. Disadvantages, other than price of the filter, include limited amount of water which can be filtered in a given period of time.
- Solar disinfection: The, so-called, SODIS [44–48] is a method of water disinfection using the sun. "SODIS" has never become popular, although the method is interesting and it has few requirements. Many variables seem to affect its efficiency and eventual safety of treated water. Nevertheless it is a very affordable method for raising water quality. Disinfection requires sunlight (UV light), a PET bottle and time.
- Other options, like using ultraviolet light or ozone [43], are sufficient but mostly too expensive for treatment of drinking water.

Water quality should be the same every day. Therefore, daily testing is necessary. If water is treated with chlorine, daily tests of its concentration in tapped water are obligatory. Microbiological testing has to be done regularly as well. Therefore, a water surveillance group should be set up from the beginning. The surveillance group should include drinking water and hygiene specialists and medical specialists. The latter can, for example, warn for cases of diarrhoea in their refugee patients, possibly caused by a lack of safe drinking water or problems with toilets/latrines.

16.6.3 Excreta Disposal

Safe disposal of excreta is very important. It is a crucial activity in order to keep water sources clean and people healthy. Otherwise, illnesses like diarrhoea, cholera, hepatitis A and others can spread very quickly within and outside the community/camp [49]. Besides general and technical provisions, information for newly arrived refugees in particular should be provided. Also, practical problems, such as lack of soap [40, 50, 51] or unhygienic practices including open defecation [51], should be recognised and addressed.

16.6.4 Toilets

The Sphere Project suggests the standard of 20 people per toilet. There should be three times more toilets for women than for men. The distance from the living quarters should not exceed 50 m.[6]

16.6.5 Children's Nappies

There should be enough clean spaces to change diapers. These spaces require trash bins and handwashing facilities with soap needed to avoid spreading of germs.

16.6.6 Personal Hygiene

There is a need, particularly at women's toilets, for garbage bins. As there are different products and habits used during menstruation and tampons are not common all over the world, a consultation with female refugee group is necessary in order to provide them with the right materials.

All toilets should have a space to wash hands with soap and water. These spots must be marked clearly. Using these facilities is essential for prevention of illnesses in the camp. Therefore, motivating people to use them must be a part of hygiene promotion campaigns [51].

---

[6] See again: The Sphere Project. Sphere Handbook 2011.

16.6.7 Hygiene of Toilets

Cleaning toilets is essential for keeping refugees healthy. Every toilet in a camp should be cleaned at least twice a day with proper material. For disinfection, a chlorine solution of 5 mg chlorine per 1 L water is the best option. One possibility is to buy a previously prepared solution. On the other side, it is possible to prepare a solution with HTH chlorine (calcium hypochlorite). Staff responsible for cleaning of toilets has an important role in assessing potential problems. They can signalise when toilets show signs of a diarrhoeal disease. Therefore, a reporting chain has to be established.

16.6.8 Showers

An important part of personal hygiene and psychological well-being is having a space to wash oneself or to take a shower. Many diseases in camps are vector born and spread due to a lack of personal hygiene (e.g. flee, lice). Poor water facilities can, for example, lead to outbreaks of diarrhoeal diseases (shigella, salmonella, hepatitis A) [52, 53]. Therefore, camps should have a specified space for personal hygiene as well as for washing clothes. The following key points should be taken into account:

- Men should be strictly separated from women.
- Respect for intimacy.
- Drainage system.
- Sewerage and waste water management.
- Protection of drinking water wells.

16.6.9 Soap and Personal Hygiene Items

Having the possibility to wash, shower or similar is essential for personal well-being and not only for physical health of refugees.

The International Community of Red Cross and Red Crescent (ICRC) provides hygiene kits for one person for 3 months. These kits include:

One bag of washing powder, 1 kg
Two pieces of soap, body soap, 100 g
One tube of toothpaste, 75 ml/100 g
One piece of toothbrush, medium
One bottle of hair shampoo, adult, normal hair, 250 ml
Two boxes of sanitary pads, normal[7]

[7] IFRC. IFRC Emergency relief catalogue. http://procurement.ifrc.org/catalogue/2002, accessed 15.06.2017

Toilet paper is not included but should be provided in the EU or similar host country settings, as well as towels or similar items. Sanitary napkins for women must be included in the package. It is important to know what kinds of products women are using in different countries. In some cultures tampons are thought to be among causes of "defloration" in young women [54, 55], and, as such, it is important to offer culturally appropriate hygiene products.

Additional items in the kits:

- Nine pieces of toilet paper
- A certain amount of sanitary napkins
- One towel

The kit for babies includes the following items:

- One blanket (70 × 95 cm)
- Three bags of washing powder, 1 kg
- Two pieces of soap, body soap, 100 g
- Two bottles of shampoo, for baby, 250 ml
- One bottle of baby lotion 250 ml
- One bottle of baby powder 250 g
- Twelve pieces of diapers, washable
- One piece of diaper pants
- One thermometer[8]

16.6.10 Waste Management[9]

It is of utmost importance to set up a sufficient waste management strategy from the beginning on when setting up a refugee camp. This strategy should be thought through stage-by-stage and consider how to get rid of garbage in rooms or houses, how to collect garbage in a camp, and how to treat the collected garbage.

One problem is the amount of plastic bottles which have to be stored, burnt or recycled. As tap water in many countries is not drinkable, drinking bottled water becomes a necessity and is a custom for many refugees.

Another problem is that water bottles are a perfect breeding space for all kinds of vectors. Mosquitos of any kind (*Anopheles*, *Aedes*, *Culex* or sandflies) can use even the smallest amount of water left in the bottles for breeding [56, 57]. This leads to a highly increased risk of vector-spread diseases, if common in the countries, and can lead to outbreaks of malaria, dengue fever, yellow fever or zika.

[8] World Health Organization. http://www.who.int/water_sanitation_health/diseases-risks/diseases/scabies/en/, accessed 15.06.2017

[9] Sanitary Guidelines for Camps and Settlements. PAHO—Pan American Health Organization. http://www.paho.org/, accessed 15.06.2017

Thirdly, other vectors like rats and rat fleas, and bugs, like cockroaches, live off garbage. Insufficient waste management can increase the vectors and a risk for spreading diseases.

If waste is burned, this should be done in a clearly defined space. In order to protect a camp from toxic fumes, burning has to be carried out at a safe distance from the living quarters. Waste management can widely differ from country to country and from continent to continent. Here, it is important to cooperate with local authorities both for permissions and for environmental protection. In larger camps it may be necessary to set up a paid waste management system to protect the camp inhabitants.

There are special needs regarding management of medical waste, like syringes or surgical blades. In addition to dangers inherent to sharp objects, a waste management plan should determine how these objects will be disposed in order to avoid potential contact with blood and a possible infection with diseases like HIV and hepatitis B or C.

16.7 Basic Medical Support

In a transitional refugee camp, medical assistance is of special importance. In a sample of refugees ($n = 724$) examined in 2015 in the reception centre in Hamburg, Germany, the most common medical problems were [58]:

- Respiratory infections due to a climate difference (103 patients)
- Pain (88 patients)
- Skin diseases (72 patients)
- "Psychosomatic" complaints or insomnia (69 patients)
- Others—not classified

Based on these findings, medical stock for a comparable group should include:

- Two different antibiotics (penicillin and one other)
- Analgesics (paracetamol and at least one stronger nonsteroidal anti-inflammatory drug (NSAID))
- Materials to treat blisters and wounds

Having the right equipment in appropriate quantities enables treatment of over roughly 75% of all potential cases, but continuous monitoring is required to identify specific needs as time passes. Further steps and selection of priorities will also depend on a number of factors, including funding and availability of drugs in a host country.

It is of great importance to establish a consensus between different refugee camps and between NGOs and other health-care stakeholders with regard to prescription of addictive medication, such as benzodiazepines or strong analgesics, like tramadol. Alternatives should be explored as, for example, benzodiazepines are not a drug of choice and are even counter-indicated in the treatment of sleeping disorders and trauma-related problems [59]. Sleeping problems can be better treated with other drugs, such as trazodone [60, 61]. Moreover, physical or psychological aetiology of the problems, like thyroid disorder [62], substance abuse, posttraumatic stress disorder (PTSD) or depression, should be explored. Further, experiencing pain is often not only a symptom of a somatic condition but may reveal a presence of psychological problems and be a cultural idiom of distress (see again [15]).

16.8 Diseases and Prevention

According to the Doctors Without Borders (MSF) handbook[10], there are three major sources of communicable diseases in a refugee population:

1. Infections which refugees may bring with from their home environment (e.g. malaria or trypanosomiasis) or from areas they have travelled through before arriving to a host country
2. Illnesses which are already present in a host environment and for which refugees have not acquired immunity (e.g. yellow fever, cholera, influenza, tick-borne encephalitis)
3. Diseases which may surface in a refugee camp as a result of overcrowding and poor sanitary conditions (e.g. tuberculosis, lice, scabies, diarrhoeal diseases, like shigella, salmonella, hepatitis A)

Depending (Fig. 16.5) on the region of origin, and of transit countries, refugee persons can encounter different problems classified with regard to the presence of vectors:

1. Illnesses which need vectors, not present in a host country, in order to be spread. As such, there is no danger of epidemic for the host population (e.g. malaria in the most parts of Europe or in the US, leishmaniasis, schistosomiasis), but illnesses are still active.
2. Illnesses which need vectors present in a host country and where a chance for spreading of a disease is present (e.g. malaria in epidemic countries).
3. Illnesses which do not need a particular vector for transmission (e.g. tuberculosis).

[10] refbooks.msf.org/msf_docs/en/refugee_health/rh.pdf, accessed 1.7.2017

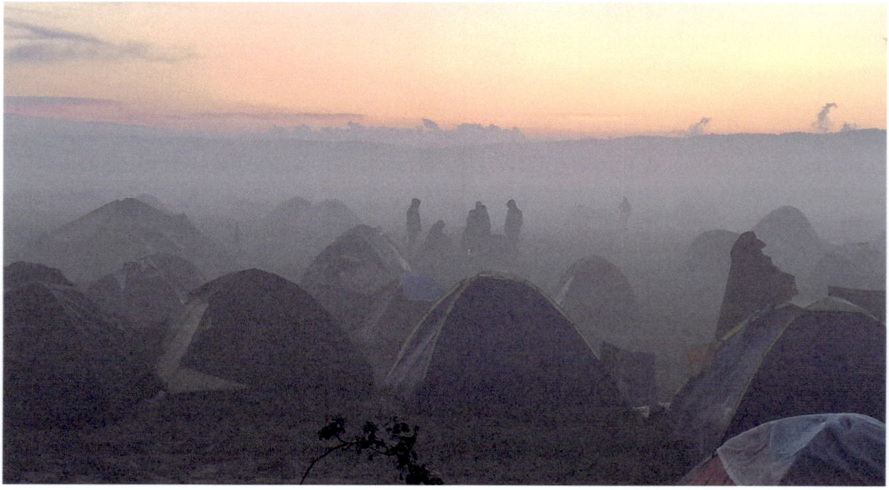

Fig. 16.5 Idomeni, Greece, February, 2016

16.9 Examples of Diseases Occurring Worldwide and Being Independent of Climate Conditions

16.9.1 Tuberculosis

Tuberculosis is one of the illnesses host countries are most afraid of because of the already mentioned droplet infections. This disease is usually included in screening procedures [63].

In 2015 in Germany, the incidence of tuberculosis (TB) has increased by 29% compared to 2014 (4533–5865 cases) due to a rising number of migrants. Of all diagnosed TB cases in 2015, 72% was found in refugees, while this percentage was 62% in 2014[11]. Migrants and refugee groups often have a significantly higher rate of tuberculosis than the host population[12], and this rate is even higher than in their countries of origin. This is due to a close contact with other refugees throughout their long journey.

Germany was, therefore, facing not only more TB cases but new types of TB as well. German health authorities were used to treat lung TB which is the main form of TB in the country. However, refugees often suffer from TB within organs, bones or joints [64]. These forms of TB are usually not contagious, as only the, so-called, "open" lung TB is dangerous for others.

[11] http://www.rki.de/EN/Content/infections/epidemiology/inf_dis_Germany/TB/summary_2015.html

[12] www.euro.who.int/__data/assets/pdf_file/0003/69024/fs07G_TBmigration.pdf accessed 1.7.2017

The cases of multidrug-resistant (MDR) TB, mainly in refugees from the eastern European countries [65] and in those originating from the Middle East [13], are rising. This is as an additional challenge and a risk for refugees.

With regard to screening of refugees for TB, the most common standard is an X-ray which can be applied in individuals aged 15 and older, but screening strategies might have to be adapted to specific situations. They should be evidence based instead of emotion guided [66]. Recent studies such as the one by Weinrich et al. [67] recommend an improved and efficient algorithm in large groups of refugees due to low prevalence of pulmonary TB in their sample (0.103%). According to this study, 1749 persons have to be screened in order to detect one case of active pulmonary TB.

Exceptions are children and (potentially) pregnant women, where a test like Mendel-Mantoux or QuantiFERON can be applied [68–70]. Another special group are HIV-positive patients where X-ray might not be sufficient.[13]

16.9.2 Scabies

Scabies is a water-related disease which is transmitted via body contact [71–73]. It can only be prevented with an adequate hygiene level, like showers, new or washed clothes, new bed sheets and medical treatment.

Options for treatment of scabies include:

- Ivermectin [74–76], a drug which has to be taken just once orally. It can be used in children >15 kg and in adults in a dosage of 200 mcg/kg. In many countries, this drug is used in the veterinary context only, and its use in human medicine is "off-label". However, this form of treatment seems less risky and easier to administer to patients than the others.
- Permethrin (5%) is applied locally as a cream. Patients have to apply it on the affected areas and leave it there for a minimum of 8 h. A disadvantage of this form of treatment is a necessity of showering after using the cream. New clothes are also needed to get rid of scabies successfully. The drug has neurotoxic side effects which have to be considered in the treatment plan, especially in (possible) pregnancy, and patients have to be informed about this risk [71, 77].
- Lindane (1%) is applied locally as well. Compared to ivermectin and permethrin, it is much cheaper, but it has more and potentially severe central nervous system side effects [78–81]. Its low price is the reason why it remains in use, but the side effects are the reason why this drug is not recommended for treatment in the EU.
- As of treatment of scabies symptoms, antihistaminic drugs are recommended against pruritus [82, 83].

[13] See again www.euro.who.int/__data/assets/pdf_file/0003/69024/fs07G_TBmigration.pdf.

16.9.3 Lice

Lice [84–86] are mainly transmitted from human to human, via direct or indirect contact between an infected and a noninfected person. Lice can be categorised in three groups:

- Head lice
- Body lice
- Pubic lice

  Head lice affect mostly children and cause itching and scratching marks on the head which can become infected [84, 87]. Treatment consists of a lotion with 1% permethrin, and it should include the patient and everyone living with him/her in the same room. Body lice are quite common where there are poor hygiene standards. It should be treated with 0.5% permethrin powder. The powder should be administered on the clothes and must stay there for at least 12 h. Pubic lice [88] are mainly transmitted via sexual contact. Marks of scratching are mostly found in the pubic area, and the disease should be treated with 1% permethrin lotion. However, the most important intervention is to increase hygiene standards in a refugee camp.

16.9.4 Measles

Measles are a highly contagious viral infection with body rash, fever and respiratory infection. Transmission occurs via droplets (e.g. coughing), contact with nasal fluids and partly airborne. Life in crowded refugee camps incurs a high risk of measles transmission, as discussed before, particularly in areas where immunisation coverage rates are low. The most vulnerable group are children under 5 years of age. The case fatality rate can be above 10% (see also [89–92]).

Currently, it is only possible to treat symptoms of this disease. Vaccination is the best and the only way to prevent an outbreak. Therefore, it is very important to start vaccination campaigns in a refugee population as soon as possible [93–100]. Immunisation of children against measles is probably the single most important (and cost-effective) preventive measure in emergency-affected populations, particularly those housed in camps and for children. Since infants as young as 6 months of age frequently contract measles in refugee camp outbreaks and are at greater risk of dying owing to impaired nutrition, it is recommended that measles immunisation programmes in emergency settings target all children between the age of 6 months and 5 years [101–104].

16.9.5 Flu

Travelling for several weeks and withstanding a variety of weather conditions, like sun, rain and snow, may raise the incidence of flu-like infections in refugees [105–108]. Symptoms, like sneezing and (sub)febrile temperature, are the signs of a viral infection.

Only symptoms can be treated. Antibiotics, which are often prescribed for flu-like diseases, do not help, as they target bacterial and not viral infections. In order to avoid a larger outbreak, patients should stay in bed.

Problems may occur if there is an outbreak of seasonal influenza, which is a viral disease as well [109–111]. Patients suffer from fever (39 °C and higher), pain in joints, severe headache and a dry cough. This condition has a higher mortality rate than the flu. There are 3–5 million cases of this severe illness worldwide, causing about 250,000–500,000 deaths.[14]

16.10 Non-communicable Diseases (NCI)

These diseases occur worldwide and are not transmitted via vectors, air or other sources. They include well-known public health challenges such as hypertension, but also "new" problems, like a non-alcoholic fatty liver disease. These diseases have to be addressed by long-term behavioural interventions [112] and they play an important role in migrant and refugee health [113].

16.10.1 Hypertension

The definition of hypertension differs between organisations and standards. MSF defines hypertension as above 160 mmHg systolic or above 90 mmHg diastolic blood pressure. The WHO defines hypertension as systolic blood pressure "equal to or above 140 mm Hg and a diastolic blood pressure equal to or above 90 mm Hg"[15]. Besides differences in definition, standardisation and implementation of measurement can be a problem in refugee camps due to a lack of equipment and opportunities.

According to the WHO fact sheet essential hypertension is related to several factors that can be partly influenced by:

- Environment and daily living conditions.
- Social determinants, like income, education and housing.
- Behavioural risks, like unhealthy diet, tobacco use and physical inactivity.

Studies with both, newly arrived but also resettled refugees, often report high rates of such risk factors and hypertension [113–119]. A larger CDC review on a group of 4923 resettled Iraqi refugees in the San Diego county, US, demonstrated that 15.2% of the sample suffered from hypertension and 24.6% were overweight or

[14] WHO—Influenza Fact Sheet. http://www.who.int/mediacentre/factsheets/fs211/en, accessed 20.1.2017

[15] WHO: A global brief of hypertension, 2013, http://www.who.int/cardiovascular_diseases/publications/global_brief_hypertension/en/, accessed 20.2.2017

obese [120]. Kumar found overweight in 52%, hypertension in 23%, vitamin B12 deficiency in 12%, diabetes in 14% and depression in 15% of Nepali Bhutanese refugee people in a US refugee clinic [121].

Factors which can reduce hypertension and might be influenced by health education are reduction of salt intake, smoking and of alcohol abuse.

In terms of medical treatment of hypertension and beyond measures like reducing weight and enhancing physical activity, the WHO recommends, depending on age or co-morbidity like cerebral vascular disease or renal insufficiency, the following drugs:

- ACE I (angiotensin-converting enzyme inhibitors)
- ARB (angiotensin receptor blockers)
- Beta blockers
- Calcium channel blockers
- Diuretics

16.10.2 Diabetes

Only approximately 5% of all diabetes cases are the "insulin-dependent diabetes mellitus" (IDDM) ones. The most common type of diabetes is the "non-insulin-dependent diabetes mellitus" (NIDDM) (approximately 95%) and it is a common challenge in refugee populations [122–125]. This illness is caused by most of the factors mentioned already with hypertension, including nutrition and tobacco use. Underestimating diabetes and its consequences can lead to secondary diseases, like heart attack, stroke or a kidney failure. Other long-term problems can be a prolonged tissue repair, vision loss or paraesthesia. Obesity and consumption of different food in a host country can speed up the process and raise the number of cases of diabetes within a refugee community.

The treatment includes:

- Lifestyle changes, like physical activity and diet with reduced sugar and salt
- Oral antidiabetics
- Combined treatment:
  Monotherapy: Metformin
  Dual therapy: Metformin and a second-line drug, like DPP-4 inhibitor or sulfonylurea
  Triple therapy: Metformin in combination with a second-line drug and insulin, though combined treatment models require further research [126]

Recommended treatment models are frequently updated [126–129], and available drugs and treatment strategies may differ from country to country.

Treatment should be carried out in coordination with local health authorities in a host country. Cultural differences, as, for example, adaptation of the treatment during the month of Ramadan in Muslim patients [127–129], or other nutrition-related habits and health belief models [130] have to be considered.

16.11 Vaccinations

The WHO recommends a minimum of the following vaccinations for adults and children[16]:

• BCG	One dose
• Hepatitis B	Three to four doses for children, for adults, if a high-risk group
• Polio	Three to four doses for children or/and adults if not vaccinated
• DTP[a]	Three doses for children, booster 1–6 years of age, adults booster every year
• *Haemophilus influenzae*	Three doses, with DTP or two to three doses with booster, at least 6 months after the last dose
• Pneumococcal	Three doses, with DTP or two to three doses with booster, at least 6 months after the last dose
• Rotavirus	Two doses with DTP
• Measles	Two doses
• Rubella	One dose
• HPV	Two doses (female)—target: 9–13-year-old girls

[a]*DTP* diphtheria, tetanus, pertussis

Even if local immunisation campaigns ask for a less comprehensive scheme, refugees should receive at least all available local vaccinations. This is the only way to avoid potential endemic outbreaks.

Addressing vaccination means addressing security and prevention for people who enter a country as well as for residents of a host country. The so-called herd immunity is a situation where most of a population is vaccinated against an illness and there is only a small percentage of risk for people who did not receive vaccination to get ill. Having a growing number of people refusing vaccination in many countries worldwide puts refugees at a higher risk as they are usually not vaccinated.

The Measles Report 2016 of the Austrian Ministry of Health shows that 1/3 of all Austrians born before 1990 have received only one vaccination against measles[17]. However, the WHO recommends a minimum of two vaccinations. Therefore, Austria has the second highest incidence rate of measles in the EU, which means that refugees hosted in Austria are also at a higher risk. Vaccination campaigns might therefore be required [131], but should consider cultural background of respective target groups [94, 132]. Working with trusted multipliers in a population might again improve acceptance of necessary vaccinations in larger groups. They also might have to counter popular or newly developing "rumour"-based health belief models that

[16]http://www.who.int/immunization/policy/immunization_tables/en/, accessed 2.3.2017; refer to recent updates.

[17]Bundesministerium für Gesundheit und Frauen (BMGF), 2016. http://www.bmgf.gv.at/cms/home/attachments/7/0/0/CH1472/CMS1473753939787/masern__kurzbericht_2016.pdf, accessed 1.3.2017

are, at present, increasingly distributed through internet and online social networks. These might create problems in vaccination campaigns [133].

16.12 Epidemic Plan

A refugee camp should always have an emergency plan in case of the outbreak of an epidemic like measles, diarrhoea (including cholera, shigellosis, norovirus), acute respiratory diseases, malaria, varicella or influenza [134]. The following considerations hereabout are taken from the Red Cross emergency plan for Vienna (Austria) [135].

Regardless of whether refugees bring a disease from a country of originy or contract it upon the flight, sick persons must be separated from the healthy ones in order to avoid spreading of an illness. Safety regulations should be adapted according to the ways an illness is transmitted. In case of a disease being transmitted via the faecal-oral route, sick people must use separate bathrooms and washing facilities. Moreover, strict hygiene regulations regarding handwashing, disinfection of rest- and bathrooms and management of faeces should be introduced. In case of an airborne or droplet disease, like measles, influenza, varicella or similar, sick individuals should be isolated, and both the cleaning and the health staff should wear personal protective equipment (PPE), like mouth masks, hand gloves and an apron. It is important to train the staff in using the equipment before an outbreak in order to familiarise them with its use and to ensure that the equipment will be used properly.

Particular attention should be paid to vulnerable groups, like pregnant women. Illnesses like varicella or rubella can cause abortion or severe malformations of the foetus. In case of an outbreak of these diseases, pregnant women must be isolated as soon as possible.

Moreover, it is of utmost importance to establish a clear communication path to local health authorities and other stakeholders. This path has to be defined in the beginning of an outbreak, and all staff working in a camp should be informed about it. Further, staff working in a camp should be vaccinated before entering a camp for the first time. This is not only for their own protection but also for protection of their relatives and friends and all refugees in a camp. Staff members who contract an illness at work should know beforehand whom to inform about being sick.

Further, cleaning should be done with bactericide substances, like chlorine or lime. For handwashing 0.05% chlorine solution which is equal to 500 mg chlorine per 1 L of water should be used. For disinfection of latrines, toilets or other contaminated materials, 0.5% chlorine solution which is equal to 5000 mg chlorine per 1 L of water should be used.

16.13 Groups with Special Needs

There are several groups within a refugee community which can be categorised as vulnerable based on medical considerations (see also other chapters in this volume). These are:

- Women and female-headed households
- Pregnant women
- Children
- Elderly
- The disabled

It is very important to address their special needs in the following ways:

- Women and female-headed households should feel safe in a refugee camp. Since refugee women are very often exposed to physical and sexual violence [11, 136], there must be safe places for unaccompanied women to live in a camp. These should include separate and guarded toilet and washing facilities to guarantee their safety.
- Pregnant women need special care and very often medical treatment [137–139]. Appropriate nutrition is essential for this group. Regular medical exams during pregnancy are useful, and a screening for diabetes in pregnancy should be administered on a routine basis.
- Children need to have opportunities to play and to "have a childhood". Moreover, school classes, including classes teaching language of a host country, should be provided as they are a very important step in education and integration of refugees in a host society.
- Elderly people may have special needs regarding their mobility. For example, using latrines can cause problems for them. Further, the elderly may be disadvantaged due to being too slow when items are distributed to large groups. They may also run a higher risk of getting infections which can cause severe health problems.
- Besides meeting medical and psychological needs of the mentally and physically disabled refugees [140, 141], it is important to protect this group from discrimination and exploitation by their surroundings.[18]

Conclusions

Humanitarian emergencies, such as the recent large influx of refugees in Europe, frequently lead to situations that cannot be immediately addressed with success and resolved using existing emergency plans and resources owned by local and international administrations or NGOs. However, basic interventions, such as those described in this chapter, modified by continuous monitoring, identification of needs and outcomes and interagency coordination can still be expected to provide at least some relief to people in need. Although the first emergency responses are usually executed by groups of international NGOs, the long-term support requires comprehensive plans by local governments and international

[18] UN Convention on the Rights of Persons with Disabilities, www.un.org/disabilities/.../convention_accessible_pdf.pdf, accessed 1.7.2017

organisations. In case of a long-lasting international crisis, coherent long-term planning between governments is necessary. Transient settlements, such as camps, must be replaced by a resettlement programme with integration of refugee services into social and health-care systems of host countries. In addition, all necessary steps should be taken in order to restore peace and enable refugees to return to their home countries.

References

1. Weissbecker I, Hanna F, El Shazly M, Gao J, Ventevogel P. Integrative mental health and psychosocial support interventions for refugees in humanitarian crisis settings. In: Wenzel T, Drožđek B, editors. An uncertain safety. Cham: Springer International; 2018.
2. Wenzel T, Völkl-Kernstock S, Wittek TU, Baron D. Identifying needs, vulnerabilities, and resources in refugee persons and groups. In: Wenzel T, Drožđek B, editors. An uncertain safety. Cham: Springer International; 2018.
3. den Otter J, Wenzel T, McGrath B, Osorio AL, Drožđek B. Special situations: places of immigration detention. In: Wenzel T, Drožđek B, editors. An uncertain safety. Cham: Springer International; 2018.
4. Escobio F, Echevarria J, Rubaki S, Viniczai V. Health assistance of displaced people along the Balkan route. Lancet. 2015;386(10012):2475.
5. Arsenijevic J, Schillberg E, Ponthieu A, Malvisi L, Ahmed WAE, Argenziano S, et al. A crisis of protection and safe passage: violence experienced by migrants/refugees travelling along the Western Balkan corridor to Northern Europe. Confl Health. 2017;11:6.
6. Pasta L, Mesa Suero LA, Farinella EM, Marchese G, Serravalle D, D'Amico N, et al. Causes of hospitalisation of migrants arrived in Lampedusa (Southern Italy) from January 2011 to June 2014. Epidemiol Prev. 2015;39(1):55–8.
7. Kulla M, Josse F, Stierholz M, Hossfeld B, Lampl L, Helm M. Initial assessment and treatment of refugees in the Mediterranean Sea (a secondary data analysis concerning the initial assessment and treatment of 2656 refugees rescued from distress at sea in support of the EUNAVFOR MED relief mission of the EU). Scand J Trauma Resusc Emerg Med. 2016;24:75.
8. Sphere Handbook 20112013 07. Available from http://www.sphereproject.org/resources/download-publications/?search=1&keywords&language=english&category=22.
9. Reed B. Technical notes on drinking water, sanitations and hygiene in emergencies. Geneva: WHO; 2013.
10. Corsellis T, Vitale A. In: Cambridge Uo, editor. Transitional settlement: displaced populations. Oxford: Oxfam; 2005.
11. Al-Modallal H, Abu Zayed I, Abujilban S, Shehab T, Atoum M. Prevalence of intimate partner violence among women visiting health care centers in Palestine refugee camps in Jordan. Health Care Women Int. 2015;36(2):137–48.
12. AlHeresh R, Bryant W, Holm M. Community-based rehabilitation in Jordan: challenges to achieving occupational justice. Disabil Rehabil. 2013;35(21):1848–52.
13. Doganay M, Demiraslan H. Refugees of the Syrian Civil War: impact on reemerging infections, health services, and biosecurity in Turkey. Health Secur. 2016;14(4):220–5.
14. Organization WH, editor. Migration and health: key issues. WHOint. Geneva: World Health Organization; 2016.
15. Kienzler H, Spence C, Wenzel T. A culture sensitive and person centred approach – understanding and evaluating cultural factors, history and social background. In: Wenzel T, Drožđek B, editors. An uncertain safety. Cham: Springer International; 2018.

16. Smith RM, Nelsen LA. Hmong folk remedies: limited acetylation of opium by aspirin and acetaminophen. J Forensic Sci. 1991;36(1):280–7.
17. Carruth L. Camel milk, amoxicillin, and a prayer: medical pluralism and medical humanitarian aid in the Somali Region of Ethiopia. Soc Sci Med. 2014;120:405–12.
18. van Andel T, Westers P. Why Surinamese migrants in the Netherlands continue to use medicinal herbs from their home country. J Ethnopharmacol. 2010;127(3):694–701.
19. Villa-Torres L, Gonzalez-Vazquez T, Fleming PJ, Gonzalez-Gonzalez EL, Infante-Xibille C, Chavez R, et al. Transnationalism and health: a systematic literature review on the use of transnationalism in the study of the health practices and behaviors of migrants. Soc Sci Med. 2017;183:70–9.
20. Ramzan S, Soelberg J, Jager AK, Cantarero-Arevalo L. Traditional medicine among people of Pakistani descent in the capital region of Copenhagen. J Ethnopharmacol. 2017;196:267–80.
21. Straka RJ, Hansen SR, Walker PF. Comparison of the prevalence of the poor metabolizer phenotype for CYP2D6 between 203 Hmong subjects and 280 white subjects residing in Minnesota. Clin Pharmacol Ther. 1995;58(1):29–34.
22. Palrasu M, Nagini S. Cytochrome P450 structure, function and clinical significance: a review. Curr Drug Targets 2017;19(1):38–54.
23. Goh LL, Lim CW, Sim WC, Toh LX, Leong KP. Analysis of genetic variation in CYP450 genes for clinical implementation. PLoS One. 2017;12(1):e0169233.
24. Cespedes-Garro C, Fricke-Galindo I, Naranjo ME, Rodrigues-Soares F, Farinas H, de Andres F, et al. Worldwide interethnic variability and geographical distribution of CYP2C9 genotypes and phenotypes. Expert Opin Drug Metab Toxicol. 2015;11(12):1893–905.
25. Mizzi C, Dalabira E, Kumuthini J, Dzimiri N, Balogh I, Basak N, et al. A European spectrum of pharmacogenomic biomarkers: implications for clinical pharmacogenomics. PLoS One. 2016;11(9):e0162866.
26. Pourgholi L, Goodarzynejad H, Mandegary A, Ziaee S, Talasaz AH, Jalali A, et al. Gene polymorphisms and the risk of warfarin-induced bleeding complications at therapeutic international normalized ratio (INR). Toxicol Appl Pharmacol. 2016;309:37–43.
27. Raguram R, Weiss MG, Channabasavanna SM, Devins GM. Stigma, depression, and somatization in South India. Am J Psychiatry. 1996;153(8):1043–9.
28. Bagayogo IP, Interian A, Escobar JI. Transcultural aspects of somatic symptoms in the context of depressive disorders. Adv Psychosom Med. 2013;33:64–74.
29. Rohlof HG, Knipscheer JW, Kleber RJ. Somatization in refugees: a review. Soc Psychiatry Psychiatr Epidemiol. 2014;49(11):1793–804.
30. Thapa TB. Living with diabetes: lay narratives as idioms of distress among the low-caste Dalit of Nepal. Med Anthropol. 2014;33(5):428–40.
31. Volpato G, Waldstein A. Eghindi among Sahrawi refugees of Western Sahara. Med Anthropol. 2014;33(2):160–77.
32. Wangdahl J, Lytsy P, Martensson L, Westerling R. Health literacy among refugees in Sweden – a cross-sectional study. BMC Public Health. 2014;14:1030.
33. Altweck L, Marshall TC, Ferenczi N, Lefringhausen K. Mental health literacy: a cross-cultural approach to knowledge and beliefs about depression, schizophrenia and generalized anxiety disorder. Front Psychol. 2015;6:1272.
34. Na S, Ryder AG, Kirmayer LJ. Toward a culturally responsive model of mental health literacy: facilitating help-seeking among East Asian immigrants to North America. Am J Community Psychol. 2016;58(1–2):211–25.
35. Kujawska M, Hilgert NI, Keller HA, Gil G. Medicinal plant diversity and inter-cultural interactions between indigenous Guarani, Criollos and Polish migrants in the subtropics of Argentina. PLoS One. 2017;12(1):e0169373.
36. The Sphere Project. Humanitarian charter minimum standards in humanitarian response, The Sphere Handbook. 3rd ed; 2011. p. 104. www.sphereproject.org July 2017.
37. Solsona F. Water disinfection. Lima, Peru: Pan American Center for Sanitary Engineering and Environmental Sciences (PAHO); 2003.

38. Doocy S, Burnham G. Point-of-use water treatment and diarrhoea reduction in the emergency context: an effectiveness trial in Liberia. Tropical Med Int Health. 2006;11(10):1542–52.
39. Roberts L, Chartier Y, Chartier O, Malenga G, Toole M, Rodka H. Keeping clean water clean in a Malawi refugee camp: a randomized intervention trial. Bull World Health Organ. 2001;79(4):280–7.
40. Mahamud AS, Ahmed JA, Nyoka R, Auko E, Kahi V, Ndirangu J, et al. Epidemic cholera in Kakuma Refugee Camp, Kenya, 2009: the importance of sanitation and soap. J Infect Dev Ctries. 2012;6(3):234–41.
41. Nimri LF, Hijazi S. Rotavirus-associated diarrhoea in children in a refugee camp in Jordan. J Diarrhoeal Dis Res. 1996;14(1):1–4.
42. Lubick N. Ceramic filter makes water treatment easy. Environ Sci Technol. 2008;42(3):650–1.
43. Aidan A, Mehrvar M, Ibrahim TH, Nenov V. Particulates and bacteria removal by ceramic microfiltration, UV photolysis, and their combination. J Environ Sci Health A Tox Hazard Subst Environ Eng. 2007;42(7):895–901.
44. Rainey RC, Harding AK. Drinking water quality and solar disinfection: effectiveness in peri-urban households in Nepal. J Water Health. 2005;3(3):239–48.
45. Oates PM, Shanahan P, Polz MF. Solar disinfection (SODIS): simulation of solar radiation for global assessment and application for point-of-use water treatment in Haiti. Water Res. 2003;37(1):47–54.
46. McGuigan KG, Joyce TM, Conroy RM, Gillespie JB, Elmore-Meegan M. Solar disinfection of drinking water contained in transparent plastic bottles: characterizing the bacterial inactivation process. J Appl Microbiol. 1998;84(6):1138–48.
47. Heri S, Mosler HJ. Factors affecting the diffusion of solar water disinfection: a field study in Bolivia. Health Educ Behav. 2008;35(4):541–60.
48. Davies CM, Roser DJ, Feitz AJ, Ashbolt NJ. Solar radiation disinfection of drinking water at temperate latitudes: inactivation rates for an optimised reactor configuration. Water Res. 2009;43(3):643–52.
49. Brown V, Jacquier G, Bachy C, Bitar D, Legros D. Management of cholera epidemics in a refugee camp. Bull Soc Pathol Exot. 2002;95(5):351–4.
50. Mubarak MY, Wagner AL, Asami M, Carlson BF, Boulton ML. Hygienic practices and diarrheal illness among persons living in at-risk settings in Kabul, Afghanistan: a cross-sectional study. BMC Infect Dis. 2016;16:459.
51. Biran A, Schmidt WP, Zeleke L, Emukule H, Khay H, Parker J, et al. Hygiene and sanitation practices amongst residents of three long-term refugee camps in Thailand, Ethiopia and Kenya. Tropical Med Int Health. 2012;17(9):1133–41.
52. Stutman HR. Salmonella, Shigella, and Campylobacter: common bacterial causes of infectious diarrhea. Pediatr Ann. 1994;23(10):538–43.
53. Afghani B, Stutman HR. Toxin-related diarrheas. Pediatr Ann. 1994;23(10):549–50, 53–5.
54. Goodyear-Smith FA, Laidlaw TM. Can tampon use cause hymen changes in girls who have not had sexual intercourse? A review of the literature. Forensic Sci Int. 1998;94(1–2):147–53.
55. Berg DH, Coutts LB. Virginity and tampons: the beginner myth as a case of alteration. Health Care Women Int. 1993;14(1):27–38.
56. Mazine CA, Macoris ML, Andrighetti MT, Yasumaro S, Silva ME, Nelson MJ, et al. Disposable containers as larval habitats for Aedes aegypti in a city with regular refuse collection: a study in Marilia, Sao Paulo State, Brazil. Acta Trop. 1996;62(1):1–13.
57. Dhar-Chowdhury P, Haque CE, Lindsay R, Hossain S. Socioeconomic and ecological factors influencing aedes aegypti prevalence, abundance, and distribution in Dhaka, Bangladesh. Am J Trop Med Hyg. 2016;94(6):1223–33.
58. Pruskil S, Quellhorst S, Diederichs-Holthusen R. Das medizinische "first-line" Versorgungskonzept von Geflüchteten in Hamburg – ein Beispiel für Integration der Geflüchteten in das Regelsystem. Gesundheitswesen. 2017;79(4):299–374.
59. Guina J, Rossetter SR, De RB, Nahhas RW, Welton RS. Benzodiazepines for PTSD: a systematic review and meta-analysis. J Psychiatr Pract. 2015;21(4):281–303.

60. Warner MD, Dorn MR, Peabody CA. Survey on the usefulness of trazodone in patients with PTSD with insomnia or nightmares. Pharmacopsychiatry. 2001;34(4):128–31.
61. Singareddy RK, Balon R. Sleep in posttraumatic stress disorder. Ann Clin Psychiatry. 2002;14(3):183–90.
62. Demet MM, Ozmen B, Deveci A, Boyvada S, Adiguzel H, Aydemir O. Depression and anxiety in hyperthyroidism. Arch Med Res. 2002;33(6):552–6.
63. Hvass AMF, Wejse C. Systematic health screening of refugees after resettlement in recipient countries: a scoping review. Ann Hum Biol. 2017;44(5):475–83. doi:10.1080/03014460.2017.1330897.
64. Kristensen KL, Podlekareva D, Ravn P. Delayed diagnosis of severe tuberculous spondylodiscitis in an asylum seeker; patient or doctors delay? Respir Med Case Rep. 2017;21:145–6.
65. Hargreaves S, Lonnroth K, Nellums LB, Olaru ID, Nathavitharana RR, Norredam M, et al. Multidrug-resistant tuberculosis and migration to Europe. Clin Microbiol Infect. 2017;23(3):141–6.
66. Seybold U, Wagener J, Jung J, Sammet S. Multidrug-resistant organisms among refugees in Germany: we need evidence-based care, not fear-based screening. J Hosp Infect. 2016;92(3):229–31.
67. Weinrich JM, Diel R, Sauer M, Henes FO, Meywald-Walter K, Adam G, et al. Yield of chest X-ray tuberculosis screening of immigrants during the European refugee crisis of 2015: a single-centre experience. Eur Radiol. 2017;27:3244–8.
68. Walters JK, Sullivan AD. Impact of routine quantiferon testing on latent tuberculosis diagnosis and treatment in refugees in Multnomah County, Oregon, November 2009–October 2012. J Immigr Minor Health. 2016;18(2):292–300.
69. Harstad I, Winje BA, Heldal E, Oftung F, Jacobsen GW. Predictive values of QuantiFERON-TB gold testing in screening for tuberculosis disease in asylum seekers. Int J Tuberc Lung Dis. 2010;14(9):1209–11.
70. Baker CA, Thomas W, Stauffer WM, Peterson PK, Tsukayama DT. Serial testing of refugees for latent tuberculosis using the QuantiFERON-gold in-tube: effects of an antecedent tuberculin skin test. Am J Trop Med Hyg. 2009;80(4):628–33.
71. Dressler C, Rosumeck S, Sunderkotter C, Werner RN, Nast A. The treatment of scabies. Dtsch Arztebl Int. 2016;113(45):757–62.
72. Carr PC, Brodell RT. Images in clinical medicine. Scabies. N Engl J Med. 2016;374(11):e13.
73. Shmidt E, Levitt J. Dermatologic infestations. Int J Dermatol. 2012;51(2):131–41.
74. Zargari O, Aghazadeh N, Moeineddin F. Clinical applications of topical ivermectin in dermatology. Dermatol Online J. 2016;22(9).
75. Sunderkotter C, Feldmeier H, Folster-Holst R, Geisel B, Klinke-Rehbein S, Nast A, et al. S1 guidelines on the diagnosis and treatment of scabies – short version. J Dtsch Dermatol Ges. 2016;14(11):1155–67.
76. Steer AC, Romani L, Kaldor JM. Mass drug administration for scabies control. N Engl J Med. 2016;374(17):1690.
77. Patel VM, Lambert WC, Schwartz RA. Safety of topical medications for scabies and lice in pregnancy. Indian J Dermatol. 2016;61(6):583–7.
78. Ramabhatta S, Sunilkumar GR, Somashekhar C. Lindane toxicity following accidental oral ingestion. Indian J Dermatol Venereol Leprol. 2014;80(2):181–2.
79. Nolan K, Kamrath J, Levitt J. Lindane toxicity: a comprehensive review of the medical literature. Pediatr Dermatol. 2012;29(2):141–6.
80. Koch E, Clark JM, Cohen B, Meinking TL, Ryan WG, Stevenson A, et al. Management of head louse infestations in the United States-a literature review. Pediatr Dermatol. 2016;33(5):466–72.
81. Goldust M, Rezaee E, Raghifar R, Naghavi-Behzad M. Ivermectin vs. lindane in the treatment of scabies. Ann Parasitol. 2013;59(1):37–41.
82. Folster-Holst R. Itch management in childhood. Curr Probl Dermatol. 2016;50:173–91.

83. Orion E, Marcos B, Davidovici B, Wolf R. Itch and scratch: scabies and pediculosis. Clin Dermatol. 2006;24(3):168–75.
84. Meister L, Ochsendorf F. Head lice. Dtsch Arztebl Int. 2016;113(45):763–72.
85. Sangare AK, Doumbo OK, Raoult D. Management and treatment of human lice. Biomed Res Int. 2016;2016:8962685.
86. Benelli G, Caselli A, Di Giuseppe G, Canale A. Control of biting lice, Mallophaga – a review. Acta Trop. 2018;177:211–9.
87. Yetman RJ. The child with pediculosis capitis. J Pediatr Health Care. 2015;29(1):118–20.
88. Galiczynski EM Jr, Elston DM. What's eating you? Pubic lice (Pthirus pubis). Cutis. 2008;81(2):109–14.
89. Zachariah P, Stockwell MS. Measles vaccine: past, present, and future. J Clin Pharmacol. 2016;56(2):133–40.
90. Kumar D, Sabella C. Measles: back again. Cleve Clin J Med. 2016;83(5):340–4.
91. Drutz J. Measles. Pediatr Rev. 2016;37(5):220–1.
92. Bester JC. Measles and measles vaccination: a review. JAMA Pediatr. 2016;170(12):1209–15.
93. Prymula R, Shaw J, Chlibek R, Urbancikova I, Prymulova K. Vaccination in newly arrived immigrants to the European Union. Vaccine. 2017. https://doi.org/10.1016/j.vaccine.2017.05.079.
94. Mipatrini D, Stefanelli P, Severoni S, Rezza G. Vaccinations in migrants and refugees: a challenge for European health systems. A systematic review of current scientific evidence. Pathog Glob Health. 2017;111(2):59–68.
95. Lee D, Weinberg M, Benoit S. Evaluation of measles-mumps-rubella vaccination among newly arrived refugees. Am J Public Health. 2017;107(5):684–6.
96. Giambi C, Del Manso M, Dente MG, Napoli C, Montano-Remacha C, Riccardo F, et al. Immunization strategies targeting newly arrived migrants in Non-EU countries of the Mediterranean Basin and Black Sea. Int J Environ Res Public Health. 2017;14(5):E459.
97. Coleman MS, Burke HM, Welstead BL, Mitchell T, Taylor EM, Shapovalov D, et al. Cost analysis of measles in refugees arriving at Los Angeles International Airport from Malaysia. Hum Vaccin Immunother. 2017;13(5):1084–90.
98. Ozaras R, Leblebicioglu H, Sunbul M, Tabak F, Balkan II, Yemisen M, et al. The Syrian conflict and infectious diseases. Expert Rev Anti-Infect Ther. 2016;14(6):547–55.
99. Jones G, Haeghebaert S, Merlin B, Antona D, Simon N, Elmouden M, et al. Measles outbreak in a refugee settlement in Calais, France: January to February 2016. Eurosurveillance. 2016;21(11):30167.
100. Jablonka A, Happle C, Grote U, Schleenvoigt BT, Hampel A, Dopfer C, et al. Measles, mumps, rubella, and varicella seroprevalence in refugees in Germany in 2015. Infection. 2016;44(6):781–7.
101. Taylor WR. Measles in Vietnamese refugee children in Hong Kong. Epidemiol Infect. 1999;122(3):441–6.
102. Joshua PR, Smith MM, Koh AS, Woodland LA, Zwi K. Australian population cohort study of newly arrived refugee children: how effective is predeparture measles and rubella vaccination? Pediatr Infect Dis J. 2013;32(2):104–9.
103. Rungan S, Reeve AM, Reed PW, Voss L. Health needs of refugee children younger than 5 years arriving in New Zealand. Pediatr Infect Dis J. 2013;32(12):e432–6.
104. Navarro-Colorado C, Mahamud A, Burton A, Haskew C, Maina GK, Wagacha JB, et al. Measles outbreak response among adolescent and adult Somali refugees displaced by famine in Kenya and Ethiopia, 2011. J Infect Dis. 2014;210(12):1863–70.
105. van Berlaer G, Bohle Carbonell F, Manantsoa S, de Bethune X, Buyl R, Debacker M, et al. A refugee camp in the centre of Europe: clinical characteristics of asylum seekers arriving in Brussels. BMJ Open. 2016;6(11):e013963.
106. Lange B, Stete K, Bozorgmehr K, Camp J, Kranzer K, Kern W, et al. Health care of refugees – a short review with focus on infectious diseases. Dtsch Med Wochenschr. 2016;141(11):772–6.

107. Mohamed GA, Ahmed JA, Marano N, Mohamed A, Moturi E, Burton W, et al. Etiology and incidence of viral acute respiratory infections among refugees aged 5 years and older in Hagadera Camp, Dadaab, Kenya. Am J Trop Med Hyg. 2015;93(6):1371–6.
108. Ahmed JA, Katz MA, Auko E, Njenga MK, Weinberg M, Kapella BK, et al. Epidemiology of respiratory viral infections in two long-term refugee camps in Kenya, 2007-2010. BMC Infect Dis. 2012;12:7.
109. Waterer GW. Community-acquired pneumonia: a global perspective. Semin Respir Crit Care Med. 2016;37(6):799–805.
110. Heron M. Deaths: leading causes for 2013. Natl Vital Stat Rep. 2016;65(2):1–95.
111. Epidemic focus: Influenza. Wkly Epidemiol Rec. 2016;91(22):285–6.
112. Romero-Gomez M, Zelber-Sagi S, Trenell M. Treatment of NAFLD with diet, physical activity and exercise. J Hepatol. 2017;67:829–46.
113. Yun K, Hebrank K, Graber LK, Sullivan MC, Chen I, Gupta J. High prevalence of chronic non-communicable conditions among adult refugees: implications for practice and policy. J Community Health. 2012;37(5):1110–8.
114. Culhane-Pera KA, Moua M, DeFor TA, Desai J. Cardiovascular disease risks in Hmong refugees from Wat Tham Krabok, Thailand. J Immigr Minor Health. 2009;11(5):372–9.
115. Dookeran NM, Battaglia T, Cochran J, Geltman PL. Chronic disease and its risk factors among refugees and asylees in Massachusetts, 2001-2005. Prev Chronic Dis. 2010;7(3):A51.
116. Drummond PD, Mizan A, Burgoyne A, Wright B. Knowledge of cardiovascular risk factors in West African refugee women living in Western Australia. J Immigr Minor Health. 2011;13(1):140–8.
117. Renzaho AM, Bilal P, Marks GC. Obesity, type 2 diabetes and high blood pressure amongst recently arrived Sudanese refugees in Queensland, Australia. J Immigr Minor Health. 2014;16(1):86–94.
118. Nelson-Peterman JL, Toof R, Liang SL, Grigg-Saito DC. Long-term refugee health: health behaviors and outcomes of Cambodian refugee and immigrant women. Health Educ Behav. 2015;42(6):814–23.
119. Mulugeta W, Glick M, Min J, Xue H, Noe MF, Wang Y. Longitudinal changes and high-risk subgroups for obesity and overweight/obesity among refugees in Buffalo, NY, 2004-2014. J Racial Ethn Health Disparities. 2017. https://doi.org/10.1007/s40615-017-0356-y.
120. Centers for Disease C, Prevention. Health of resettled Iraqi refugees – San Diego County, California, October 2007-September 2009. MMWR Morb Mortal Wkly Rep. 2010;59(49):1614–8.
121. Kumar GS, Varma S, Saenger MS, Burleson M, Kohrt BA, Cantey P. Noninfectious disease among the Bhutanese refugee population at a United States urban clinic. J Immigr Minor Health. 2014;16(5):922–5.
122. Yusef JI. Management of diabetes mellitus and hypertension at UNRWA primary health care facilities in Lebanon. East Mediterr Health J. 2000;6(2–3):378–90.
123. Wagner J, Berthold SM, Buckley T, Kong S, Kuoch T, Scully M. Diabetes among refugee populations: what newly arriving refugees can learn from resettled Cambodians. Curr Diab Rep. 2015;15(8):56.
124. Strong J, Varady C, Chahda N, Doocy S, Burnham G. Health status and health needs of older refugees from Syria in Lebanon. Confl Health. 2015;9:12.
125. Shahin Y, Kapur A, Seita A. Diabetes care in refugee camps: the experience of UNRWA. Diabetes Res Clin Pract. 2015;108(1):1–6.
126. Downes MJ, Bettington EK, Gunton JE, Turkstra E. Triple therapy in type 2 diabetes; a systematic review and network meta-analysis. Peer J. 2015;3:e1461.
127. Ilkilic I, Ertin H. Ethical conflicts in the treatment of fasting Muslim patients with diabetes during Ramadan. Med Health Care Philos. 2017;20:561–70.
128. Hassanein M, Al-Arouj M, Hamdy O, Bebakar WMW, Jabbar A, Al-Madani A, et al. Diabetes and Ramadan: practical guidelines. Diabetes Res Clin Pract. 2017;126:303–16.

129. Almansour HA, Chaar B, Saini B. Fasting, diabetes, and optimizing health outcomes for Ramadan observers: a literature review. Diabetes Ther. 2017;8(2):227–49.
130. Chau P, Lee HS, Tseng R, Downes NJ. Dietary habits, health beliefs, and food practices of elderly Chinese women. J Am Diet Assoc. 1990;90(4):579–80.
131. Das JK, Salam RA, Arshad A, Lassi ZS, Bhutta ZA. Systematic review and meta-analysis of interventions to improve access and coverage of adolescent immunizations. J Adolesc Health. 2016;59(4S):S40–S8.
132. Hasahya OT, Berggren V, Sematimba D, Nabirye RC, Kumakech E. Beliefs, perceptions and health-seeking behaviours in relation to cervical cancer: a qualitative study among women in Uganda following completion of an HPV vaccination campaign. Glob Health Action. 2016;9:29336.
133. Kaler A. Health interventions and the persistence of rumour: the circulation of sterility stories in African public health campaigns. Soc Sci Med. 2009;68(9):1711–9.
134. Kuehnel MVsn, 2016. Epidemieplan des Wiener Roten Kreuzes. Vienna: Wiener Roten Kreuz; 2016.
135. Kuehnel M, Notfallplan des Rotes Kreuz beim Auftreten von hochkontagiösen Erkrankungen, (intern paper); 2016.
136. Al-Modallal H, Hamaideh S, Mudallal R. Mental health status of women in Jordan: a comparative study between attendees of governmental and UN relief and works agency's health care centers. Issues Ment Health Nurs. 2014;35(5):386–94.
137. Vasilevski V, Carolan-Olah M. Food taboos and nutrition-related pregnancy concerns among Ethiopian women. J Clin Nurs. 2016;25(19–20):3069–75.
138. Alnuaimi K, Kassab M, Ali R, Mohammad K, Shattnawi K. Pregnancy outcomes among Syrian refugee and Jordanian women: a comparative study. Int Nurs Rev. 2017;64:584–92.
139. Simsek Z, Yentur Doni N, Gul Hilali N, Yildirimkaya G. A community-based survey on Syrian refugee women's health and its predictors in Sanliurfa, Turkey. Women Health. 2017. https://doi.org/10.1080/03630242.2017.1321609.
140. Moszynski P. Needs of disabled refugees are "routinely ignored". BMJ. 2008;337:a620.
141. Mirza M, Heinemann AW. Service needs and service gaps among refugees with disabilities resettled in the United States. Disabil Rehabil. 2012;34(7):542–52.
142. Zonszein J, Groop PH. Strategies for diabetes management: using newer oral combination therapies early in the disease. Diabetes Ther. 2016;7(4):621–39.
143. Wise J. NICE recommends new triple therapy option for type 2 diabetes. BMJ. 2016;355:i5472.
144. Scheen AJ. Pharmacotherapy of 'treatment resistant' type 2 diabetes. Expert Opin Pharmacother. 2017;18(5):503–15.
145. Cornell S. Comparison of the diabetes guidelines from the ADA/EASD and the AACE/ACE. J Am Pharm Assoc (2003). 2017;57(2):261–5.

Medical Aspects of Care in Host Countries: Embedding Refugees in Healthcare Systems

17

Maria van den Muijsenbergh

Abstract

Health of refugees and other migrants tends to deteriorate upon arrival in a host country. Also, outcomes of care are less favourable for this in comparison with a host population. Hereby, social determinants of health, such as a lack of social participation, poverty, discrimination and a lack of accessible, good quality of healthcare, play a decisive role.

Access to and good quality of healthcare are hampered by limited health literacy and lack of resources in migrant patients; lack of cultural competency in healthcare providers, resulting in inadequate communication and care which is not tailored to the needs of the patient; and financial, organisational and informational barriers in healthcare systems.

In order to realise the universal right to access affordable, good quality healthcare and to establish equity in healthcare, migrants should receive information on local healthcare systems and on health promotion. Further, healthcare providers should be trained in providing compassionate, person-centred culturally competent healthcare, interpreter services and cultural mediation services should be available, and financial and organisational barriers should be limited. Besides, probably the most important is to create jobs, good housing and a migrant-friendly environment for all refugees.

M. van den Muijsenbergh
Pharos, Centre of Expertise on Health Disparities, Utrecht, The Netherlands

Department of Primary and Community Care, Radboud University Medical Centre, Nijmegen, The Netherlands
e-mail: M.Muijsenbergh@pharos.nl

T. Wenzel, B. Drožđek (eds.), *An Uncertain Safety*,
https://doi.org/10.1007/978-3-319-72914-5_17

17.1 Introduction: Health of Refugees and Other Migrants—Social Determinants of Health

Refugees who are able to undertake the, sometimes dangerous and difficult, journey to a safe country are often relatively healthy compared to the general population in their countries of origin. This is called the 'healthy migrant effect' [1, 2]. However, after arrival in the host country, refugees' health often deteriorates. Compared to the population of the host country, refugees and other migrants rate their own health as being worse [3], and the older they become, the larger this difference gets [4, 5]. Several social determinants of health play an important mediating role hereby: length of asylum procedure (the longer the procedure, the more mental health problems surface) [6], opportunities for family reunion (the sooner refugees can be reunited with their families the better) [7] and, most importantly for a healthy life, social support in their new environment, as well as opportunities to obtain employment commensurate with their abilities and experience [8]. Highly educated and young refugees (with exception of unaccompanied minors) have better health prospects than less-educated or older refugees [5].

Similar ethnic minority groups living in different countries differ in mortality rates, possibly reflecting local context [9, 10]. However, mental health problems, cardiovascular diseases, being overweight, diabetes mellitus, some infectious diseases and reproductive health problems are much more prevalent amongst refugees and other migrants, especially amongst those originating from South Asia, Africa and the Caribbean, than amongst the host population [5, 11, 12]. Whilst genetically based differences in morbidity, violence and other unfavourable life experiences contribute to this high incidence, there is also growing evidence of the relationship between migration-related social problems and chronic stress and the rapid development of metabolic diseases, such as hypertension, overweight and diabetes in migrants, particularly in refugees [13–16]. So the actual development of many of these health problems depends on social determinants, like participation in society, social support and health literacy [17]. Moreover, it depends also on preventive measures, timely diagnosis and treatment, for which access to and a good quality of healthcare are prerequisites. Healthcare systems are, therefore, also a crucial social determinant of health [18]. In general, health problems often overlap with deprivation and poor living conditions, highlighting the relationship between poverty, poor health and a lack of access to healthcare [19, 20]. In addition, a direct relation between discrimination and poor health has also been documented [21, 22].

The important role of social determinants in health is best illustrated with the example of diabetes mellitus. Refugees residing for a longer period of time in host countries, like the Netherlands, develop diabetes twice as often as other people of the same age [23]. This is attributed to their physical inactivity, overweight, chronic stress and mental health problems. Asylum seekers with a posttraumatic stress disorder (PTSD) diagnosis develop diabetes 1 four times more often than asylum seekers without PTSD [14, 15]. Diabetes is also more prevalent amongst lower-educated persons, and the outcome of diabetes care is worse amongst non-Western immigrants than amongst other inhabitants of the same education and socio-economic status [24]. These poor health outcomes are caused by limited health literacy, language barriers and a lack of culturally competent healthcare.

Unintended pregnancies, teenage pregnancies, induced abortion and maternal morbidity are more prevalent amongst refugees, especially those from Africa [25, 26]. Postpartum maternal morbidity and mortality rates amongst foreign women in France, the UK and the Netherlands are significantly higher compared to non-foreigners [27–29]. Causes of these elevated reproductive health risks include sexual violence, a general lack of knowledge about contraception, unfamiliarity with the local healthcare system and a later engagement with maternity services in case of pregnancy. On top of this, these studies suggest that inferior medical attention may have also played a role herein. Substandard perinatal care included the lack of or late attention to specific conditions more common in migrant women (like preterm birth) [30].

In general, poor health outcomes in refugees are caused by limited health literacy, language barriers and a lack of culturally competent healthcare. Despite the fact that everyone has a fundamental right to health and to access healthcare, actual access and quality of care are often hampered in migrants in vulnerable situations [31].

In this chapter we will discuss the use of healthcare services, differences between countries in healthcare systems and entitlements of refugees and barriers in access and quality of care. We will conclude pointing out the need for person-centred, integrated healthcare services and discuss how to create them.

17.2 Use of Healthcare Services

The ability to access healthcare is influenced by many different factors, including legal entitlement, organisation of the health system in the host country, knowledge about and awareness of this health system [32], previous experiences with healthcare [33], language and cultural barriers [34] and health beliefs and attitudes [18, 35]. The ability to find, understand and apply knowledge about health and healthcare is called health literacy, which is often found to be low in refugees [36]. Availability of services and healthcare insurance, extent of a healthcare coverage and out-of-pocket payments can all impact access to and use of healthcare. This is particularly documented in individuals with low health literacy and a different cultural background and those facing language barriers which lessen their capacity to cope with such demands [18].

In most countries documented or regular migrants and asylum seekers are entitled to some form of healthcare insurance that covers most of the costs in primary care or, at least, basic treatment for acute diseases and antenatal care [19]. Although the right to medical care for all is an acknowledged human right [37], and medical professionals are bound to deliver all necessary medical care irrespective of finances or one's legal status [38], rejected asylum seekers and other undocumented migrants face substantial financial and administrative barriers in accessing healthcare [39–41]. In most countries they have no right to health insurance and are required to cover costs of healthcare by themselves. However, some form of 'emergency' care is provided for them, and, in some situations, healthcare workers can get some reimbursement of costs if the migrants are unable to pay.

Migrants make less use of public health facilities, screening and preventive programmes, antenatal services and homecare provisions [42–45], than a general population. Avoidance of mental healthcare often occurs due to taboos and stigma for having mental health problems, and mistrust or lack of knowledge about the local healthcare system [46]. On the other hand, the use of general practice care and of emergency services is generally higher amongst migrants, even when compared with native patients of a same socio-economic level and health status [47, 48]. This has been related to inadequate access to other health services.

As mentioned before, there are indications that not only access but also effectiveness of care in some medical fields is lower for migrants [45, 49, 50]. On top of other factors, language and cultural barriers play here a decisive role [51, 52].

17.3 Barriers in Access and Quality of Healthcare

Many refugees and other migrants have been found to have inadequate access to health services [10, 53]. Barriers to access care and to receive good quality of care occur at three different levels: the patient, the provider and the system.

At a patient level, access and adequate use of care are hampered by a lack of knowledge of the healthcare system [54], language barriers [55] as well as cultural beliefs which impact communication and health-seeking behaviour [56]. For instance, refugees and other migrants often do not take initiative to talk about mental health problems or about war trauma with their doctor. Common reasons for this are taboo for sharing mental health issues with a health professional, not knowing if this professional would be the appropriate person to speak about it or not considering the impact of war or mental health problems as a health-related issue or as a relevant topic during clinical visits. Besides, some refugees also do not want to raise bad memories whilst sharing their difficult past [46, 57, 58].

Moreover, lack of social support and other social problems adversely affect the capacity of vulnerable migrants to successfully navigate the complex healthcare system [18]. Financial barriers play here a role as well, for example, having to deal with out-of-pocket money or with services that are not included in health insurance, like dental care. However, communication difficulties have been identified by many scholars as a primary barrier [59–63].

At a provider level, weak communication skills and a lack of cultural competence, including the lack of knowledge about rights and needs of refugees and their complex medical and social history, act as a major barrier [59, 60, 63, 64]. Moreover, health providers make seldom use of formal interpreters in their daily work [62]. An example of cultural insensitivity of practitioners is not engaging family in maternal care even though this is a part of culture and is expected by patients [61, 63]. Health professionals themselves also mention lack of time as an important barrier to addressing the needs of migrants in an adequate way [65].

At a system level several barriers are also present.

There are enormous differences in the 'diversity sensitivity' of health systems. In many countries, this principle seems to be unknown [66]. 'Diversity sensitivity' means that the system acknowledges the fact that migrants may need additional or different things to achieve access to good quality healthcare, for instance, the availability of interpreter services, cultural mediators and cultural sensitive health information materials, training of professionals in culturally competent care, etc. Very often, these are countries with little experience of migration, but this is by no means always the case. An important variable influencing overall 'migrant-friendliness' of health systems is the GDP per capita. Poor countries give migrants fewer entitlements and make less effort to adapt services to migrants' needs [66]. These differences in 'diversity sensitivity' are also reflected by the Migrant Integration Policy Index (MIPEX) that provides information on the level of migrant-friendliness of a specific country. It is a tool which measures policies to integrate migrants in all EU member states, Australia, Canada, Iceland, Japan, South Korea, New Zealand, Norway, Switzerland, Turkey and the USA (http://www.mipex.eu/what-is-mipex accessed May 6, 2017). Concerning health, their key findings are that major differences between countries emerge in immigrants' healthcare coverage and their ability to access services. Policies often fail to take migrants' specific health needs into account (http://www.mipex.eu/health).

Since primary care is in many countries the first or main entrance to healthcare, O'Donnell et al. [18] explored the impact of a strong or a weak primary healthcare system on migrants' access to healthcare using Kringos's framework of primary care [67]. They have mapped the key barriers and facilitators to migrants' access to primary care. These authors concluded that 'national level system and political decisions, which limit rights to entitlement and access and lead to a reliance of out-of-pocket payments, reduce the capacity of migrants to access primary care and—importantly—hamper professionals to respond to such patients. For example, in the Netherlands, a change in government has resulted in a policy retraction from migrant health, including the dissolution of paid interpreter services' ([18], p. 10, par. 4.1.1). Registration procedures, appointment systems and a need to negotiate access with reception staff at health offices, all add to a burden of accessing care in refugees [18]. On top of this, social stigma and discrimination towards the target groups constitute another profound barrier [68].

17.4 The Need for a Person-Centred Integrated Care

When a refugee who has obtained asylum in the Netherlands was interviewed, he said 'Show me the way, explain how things work over here, teach me the language, and give me a job'. This person emphasised integration into Dutch society as his main concern. And indeed, social participation appears to be a major facilitator of good health in refugees in the long term [23]. Improving social determinants of health amongst refugees should therefore be the first priority. Governments should provide appropriate housing, access to employment and other aspects for a good habitat [69]. Also, in order to prevent the health of refugees from deteriorating and treat conditions from which they suffer adequately, the healthcare system of a host country and healthcare professionals, in particular, need to better adjust their care to needs and concerns of refugees.

This requests integrated actions of healthcare professionals, community workers, municipalities, social workers and schools. An integrated, community-oriented approach, which actively involves refugees, is needed to inform them about a host society and healthcare as well as about healthy lifestyle. Activities designed to improve refugees' health literacy should be applied, aiming at strengthening their resilience and reducing mental stress [59]. Refugees should themselves be involved in the organisation of healthcare as to clearly identify their needs and tailor interventions according to them. Involvement of migrants and refugees in design and delivery of services is seen as a key tool for improving access and quality of health services [70]. Unfortunately, these groups are usually poorly represented [71, 72]. Community-based approaches aiming at mobilising health resources already present in communities seem to be promising [70, 72]. For instance, in the Netherlands, Syrian and Eritrean refugees with a medical background are often asked for medical advice by other refugees from their country, especially when Dutch medical practices differ from those in their country of origin (e.g. the limited prescription of antibiotics in the Netherlands). As the information from their compatriots is more trusted than the information of the Dutch healthcare workers, the Dutch health information and promotion organisations, together with these refugee health professionals, introduced a health information page on Facebook and a website written by the refugee professionals in the local languages (Arab and Tigrinya), which provide health information and answers to questions of refugees. These refugee professionals are informed about the Dutch healthcare system by the Dutch professionals (Facebook page 'Syriërs gezond' (Healthy Syrians) and www.gezondinnederland.info (Healthy in the Netherlands)).

Refugees, like anybody else, benefit from person-centred care [73], a care that is tailored to their needs and background. To be able to deliver such care, healthcare professionals need cultural competencies [74]. These include an open, nonjudgemental, curious and compassionate attitude and a basic knowledge of ethnic and socio-economic health differences and conditions that often occur amongst migrants. Also, cultural competence is about knowing refugees' entitlements, possessing a basic understanding of the political situation in their country of origin and having good communication skills to overcome linguistic and cultural differences and to interact with low-literate persons [62, 75–77]. Training of professionals in cultural sensitive aspects of their work is a core enabler [69, 78]. However, as the composition of migrant populations varies from country to country, as does the degree of integration of migrants within the host society and their adherence to traditional or cultural practices, health professionals should avoid relying on cultural stereotypes [66]. Recently, more attention is paid to the importance for professionals to understand their own culture, as little use can be learned about a patient's culture from books. This way, one can improve acceptance and understanding of others. In patient-centred care, the way to overcome cultural barriers is to take time to get to know a patient better [66].

Another very important aspect is availability and use of professional interpretation services in healthcare delivery [34, 79]. The use of these services has proved to be cost-effective and to improve patients' satisfaction and outcome of care [80, 81]. Many health professionals and migrants tend to rely for interpretation on family, friends or migrant workers. Although the presence and involvement of family can empower a patient [82, 83] and advocate his interests, it is more often causing problems. Many family members lack skills to translate medical terms or choose not to translate when they judge that a message would be painful or harmful for a patient, for instance, when it comes to bringing bad news [84–86]. On the other hand, it is important to explore quality, professionality and appropriateness of a professional interpreter service, as sometimes refugees may fear (not always unfunded) that interpreters from the same background as their own may be connected with a suppressive regime that a refugee has escaped from.

Obviously, when sensitive topics, like violence and reproductive or mental health, have to be addressed, the presence of a family member as interpreter can be an obstacle for patients to disclose their problems. Even in the presence of professional interpreters, many refugees seldom mention these topics spontaneously to a health professional. Instead, they prefer a professional to inquire into their mental health, experiences with violence or reproductive health issues proactively [46, 57, 87].

In many countries cultural mediators are available. These are migrants who know how the local healthcare systems work, speak the local language and support other migrants in their interactions with a healthcare system and professionals. The use of cultural mediator services can support migrants navigating through a healthcare system effectively, if one assures that the mediator's gender and age fits with the patient's expectations. Women may, for example, feel uncomfortable sharing sensitive issues with male cultural mediators. The continuous presence of the same cultural mediator throughout a treatment process can help in building trust and prevent patients from having to share their private stories with different mediators [63].

The same importance of personal continuity of care has been found for the role of health professionals: seeing as much as possible the same doctor or nurse [63, 64] increases satisfaction, trust and confidence and improves communication with a patient [63, 88].

Last but not least, the main ingredient of a good healthcare for refugees is something all health professionals should be able to provide—a smiling face, a welcoming gesture and sufficient time, compassion with and respect for a refugee patient.

References

1. Kennedy S, McDonald JT, Biddle N. The healthy immigrant effect and immigrant selection: evidence from four countries. In: Social and economic dimensions of an aging population research papers 164; 2006. Hamilton: McMaster University. http://ideas.repec.org/p/mcm/sedapp/164.html.
2. Razum O, Zeeb H, Rohrmann S. The 'healthy migrant effect'- not merely a fallacy of inaccurate denominator figures. Int J Epidemiol. 2000;21:199–200.

3. Nielsen SS, Krasnik A. Poorer self-perceived health among migrants and ethnic minorities versus the majority population in Europe: a systematic review. Int J Public Health. 2010;55:357–71.
4. Rechel B, Mladovsky P, Ingleby D, Mackenbach JP, McKee M. Migration and health in an increasingly diverse Europe. Lancet. 2013;381:1235–45.
5. Hadgkiss EJ, Renzaho AM. The physical health status, service utilisation and barriers to accessing care for asylum seekers residing in the community: a systematic review of the literature. Aust Health Rev. 2014;38:142–59.
6. Laban CJ, Komproe IH, Gernaat HB, de Jong JT. The impact of a long asylum procedure on quality of life, disability and physical health in Iraqi asylum seekers in the Netherlands. Soc Psychiatry Psychiatr Epidemiol. 2008;43(7):507.
7. Gerritsen AA, Bramsen I, Deville W, van Willigen LH, Hovens JE, van der Ploeg HM. Physical and mental health of Afghan, Iranian and Somali asylum seekers and refugees living in the Netherlands. Soc Psychiatry Psychiatr Epidemiol. 2006;41(1):18–26. https://doi.org/10.1007/s00127-0050003-5.
8. Schellingerhout R. Self-experienced Health, lifestyle and healthcare use (Ervaren gezondheid, leefstijl en zorggebruik). In: Dourleijn E, Dagevos J, editors. Refugees groups in the Netherlands (Vluchtelingengroepen in Nederland). Den Haag: Dutch Social Cultural Planning Agency (SCP); 2011.
9. Bhopal R, Rafnsson S, Agyemang C, Fagot-Campagna A, Giampaoli S, Hammar N, Harding S, Hedlund E, Juel K, Wild S, Kunst A. Mortality from circulatory diseases by specific country of birth across six European countries: test of concept. Eur J Public Health. 2012;22(3):353–9.
10. Rafnsson SB, Bhopal RS, Agyemang C, Fagot-Campagna A, Giampaoli S, Hammar N, Hedlund E, Juel K, Primatesta P, Wild S, Mackenbach JP. Sizable variations in cardiovascular mortality by country of birth in five European countries: implications for measuring health inequalities in the region. Migrant and Ethnic Health Observatory. 2009. http://www.meho.eu.com/Upload/15WP6%20-%20annex%20deliverable%206.4c%20sizeable%20variations%20in%20cardiovascular%20mortality.pdf.
11. European Centre for Disease Prevention and Control. Communicable disease risks associated with the movement of refugees in Europe during the winter season. Stockholm: ECDC; 2015.
12. Vandenheede H, Deboosere P, Kunst AE. Migrant mortality from diabetes mellitus across Europe. Migrant and Ethnic Health Observatory. 2009. http://www.meho.eu.com/Upload/7WP5%20-20annex%20deliverable%205.1%20mortality%20diabetes.pdf.
13. Schulz AJ, House JS, Israel BA, Mentz G, Dvonch JT, Miranda PY, Kannan S, Koch M. Relational pathways between socioeconomic position and cardiovascular risk in a multiethnic urban sample: complexities and their implications for improving health in economically disadvantaged populations. J Epidemiol Community Health. 2008;62:638–46. https://doi.org/10.1136/jech.2007.063222.
14. Pyykkönen AJ, Räikkönen K, Tuomi T, Eriksson JG, Groop L, Isomaa B. Stressful life events and the metabolic syndrome. The Prevalence. Prediction and Prevention of Diabetes PPP: Botnia Study. Diabetes Care. 2010;33(2):378–84.
15. Agyemang C, Goosen S, Anujo K, Ogedegbe G. Relationship between post-traumatic stress disorder and diabetes among 105.180 asylum seekers in the Netherlands. Eur J Pub Health. 2011: 1–5. https://doi.org/10.1093/eurpub/ckr138.
16. Murray KE, Davidson GR. Review of refugee mental health interventions following resettlements: best practices and recommendations. Am J Orthopsychiatry. 2010;80(4):576–85.
17. Hirani K, Payne D, Mutch R, et al. Health of adolescent refugees resettling in high-income countries. Arch Dis Child. 2015;101:670–6. https://doi.org/10.1136/archdischild-2014-307221.
18. O'Donnell CA, Burns N, Mair F, Dowrick C, Clissmann C, Van den Muijsenbergh M, Van Weel-Baumgarten E, Lionis C, Papadaki M, Saridaki A, de Brun T, O'Reilly de Brun M, MacFarlane A. Reducing the health care burden for marginalised migrants: the potential role for primary care in Europe. Health Policy. 2016;120:495–508. https://doi.org/10.1016/j.healthpol.2016.03.012.

19. Stanciole AE, Huber M. Access to health care for migrants. Ethnic minorities and asylum seekers in Europe. Policy Brief May 2009. European Centre for Social Welfare Policy and Research, Vienna; 2009.
20. Ingleby D. Ethnicity, migration and the "Social Determinants of Health" agenda. Psychosoc Interv. 2012;21(3):331–41.
21. Pascoe EA, Smart Richman L. Perceived discrimination and health: a meta-analytic review. Psychol Bull. 2009;135(4):531–54.
22. Ikram UZ, Snijder MB, Agyemang C, Schene A, Peters RJ, Stronks K, Kunst AE. Perceived ethnic discrimination and the metabolic syndrome in ethnic minority groups: the Healthy Life in an Urban Setting study. Psychosom Med. 2017;79:101–11.
23. Lamkaddem M. Explaining health and healthcare utilisation of ethnic minorities in the Netherlands. Thesis. Amsterdam University; 2013.
24. Lanting LC, Joung IM, Mackenbach JP, Lamberts SW, Bootsma AH. Ethnic differences in mortality, end-stage complications, and quality of care among diabetic patients: a review. Diabetes Care. 2005;28:2280–8.
25. Hynes M, Sheik M, Wilson HG, Spiegel P. Reproductive health indicators and outcomes among refugee and internally displaced persons in postemergency phase camps. JAMA. 2002;288(5):595–603.
26. Aptekman M, et al. Unmet contraceptive needs among refugees. Can Fam Physician Med Fam Can. 2014;60(12):e613–9.
27. Philibert M, Deneux-Tharaux C, Bouvier Colle M. Can excess maternal mortality among women of foreign nationality be explained by suboptimal obstetric care? BJOG. 2008;115:1411–8.
28. Centre for Maternal and Child Enquiries. Saving Mothers' lives: reviewing death to make motherhood safer: 2006–2008. BJOG. 2011;118(s1):1–203.
29. Boerleider AW. Non-western women in maternity care in the Netherlands. Thesis. Amsterdam University; 2015.
30. Alderliesten ME, Stronks K, van Lith JM, Smit BJ, van der Wal MF, Bonsel GJ, Bleker OP. Ethnic differences in perinatal mortality: a perinatal audit on the role of substandard care. Eur J Obstet Gynecol Reprod Biol. 2008;138(2):164–70.
31. Pace P. The right to health of migrants in Europe. In: Rechel B, Mladovsky P, Deville W, Petrova-Benedict R, McKee M, editors. Migration and health in the European Union. 1st ed. Maidenhead: McGraw Hill; 2011. p. 55–66.
32. O'Donnell CA, Higgins M, Chauhan R, Mullen K. "They think we're OK and we know we're not". A qualitative study of asylum seekers' access, knowledge and views to health care in the UK. BMC Health Serv Res. 2007;7:75.
33. O'Donnell CA, Higgins M, Chauhan R, Mullen K. Asylum seekers' expectations of and trust in general practice: a qualitative study. Br J Gen Pract. 2008;58(12):870–6.
34. Bischoff A. Do language barriers increase inequalities? Do interpreters decrease inequalities? In: Ingleby D, Chiarenza A, Deville W, Kotsioni I, editors. Inequalities in health care for migrants and ethnic minorities. 1st ed. Antwerp: Garant; 2012. p. 128–43.
35. Cooper M, Harding S, Mullen K, O'Donnell C. 'A chronic disease is a disease which keeps coming back?…?it is like the flu': chronic disease risk perception and explanatory models among French- and Swahili-speaking African migrants. Ethn Health. 2012;17(6):597–613.
36. Wangdahl J, et al. Health literacy among refugees in Sweden – a cross-sectional study. BMC Public Health. 2014;14:1030.
37. UN economic saCRC. 2000: General comment No. 14. The right to the highest attainable standard of health. UN Doc E/C. 12/2000/4. 2000; 2000.
38. World Medical Association WMA. International code of medical ethics; 2006.
39. Chauvin P, Parizot I, Simonnot N. Access to health care for undocumented migrants in 11 European countries. Medicins de Monde Observatory on Access to Health Care. Medicins du Monde; 2009.
40. Cuadra CB. Right of access to health care for undocumented migrants in the EU: a comparative study of national policies. Eur J Pub Health. 2011;22(2):267–71.

41. Suess A, et al. The right of access to health care for undocumented migrants: a revision of comparative analysis in the European context. Eur J Pub Health. 2014;24(5):712–20.
42. Nørredam M, Nielsen S, Krasnik A. Migrants' utilization of somatic healthcare services in Europe – a systematic review. Eur J Pub Health. 2010;20(5):555–63.
43. Berens E-M, Spallek J, Razum O. Breast cancer screening among immigrant women: do we need specific approaches in risk communication? In: Ingleby D, Krasnik A, Lorant V, Razum O, editors. Health and health inequalities and risk factors among migrants and ethnic minorities. COST series diversity, vol. I. Antwerp: Garant; 2012. p. 304–18.
44. Alderliesten ME, Vrijkotte TG, van der Wal MF, Bonsel GJ. Late start of antenatal care among ethnic minorities in a large cohort of pregnant women. Int J Obstet Gynaecol. 2007;114(10):1232–9.
45. Denktaş S, Koopmans G, Birnie E, Foets M, Bonsel G. Ethnic background and differences in health care use: a national cross-sectional study of native Dutch and immigrant elderly in the Netherlands. Int J Equity Health. 2009;8:35.
46. Teunissen E, Sherally J, van den Muijsenbergh M, Dowrick C, van Weel-Baumgarten E, van Weel C. Mental health problems of undocumented migrants (UM) in the Netherlands: a qualitative exploration of help-seeking behaviour and experiences with primary care. BMJ Open. 2014;4(11):e005738.
47. McMahon J, MacFarlane A, Avalos G, Cantillon P, Murphy AW. A survey of asylum seekers' general practice GP: service utilisation and morbidity patterns. Ir Med J. 2009;1005:461–4.
48. Uiters E, Devillé W, Foets M, Spreeuwenberg P, Groenewegen PP. Differences between immigrant and non-immigrant groups in the use of primary medical care; a systematic review. BMC Health Serv Res. 2009;9:76.
49. Huber M, Stanciole A, Bremner J, Wahlbeck K. Quality in and equality of access to healthcare services: HealthQUEST.Brussels: DG Employment. Social affairs and equal opportunities. 2008. http://www.euro.centre.org/detail.php?xml:id=866.
50. Lanting LC, Joung IM, Vogel I, Bootsma AH, Lamberts SW, Mackenbach JP. Ethnic differences in outcomes of diabetes care and the role of self-management behavior. Patient Educ Couns. 2008;72(1):146–54.
51. Smedley B, Stith A, Nelson A. Assessing potential sources of racial and ethnic disparities in care: the clinical encounter. In: Unequal treatment: confronting racial and ethnic disparities in health care. Washington DC: The National Academies Press; 2003. p. 160–79.
52. Sievers E. Perinatal morbidity and mortality among migrants in Europe. In: Ingleby D, Krasnik A, Lorant V, Razum O, editors. Cost series on health and diversity 2012. Volume 1. Health inequalities and risk factors among migrants and ethnic minorities. Antwerp: Garant; 2012. p. 180–92.
53. Fundamental Rights Agency FRA. Inequalities and multiple discrimination in access to and quality of health care. Vienna: Fundamental Rights Agency; 2013.
54. Otoukesh S, Mojtahedzadeh M, Figlin RA, Rosenfelt FP, Behazin A, Sherzai D, et al. Literature review and profile of cancer diseases among Afghan refugees in Iran: referrals in six years of displacement. Med Sci Monit Int Med J Exp Clin Res. 2015;21:3622.
55. Wagner J, Berthold SM, Buckley T, Kong S, Kuoch T, Scully M. Diabetes among refugee populations: what newly arriving refugees can learn from resettled Cambodians. Curr Diab Rep. 2015;15(8):1–14.
56. Modesti PA, Bianchi S, Borghi C, Cameli M, Capasso G, Ceriello A, et al. Cardiovascular health in migrants: current status and issues for prevention. A collaborative multidisciplinary task force report. J Cardiovasc Med. 2014;15(9):683–92.
57. Shannon P, O'Dougherty M, Mehta E. Refugees' perspectives on barriers to communication about trauma histories in primary care. Ment Health Fam Med. 2012;9:47–55.
58. Schoevers MA, Loeffen MJ, van den Muijsenbergh M, Lagro-Janssen AL. Health care utilisation and problems in accessing health care of female undocumented immigrants in the Netherlands. Int J Public Health. 2010;55:421–8.
59. Casey SE, Chynoweth SK, Cornier N, Gallagher MC, Wheeler EE. Progress and gaps in reproductive health services in three humanitarian settings: mixed-methods case studies. Confl Heal. 2015;9(1):S3.

60. Krause S, Williams H, Onyango MA, Sami S, Doedens W, Giga N, Stone E, Tomczyk B. Reproductive health services for Syrian refugees in Zaatri Camp and Irbid City, Hashemite Kingdom of Jordan: an evaluation of the minimum initial services package. Confl Heal. 2015;9(1):S4.
61. Boerleider AW, Francke AL, van de Reep M, Manniën J, Wiegers TA, et al. "Being flexible and creative": a qualitative study on maternity care assistants' experiences with non-western immigrant women. PLoS One. 2014;9:3.
62. van den Muijsenbergh M, van Weel-Baumgarten E, Burns N, O'Donnell C, Mair F, Spiegel W, Lionis C, Dowrick C, O'Reilly-de Brún M, de Brun T, MacFarlane A. Communication in cross-cultural consultations in primary care in Europe: the case for improvement. The rationale for the RESTORE FP 7 project. Prim Health Care Res Dev. 2014;15:122–33.
63. Correa-Velez I, Ryan J. Developing a best practice model of refugee maternity care. Women Birth. 2012;25:13–22.
64. Hoogenboom G, Thwin MM, Velink K, Baaijens M, Charrunwatthana P, Nosten F, McGready R. Quality of intrapartum care by skilled birth attendants in a refugee clinic on the ThaiMyanmar border: a survey using WHO Safe Motherhood Needs Assessment. BMC Pregnancy Childbirth. 2015;15:17.
65. Teunissen E, Gravenhorst K, Dowrick C, Van Weel-Baumgarten E, Van den Driessen Mareeuw F, de Brún T, Burns N, Lionis C, Mair FS, O'Donnell C, O'Reilly-de Brún M. Implementing guidelines and training initiatives to improve cross-cultural communication in primary care consultations: a qualitative participatory European study. Int J Equity Health. 2017;16(1):32.
66. Mock-Muñoz de Luna C, Ingleby D, Graval E, Krasnik A. Synthesis report Work- package 1. Training packages for health professionals to improve access and quality of health services for migrants and ethnic minorities, including the Roma. MEM-TP. Kopenhagen: Europese Unie; 2015.
67. Kringos D, Boerma W, Bourgueil Y, et al. The strength of primary care in Europe: an international comparative study. Br J Gen Pract. 2013;63(616):e742–e50.
68. Kärki T, Napoli C, Riccardo F, Fabiani M, Dente MG, Carballo M, Declich S. Screening for infectious diseases among newly arrived migrants in EU/EEA countries – varying practices but consensus on the utility of screening. Int J Environ Res Public Health. 2014;11(10):11004–14.
69. Mollica RF, Brooks RT, Ekblad S, McDonald L. The new H5 model of refugee trauma and recovery. In: Lindert J, Levav I, editors. Violence and mental health. Dordrecht: Springer Science+ Business Media; 2015. p. 341.
70. Garcia Ramirez M, Hatzidimitriadou E. User involvement and empowerment in health care. Practices with ethnic minority groups. A community approach. Int J Migr Health Soc Care. 2009;5:2–5.
71. Van den Muijsenbergh M, Teunissen E, van Weel-Baumgarten E, van Weel C. "Giving voice to the voiceless." How to involve vulnerable migrants in healthcare research. Br J Gen Pract. 2016;16:284–5.
72. O'Reilly-de Brún M, de Brún T, Okonkwo E, Bonsenge-Bokanga JS, De Almeida Silva MM, Ogbebor F, Mierzejewska A, Nnadi L, van Weel-Baumgarten E, van Weel C, van den Muijsenbergh M, MacFarlane A. Using participatory learning & action research to access and engage with 'hard to reach' migrants in primary healthcare research. BMC Health Serv Res. 2016;16:25. https://doi.org/10.1186/s12913-015-1247-8.
73. Zandbelt LC, Smets EM, Oort FJ, Godfried MH, de Haes HC. Patient participation in the medical specialist encounter: does physicians' patient-centred communication matter? Patient Educ Couns. 2007;653:396–406.
74. Saha S, Beach MC, Cooper LA. Patient centeredness, cultural competence, and healthcare quality. J Natl Med Assoc. 2009;100(11):1275–85.
75. Seeleman C. Cultural competence and diversity responsiveness: how to make a difference in healthcare? Thesis Amsterdam University; 2014.
76. Pottie K, Greenaway C, Hassan G, Hui C, Kirmayer LJ. Caring for a newly arrived Syrian refugee family. Can Med Assoc J. 2016;188:207–11.
77. Andrulis DP, Brach C. Integrating literacy, culture and language to improve health care quality for diverse populations. Am J Health Behav. 2007;31(1):S122–33.

78. Van Melle M, Lamkaddem M, Stuiver MM, Gerritsen AAM, Devillé WLJM, Essink-Bot ML. Quality of primary care for resettled refugees in the Netherlands with chronic mental and physical health problems: a cross-sectional analysis of medical records and interview data. BMC Fam Pract. 2014;15:160.
79. de Maesschalck S. Linguistic and cultural diversity in the consultation room: a tango between physicians and their ethnic minority patients. (Academisch Proefschrift). Gent: Ghent University, Department of Family Medicine and Primary Health Care; 2012.
80. Karliner LS, Jacobs EA, Hm Chen A, Mutha S. Do professional interpreters improve clinical care for patients with limited English proficiency? A systematic review of the literature. HSR Health Serv Res. 2007;42:727–54.
81. Bischoff A, Denhaerynck K. What do language barriers cost? An exploratory study among asylum seekers in Switzerland. BMC Health Serv Res. 2010;10:248. https://doi.org/10.1186/1472-6963-10-248.
82. Rosenberg E, Seller R, Leanza Y. Through interpreters' eyes: comparing roles of professional and family interpreters. Patient Educ Couns. 2008;70:87–93.
83. Green J, Free C, Bhavnani V, Newman T. Translators and mediators: bilingual young people's accounts of their interpreting work in health care. Soc Sci Med. 2005;60:2097–110.
84. Aranguri C, Davidson B, Ramirez R. Patterns of communication through interpreters: a detailed sociolinguistic analysis. J Gen Intern Med. 2006;21(6):623–9. https://doi.org/10.1111/j.1525-1497.2006.00451.x.
85. Flores G. The impact of medical interpreter services on the quality of health care: a systematic review. Med Care Res Rev. 2005;62(3):255–99. https://doi.org/10.1177/1077558705275416.
86. Messias DKH, McDowell L, Estrada RD. Language interpreting as social justice work: perspectives of formal and informal healthcare interpreters. Adv Nurs Sci. 2009;32(2):128–43.
87. Schoevers MA, van den Muijsenbergh M, Lagro-Janssen AL. Illegal female immigrants in The Netherlands have unmet needs in sexual and reproductive health. J Psychosom Obstet Gynecol. 2010;31(4):256–64.
88. Razavi MF, Falk L, Wilhelmsson S. Experiences of the Swedish healthcare system: an interview study with refugees in need of long-term health care. Scand J Public Health. 2011;39:319–25.

Index

T. Wenzel, B. Droždek (eds.), *An Uncertain Safety*,
https://doi.org/10.1007/978-3-319-72914-5

C

Q

R

MIX
Papier aus verantwortungsvollen Quellen
Paper from responsible sources
FSC® C105338

If you have any concerns about our products,
you can contact us on
ProductSafety@springernature.com

In case Publisher is established outside the EU,
the EU authorized representative is:
Springer Nature Customer Service Center GmbH
Europaplatz 3, 69115 Heidelberg, Germany

Printed by Libri Plureos GmbH
in Hamburg, Germany